Information Technology in Health Science Education

COMPUTERS IN BIOLOGY AND MEDICINE

Series Editor: George P. Moore

University of Southern California, Los Angeles

COMPUTER ANALYSIS OF NEURONAL STRUCTURES
Edited by Robert D. Lindsay

ANALYSIS OF PHYSIOLOGICAL SYSTEMS
 The White-Noise Approach
Panos Z. Marmarelis and Vasilis Z. Marmarelis

INFORMATION TECHNOLOGY IN HEALTH SCIENCE EDUCATION
Edited by Edward C. DeLand

Information Technology in Health Science Education

Edited by
Edward C. DeLand
University of California at Los Angeles

PLENUM PRESS · NEW YORK AND LONDON

Library of Congress Cataloging in Publication Data

Main entry under title:

Information technology in health science education.

    (Computers in biology and medicine)
    Bibliography: p.
    Includes index.
    1. Medicine–Computer-assisted instruction. I. DeLand, Edward Charles, 1922-
        II. Series: Computers in biology and medicine (New York, 1977-   )
[DNLM: 1. Computer assisted instruction. 2. Health occupations–Education–United
States. W18.3 I43]
R837.C6I53   610'.7'8   78-7201
ISBN-13: 978-1-4684-2462-1   e-ISBN-13: 978-1-4684-2460-7
DOI: 10.1007/978-1-4684-2460-7

© 1978 Plenum Press, New York
Softcover reprint of the hardcover 1st edition 1978
A Division of Plenum Publishing Corporation
227 West 17th Street, New York, N.Y. 10011

To

my dear wife, Janet,

and

my darling daughter, Katherine

Contributors

R. A. Avner, Computer-Based Education Laboratory, University of Illinois, Urbana, Illinois

G. Octo Barnett, Massachusetts General Hospital and Harvard Medical School, Boston, Massachusetts

Howard L. Bleich, Thorndike Memorial Laboratory and Department of Medicine, Harvard Medical School and Beth Israel Hospital, Boston, Massachusetts

D. K. Bloomfield, School of Basic Medical Sciences, University of Illinois College of Medicine, Urbana, Illinois

Christopher R. Brigham, Family Practice Center, Eastern Maine Medical Center, Bangor, Maine

Jeanne L. Burson, Division of Computing Services for Medical Education and Research, Ohio State University, Columbus, Ohio

John Casbergue, Office of Medical Education Research and Development, Michigan State University, East Lansing, Michigan

Ralph E. Cutler, Department of Medicine, Harborview Medical Center, University of Washington School of Medicine, Seattle, Washington

Edward C. DeLand, Division of Thoracic Surgery, Health Science Center, University of California, Los Angeles, California

R. B. Dell, Columbia College of Physicians and Surgeons, Babies Hospital, New York, New York

John Doull, Department of Pharmacology, University of Kansas Medical Center, Kansas City, Kansas

Karen A. Duncan, Director, Office of Computer Resources, College of Dental Medicine, Medical University of South Carolina, Charleston, South Carolina

Kathleen T. Famiglietti, Laboratory of Computer Science, Massachusetts General Hospital, Boston, Massachusetts

Barbara B. Farquhar, Educational Computer Group, Digital Equipment Corporation, Marlboro, Massachusetts

Nancy A. Farr, University of the Pacific, Pacific Medical Center, San Francisco, California

William F. Fitzgerald, Director of Education, Menequil Corporation, Alexandria, Virginia

Mark H. Forman, Division of Computing Services for Medical Education and Research, Ohio State University, Columbus, Ohio

Arden W. Forrey, Department of Medicine, Harborview Medical Center, University of Washington School of Medicine, Seattle, Washington

Alan B. Forsythe, Health Sciences Computing Facility, Department of Bio-mathematics and School of Dentistry, University of California, Los Angeles, California

James R. Freed, Health Sciences Computing Facility and Department of Bio-mathematics, University of California, Los Angeles, California

Richard B. Friedman, Department of Medicine, University of Wisconsin, Madison, Wisconsin

John R. Gamble, University of the Pacific, Pacific Medical Center, San Francisco, California

Wilbur D. Hagamen, Department of Anatomy, Laboratory of Computer Science, Cornell University Medical College, Ithaca, New York

William G. Harless, University of the Pacific, Pacific Medical Center, San Francisco, California

Jane B. Hirsch, Department of Anatomy, Laboratory of Computer Science, Cornell University Medical College, Ithaca, New York

Edward P. Hoffer, Massachusetts General Hospital and Harvard Medical School, Boston, Massachusetts

G. L. Hody, School of Basic Medical Sciences, University of Illinois College of Medicine, Urbana, Illinois

Beverly Hunter, Human Resources Research Organization, Alexandria, Virginia

Gary S. Kahn, Educational Research and Evaluation Branch, National Medical Audiovisual Center, Atlanta, Georgia

M. Kamp, Chief, Scientific Computing Services, University of California School of Medicine, San Francisco, California

Marilyn Knetsch, Human Resources Research Organization, Alexandria, Virginia

Leo L. Leveridge, Department of Continuing Medical Education, American Medical Association, Chicago, Illinois

A. H. Levy, School of Basic Medical Sciences, University of Illinois College of Medicine, Urbana, Illinois

A. John Merola, Independent Study Program, Division of Computing Services for Medical Education and Research, College of Medicine, Ohio State University, Columbus, Ohio

Suzanne S. Murphy, Department of Anatomy, Laboratory of Computer Science, Cornell University Medical College, Ithaca, New York

Theodor H. Nelson, Project Xanadu, Swarthmore, Pennsylvania

Ruann E. Pengov, Director, Division of Computing Services for Medical Education and Research, College of Medicine, Ohio State University, Columbus, Ohio

Douglas Porter, Thorndike Laboratory, Department of Medicine, Harvard Medical School and Beth Israel Hospital, Boston, Massachusetts

R. Ramakrishnan, Columbia College of Physicians and Surgeons, Babies Hospital, New York, New York

Craig J. Richardson, Digital Equipment Corporation, Marlboro, Massachusetts

Martin L. Rubin, Human Resources Research Organization, Alexandria, Virginia

Charles W. Slack, Thorndike Laboratory, Department of Medicine, Harvard Medical School and Beth Israel Hospital, Boston, Massachusetts

Warner V. Slack, Thorndike Laboratory, Department of Medicine, Harvard Medical School and Beth Israel Hospital, Boston, Massachusetts

J. A. Starkweather, Department of Psychiatry, University of California, San Francisco, California

Bradford T. Stokes, Independent Study Program, Division of Computing Services for Medical Education and Research, College of Medicine, Ohio State University, Columbus, Ohio

Charles S. Tidball, Director, Computer Assisted Education and Services, George Washington University Medical Center, Washington, D.C.

Edward J. Walaszek, Department of Pharmacology, University of Kansas Medical Center, Kansas City, Kansas

Richard F. Walters, Medical Learning Resources, School of Medicine, University of California, Davis, California

John C. Weber, Department of Anatomy, Laboratory of Computer Science, Cornell University Medical College, Ithaca, New York

Harold Wooster, Special Assistant for Program Development, Lister Hill National Center for Biomedical Communications, National Library of Medicine,

National Institutes of Health, Public Health Service, Department of Health, Education, and Welfare, Bethesda, Maryland

Eric D. Zemper, Office of Medical Education Research and Development, Michigan State University, East Lansing, Michigan

Marcia A. Zier, University of the Pacific, Pacific Medical Center, San Francisco, California

Preface

This first volume is but an introduction to the growing use of computer-based systems in health-science education. It is unlikely that the intellectual or applied system constructs herein are either exhaustive of the field or immutable; growth is inevitable. For one thing, the field is still fractured and loosely organized, which is an inevitable description of an adolescent science in a rich mine of ideas.

There is emerging, however, an organizing concept. A short look into the future indicates that educational system design will be dominated by a concept which, for want of a better term, we may call an "information system." Actually, this term derives from an early New York World's Fair exhibition designed by Charles Eames entitled the "Informational Machine," in which the designer illustrated once again his insight into the future by showing how in a fundamental manner the digital computer promised to affect and to change our lives; and this change is by no means completed. Even during the publication of this volume, the basic sciences requisite to the development of an information machine have evolved significantly. The three intellectual areas to watch are developments in artificial intelligence, graphics and man/machine interaction, and basic component and computer system design.

No doubt, as in biological systems, the highest rates of growth and change occur in the early years. But the stored-program digital computer is about 30 years old, and, consequently, many of the observers of the field have expected to find the rates of growth and development beginning to taper off. In fact, they have not. Anyone conversant with computer-system design can describe dramatic developments that are just around the corner. What this means simply is that authors of future user systems are being presented with new freedoms and with speed and power for design and implementation of creative ideas. I believe that these phenomena will continue to have profound effects for some time, particularly for such challenging problems as automated systems for teaching and learning. In short, the exciting part of this business is still unfolding.

I should like to take this opportunity to express, however inadequately, my thanks to the many authors for their dedication, diligence, and patience. It is no easy task to write a chapter for such a book since much of the manuscript is necessarily descriptive and narrative rather than technical. I very much appreciate the efforts of this highly skilled and technical group and thank them for their time and effort. In addition, I wish to thank Dr. George Moore, the series editor, for the opportunity to present this material. It marks a plateau of progress. The volume finally came together under the sure hand of Harvey Graveline, senior production editor of Plenum Publishers, whose remarkable forbearance allowed us to conclude.

EDWARD C. DELAND

Contents

Introduction

Edward C. DeLand

History will undoubtedly record that the development of the digital computer marked a major turning point in the stormy course of human welfare; whether for better or worse is not yet settled. Over the past 25 years the computer and its attendant technology have, in any case, become the basis, if not the cause, for some rather remarkable changes in our intellectual environment. Perhaps the most important of these changes has been the opportunity for the human mind to express itself in a new medium and to experiment with new and novel ideas. And, even if the development has had no other effect, the computer has certainly expanded our concept of what a machine is, or more accurately, what a machine can do.

Most of us carry a deep suspicion that a machine — however complexly organized — is but a machine; that it cannot, by some basic law, be used to teach our young. Common experience teaches us that human behavior and machine behavior are fundamentally disparate, and that the functions associated with teaching and learning are in some way intrinsic to one but not to the other. It therefore sometimes requires an effort of the mind to perceive the large areas of potential becoming available with the new computers wherein the functions of the machine can be designed to complement and support human intellectual processes.

Some of this potential has been exploited in recent computer-assisted instruction systems where new concepts of man—machine interactions are becoming apparent. There are computer system arrangements in which the machine acts as a fast and efficient information resource in a particular subject matter, flexible enough to skip material or to branch, to dwell on a subject or to pursue a tangential concept in response to student interest. There may be interaction in which the machine asks questions and keeps score, as well as acting as a resource, or where the student, growing bored with a particular subject matter, follows his curiosity by directing the machine into new subject areas. The system may provide rote memory work, drill and practice, or, at another extreme, abstract simulations of real systems for the student to manipulate or to design, but in any case to learn from.

This volume will review many such CAI (computer-assisted instruction) systems. The objective is to show a carefully selected variety of such systems in order to exemplify the range and depth of activity in this field. The volume began in

Edward C. DeLand • Division of Thoracic Surgery, Health Science Center, University of California, Los Angeles, California.

response to a question from a Dean for Curricular Affairs regarding the activity, and it is designed to respond to similar questions from similar deans whose responsibilities recently have expanded to include, among other things, a computer.

This question occurred in a medical school, but while the response would not be identical in another school, it would be the same in spirit: There is a very substantial effort afoot to investigate the ways that an interactive computer information system can be of service to students and faculty alike. This effort is not always well or dependably funded, but it has nevertheless over the years engaged the curiosity and talent of an impressive list of perceptive and reliable investigators. The results have been up and down; sometimes the task is underestimated, sometimes the cost, but, the historical examples of classic failures in this field notwithstanding, the effort is beginning to pay off. This volume is a report on the current activity and use of CAI in the health sciences. We have chosen to discuss only systems that are in use every day and whose user lists are growing. Perhaps this is a mistake, particularly in an experimental educational field, where we often learn useful lessons from the failures. Nevertheless, there were more than enough running systems to supply a variety of concepts for one volume.

It turns out that the precise design of such interactive human/computer systems is very critical. Students are quick to reject and turn away from trivial or irrelevant subject matter, or from a control system that gets in the way of the learning process, for example, one that requires complex typing. On the other hand, students readily embrace a resource that leads them through an intellectual process that may have surprises in store, that is apparently correct and to the point, and that provides either an efficient or a fulfilling way to spend their limited time.

The ideal system has a compelling quality. Students get remarkably involved, as in playing a game. They may see their skill improving and try again and again. The CASE (Harless *et al.*, 1971) system is one of the earliest successful, self-motivating CAI systems in the health sciences. Observers are inevitably struck by the way a CASE terminal will attract bunches of students, each involved and arguing his point among the others, hour after hour.

The easily imagined benefits anticipated from an ideal information machine are a good deal more difficult to accomplish than was presumed some 20 years ago when the first CAI systems were designed. Subtle nuances may motivate a student or capture his attention, but only when this occurs can the magic chemistry of learning proceed. Over the years, a good many CAI systems have been designed, and many have fallen by the wayside for reasons that will be discussed later in this book. Mostly they have failed to have any semblance of this subjective compelling quality. Neither students nor faculty cared, and therefore the system cost was too high by any measure of benefit that could be applied.

There are three major objective criteria that a CAI system must satisfy in order to survive: User acceptance; a reasonable costs/benefits ratio, and goal fulfillment. A system may satisfy one or two of these requirements, but if it does not satisfy the third it will not succeed. Also, the standards by which a computer-based instructional system is judged are automatically higher than those for conventional systems, particularly since for conventional teaching systems the standards of quality or performance are either nonexistent or seldom measured.

This volume will review a broad sample of computer-based systems that have survived all three of the primary tests and are in use every day. Several are very widely used; more than 40 medical schools have local copies or access to them remotely. There are very few systems that are used at only one university.

This volume deals specifically with health science education, but many of the systems described are used in other domains and education disciplines. We have by no means been able to show all of the important computer-assisted or computer-managed instructional systems in health science education even in the United States. Many important systems do not appear here for one mechanical reason or another, such as lack of space or time. We hope, however, to have covered the concepts of CAI and in so doing have separated these concepts along three axes: the hardware axis, the user axis, and the task axis. In the first of these, the concept of the CAI program will vary if the program is designed for local use only on an independent cassette terminal, or if it is designed for campuswide use or for nationwide use on a network. With respect to the user community, the programs may range from a prophylaxis program for the layman through basic science for the undergraduate to patient management for graduate and continuing education audiences. Finally, along the third axis, the concept of a CAI program will vary with the authors' intent. The task requirement may be for drill-and-practice or exercises, for tutorial or self-evaluation, or for problem solving and simulation, each a distinct category and type of CAI program.

Programs from each of these three axes have been chosen for this book – at the expense, in some instances, of omitting other representative, successful CAI systems. For any such omissions, the editors are deeply regretful. There are certain other omissions as well, three of which should be mentioned. The first omission is a chapter on the CASE system which was developed around 1969 by William G. Harless and his colleagues at the University of Illinois. This was a benchmark program in at least two respects: It allowed the use of natural language across the interface by both the computer and the student, and it provided a remarkably credible patient simulation. However, Appendix A describes an application of the CASE system which is equally important for the goals of this volume, since it consists of a computer-based instructional and testing system for continuing education. The second necessary omission occurs in the loss of a chapter from the American Association of Medical Colleges, an institution that has for many years been a leader in the development and study of the application of educational technology in medical sciences. Typical of their work was a remarkable publication in volume 46 of their journal, *The Journal of Medical Education*, entitled "Educational Technology for Medicine: Roles for the Lister Hill Center" (Stead *et al.*, 1971). This study departs from the tradition of the work of federal study committees in that it was then and still remains the outstanding review and summary of the problems of educational technology in medicine. Unfortunately, it was too long to include as an appendix here, but it certainly should be read by anyone aspiring to be conversant with health science education. Finally, the third omission is not so much an omission as giving a subject short shrift. This concerns the problem of evaluation of CAI systems. This is not the place to go into great detail defining "evaluation" and "appraisal," particularly since these tasks are handled well in the text; however, a few comments may be in order. We have alluded above to the requirement for evaluation of computer-based instructional systems. Unfortunately, no one knows quite how to go about this beyond the trivial step of giving students an objective examination at the end of a course. After designing controls, before-and-after examination protocols, and the other paraphernalia of a controlled experiment, there still remains the question of measuring the quality of a human learning experience. Certain steps have been made in that direction, as will be seen in various chapters of the book, and certain "use tests" have been applied to determine the popularity of CAI systems, but no thoroughgoing, full-blown educational experiment has been reported with proper statistical controls. In addition to several partial experiments described in several chapters in the book, Appendix B summarizes the use and evaluation of a national network implemented by the National Library of Medicine, Lister Hill Center. The network was established as a direct consequence of the previously cited report by the Association of American Medical Colleges. The entire report is quite long, but we believe it is important enough to excerpt portions for reference here.

Appendix C is a bibliography for medical science CAI systems. It is a collection from several sources and is intended to be thorough. Continuing bibliographies are kept, for example, by the University of Wisconsin (Leakan, 1971; Hoye and Wang, 1974) and the Lister Hill Center, National Library of Medicine.

Investigators at the Lister Hill Center are continuing their researches on the application of CAI and automated information dissemination in the health sciences (a chapter describing this work was unfortunately delayed), and visitors are invited to the Learning/Resource Center in Bethesda to be apprised of these activities. A direction of their efforts that should be mentioned is the development of computer graphics applications. A very large gap in CAI systems has been the failure to provide easily presentable visual, analog, and other multimedia information. These developments will help to close that gap. It is to be hoped that Lister Hill will also continue development of television information distribution and, in particular, closed-circuit and cable television two-way training networks.

Finally, a note on the future. To the perceptive citizen, there is a certain inevitability about the way computers and computer systems insinuate themselves into ordinary life activities. If at first the computer appears clumsy in handling bills and accounts and reservations, it is only because it is learning how. With time the complaints decrease and we come to expect that the telephone calls will be billed correctly and that the reservations can be made instantaneously for any theater or airplane in the country. This quality is dependent upon the fact that computer programs, if they grow at all, can only become more sophisticated, less error prone, and more dependable. The same characteristic applies to CAI programs as well. Given the time, the money, and the perception of the problem, the computer system will inevitably grow to better serve the needs of the user. It may be that the computer system could grow to be costly, but it could not, by definition, perpetuate malfunctions, mistakes, or poor design; these errors are eventually worked out, never to recur. This leaves us with the probability that given time, even a small effort would succeed, let alone the substantial effort in CAI.

This is not to say that all problems are necessarily solvable. Some problems and tasks set for the computer are exceedingly complex and difficult, as difficult as anything the human mind has previously attempted, for example, the task of discovering the meaning of the phrase "artificial intelligence." It is possible that a CAI system, in order ultimately to be "successful," will have to solve similar profound problems. It appears, however, that there is yet a great deal of room for work between where we are now and such difficult future considerations. True, it would be convenient to find sophisticated solutions to the "pattern recognition" problem, since this would have direct applications in diagnostic as well as physician-training programs, but it is not necessary to solve that problem for a computer to play an effective role in physician training.

Any role that an information-handling system does play in health sciences eventually devolves from the fact that medicine is an information intensive science. The timely and reliable gathering, organization, and distribution of information, whether from a library or a patient, whether to an archive or a ward, is essential to every activity of health science. The primary skill of a physician could, in fact, be described as information organization and management. A remarkable range of information, ideally, is arranged and reviewed for each decision. Can an information machine be designed to slip into this activity, to support and supplement the training and even the patient management? Such a machine would be the ideal CAI system, and in its potential development lies the value of CAI research.

References

Harless, W. G., Diennon, G. G., Marxer, J. J., Root, J. A., and Miller, G. E., 1971. CASE: A computer-aided simulation of the clinical encounter, *J. Med. Educ.*, **46**: 443.

Hoye, R. E., and Wang, A. C., (Eds.), 1974. *Index to Computer Based Learning, Instructional Media Laboratory, University of Wisconsin*, Educational Technology Publications, Englewood, N.J.

Lekan, H. A. (Ed.), 1971. *Index to Computer Assisted Instruction, Instructional Media Laboratory, University of Wisconsin*, 3rd ed., Harcourt Brace Jovanovich, New York.

Stead, E. A., Jr., Smythe, C. McC., Gunn, C. G., and Littlemeyer, M. H. (Eds.), 1971. Educational technology for medicine: Roles for the Lister Hill Center, *J. Med. Educ.*, **46** (7), Part 2: 97 (July).

2

CAIDENT: Dental Education Marching to the Beat of a Different Drummer

William F. Fitzgerald

Introduction

A broad survey by Dr. Martin Kamp (1975) indicates that approximately 15% of the instructional computer programs and 11% of the student-access computer program hours in computerized health science teaching are specifically identified for dentistry. Why would a profession that is viewed by the public as "drilling and filling teeth" make use of computers to teach? Certainly, the historical method of training dentists by apprenticeship prior to the middle of the nineteenth century was sufficient then. What has happened to make it attractive to use computer technology in the dental educational process now?

The first dental school was founded in 1839 (Bremner, 1959), and for almost 90 years, schools which were organized primarily for profit flourished in the United States. In 1926, standards for education were imposed by the American Dental Association, and many of those proprietary schools closed. Since then, standards have been raised, and the amount of material to be mastered has increased by several magnitudes. Currently, 60 dental schools in the United States accept students to study for the dental doctoral degree.

Dentistry is one of the few professions or vocations which places an extremely high demand on the three basic domains of human performance: cognitive, affective, and psychomotor. The dental practitioner must have substantial knowledge of what must be done to deliver optimum oral health care. In addition, he or she must be skilled in the affective, or emotional domain, because many patients bring anxieties and unrealistic expectations to the dental situation, and the dentist must be able to motivate patients to accept oral health care and to maintain oral health care. Finally, all areas of dentistry require fine muscle coordination, whether the procedure is drilling a tooth, wiring braces, or extracting a molar. This need for a high degree of competence in these three areas of human performance places a significant demand on the admissions process. Dental education is very expensive, and it is important to both the applicants and the admissions officers to minimize attrition and to maximize successful completion of the curriculum. The philosophy,

William F. Fitzgerald · Director of Education, Menequil Corporation, Alexandria, Virginia.

somewhat simply stated, is to select the best possible applicants, to provide the best possible education and training, and to graduate the best possible dental practitioners. While instructional technology comes into play in the second phase, providing the best possible education, its role and relationship to other learning opportunities must be interpreted in the context of the nature of the target population — the student who is admitted.

It has been well documented that humans vary remarkably in their achievement and aptitude of the three primary areas of human performance. Dental students are no exception in this regard, and despite rigorous screening and admissions assessment, there is variance in their achievement and aptitude in these three domains.

In the first half of the twentieth century, applicants to dental schools were admitted based on the evaluation of each school's admissions officer. Accurate summaries of the dropout rate then are not now available, but the attrition is reported to have been approximately 25% from entrance to graduation. In 1946, the dental admissions test was introduced, and largely because of that the first-year attrition has been reduced to only 3.72% for the entering class of 1974—75, and for the entire curriculum, dentistry now graduates 92.6% of those who enter school. This historical perspective is germane because the use of instructional technology must be conditioned by an appreciation of the extreme selectivity with which students enter dental school. The assessment of applicants to dental school in the cognitive domain is more precise than similar measurement in the psychomotor and affective domains, and while this is a relative statement, it nonetheless emphasizes the role of individualized instruction, which is considered to be most appropriate in target learner populations in which the aptitude and achievement variance is relatively great.

Why CAI in Dentistry?

What is the problem for which computer-assisted instruction is the solution in dental education? Although dental students are rigorously screened so that they are remarkably homogeneous in their intellectual aptitude and achievement, there still remains a significant interaction among the domains of human performance. Some students are extremely interested and competent in fine muscle skills but are bored by the more traditional textbook courses; others have arrived in dental school through successful competition in the undergraduate educational arena which typically measures more purely cognitive functioning to the exclusion of psychomotor skills. Although there is an emphasis in the first half of the dental curriculum on basic science, hence, lecture—textbook courses, material which appeals principally to the cognitive domain is presented continuously throughout the curriculum. Furthermore, there is a progressive emphasis on the integration of information learned in earlier stages, to a point later in the curriculum where more hours are spent in psychomotor activities, but the hours spent in decision making and integration of scientific material assumes cumulative importance.

The public perception of the dentist as the health care practitioner who drills and fills teeth focuses on the end product of substantial decision making. The majority of the treatment-plan decisions are achieved through a scientific model tersely summarized as identifying the problem exhaustively, entertaining a variety of hypotheses that will account for the nature of the problem, identifying solutions or actions that will address the problem, and formulating the treatment strategy with the highest probability of success. In the course of reaching a decision, the dentist must call upon a large body of knowledge that correlates the patient's medical history, current disease manifestation, and receptivity to various forms of therapy. Because of the essentially infinite combinations of patient situations and treatment possibilities, it would be impossible and unrealistic to confront the dental student with all possible combinations of patient medical histories, patient disease manifestations, and patient acceptance of treatment. And yet, the standards of dental education and of the profession require that the successful graduate be competent to perform in extraordinarily heterogeneous situations. And here, specifically, is where teacher-absent, mediated instruction, in general, and computer-assisted instruction, in particular, play their most important role: simulating a wide variety of circumstances in which the student is confronted with data that require diverse decisions and, as an essential adjunct, presenting these data in an environment in which the student is free to pursue different courses of action.

The health professions student develops confidence as a function of his or her sense of certainty, and as a result of interaction with faculty. Although students present diagnoses and proposed treatment plans to faculty, there is an expectation that the proposal of an inappropriate plan will be met with overt or unspoken criticism and judgment. The opportunity to simulate the consequences of inappropriate courses of action, or more importantly, courses of action which are believed to be correct by the student at that time, is a significant contribution of instructional technology.

These, then, are the two most important roles for mediated instruction in dentistry: (1) the simulation of case presentations that are not available during his relatively brief tenure in the educational system, and (2) the opportunity to experimentally and artificially manipulate the environment to investigate the consequences of various decision paths. In addition, however, dentistry is similar to other educational environments in that it involves a certain amount of rote memorization and the requirement of learning mastery in which the options are narrowly constrained. Because students learn at different rates, and because dentistry involves some memorization and mimicry, dental education makes use of a variety of teacher-absent learning devices, including videotapes, slides, audio tapes, and other media, as well as CAI.

Specific Uses of CAI in Dentistry

Dental CAI programs currently in use reflect the biases of both the producer and the instructor. Most, however, conform to general guidelines or conditions that describe the appropriate application of CAI. These conditions will be described abstractly and specific examples of dental CAI will be presented. CAI is particularly appropriate in response to these eight conditions:

1. Students require substantially different amounts of time to learn. It has been indicated above that, despite precise assessment of dental school applicants, there is still an appreciable heterogeneity of aptitude on the part of dental students, especially considering the mix of cognitive, psychomotor, and affective attributes required.

2. Different responses are made by students to the same question. In dentistry, as in all other education, student response to a question will vary.

3. Students need to explore the effects of various decision strategies. Because of the complex mixture of patient characteristics (medical history, disease manifestation, and receptivity to treatment), students need to simulate the differential success of alternative treatment plans in order to develop a firm foundation for decision making.

4. Actions taken on the basis of student response can be identified. It is possible to achieve a respectable consensus of opinion from dental educators on the question of the relative value of different decisions or proposed actions in the face of patient characteristics.

5. Each student is required to participate actively in the specification of or commitment to a particular decision. Since dentistry is practiced in a solo environment by a majority of dentists, eliciting a student commitment to a decision or opinion during dental school does simulate the practice environment. Significant prior research in what is called "transfer of training" endorses the value of this simulation during dental school.

6. It is cumbersome, difficult, or unnecessary to present all cues which comprise a particular problem situation. Since a dental student's clinical experience is tautologically limited to the cases that are presented to him during dental school, it would be impossible to confront him with the infinite variety and combination of patient characteristics. Both because of the interaction among patient characteristics and because of the infrequency of certain cases, the simulation of diverse cases is justified.

7. Material is substantially repetitive. As has been indicated earlier, dentistry contains some material that requires rote memorization or few decisions.

8. The alternatives are costly or unacceptable. Cost is used here, in the broadest sense, to include patient satisfaction, instructor time, and student confidence. If it is deemed important for the student to develop an understanding of the effect of drug dosage, overdosing a real patient is unacceptable, but that is an error that can be richly simulated by a computer.

In the context of these dimensions, the following illustrative examples reflect material that has been presented or proposed for presentation by means of a CAI format. In the following illustrations, three modes or types of CAI will be referenced: drill and practice, tutorial CAI, and environment simulation. Drill and practice refers to the mode of CAI in which the computer presents multiple choice, true or false, or fill-in-the-blank questions to the student. The student's response is evaluated by the computer and he or she is told if the response is correct or incorrect. In tutorial CAI, there is an attempt to establish a dialogue with the student so that the nature of the response to computer-proposed questions causes additional dialogue that can be unique for each student. In this mode of CAI, an incorrect or inefficient response by the learner may be met with an explanation of why the choice was inappropriate, followed by an invitation for the student to choose another alternative, or by the presentation of remedial instruction. Environment simulation, the third mode of CAI which will be cited in the following illustrations, is considered by many to be the most sophisticated use of instructional computer technology. In this mode, the learner is presented with a rich variety of stimuli and is frequently required to make a number of choices or decisions simultaneously. Since it is difficult to explain completely environment simulation in the absence of a specific example, the following illustrations may serve to explain this mode.

The general conditions presented above apply abstractly to CAI, regardless of content area. For example, foreign language learning illustrates a situation in which students vary in their aptitudes, and the material is repetitive. Similarly, CAI in the training of airline pilots is adequately justified by the eighth principle, concerning alternatives that are costly or unacceptable: the simulated crash landing of an airplane is preferable to the real event. The following illustrative examples are presented to indicate the relevance of these conditions to the context of dental education.

Basic Science. CAI programs in various modes have been written on the subjects of acid—base balance, anesthesia, anatomy, physiology, histology, and numerous other basic science areas. The predominant use of CAI in basic science dental education has been in drill-and-practice and tutorial modes, primarily because the complex decision-making aspects of basic science are most frequently integrated with the clinical applications of these sciences. Many dental students have anecdotally reported appreciation for the substantial reduction of anxiety by taking a computer simulation of part one of the National Boards. By alternating between studies and the simulated national boards, dental students can identify their own areas of weakness and focus their energies on their weak subjects.

Patient-History Taking. For first-year dental students, whose dental education to date has been rigorous course work, the prospects of their first interaction with a patient is intimidating. To complicate the interpersonal anxiety, the student is experientially ill-equipped to probe for a complete answer from the response of a patient to a medical history form. There are CAI programs that simulate the response of an inarticulate patient to questions on a medical history form. These programs contain a number of "trap" conditions and at the completion of the interview provide the student with a count of the number of probes he made which were unnecessary, and the number of responses he received which were not probed. Some programs then advise the student of the ramifications of his incomplete information. Students frequently report an appreciation of the relevance and importance of that experience.

Oral Diagnosis. One of the most challenging and important areas for a dental student is the oral diagnosis. It is in this area that the student must correlate vast quantities of basic and clinical science instruction, and in which errors are significant. One program in oral diagnosis focuses on the quantitative aspects of laboratory tests and presents a brief résumé of the patient, along with a medical history which includes systematic complications. The program then asks the student if he or she would order any laboratory tests for the patient. Following the choice of laboratory tests, the student is told whether the test would be appropriate or not, or is interrogated for the rationale for ordering a test, following which the laboratory results are presented. In the case of some of the tests, such as the complete blood count, the student is asked to identify the value(s) that exceed the normal range. The student may ask the computer for a specification of the normal ranges. After a series of tests have been requested by the student, the program demands a diagnosis. If the diagnosis required the interpretation of a test that was not requested, the student is so advised. This environment simulation is one of the more dramatic examples of the variety of cases that exist in the private dental practice which may not be seen by a student during his or her educational tenure. While it would be possible to present unusual cases in a lecture format, the amount of individualized instruction and the degree of long-term retention is questionable in that educational method. By using a computer program, the student is free from both peer pressure and the anticipation of instructor criticism if he chooses to make an incorrect response.

Craniofacial Growth and Occlusion. A program has been proposed which would simulate the orthodontic treatment plan of a simulated patient based on a computer-generated television display of the cranial bone structure, including the teeth. The proposal involves digitizing craniofacial cephalometric radiographs. Once communicated to a computer in digital form, the radiographic information could be displayed to a student on a cathode ray tube (basically, a television set; called a "CRT" by computer personnel). By use of simple commands, a student could rotate the image on the television screen to determine the extent and nature of the malocclusion. The student could then simulate the placement of orthodontic appliances, and, with mathematical projection models, craniofacial growth could be simulated. In this way, students could simulate a variety of orthodontic treatment plans to develop a better understanding of the cause-and-effect relationships between occlusal development and orthodontic intervention. No method other than the computer can provide this type of individual experience for each student.

Oral Cancer Recognition. The ability to detect the pathology of oral cancer is an important perquisite of dental education. Because the student's education is essentially limited to the patient case load during dental school and the educational material presented by faculty, it is important to simulate the manifestations of a variety of cancer patients as richly as possible. Although it is possible to show photographs of lesions and histologic slides, the importance of this subject warrants substantial assurance that the student is competent in this area of diagnosis. Such assurance can be provided by a computer program that requires increasingly more subtle discriminations on the part of a student.

The preceding applications of CAI in dentistry have been presented as illustrative examples. Essentially, any information can be taught using CAI if the content material can be portrayed by existing computer output devices, if the range of student responses can be anticipated, and if predictable actions can be taken based on student response.

Factors Facilitating Dental CAI

Factors that have encouraged the use of computer-assisted instruction in dentistry are not unique to dental education. In general, these factors are administrative support, an increasing commitment to educational resources, the evaluation of this medium, faculty involvement and reaction, and student reaction. These factors will now be discussed in detail.

Administrative Support

First and foremost, the support and commitment of the administrators of dental schools have played a major role in initiating and perpetuating projects involving computers for teaching purposes. Although computer technology is currently used in dental schools for research and administrative purposes, the use of this technology for instructional purposes is relatively recent. A few projects have been initiated on school budgets, and the majority of the others have received significant assistance from the federal government in one form or another. Independent of the funding source, however, it has been the progressive thinking of dental administrators that has allowed this innovative technology to be used. The role of the dean of a professional school is a difficult one. The dental dean is required to have skills in business management, public relations, and other areas, and most deans have not had the opportunity of a rich involvement in educational psychology, in general, and technological advances in educational delivery systems, in particular.

Commitment to Educational Resources

The last decade has seen a dramatic increase in the commitment of dental schools to departments of educational resources. Historically, dental education has relied heavily on photographic slides, and from those initial activities have come major, expensive, and substantial commitments to television, videotape, programmed instruction, graphic illustration, and computer-assisted instruction. With this increase in the use of instructional media has come a growing awareness of the need for advice and direction from professionals trained in communications and learning media, and these professionals have proposed increasingly effective approaches to learning problems. Of significant note in this regard is a resolution of the House of

Delegates of the American Association of Dental Schools urging all member institutions of the association to establish an administrative unit charged with educational devolopment that would include the provision of both instruction for faculty in teaching methodology and appropriate educational resources. Such a recommendation by the representatives of all dental schools in the United States reflects the increasing awareness of the advantages that accrue from educational methodology.

Evaluation

Numerous CAI projects in dental schools include evaluation of the learning effectiveness of such efforts, and the results of evaluation studies are confirming the hypotheses related to learning effectiveness and student performance.

Faculty Involvement

There are many ways in which faculty can be motivated (in the broadest sense) to serve as content experts in the development of CAI materials, and these will be presented with comments on their value and effectiveness.

Walk-In. This method is usually best if it results from personal interest or initiative. Typically, a faculty member finds that some educational problems do not seem to respond to his efforts, which motivates him to contact a member of the instructional development staff who assists in analyzing the problem and suggesting solutions. Although faculty initiative does have some occasional problems ("I want to put something on computer" [sic]), it is frequently the reflection of some familiarity with the advantages of CAI and a suspicion that CAI may be an appropriate solution.

Pyramid Subscription. This technique is expressed concisely in the words of an instructional programmer as spoken to a faculty member: "Don't thank me; just advertise what you've done and get two of your colleagues to help us develop materials." This technique can be very effective if adroitly but sincerely handled.

Executive Mandate. Mandates come from department chairmen, heads of curriculum committees, and deans, and have mixed results. Since there is often some degree of suspicion, defensiveness, or resentment, initial communications are peppered with explanations and demonstrations. Usually, there are more subtle but more effective ways to express the same message.

Competition. Occasionally there is the faculty member whose self-image contains such descriptors as innovative, flexible, experimental, a leader, etc. While an overture from a person such as this may not be based on the "right" reasons, there is, nonetheless, an eagerness which should not perish. Above all, faculty interest is a perishable commodity.

Promotion Incentive. The vast majority of professional faculty are promoted and otherwise recognized on the basis of research and publications. It is difficult, if not impossible, to answer satisfactorily the question, "Why should I spend time developing an instructional package when that will reduce my research/writing/publishing time and hence potentially slow down my promotions?" Even if appropriate recognition is provided within a single institution, there still remains the problem of positions in other schools if transfer is considered. Clearly, this lack of recognition will not be rectified quickly nor will appropriate recognition receive universal acceptance. And it certainly will not happen until some faculty add a section to their curicula vitae titled "Instructional Programs Produced" and describe these efforts proudly to reflect the extensive time and energy spent.

Student Reaction

In general, student reaction to CAI raises only the problem of restricting access by one student for extensive lengths of time so that many students may be accommodated. Most dental students are extremely eager to assess and predict their achievements. Consequently, drill-and-practice CAI courses on part one of the National Boards, and simulations of course final examinations are extremely popular. In addition, this author has had the pleasurable experience of overhearing dental students discuss various alternative strategies in response to an environment simulation program in which the stimulus distinctions were subtle, and incorrect treatment plans or actions produced "untoward" results. As has been indicated above, the opportunity to pursue the consequences of an obviously incorrect choice can teach a student "why not" as well as "what not." In general, dental students perceive their education to contain significant pressures due primarily to the novelty of what they are learning, and they frequently express profound appreciation for the opportunity to proceed through instructional material at their individual pace and to receive the immediate diagnostic feedback provided by a computer program that is presented in the absence of instructor evaluation and peer pressure.

Factors Inhibiting the Use of CAI in Dental Education

Computer-assisted instruction has not received universal acceptance and utilization in dental education. Although there are many reasons for this, the overwhelming majority of them fall into the two categories of cost and conviction. The prominent cost categories are administrative and technical personnel, faculty time, physical space, and equipment expense. Computers require a variety of specialized personnel, and for even a small computer housed within the school, numerous personnel can be required. Space is at a premium in most schools, and a CAI project may pale in comparison with the competitive demands for more clinic, library, research, or faculty office space. In addition, although many dental schools were built with the expectation of installing a computer, if the computer is assigned to undeveloped space, it can be a rude shock to be confronted with the hidden cost of raised flooring or special air conditioning.

The category of lack of conviction ranges from being unaware of CAI as an instructional delivery mechanism to having substantial familiarity with this medium but conservative suspicion that CAI is not appropriate to the educational needs of the particular institution.

The Future of CAI in Dental Education

The future of CAI in dental education is best predicted from an analysis of its past and its current status. It has been used to good advantage where resources were available to implement and support its use. The methodology is proven effective in a wide variety of learning environments, and dental education is among them. Although it is considered too discretionary or not essential when compared with clinic operatories and lecture space, those aspects are a function of cost, and as the cost of CAI continues to decline and as resources increase, a prediction can be made that the use of CAI will expand.

References

Bremner, M. D. K., 1959. *Story of Dentistry.* Dental Items of Interest Publishing Company, Brooklyn, New York.

Kamp, M., 1975. *Index to Computerized Teaching in the Health Sciences*, Association for the Development of Computer-Based Instructional Systems, San Francisco.

3

Computer-Supported Independent Study in the Basic Medical Sciences

A. John Merola, Ruann E. Pengov, and Bradford T. Stokes

Independent study at The Ohio State University College of Medicine had its beginnings approximately fifteen years ago in the Department of Anatomy largely due to the energy and interest of Professor Grant O. Graves. Successful programs in that department were followed by experimental approaches in this direction by some members of the Department of Physiological Chemistry, who employed biochemistry discussion groups instead of a traditional lecture program to cover first-year medical biochemistry. Both of these experiments retained a significant lock-step feature with respect to the total elapsed time allowable to each student. This time constant was forced on the students in these programs due to the necessity of remaining in step with other disciplines which continued to be presented by the traditional lecture mode. Still, these programs led to several valuable conclusions. The principal findings of these experiments were these:

1. One need not expose medical students to a series of expert lectures in order for students to meet predetermined acceptable standards in the medical sciences. Parenthetically, students found it to be enjoyable to learn by discovering *with* a faculty member as well as *from* a faculty member.

2. Volunteer students in experimental programs tended to score slightly higher than their counterparts in a combination of criteria generally accepted to be predictors of preclinical performance at our college, i.e., MCAT science and premedical point–hour ratio.

3. The entering medical student who opted for independent study was generally mature and secure enough to be given substantial responsibility for his learning, provided he was afforded clear objectives to guide his study and a tutorial evaluation to evaluate his progress periodically.

In spite of these successful ventures on the departmental level, it was not until 1969 that a major effort was launched to develop a self-contained independent study program covering the *entire* basic science curriculum. In retrospect, it is clear that several factors made this effort possible. There was the leadership of the

A. John Merola, Ruann E. Pengov, and Bradford T. Stokes · Independent Study Program, Division of Computing Services for Medical Education and Research, College of Medicine, Ohio State University, Columbus, Ohio.

Anatomy group who established the feasibility of independent study and whose innovations whetted the appetite of others to innovate. There was an aggressive Division of Research and Evaluation in Medical Education that expressed a belief in the wisdom of independent study, as well as a small core of faculty willing to commit a large portion of their time and effort to the development of the program. There was also developing at the College of Medicine a group in the Division of Computing Services for Medical Education and Research committed to the development of computer-assisted instruction who were willing and able to relieve the faculty of the necessity of mastering instructional programming. These factors, present in an arena in which students were expressing strong feelings about so-called relevance in medical education, catalyzed a proposal subsequently funded by the U.S. Public Health Service, Bureau of Health Manpower, to design, test, and evaluate an indpendent study program that was to feature an integrated curriculum, modular student study objectives, and a computer-based tutorial evaluation system, together with some means of managing a student population progressing at independent rates. The principal departure from the traditional system was clearly the commitment to accept a prescribed level of mastery as a constant with time a variable in the learning equation. This commitment was made possible by designing the program to include the entire basic science portion of the medical curriculum and to allow students completing their basic science studies to enter their clinical clerkships at any month of the year. Flexibility, therefore, is a very positive feature of independent study, and it is remarkable that the clinical educators in our college responded to the needs of the Independent Study Program (ISP) in such a positive manner.

Earlier descriptions of the Independent Study Program and its predecessor, the Pilot Medical School have appeared (Griesen et al., 1973; Beran *et al.*, 1976). In this chapter, we shall emphasize changes that have risen in the evolution of the program as well as describe some of the results that have been observed since these earlier reports have appeared.

The Curriculum

The regular curriculum at The Ohio State University College of Medicine is a lecture-based, 15-month program composed of 6 months of Normal Man and 9 months of Pathophysiology. Following this preclinical phase, all students are required to spend 20 months in their clinical clerkships. The entire curriculum is designed to be a minimum 3-year program. It is the first 15 months of the regular curriculum that corresponds to the ISP. Both programs were designed to fulfill requirements previously met by the traditional first 2 years of basic medical sciences, i.e., Anatomy, Biochemistry, Physiology, Microbiology, Pathology, and Pharmacology. Both programs have weak and strong points, but, for the sake of brevity, we will describe only the Independent Study Program.

The curriculum in use in the ISP in 1976 resembles to a great extent that developed for the first class which entered in 1970. For example, the three main areas covered were Normal Man, Introduction to Pathophysiology and Therapeutics, and

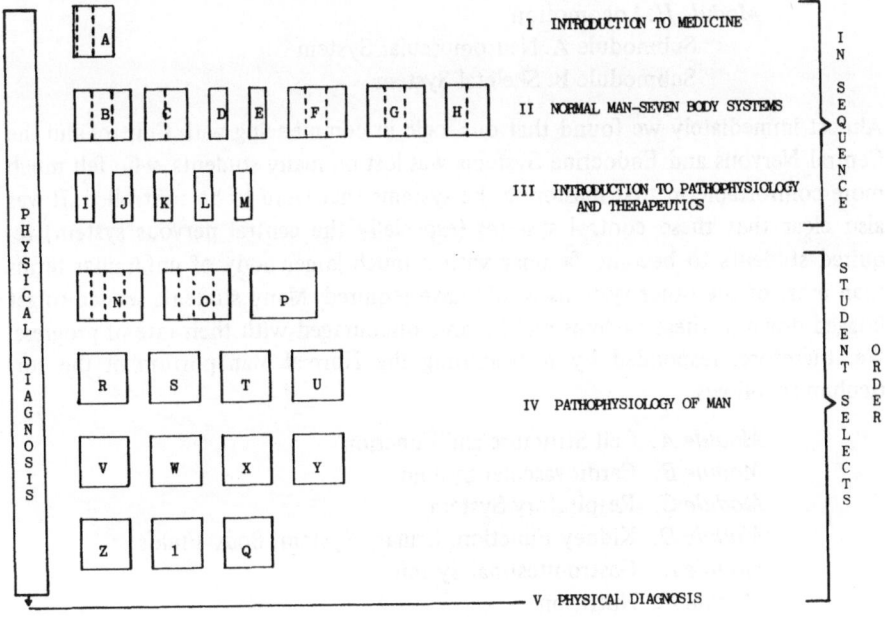

Figure 1. Curricular design, 1970.

Pathophysiology. A closer look at these main areas reveals subtle changes that have taken place over the ensuing years. In 1970, the curriculum was divided as shown in Figure 1.

In 1970, the Normal Man portion was composed of seven modules that were presented in a seemingly logical order. Specifically these were:

Module A. Introduction – Nature of Life Processes
Module B. Control Systems
        Submodule A. Central Nervous System
        Submodule B. Endocrine–Metabolic System
        Submodule C. Psychosocial System
Module C. Transport
        Submodule A. Cardiovascular System
        Submodule B. Respiratory System
Module D. Excretion–Renal System
Module E. Nutrition–Gastrointestinal System
Module F. Reproduction and Growth
        Submodule A. Genetics
        Submodule B. Reproductive System
        Submodule C. Growth and Development
Module G. Defense
        Submodule A. Hematologic System
        Submodule B. Immunology
        Submodule C. Skin

Module H. Locomotion
    Submodule A. Neuromuscular System
    Submodule B. Skeletal System

Almost immediately we found that our logic in commencing with Control and the Central Nervous and Endocrine Systems was lost on many students, who felt much more comfortable in first mastering the systems that were to be controlled. It was also clear that these control systems (especially the central nervous system) required students to become familiar with a much larger body of unfamiliar terms than most of the other systems would have required. Many students tended to get bogged down in these systems and became discouraged with their rate of progress. We, therefore, responded by restructuring the Normal Man portion of the curriculum as follows:

Module A. Cell Structure and Function
Module B. Cardiovascular System
Module C. Respiratory System
Module D. Kidney Function, Urinary System, Body Fluids
Module E. Gastrointestinal System
Module F. Nutrition

Posttest I

Module G. Skin and Supporting Tissues
Module H. Muscle, The Spinal Cord, and Peripheral
             Nervous System
Module I. Central Nervous System
Module J. Endocrine–Metabolic System
Module K. Genetics

Posttest II

Module L. Reproduction
Module M. Growth and Development
Module N. Psychosocial Development
Module O. Hematology
Module P. Immunologic System

Posttest III

Following Normal Man there are three modules designed to introduce the students to Pathophysiology of the Body Systems. These modules, which need not be taken in sequence, are: the Principles of Pathology, Principles of Microbiology, and Principles of Pharmacology. They represent surveys of each of these specialities, not exhaustive treatments.

The third major phase of the curriculum is the Pathophysiology of the Body Systems. There has been substantial change in the content of these modules over the years, but the main procedural change has been one from student-selected order to faculty-selected order. This was a decision based on the observation that many of the modules were only partially self-contained and that successful completion of one body of information (e.g., Acid–Base Balance in Module 5, the Endocrine– Metabolic System) depended to a great extent on knowledge gained in the Respiratory Pathophysiology and Renal Pathophysiology modules (Modules Y and Z, respectively). Furthermore, it was found that students did not find it particularly advantageous to order their own sequence. For these reasons, together with the desirability of monitoring student progress, a process that is best achieved if students follow a set sequence of modules, we decided to abandon the policy of student-directed sequencing except to a very limited extent. The Pathophysiology portion of the curriculum is now structured as follows:

Module U. Hematology
Module V. Infectious Diseases
Module W. The Gastrointestinal System

Posttest V

Module X. The Cardiovascular System
Module Y. The Respiratory System
Module Z. The Renal System

Posttest VI

Module 1. Central and Peripheral Nervous System
Module 2. Musculoskeletal System

Posttest VII

Module 3. The Diseases of Infants and Children
Module 4. Abnormal Psychology
Module 5. The Endocrine System
Module 6. The Reproductive System

Posttest VIII

A second major change in the nature of the curriculum involves Physical Diagnosis, which was originally designed to be covered "from day one" in the student's academic career. Logistical difficulties in scheduling students with varied backgrounds and at different stages of their medical careers induced the change to a more compressed exposure to physical diagnosis following Posttest IV. ISP students who are progressing at a rate comparable to students in the Lecture– Discussion Program take this course together with the Lecture–Discussion students. Early and late ISP students who cannot take this course receive this portion of their physical diagnosis training in the Family Practice Clinic at the University Hospitals Clinic.

The Faculty

Active faculty participation has been and remains the major asset of the ISP. The creation of this curriculum under the original NIH grant (1969) involved nearly a year of release time for many of the faculty involved. Although many of the original faculty remain, rotations into the program continue to bring new ideas into an already innovative curriculum.

Faculty members in a specific discipline (clinical or basic science) are responsible for the preparation of the individual aspects of each module (tutorial evaulation system, objectives, learning resources). The review of these materials with colleagues in the same or similar areas of specialization (e.g., acid–base chemistry between Departments of Physiology, Biochemistry, and Pharmacology) early in the developmental process insured that materials were minimally redundant and up to date. The size of these faculty groups range from a single author from each discipline to as many as four per module (e.g., Infectious Diseases involves four faculty from the Microbiology Department alone).

The review process involves initially discussions on the selection of appropriate learning resources and the revision and/or pagination required to match the stated objectives with both the resources and the tutorial evaluation system (TES). In this regard, we have recently begun to identify specifically each TES item on the computer printout with its matching objective from the modular handout. The final phase of the review process is concerned with the revision of the TES itself.

TES revision and design changes are the prerogative of individual faculty members on each module. The almost infinite variety of question types that involve both corrective feedback, coaching statements, and immediate reinforcement allows for the individual expression of different approaches to the same material. Examples of problem types utilized include everything from the simplest true–false questions to problems requiring analytical and quantitative manipulations. The capacity to make constant changes in TES design affords each faculty member the opportunity to correct errors or emphasis instantly in his original system.

The authorship of the TES has, of course, changed as new faculty are rotated into the program. The design of individual TES material is then modified and revised by new faculty concomitantly with changes in source and objective materials. It is during the TES revision process that each new faculty member is encouraged to collaborate with the instructional programmers for his module. Such collaboration can take the form of correcting obvious problem areas in the TES or discussing and implementing formats for new material.

Faculty responsibilities are, therefore, somewhat different in the ISP than in a traditional lecture curriculum. Instead of designing and presenting lectures, emphasis is placed upon integration of material into modules prepared by an interdisciplinary team of faculty. The scheduling of individual, small-group, discussion sessions by a faculty member when students are taking his module allows him to assess directly the depth with which they grasp his material. Occasional clinical correlation sessions conducted with both basic science and clinical faculty serve to facilitate the extension

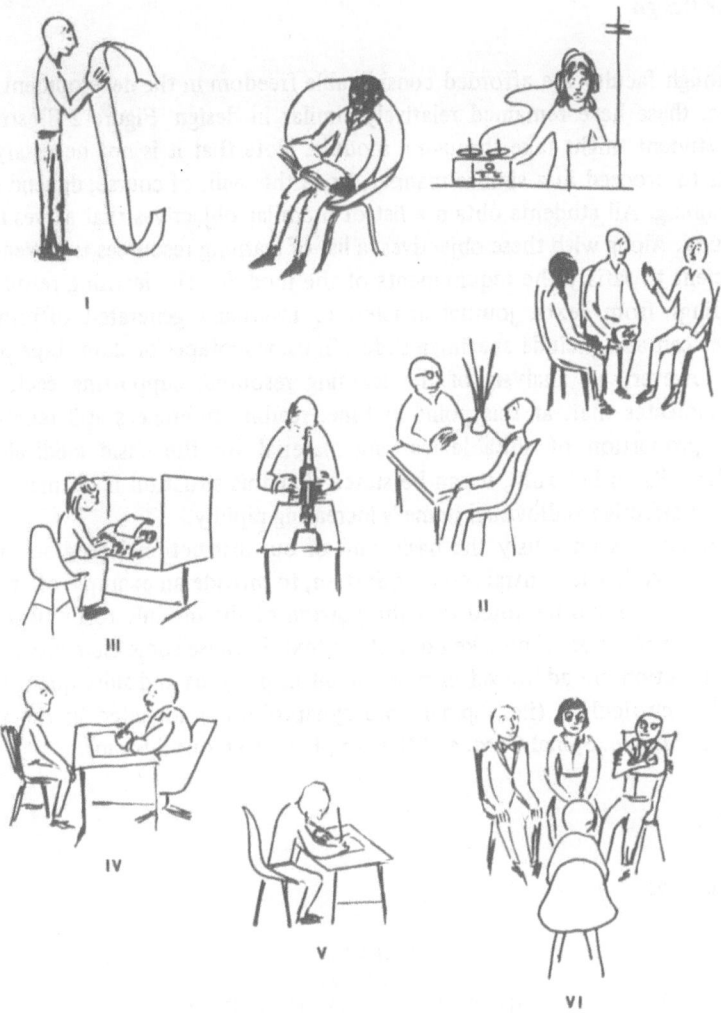

Figure 2. Student flow in a typical module. In Step I each student receives and examines the modular objectives and learning resource list. Step II represents the student's use of the learning resources to satisfy the learning objectives. These can include readings, audiovisuals, small group discussions, faculty conferences, and laboratory exercises. Following Step II the student tests his learning by accessing the tutorial evaluation system (TES) (Step III). He may then opt for further faculty conferences (Step IV). At specified points in the curriculum he must take a written examination covering several modules (Step V) and demonstrate his ability to transmit information orally in prescheduled oral exercises (Step VI).

of concepts of normal function to those of pathophysiology. The emphasis placed on curriculum development within an interdisciplinary team rather than lecture preparation has created a curriculum that is constantly changing as faculty receive helpful suggestions from both their peers and their students.

Modular Design

Although faculty are afforded considerable freedom in the development of their modules, these have remained relatively similar in design. Figure 2 illustrates the path a student might take through a module. Note that it is not necessary for all students to proceed in a similar manner, since this will, of course, depend on their prior training. All students obtain a list of modular objectives that serves to direct their study. Along with these objectives, a list of learning resources is presented that is sufficient to satisfy the requirements of the module. The learning resources can be readings from texts, journal articles, or internally generated offprints. The resources can also include specimen slides, films, videotapes or slide—tape presentations. However, an analysis of the learning resources supporting each module clearly indicates that, at this point in time, reading references still represent the greatest proportion of suitable learning material for the basic medical science curriculum. Parenthetically, it can be stated that this situation is changing and the number of effective audiovisual items is increasing rapidly.

The module is obviously the basic unit of our instructional program. We have chosen Module I, The Central Nervous System, to provide an example of an instructional unit. It should be noted that the portion of the module to be illustrated is only an example, not to be taken out of context, because some elements of central nervous function are addressed in more detail in previous and subsequent modules within the curriculum (i.e., spinal cord synaptology is included in the previous module on Muscle, Spinal Cord, and the Peripheral Nervous System).

Example I

The Objectives

MODULE I
1975–76
THE CENTRAL NERVOUS SYSTEM
(Drs. Stokes and King)

I. Scope and Objectives

The major purpose of this module is to attempt an integration of the bodily processes and anatomical constructs you have studied so far with the physiology and anatomy of the central nervous system. You have already encountered a number of the basic principles of spinal cord neurophysiology in Module H. It is necessary that you review these principles in a more refined way as you begin a study of the basic structures of the CNS, i.e., eliminate the black-box approach and learn the functional anatomy.

You can neither memorize tracts nor isolated potential changes if you wish to achieve the synthesis of neuroscience concepts we expect of you.

A. Basic structures and physiological principles of the central nervous system.

1. Structural Relationships

   The basic objective of your initial encounter with the brain and spinal cord is to localize their structural features and to learn the vocabulary needed to discuss the physiology and anatomy of individual functional systems.

   a. Neurohistology and Ultrastructure

      Identify the structural features (e.g., all terms in italics in A, pp. 41–76) of the cellular components of the CNS and their roles in synaptic transmission, axoplasmic flow, myelin formation, brain barriers, and injury. (See J)

   b. Spinal Cord Anatomy (A, pp. 133–146, all terms in italics)

      Identify and describe the gross features of the spinal cord and the distinguishing appearance of the cord sectioned at cervical, thoracic, lumbar, and sacral levels, and the organization of gray and white matter.

   c. Brainstem and Forebrain Anatomy (C; K and H)

      Identify and recognize the structures on the Weigert stained sections that are labeled in sections 1–3 in the handout entitled, "Cross-sectional Anatomy of the Brainstem and Forebrain." Identify the structures on the gross brain described and labeled in the handout on the "Gross Brain and Vascular Patterns." (E) View audiovisual I after this handout.

   d. Cranial Nerves (D)

      Describe the functional components (e.g., cranial nerve III has two components – motor to striated voluntary muscle – autonomic to constructor muscle of the eye) in each of the cranial nerves and identify each of the brainstem nuclei that give rise to the components.

   e. Blood Supply and Cerebrospinal Fluid (A, pp. 25–40; A, pp. 282–283; Fig. 8–21)

      Describe the major arterial trunks that supply the spinal cord brainstem and forebrain. This will be of particular importance in future considerations of functional deficits as a result of vascular insult to the hemispheres and brainstem. Describe the venous drainage of the brain (A, p. 32; Fig. 1–26). Describe the formation and circulation of cerebrospinal fluid (A, p. 36; Fig. 1–29).

2. Physiological Relationships

   a. Review the evidence for the different types of central synaptic events in the central nervous system (B, pp. 193–206). Can you describe the processes involved in the initiation of impulses, different types of synaptic interaction, and the role of interneurons in the CNS?

   b. Consider the elements and candidates for different synaptic transmitter agents in the CNS (B, pp. 206–215 and McGeer). Can you describe the potential functional role that each of the following play in synaptic transmission and/or behavior:

acetylcholine   glutamate
norepinephrine   GABA
dopamine   glycine
serotonin

Review the above material using the McGeer article (Learning Resources, G).

c. Contrast the principles of synaptic transmission in cerebral cortex with those in spinal cord (B, pp. 237–243). Include in your study the roles of postsynaptic potentials in action potential initiation, the relationship of cellular activity (postsynaptic potentials, action potentials) to surface potential changes (the evoked potential, the electroencephalogram). Be able to relate to an examiner the frequency spectrum of the EEG and how it changes with different incoming sensory stimuli.

d. Consider some of the basic physiologic anatomy of the cerebrospinal fluid. Include in your study:

1. The basics of the ventricular system (B, pp. 1116–1119; review audiovisual I in detail).
2. What is the blood–brain barrier?
3. A review of the CSF role in respiratory control (B, pp. 1131–1133).

e. Before you begin your study of CNS systems, consider the major functions of the central nervous system in the "overview" handout (F).

The Learning Resources

Note that each of the learning resources is identified in the objectives by a specific letter and pagination throughout the objectives.

Texts and Handouts

A. Noback, C.R. and R.J. Demarest, *The Human Nervous System, Basic Principles of Neurobiology*, 2nd ed., New York; McGraw-Hill, 1975.
B. Mountcastle, V.B., *Medical Physiology*, 13th ed., St. Louis; C.V. Mosby Co., 1974.
C. King, J.S., "Cross Sectional Anatomy of the Brainstem and Forebrain." (Handout).
D. King, J.S., "Cranial Nerves" (handout).
E. King, J.S., "Brain and Vascular Patterns" (handout).
F. Stokes, B.T., "Overview of the Central Nervous System" (handout).

Articles

G. McGeer, Patrick, "The Chemistry of Mind" from *Audiovisual Materials* The American Scientist, 1971.

Slides To Be Used with Handout C. Copied from:

H. Frontal Sections of the Brain in "The Atlas," from Hall, J.L., and Humbertson, A.O., *A Correlative Study Guide for Neuroanatomy*, 2nd ed., New York; Harper and Row, 1970. Plates 3, 4, 7, 9, 10, 13, 18, 21, 24, 25, 28, 29, 32.

Cassettes

I.   "3-D Dissection of the Brain" (good for ventricular anatomy)

Slide and Audio Tapes

J.   "Neurohistology" (audio tape)
K.   "Overview of the Gross and Cross Sectional Anatomy of the Brain and Brainstem"

Conferences

An integral part of many modules are the small group laboratory/conference sessions such as the following listed for Module I. These occur at a time in the curriculum when most students are well into their study of this module and are occasionally repeated if student time spread warrants.

Neuroanatomy Discussion Sessions

1–3	9/18/76	(Th)	Mind of Man, Introduction to Module
1–3	9/23/76	(T)	Neurohistology, Ultrastructure and Spinal Cord Anatomy
9–11 & 1–3	9/25/76	(Th)	Brainstem (½ Class) and Forebrain Sectional Anatomy (½ Class)
9, 10, 11	9/30/76	(T)	Gross Brain Demonstrations
9, 10, 11	10/1/76	(Th)	Gross Brain Demonstrations
1–3	10/7/76	(T)	Cranial Nerves, Blood Supply, CSF (½ Class)
1–3	10/9/76	(Th)	Cranial Nerves, Blood Supply, CSF (½ Class)

Neurophysiology and Neuroanatomy Discussion Sessions

1–3	10/14/76	(T)	Visual System
1–3	10/16/76	(Th)	Auditory System
1–3	10/21/76	(T)	Somatosensory System
1–3	10/23/76	(Th)	Vestibular System
1–3	10/28/76	(T)	Pyramidal System
1–3	10/30/76	(Th)	"Extraphyramidal" System
1–3	11/7/76	(F)	Cerebellum
1–3	11/7/76	(T)	Higher Nervous Control, Cerebral Hemispheres, and Thalamus
1–3	11/14/76	(F)	Limbic System and Hypothalamus
1–3	11/18/76	(T)	Reticular Formation

Following a variable period of study of the modular material, the student is afforded an opportunity to assess the effectiveness of his endeavors. Each module is supported by the computer-based Tutorial Evaluation System. This system is designed to be a nonpunitive measure of the student's degree of mastery of the subject. If no glaring weaknesses are perceived, the student moves on to the next module. The TES has characteristics of an examination and of computer-assisted instruction, but is not intended to be either. It lacks the punitive aspect of a certifying examination and, unlike, programmed instruction it makes no attempt to be all inclusive. Rather, it samples the much larger body of knowledge addressed in the modular objectives. An example of the TES as it appears to the student might be as follows (sample from Module I TES).

Example II

MODULE I: CENTRAL NERVOUS SYSTEM

T, terminal; S, student

(T) 1. Where is the first synapse in the pathway relaying impulses of pain from the skin of the extremities located?

(S)   Thoracic nucleus

(T)   The thoracic nucleus (Clarke's column) is not primarily concerned with the relay of superificial peripheral pain modalities. It is concerned with modalities relayed to the cerebellum. Reconsider and try again.

(S)   Dorsal root ganglion

(T)   The dorsal root ganglion is not a synaptic station. Consider a single neuron relaying any peripheral sensory impulse to the central nervous system.

Which of the following parts of the neuron is housed in the dorsal root ganglion?

peripheral fiber
cell body
proximal fiber

(S)   Proximal fiber

(T)   You are overlooking a very important fact of the neuron. Try to reason it out.

(S)   Cell body

(T)   O.K. Now consider the proximal fiber of this cell body and go back and answer the original question.

(S)   Nucleus proprius

(T)   Right. The synapse here is by the proximal fiber with its cell body located in the root ganglion.

(T) 2. O.K. Let's follow the pain impulse. Beginning with the second order neuron, which you just stated was in the nucleus proprius, follow the impulse to the cerebral cortex by choosing the correct statements and arrange them in their correct sequence.

NOTE: Do not use any punctuation to separate the letters you select.

TYPE IN ANSWERS YOU CHOOSE ALL AT ONCE.

A. Second order neuron crosses midline in ventral commisure and ascends in lateral funiculus.

B. Third order neuron originating in thalamus, crosses to opposite cerebral cortex.

C. Second order neuron ascends in lateral funiculus ipsilateral to its origin in the nucleus proprius.

> D. Synapse in the thalamus on the side ipsilateral to origin of second order neuron.
> E. Third order neuron, originating in thalamus, ascends to the ipsilateral cerebral cortex.
> F. Synapse in the thalamus on the side opposite to the origin of second order neuron.

(S)   CFE.

(T)   Incorrect. Think of what the second order neuron always does in a sensory pathway to the thalamus.
Reconsider and try again.

(S)   AFE.

(T)   Very good! You have completed a three neuron sensory pathway to the cerebral cortex.

(T) 3. Identify the tracts which would be interrupted by a hemisection of the spinal cord (Brown–Sequard Syndrome) caused by a bullet or knife wound and would be responsible for the following findings.

> A. Pyramidal paralysis below the level of the lesion
> B. Ipsilateral loss of proprioception (at the unconscious level)
> C. Contralateral loss of pain and temperature sensations beginning one or two segments below the lesion
> D. Sensory ataxia

LET'S TAKE THEM ONE AT A TIME.

> A. Pyramidal paralysis below the level of the lesion.

(S)   Corticospinal tract

(T)   Which corticospinal tract is it?

(S)   Lateral

(T)   That's right. Note that it is evident below the level of the lesion and is ipsilateral

> B. Ipsilateral loss of proprioception (at the unconscious level):

(S)   Anterior spinocerebellar tract

(T)   No. Keep in mind that anterior spinocerebellar tract contains both CROSSED and uncrossed fibers. We are looking for an ipsilateral loss. Now what do you say?

(S)   Lateral spinocerebellar tract

(T)   I know of a dorsal and ventral spinocerebellar tract – not a lateral. Are the spinocerebellar tracts located superficial or deep in the lateral funiculus?

(S)   Superficial

(T)   Good! In the upper thoracic and cervical cord, the spinocerebellar tracts occupy the entire extent of the superficial portion of the lateral funiculus.

> C. Contralateral loss of pain and temperature sensation beginning one or two segments below the lesion.

(S)   Spinothalamic tract

(T)   There are two of these tracts, to which you are referring?

(S)   Lateral spinothalamic tract

(T)	Correct! Can you recall why the effects may be one or two segments away from the lesion; in other words, what tract is utilized by all incoming fibers that bifurcate and ascend or descend one or two segments?
(S)	Lissauer tract
(T)	Very good! This is an important point to remember in evaluation of clinical findings.
(T)	Sensory ataxia
(S)	Fasciculus gracilis
(T)	Correct. Practically all tactile sensation is absent on one side. What is the clinical syndrome resulting from a degenerative disease that affects the dorsal columns of the spinal column?
(S)	Tabes dorsalis.
(T)	Very good! The pathological process may begin in the dorsal roots and spread to the posterior funiculus of the cord.

Note that an immediate response is obtained whether the student's attempt was correct or incorrect. Correct responses are supported by feedback designed to increase the student's insight into the problem. Incorrect responses trigger a comment which very often contains clues to direct the student to a more acceptable answer.

Posttest. Following the completion of a specified block of modules each student must take a written objective posttest. This examination, unlike the TES, is intended to certify the student's mastery of the modular objectives and posttest items are prepared on the basis of specific objectives. The number of questions per module will, of course, vary with student time needed to complete the unit. Grades on such posttests are used by the faculty to make "GO–NO GO" decisions on each student with 70% set as a cutoff point for required remedial work. An example of posttest questions covering Module I is as follows:

Example III

1. Surgical transection of the descending (spinal) trigeminal tract on the right side caudal to the root entry zone of C.N.V. would produce loss of:
   A. Pain and temperature on the same side of the face – excluding angle of the jaw
   B. Pain and temperature on the opposite side of the face
   C. Proprioception on the same side of the face
   D. Light touch on the same side of the face – excluding the angle of the jaw
   E. Movements of the muscles of mastication

2. If as the result of an automobile accident an individual suffered a cord hemisection on the right side at a T-4 cord level, which of the following would be true one month after the accident?
   A. Some flaccid paralysis of the right upper extremity
   B. Loss of pain and temperature on the side of the lesion below T-4

C. Loss of position sense in the lower extremity on the side opposite the lesion

D. A spastic paralysis of the musculature on the side of the lesion

E. A flaccid paralysis of the musculature on the side of the lesion

3. The ability of ballet dancers and sailors to control the nystagmus and visceral reactions to repeated motion is an example of:

A. Vestibular neuropathy

B. Cerebellar damping

C. Spinal shock syndrome

D. Vestibular habituation

4. A washed out appearance of the substantia nigra as in Parkinson's disease results from:

A. An enhanced dopamine synthesis in the striatum

B. A depletion of norepinephrine in the subthalamic region

C. An increase in serotonin activity in the striatum

D. Enhancement of ascending reticular input

E. A decrease in dopamine in nigrostriatal pathways

Oral Exercises. Originally the oral examination took the form of a faculty board examining each student in a question-and-answer format. Over a period of time, it became clear that we could not expand the class and continue this practice without a constant problem of scheduling physicians. Furthermore, it was apparent that we were measuring parameters that could just as easily be measured in the written examination, whereon the major objective of the oral was intended to be an assessment of verbal communicative skills. We have, therefore, eliminated the oral examination in favor of an exercise that is intended to concentrate on communicative skills with very little emphasis on factual recall. These exercises are given at least twice during the curriculum; once by a basic scientist during Normal Man and once during the Pathophysiology phase of the program by a physician. Emphasis is placed on communication, and every attempt is made to neutralize effects a deficit in factual knowledge might have on communicative skills. Indeed, some faculty give the students advance notice of the topic to be discussed and choose an unfamiliar area to avoid covering topics that are areas of expertise of the faculty. The exercise then serves as a gross screen to discover students who could use practice and guidance in delivery of a verbal information. Students experiencing difficulty in this area are given further opportunities to practice their skills with other members of the faculty.

Management of the System

The highly individualized nature of the ISP could cause logistical problems in monitoring student progress and scheduling of resources. To help meet these needs, an ISP extension of the college's computerized management system is provided.

The college's Computer-Assisted Instruction Reporting System (CAIRS)* was developed to help monitor the usage of, evaluate the effectiveness of, and upgrade the efficiency of the CAI system which supports the college's 3000 to 5000 hours of student usage per month. CAIRS is an extensive series of reports and the computer programs that generate and maintain them; the reports provide feedback regarding CAI utilization and effectiveness to students, faculty advisers and tutors, authors of CAI materials, educators, programmers and analysts, managers of CAI operations, and administrators.

Data generated by student interaction at a CAI terminal are stored by CAIRS for later retrieval. The modular design of the daily, weekly, monthly, and on-demand subsystems of the CAIRS gives the user great flexibility in selecting and obtaining only those outputs that are of interest at a particular point in time. A schematic of the CAIRS system flow is shown in Figure 3. At the heart of the system are three types of data that are generated by the on-line CAI system, in real time.

Line activity (LA) records are automatically generated when the on-line system is initiated, when a user signs on or off, when operator messages are sent to users, and when certain error conditions occur in the system.

Student response (SR) records are generated as requested by authors, faculty or staff. (a) each time a student enters a response or a comment at a terminal, and (b) when an author triggers the storage of information regarding student performance in a course.

System control records are generated for use by system programmers in monitoring system operation.

Operationally, the background system is divided into four subsystems (see Figure 3) on the basis of frequency of operation. Each subsystem processes the three types of data described above.

1. *Daily Processing Subsystem.* This subsystem

    a. Transfers from temporary disc storage to semi-permanent tape storage all records generated from around-the-clock operation of the CAI on-line system.
    b. Generates a backup copy of all CAI course material files.
    c. Lists system control counts and records for use in monitoring line errors, system problems, and efficiency factors (i.e., response time) of the on-line software.

2. *Weekly Processing Subsystem.* This subsystem consolidates the daily data (LA and SR) onto month-to-date tapes and produces the following reports:

    a. A composite listing of all LA records for the week.
    b. A chart showing the total student load on the system day-by-day and hour-by-hour divided by major user groups (Figure 4).

---

* Only the ISP portion of the CAIRS system is described herein. Full discussion of the CAIRS system is offered in Pengov, R.E., 1974, A Modularly-Designed Computer Assisted Instruction Reporting System (CAIRS), *MEDINFO* 74, North Holland Publishing Co., Amsterdam; and in *The Computer-Based Management System for Support of Computer Assisted Instruction at The Ohio State University College of Medicine,* 1973, available from the Division of Computing Services for Medical Education and Research.

c. A listing by day of the individual time periods when the system was up and down (Figure 5).

d. A usage and stability report (Figure 6). This report gives a weekly summary of the load on the CAI system. Note that actual line-hour availability may exceed that guaranteed and that the system can accommodate considerably higher usage as evidenced by the percent of available time used.

These reports are particularly important in monitoring the availability and stability of both the CAI student usage terminals and the CAI System itself.

3. *Monthly Processing Subsystem*. This subsystem transfers the LA and SR records to long-term storage media and produces the following reports:

a. A detailed listing of all student responses to individual questions within a course.

b. A detailed listing recreating an individual student's flow through a course. (Very fine-grain student data are available but are used only when the adviser wishes to pursue a difficulty being encountered by a student in a particular area. Sometimes essay question response is recreated via this mechanism.)

c. A listing of all unanticipated responses to questions within a course

d. An "item statistics" summary of student answers to questions which cross tabulates type of answer (i.e., correct, incorrect, unanticipated) with attempt number (Figure 7).

e. A summary of unsolicited comments entered at the terminal and arranged by course, student, and time.

(Reports c, d, and e are invaluable in updating and revising TES modules and in insuring that the CAI materials remain "viable" and responsive to

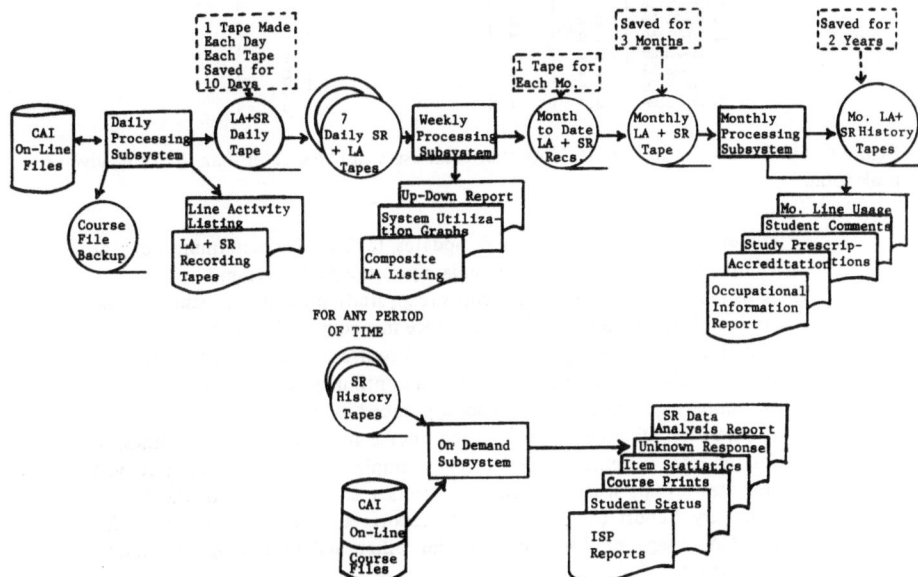

Figure 3. System flow chart of the CAIRS. Note the temporal relationships of the *daily, weekly, monthly,* and *on-demand* subsystems. Copyright 1974, Ohio State University College of Medicine CAIRS.

ROTARY USAGE REPORT FOR 01/14/76

TIME	MEAN USAGE	PEAK TOTAL	DISTRIBUTION AT PEAK USAGE MAIN DCS	CRN	SU	COM	TYMSHAR HEN	UNDEF
00:00–00:29	.5	1					1	
00:30–00:59								
01:00–01:29								
01:30–01:59								
02:00–02:29								
02:30–02:59								
03:00–03:29								
03:30–03:59								
04:00–04:29								
04:30–04:59								
05:00–05:29								
05:30–05:59								
06:00–06:29								
06:30–06:59								
07:00–07:29								
07:30–07:59	1.5	2		1		1		
08:00–08:29	5.0	7		2		5		
08:30–08:59	8.5	11		3		7	1	
09:00–09:29	13.5	15		3		10	2	
09:30–09:59	14.0	16	2	3		9	2	
10:00–10:29	17.5	20	2	3	1	13	1	
10:30–10:59	16.0	18	1	3	1	11	2	
11:00–11:29	11.0	15	1	3	1	8	2	
11:30–11:59	10.0	11		3	1	6	1	
12:00–12:29	9.0	12		4		7	1	
12:30–12:59	13.5	15	1	5		8	1	
13:00–13:29	12.5	15	1	4	1	8	1	
13:30–13:59	15.0	18		3	1	11	3	
14.00–14:29	18.0	20		4	1	12	3	
14:30–14:59	15.5	19		4	1	11	3	
15:00–15:29	16.5	21		4	1	13	3	
15:30–15:59	20.0	22	1	4	1	13	3	
16:00–16:29	20.5	23	2	2	1	13	5	
16:30–16:59	20.5	24	1	3	1	13	6	
17:00–17:29	16.0	20	1	3		12	4	
17:30–17:59	11.0	13		2		8	3	
18:00–18:29	11.5	13	1	3		6	3	
18:30–18:59	10.0	13	1	1		7	4	
19:00–19:29	9.0	11		1		6	4	
19:30–19:59	10.5	12		2		7	3	
20:00–20:29	9.5	11		3		5	3	
20:30–20:59								
21:00–21:29	2.0	3				2	1	
21:30–21:59	1.0	2				2		
22:00–22:29	2.0	3		2			1	
22:30–22:59	2.5	3		1			2	
23:00–23:29	2.5	3		1			2	
23:30–23:59	3.0	4		1			3	

Figure 4. The Rotary Usage Report. Note that total users can be greater than the value given for peak total.

student flows. Corrections and updates to TES [as determined by the faculty member] are added immediately to the TES program.)

   f. A listing of author-triggered records (e.g., study prescriptions and question statistics) regarding student performance in a course (Figure 8).

   g. A listing by accrediting orgnization and course of students who have completed courses or sections of courses for continuing education credit.

   h. A summary of CAI user occupations, grouped by course.

   i. A summary of usage hours of each course for a line, groups of lines, or for the total system; Figure 9 offers a sample CAI Usage Summary Report (by user group) whereas Figure 10 offers a sample portion of the Course Summary Report (by course). Both reports are important in monitoring the CAI usage of ISP students and other audiences (e.g., continuing education).

  4. *On-Demand Subsystem.* This subsystem provides all reports decribed under "monthly processing subsystem," but covers varying time periods. It retrieves information as desired from the month-to-date and/or monthly history tapes for specific courses, time periods, student numbers, and lable ranges (within a

```
CAI WEEKLY DOWN TIME REPORT FOR 03:22 ON 03/28/76 - 02:59 ON 04/04/76


03/29/76    02:59-03:28 = .5 HR*
TOTAL HOURS OF SYSTEM DOWN TIME = .5

03/30/76    02:59-03:44 = .7 HR*
            05:51-07:14 = 1.4 HR*
            07:47-07:48 = .0 HR*
            08:00-08:01 = .0 HR*
TOTAL HOURS OF SYSTEM DOWN TIME = 2.2

03/31/76    03:09-03:36 = .4 HR*
            05:27-07:39 = 2.2 HR*
            15:27-15:32 = .1 HR**
TOTAL HOURS OF SYSTEM DOWN TIME = 2.7

04/01/76    03:02-03:25 = .4 HR*
TOTAL HOURS OF SYSTEM DOWN TIME = .4

04/02/76    02:58-03:38 = .7 HR*
            05:29-07:24 = 1.9 HR*
            10:49-10:54 = .1 HR**
TOTAL HOURS OF SYSTEM DOWN TIME = 2.7

04/03/76    03:03-03:39 = .6 HR*
            19:36-19:42 = .1 HR**
TOTAL HOURS OF SYSTEM DOWN TIME = .7


* SCHEDULED DOWN TIME

** SYSTEM CRASH.  DOWN TIME COULD BE LESS THAN SHOWN


NOTE:  PRIME TIME IS 9:00 AM - 12 MIDNIGHT EST
```

Figure 5. Weekly Down Time Report. This report gives the daily down time by specific times and the total daily down time.

course). Two reports produced from the "on-demand" subsystems are of particular importance to ISP faculty:

a. *Course Prints.* Several different types of prints of CAI course statements are provided to faculty for review and revision of the TES modules and for use in answering student questions about the content and flow of the TES. These prints are like shelf copies of books except that new versions of them are needed much more frequently (each time a module is revised).

b. *Student Status Report.* This report is an abbreviated form of the Student Progress Report (see below) and is available at the CAI terminal any time a faculty adviser needs an up-to-the-minute report on student progress. The adviser need only type in the course name and his initials to receive a current status report for each of his advisees or for the entire class (Figure 11).

In addition to the reports described above, two special reports are provided to ISP faculty and administrators.

1. *Individual Student Progress Report.* This report is generated weekly for each student in the ISP. Figure 12 offers an example of this report which shows the student's name, access number, class, adviser, date of last usage on TES, and current module/submodule location within the ISP curriculum. The report charts the students' weekly progress through the curriculum by noting modules actually completed (line marked COMP) compared to a schedules progress plan

USAGE AND STABILITY REPORT FOR 03/28/76 TO 04/04/76

	MAIN	TYMSHAR	TOTAL
GUAR LINE-HR AVAIL			
TOTAL	2,800	700	3,500
PRIME	2,100	525	2,625
ACTUAL LINE-HR AVAIL			
TOTAL	3,236	809	4,046
PRIME	2,094	523	2,618
% OF POTENTIAL AVAIL			
TOTAL	115	115	115
PRIME	99	99	99
ACTUAL LINE-HR USED			
TOTAL	473	273	646
PRIME	428	161	589
% OF AVAIL TIME USED			
TOTAL	14	21	15
PRIME	20	30	22
# OF SIGN-ONS			
TOTAL	813	408	1,221
PRIME	757	385	1,142
MEAN/SESSION (MIN)			
TOTAL	34	25	31
PRIME	33	25	30

NOTE: PRIME TIME IS 9:00 AM - 12 MIDNIGHT EST

Figure 6. Usage and Stability Report. Note that in this case actual line hours available exceeded the total guaranteed time available and that 99% of potential prime time was available during this period. Also note that only 20% of available prime time is actually being used at the present time.

(line marked SCHED). This scheduled progress plan is set individually for each student; it can be the previous class' average time, or a special progress plan mutually set by the student and his adviser.

2. *Student Cluster Report.* This report provides faculty and directors with a point-in-time picture of how students are dispersed throughout the curriculum. Figure 13 shows a portion of the Cluster Report which maps all ISP students by their location within the module and submodules of the ISP. This report is particularly valuable in monitoring student dispersion in that it gives the ISP director knowledge of where all students are in the curriculum at any point in time. It also facilitates faculty scheduling of small groups of students for group discussions, lab exercises, enrichment sessions, testing, or other purposes.

Results and Discussion

The ISP has proven to be an attractive alternative to the more traditional lecture system in the study of the preclinical medical sciences for some medical students. Many undergraduate programs now include some experiences in independent study so that students entering our college have very often been exposed to some aspects of this type of curriculum. For this reason, independent study might be expected to appeal to entering medical students. The volunteer rate per class has stabilized at approximately 40% of all students afforded the choice between independent study and the more traditional lecture—discussion programs. The overall results of the past 7 years show a volunteer rate of 36% for all classes. We believe our class to be somewhat typical of entering classes in larger, state-supported, medical schools; therefore, for planning purposes, one might expect a comparable rate in similar institutions.

ITEM STATISTICS FOR QUESTION, IA1106- 1   COURSE: PILOT

TIME PERIOD: 10/01/75 - 12/29/75   DATA COVERS   47 STUDENTS USAGE

RESPONSE	ATTEMPT NUMBER 1	2	3	4	>4	RESPONSE TOTALS	% OF TIME WA LEAD TO UN	% OF TIME UN LEADS TO UN
1- 2 CA	4	19	9	3		35		
1- 3 CA	1					1		
1- 9 WA		2	1			3	33%	
1- 14 WA			1			1	100%	
1- 18 WA	2	3				5	60%	
1- 24 WA	14	3				17	71%	
99- 99 UN	26	15	3			44		14%
ATTEMPT TOTALS	47	42	14	3		106		

UNANTICIPATED RESPONSES MADE ON FIRST AND SECOND ATTEMPTS:

1. NUCLEUSRUBRUM
    INFERIORCEREBELLARPEDUNCLE

    MLF
    BASESPEDUNCULI
    MLF
    REDNUCLEEI

    MIDDLECEREVELLARPEDUNCLE
    *** ALL UNS NOT LISTED ***

2. BRACHIUMPONTIS
    REDNUCLEUS
    NO

    TECTUM
    CEREBRALPEEDUNCLE
    CERBRALPEDUNCLE
    RETICULARFORMATIONN
    TEGMENTUM
    *** ALL UNS NOT LISTED ***

STATISTICS FOR NUMBER OF RESPONSES
RANGE   1- 4
MEAN   2
MODE   1

Figure 7. Item Statistics for a Single Question. Correct answer is designated CA and unanticipated responses are designated UN. In this example "define hemolyze" and "define RBC's" were common unanticipated responses, therefore these would be logical suggestions for additions to the bank of anticipated responses in the computer program.

One question that arises in a time-independent study program such as ours concerns student rate of progress through the curriculum. Since we had no prior experience to draw on, we did not know what to expect from our first class entering in 1970. As previously reported (Beran *et al.*, 1976) and shown in Table 1, this class proceeded in a tight group through the program with only a 4-month period elapsing from the earliest to the latest student. This could have been due to the small class or to the fact that it was very clear that the program was an experimental one, and the students tended to study with each other because they had a rather common identity. The class entering in 1971 took a mean time of 17.5 months with a spread of 10 months to 29 months. Roughly 39% of the class graduated at least one quarter later than the projected date. Similar results have been obtained for the 1972 and 1973 entering classes with a notable compression of the progress of the 1972 class. For reasons that are still unclear, there has been a large difference in the progress of the 1974 class. While the early students are completing their studies normally, over 40% of this class will be graduating at least one quarter later than the date normally expected of them. Anecdotally, it appears that a higher proportion of each class enters the ISP with the intention of spending more time than

RX INFORMATION   STUDY PRESCRIPTION LISTING PRINTED ON 03/04/74   COURSE: PILOT

STUDENT	STUDENT #	DATE	LABEL-PROB #		COMMENT
S 110		02/15/74	EA8889-	2	7 OF 54 IN 15 QUES IN THE ESOPHAGUS
		02/16/74	EB8888-	2	13 OF 60 IN 24 QUES IN STOMACH AND DUODENUM
		02/19/74	EC2999-	2	21 OF 81 IN 21 QUES IN THE COLON
S 144		02/04/74	EA8889-	2	7 OF 54 IN 15 QUES IN THE ESOPHAGUS
		02/04/74	EB8888-	2	10 OF 60 IN 24 QUES IN STOMACH AND DUODENUM
		02/11/74	EC2999-	2	25 OF 81 IN 21 QUES IN THE COLON
		02/11/74	ED2888-	2	8 OF 64 IN 21 QUES IN THE LIVER
		02/11/74	EE9888-	2	18 OF 38 IN 11 QUES IN PANCREAS AND BILIARY TREE
S 146		02/08/74	EA8889-	2	10 OF 54 IN 15 QUES IN THE ESOPHAGUS
		02/08/74	EB8888-	2	12 OF 60 IN 24 QUES IN STOMACH AND DUODENUM
		02/08/74	EC2999-	2	18 OF 81 IN 21 QUES IN THE COLON
		02/08/74	ED2888-	2	7 OF 64 IN 21 QUES IN THE LIVER
		02/08/74	EE9888-	2	14 OF 38 IN 11 QUES IN PANCREAS AND BILIARY TREE
S 338		02/18/74	EA8889-	2	9 OF 54 IN 15 QUES IN THE ESOPHAGUS
		02/20/74	EB8888-	2	15 OF 60 IN 24 QUES IN STOMACH AND DUODENUM
		02/20/74	EB8888-	2	15 OF 60 IN 24 QUES IN STOMACH AND DUODENUM
S 5711		02/12/74	DA3399-	2	3 OF 9 IN 3 QUES IN BODY FLUID COMPARTMENTS
		02/13/74	DB3398-	2	0 OF 11 IN 4 QUES IN RENAL MECHANISMS
		02/13/74	DC3390-	2	5 OF 40 IN 5 QUES IN REGULATION OF SALT AND WATER EXCRETION
		02/26/74	DD3396-	2	3 OF 16 IN 6 QUES IN RENAL ACID-BASE REGULATION

ETC.

Figure 8. A Study Prescription Listing. Each faculty member may set a minimum level of performance expected from the students on the TES. Performance below this minimum triggers a study prescription received by the student at the terminal.

CAI USAGE SUMMARY   02/29/76-03/31/76

GROUP	PRIME HOURS	TOTAL HOURS	TERMINALS	SIGN-ONS	MIN/ SESS	% OF CAI
CAIREN	483.6	530.4	16	1,029	30.9	23.3
COLL OF MED	746.8	762.1	19	1,020	44.8	33.5
DCS	240.7	260.3	15	936	17.0	11.7
HENUG	601.0	624.7	94	1,322	28.3	27.5
SPECIAL USER	88.5	90.9	5	196	27.8	4.0
UNDEFINED USERS	0.2	0.2	1	1	14.0	0.0
TOTAL	2,160.8	2,274.9	150	4,504	30.3	100.0

PRIME HRS= 2,160.8   NON-PRIME HRS= 114.1   % PRIME= 95.0
(PRIME TIME IS 9 AM TO 12 MIDNIGHT E.T.)

Figure 9. CAI Usage Summary. This monthly report shows at a glance the use by major users of the OSU CAI System. Main users are the Regional Educational Network, the OSU College of Medicine, the OSU Division of Computing Services, and the Health Education Network Users Group.

the 15 months normally afforded the Lecture—Discussion students to complete their basic science studies. It will be interesting to note if this trend continues. Nevertheless, it is clear that the ISP appeals to some students who wish to accelerate and to others who wish to decompress their medical studies. In any case, with the possible exception of one or two students, all of the ISP students will complete their training in four years or less.

COURSE SUMMARY REPORT   02/29/76 - 03/31/76

COURSE	STUDENT HRS	AUTHOR HRS	PRIME TOTAL	TOTAL HRS	SIGN ONS	MIN/ SESS	% OF TOTAL
ABANG	0.2	0.1	0.2	0.2	3	4.3	0.0
ABBREV	2.1	0.1	1.8	2.2	10	13.3	0.1
ABEL	14.9	0.0	14.4	14.9	22	40.6	0.7
ACIBA	51.7	0.0	51.5	51.7	86	36.1	2.3
AGENT	21.5	0.0	20.0	21.5	34	38.0	0.9
ALTRAC	2.9	0.0	3.0	3.0	5	35.6	0.1
ASSESS	5.1	0.1	5.2	5.2	12	26.2	0.2
BLOOUT	0.2	0.0	0.2	0.2	3	4.3	0.0
BOTTLE	7.5	0.0	7.5	7.5	11	40.9	0.3
BREECH	5.6	1.1	5.7	6.7	20	20.9	0.3
BUGOUT	9.4	0.0	9.2	9.4	15	37.7	0.4
CAI	29.6	0.3	21.1	29.9	112	16.0	1.3
CALC	1.1	0.0	1.1	1.1	12	5.4	0.0
CAMEO	0.0	3.7	3.7	3.7	6	36.8	0.2
CASE	172.7	208.6	365.2	381.3	809	28.3	16.8
CCNUR	23.2	0.0	21.8	23.2	27	51.6	1.0
CETEST	1.7	0.0	1.7	1.7	37	2.7	0.1
CVTERM	3.2	0.1	2.5	3.2	10	19.3	0.1
DIETAN	3.2	0.3	3.2	3.5	9	23.2	0.2
ELBOW	2.4	0.0	2.5	2.5	6	24.5	0.1
ENDO	18.9	0.1	19.0	19.0	34	33.5	0.8
ENZICS	3.7	0.3	3.9	3.9	7	33.4	0.2
FAMMED	1.3	0.1	1.4	1.4	3	27.0	0.1
FCODS	29.4	1.0	30.3	30.4	74	24.6	1.3
FUNDUS	9.4	0.2	9.6	9.6	19	30.4	0.4
GAMES	26.2	0.0	26.1	26.2	84	18.7	1.1
GANAT1	10.0	1.8	11.5	11.8	33	21.4	0.5
GANAT2	1.3	1.0	1.2	2.3	10	13.9	0.1
GLOSSR	0.1	0.7	0.8	0.8	4	12.0	0.0
GROUP	4.7	0.0	4.7	4.7	9	31.4	0.2
ETC.							
MONITOR			4.2	4.5	126	2.1	0.2
SUPERVISOR			35.7	42.7	92	27.9	1.9
TOTAL	1,903.0	324.7	7.0	2,274.9	4,504	30.3	100.0

PRIME HRS = 2,160.8   NON-PRIME HRS = 114.1   % PRIME = 95.0

(PRIME TIME IS 9 AM TO 12 MIDNIGHT E.T.)

Figure 10. A portion of the Course Summary Report. Only a small number of the total courses loaded on the system are shown. A glance at the total hours and sign ons gives a quick impression of the popularity and use of a particular course.

STUDENT STATUS - - PILOT
DATE 04/07/76 TIME 4:57 SELECTION=ALL

STUDENT NAME	STUDENT NO.	GROUP	AREA	TYREC	START DATE	LAST DATE	TIME	SEG	LABEL-PROB-SEQ	030
CHARLES JONES	339	75	0	15	7/17/75	3/04/76	22:00	QW	UAOOOT-	3- 0
PHYLLIS SMITH	340	75	0	15	7/14/75	3/20/76	32:14	QW	UAOOOT-	3- 0
DALE WITHE	341	75	0	15	7/18/75	1/14/76	27:52	QW	QAOOOT-	1- 0
SCOTT GREEN	342	75	0	15	7/14/75	4/03/76	42:22	QW	WG999Z-	1- 0
JOANN BROWN	344	75	0	15	7/22/75	3/04/76	15:57	AP	LAOOOT-	1- 0
ROSALIND DOE	171	73	0	15	7/19/73	8/20/75	35:16	QW	WF100S-	1- 0
TONI BLACK	345	75	0	15	7/14/75	3/01/76	57:55	QW	UAOOOT-	3- 0
JAMES DILL	351	75	0	15	7/14/75	4/02/76	36:50	QW	WAOOOT-	1- 0
MARY HILL	352	75	0	15	7/11/75	4/01/76	32:03	QW	WA060S-	1- 0
DOUGLAS HALL	231	74	0	15	7/12/74	1/16/76	02:47	36	5BUIOS-	1- 0
JOHN DORN	353	75	0	15	7/21/75	4/03/76	19:03	QW	QA020S-	1- 0

etc.

Figure 11. A portion of the Student Status Report. (Student names are fictitious.) This report gives the location of each student in the curriculum (label), when each student started in the program, and the last date that student had any activity at the terminal.

```
ISP PROGRESS REPORT ON COURSE PILOT FOR JOHN DOE

PRINTED ON MAY 5, 1976 AT 17:44

STUDENT  NBR/0316          CLASS/75          PERSONAL CHART/75
FACULTY ADVISOR/AJM        TYPE/LINEAR       LAST USAGE/MAY 3

PROGRESS CHART USED FOR THIS REPORT/75

 7/09/75
SCHED-   -   A   A   B   C   D   D   F   F   G   G   H   H
COMP-    A   AB  BC  CD  DE  EF  F   FG  G   GH  H   H   H

10/08/75
SCHED-   I   J   K   L   M   N   O   O   P   P   P   P   P
COMP-    HI  IJK K   K   KL  LM  MNO OP  P   P   P   P   P

 1/07/76
SCHED-   P   P   Q   Q   R   R   R   R   ST  T   T   U   U
COMP-    P   PQ  Q   Q   QR  RS  S   S   S   S   S   S   SJ

 4/07/76              *CURRENT WEEK
SCHED-   U   V   V   V   W   W   W   X   X   Y   Y   Z   Z
COMP-    U   UV  V   VW  W   W   W   W
                      *CURRENT WEEK

NOTE:  CHART SHOWS ONLY MODULES COMPLETED - STUDENT CURRENTLY AT XA
```

Figure 12. A Student Progress Report. This report gives a linear view of an individual student's progress as compared to a projected rate of progress through the entire curriculum. It also gives the faculty adviser and the last date of usage.

Table 1. Rate of Student Progress through Curriculum

Year	Mean completion time (months)	First student completes	Last student completes	% Late grads[a]
1970	16.8	15	22	30%
1971	17.5	10	32	39%
1972	15.4	13	23	8%
1973	16.3	12	24	27%
1974	18+	13	_[b]	40+%

[a]Percentage of the class graduating one quarter or more later than the projected date for the entering class.
[b]At the time this was written, there were still students in the ISP from the entering class of July 1974.

    Performance comparisons between classes and between schools are difficult to achieve in medical education. Even when different classes use the same instrument (e.g., Part I of the National Board Examination) rarely do comparisons consider ability and background of the students at the time of entry into the medical school. This difficulty is compounded when one attempts comparisons using performance in the clinical clerkships where a large part of the evaluation criteria is subjective in nature. For this reason, caution should be exercised in interpreting performance data obtained on the ISP students thus far. These data do indicate that ISP students perform as well as, or better than, the Lecture—Discussion students on standard examinations, such as Part I and Part II of the Medical Examiners Examination. Furthermore, there has been a gradual improvement in student performance on Part I of this examination for each of the classes entering since 1970 through 1973 with a slight drop in the 1974 class (Figure 14). Each of the classes since 1972 has scored significantly higher than the National Candidate Mean. The extraordinarily

FOLLOWING IS ISP CLUSTER REPORT PRINTED ON APR. 7, 1976 AT 16:57

MODULE/SUBMODULE/STUDENT NAME	CLASS	PROGP-CHRT	FACULTY-ADV
HEMATOLOGY			
DISEASES OF THE RED CELL			
......JAMES SMITH	75	75	KC
......REBECCA JONES	75	75	JK
......THOMAS HILL	75	75	VVH
......RICHARD HARRIS	75	75	AJM
......JOHN MILLS	75	75	BS
......EDGAR BERGEN	75	75	AD
......DIANE VARSO	75	75	NS
......MICHAEL LONG	75	75	MA
......DANNY RHODES	75	75	EPH
......GRANT WHITE	74	74	RLF
......RALPH BENNETT	74	74	JDB
......EDWARD BROOKS	74	74	PDB
......DAVID HARRISON	75	75	TK
......ANTHONY PERKINS	75	75	NS
......TONI GIOVANNI	75	75	KC
......PHYLLIS KIRK	75	75	MBF
......CHARLES LITTLE	75	75	MBF
COAGULATION AND BLEEDING			
......GARY HENDERSON	74	74	RHN
DISEASES OF MYELOID ELEMENTS			
......LEON EARLE	74	74	NRL
LYMPHORETICULAR DISEASES			
......PAMELA BROWN	74	74	JHX
FUNC DIS OF IMMUNE ORGANS			
IMMUNOHEMATOLOGY & BLOODBANK			
......RONALD COLEMAN	75	75	RL
......RICHARD BOONE	74	74	VVH
INFECTIOUS DISEASES			
BASIC CONSIDERATIONS			
......LEONARD NIMOYER	75	75	AJM
......RICHARD BLAKE	75	75	JH
......JACK POLARI	75	75	VVH
......AARON BERNSTEIN	75	75	AJM
......MARIE MILLIKEN	75	75	JR
......MARK DENNIS	74	74	KPC
......MELISSA DRAKE	75	75	BS
ANTIBIOTIC & CHEMOTHERAGENTS			
SYNDROMES & CAUSATIVE AGENTS			
......DAVID ALAN	75	75	EPH
......GREGORY SUMMERS	75	75	NRL
......CARMEN ESTABAN	74	74	RLF
......ROMAINE DAVIS	74	74	TLK
VIRUSES & ONCOGENEIS			
PARASITES			
THE GASTROINTESTINAL SYSTEM			
ESOPHAGUS			
......AL ROBINSON	75	75	EPH
......JAMES BAKER	75	75	TK
THE STOMACH AND DUODENUM			
SMALL BOWEL			

Figure 13. Student Cluster Report. Only a portion of this report is shown. This report shows the location of all students in the curriculum. This particular example indicates that students in the class entering in 1974 have been overtaken by many members of the class entering in 1975. Initials in right hand column are those of the faculty adviser.

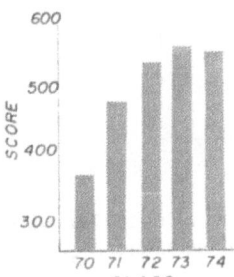

Figure 14. National Board scores of classes entering the ISP from 1970 through 1974. Scores reported are standard scores (National candidate mean = 500). The class entering in July of 1970 took the examination prior to the completion of their basic science studies.

low score for the first class was due, in part, to the fact that this class took the examination before the completion of the basic science curriculum and that there was, in fact, very little advance notice that they were to take the examination. These data are probably not valid for comparison purposes and are included for the purposes of completeness only.

As stated above, ISP students have tended to score higher on Part I of the National Board Examination. It should be noted, however, that ISP students are *required* to pass this examination, whereas it is used only as part of the overall evaluation of the Lecture–Discussion students. A second consideration is that past ISP volunteers have tended to score slightly higher on the science portion of the MCAT science test; and this factor, along with undergraduate grade point ratio, has proven to be a highly significant predictor of preclinical academic performance in our college. Recently comparisons were made on Part II of the National Board Examination of the combined 1970 through 1972 entering classes with much the same results (Figure 15). ISP students scored higher on the overal examination and significantly higher on the Obstetrics and Gynecology, Public Health, and Psychiatry portions. There were also smaller positive differences in the Surgery and Pediatrics sections of this examination. We do not know the factors which led to these results. Perhaps the ISP students develop study habits that help in their approach to the relevant clinical material, or it may simply be that these particular ISP students are good objective test takers. Further analyses will be necessary to determine if these trends will continue and to what extent an experience in the ISP contributes to these trends. We should, therefore, conclude only that ISP students compare favorably with their Lecture–Discussion counterparts; but at the same time, we should not minimize this accomplishment. It should be borne in mind that for the first time large numbers of students have studied the entire basic science portion of the curriculum by independent study techniques. The successes that we

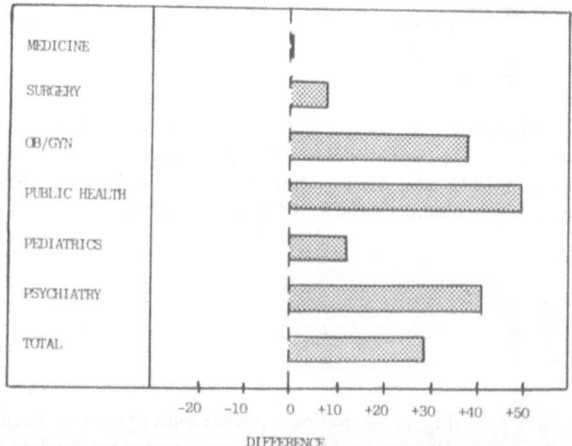

Figure 15. Comparison of National Board Part II scores for the combined 1970–1972 entering classes. Differences are expressed as ISP means minus Lecture–Dimension means. N_{ISP} = 96; N_{PHASE} = 464.

have experienced, together with the management techniques that have been developed at The Ohio State University, should lend us and others the confidence to develop curricula that are truly flexible and directed to the needs of each student who enters into the study of medicine.

ACKNOWLEDGMENT

We wish to acknowledge the expert assistance of The Ohio State University College of Medicine Division of Research and Evaluation in Medical Education in testing and maintenance of records for the Independent Study Program.

References

Griesen, J. V., Beran, R. L., Folk, R. L., and Prior, J. A., 1973. A pilot program of independent study in medical education in *Instruction Technology in Medical Education*. University of Rochester Press, New York.

Beran, R. L., Folk, R. L., Driesen, J. V., and Camiscioni, J. S. (Eds.), 1976, *Individualizing the Study of Medicine*, Westinghouse Learning Corporation, New York.

Dental Education

Karen A. Duncan

Introduction

The Educational Computer System of the College of Dental Medicine in Charleston, South Carolina is an example of a rather unusual type of design philosophy. In keeping with the national trend toward increased use of computers both directly and indirectly in the educational process, the decision to acquire a computing capability was part of a general plan to improve the learning experience of the dental students. The college is a small school, with a total enrollment of 150 dental students, so the question of acquiring a large system for the purpose of implementing computer-assisted instruction was never raised. Of the two alternatives, time-sharing on someone else's machine or acquisition of a minicomputer system in-house, the minicomputer system was selected. The challenge became to prove that effective computer-assisted instruction (CAI) could indeed be done inexpensively with the limited resources which would be available. This meant that it had to be done with an off-the-shelf hardware system, a standard operating system and language, and with relatively unskilled personnel. Clearly, special hardware, software modification, and highly trained personnel would necessitate an increase in costs which could not be justified by the small size of the student body. This chapter will present the rationale for selecting the minicomputer option and the ways in which the challenge was met to make the system a success. Most importantly the lessons learned and the pitfalls and problems of this approach will be described.

Background

Medical University

The College of Dental Medicine is one of six colleges of the Medical University of South Carolina. The Medical University, situated in Charleston, is a state institution but is separate administratively from any undergraduate campus. The other

---

Karen A. Duncan · Office of Computer Resources, College of Dental Medicine, Medical University of South Carolina, Charleston, South Carolina.

five colleges are Medicine, Nursing, Graduate, Pharmacy, and Allied Health. The total enrollment of the Medical University is less than 2000 students. In spite of its small student body, the computing problems and activities of the Medical University are myriad and complex, primarily because of the five teaching hospitals and their attendant staff and clinics.

Administrative computing utilizes about 93% of the capabilities of an IBM 370/145 computer. Another 5% of the utilization is by the Biometry Department of the University. There are about a dozen minicomputer systems scattered around the campus serving specialized needs, such as treatment planning in the Radiology Department or monitoring analog signals in the Physiology Department.

College of Dental Medicine

As is often the case, the decision to develop a CAI capability was predicated on the availability of funds for the purpose of enhancing the educational process at the school and the availability of faculty to begin the development. In mid-1972 when this project began, the options for CAI in dentistry were considerably more limited than they are today. PLATO had not yet implemented its philosophy of sharing health sciences materials with other institutions in exchange for authoring. The Health Education Network (formerly, Lister Hill National Center for Biomedical Communications Network) was on the verge of becoming a reality, but that system in its infancy did not address CAI in clinical dentistry.

An exploration of the possibility of time-sharing with our university computer or at a nearby campus revealed that our own facilities were already too crowded and that communication costs and other associated charges to a distant campus would be prohibitive. Although this factor did not come greatly into play, another very important consideration at this stage was one of control over and priority usage of the selected system facilities.

In a consideration of minicomputer systems, there were very few available which would fit the requirement of being off-the-shelf and which would allow easy software development suitable for educational applications. The College of Dental Medicine computing staff wished to begin producing immediately usable courseware and had no interest in becoming expert at system development, since this expertise would not in any way enhance the process of dental education. The minicomputer systems considered were an IBM 1130, Hewlett-Packard 2000, and Digital Equipment Corporation PDP-11 RSTS. Another consideration arose at this point: a CAI system, no matter how well developed, would not utilize the full capability of these machines. At this point, we began to consider other dental school computing needs which would utilize a system more fully.

Concurrently with the planning of a computing resource for educational purposes was the planning of the development of an Office of Education for the Dental School. It was the philosophy of the college administration that a great deal of the didactic material required of a dental student could be made self-instructional on one of the many media available to us today. It was evident therefore that a computer system to manage and monitor the use of these self-instructional units would become highly desirable. It was only a short mental step from this consideration to the recognition that if teaching resources in the learning center could be considered manageable by a computer, then so could patients in a clinic, which could also be managed, monitored, and scheduled, be considered learning units for the student. Thus, the idea was born of a complete automated management system that would direct the student through his or her didactic and clinical assignments.

Goals

Because of the storage limitations of a minicomputer, it was envisioned that the many potential elements of the total system, now called the Educational Computer System (ECS), would have to be unified. The various elements of the system are described here and some interrelationships are shown in Figure 1.

The structure of the original system was planned as follows:

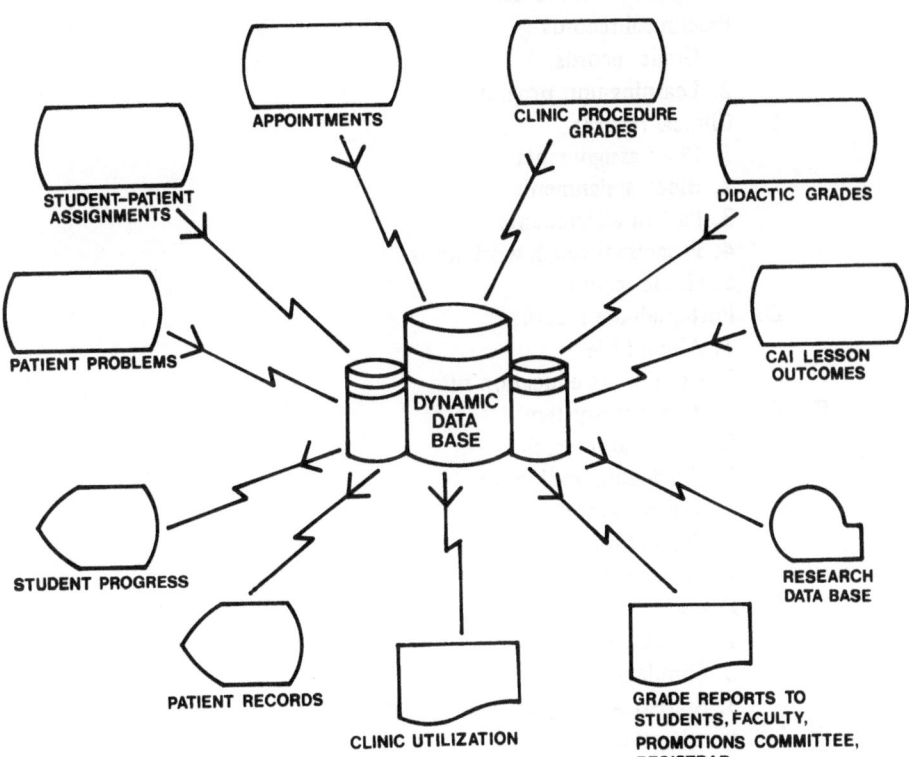

Figure 1. Flowchart of proposed system.

I. Instructional subsystem
   A. Preclinical instruction
      1. Specific didactic programs
      2. Interdepartmental coordinator review
   B. Clinical instruction
      1. Simulation of dental clinic situation
      2. Specific tutorial programs
   C. Continuing education
      1. In-house workshops
      2. Remote workshops
   D. Other educational applications
      1. Review for Dental Board programs
      2. Reinforcement programs
      3. Enrichment programs
II. Student management subsystem
   A. Admission records
      1. Personal data
      2. Scholastic data
      3. Aptitude test scores
   B. Preclinical records
      1. Grade records
      2. Learning-unit progress
   C. Clinical records
      1. Chair assignments
      2. Block assignments
      3. Patient assignments
      4. Progress through work units
      5. Grade records
   D. Post-graduate records
      1. Alumni file
      2. Continuing education file
III. Basic research subsystem
   A. Educational research
      1. Curriculum evaluation
      2. Teaching models
      3. Simulation
      4. Statistical analysis
   B. Dental research
      1. Data banks
      2. Simulation models
      3. Statistical analysis
IV. Utility subsystem

It is evident that the objectives of the system were to serve the educational needs of the college in three areas. The direct educational goals would be served through

CAI, and indirect goals would be served through programs for maintaining grades and for managing student clinical activities. The goals of research would be met through the maintenance of educational data bases of student information from registration through graduation. It was further anticipated that the staff of the Educational Computer System would facilitate faculty use of such educational data by recommending statistical analyses that were available through the Biometry Department. The unstated and most subtle goal was proving that effective computer-assisted and -managed instruction could, in fact, be done with off-the-shelf components.

Rationale for Implementation

It can be seen from Figure 1 that data from all aspects of a student's career will funnel into the same conceptual storage area and be recorded for wide report distribution. As an example of how this might work, consider a third-year student who is taking a clinical dentistry course in which he or she has patients in the clinic as well as didactic material to learn. It is possible that a considerable portion of the didactic material would be located in the learning center. Accordingly, the computer will keep track of the student's utilization of these self-instructional packages and evaluate the amount of learning that took place in this didactic portion of the course. At the same time, the computer will already have had a record of the patient's problems and the fact that they have been assigned to this particular student. All of the student's appointments will be kept on the computer through entry in the appointment center. Each time the student is scheduled to see a patient this fact is reported at the cathode-ray tube (CRT) terminal in the particular clinic. The outcome of the student—patient encounter is recorded in the clinic at the CRT. It may be recorded, for example, that the patient did not arrive, that the instructor asked the student to do a procedure other than the planned one, or that the work was satisfactorily completed. The student may receive an appropriate grade as well, also assigned at the CRT in the clinic at the time that the student sees the patient. At the end of the course, the instructor will want a summary of the student's work. The data that will be summarized have been entered at many different times during the term by many different people in a variety of locations. Since all applications for the entire Educational Computer System are coordinated, the relevant information is easily retrieved and reported concisely to the instructor. As each student completes the work required for the course (which may very well have been self-paced), the final grade is entered in the computer for retrieval by the Admissions Office.

It should be evident that this is descriptive of a miniature time-shared system. In point of fact, this design feature has many desirable spin-offs. Eliminating card readers and making all data entry the responsibility of the department or group that generates the data eliminates the need for acquisition of any card-processing equipment in the minicomputer center itself, and eliminates as well the need for the attendant keypunch and machine operators. This has the additional benefit that editing and, by extension, quality control of the data is done by the individuals most concerned. Thus, in addition to timely updating and report generation, time and costs are saved through reduction of computing equipment and personnel, and the appropriate level of quality control of the data is assured because the control rests with those concerned. Personnel reduction is further achieved by the fact that relevant departments can generate their own reports on demand at their own CRTs, rather than having to send a request to the computer center.

It should be noted, and this is more important, that this degree of user freedom can only be achieved through a careful control of the applications that will be using the system in prime time. This means that there cannot be unmonitored users running process control or heavily computationally oriented programs during the hours when the clinics are in operation or when the students are running their instructional programs. This sort of tie-up of the CPU will devastate a time-shared operation of such a small scale. A maximum response time of 2 seconds under moderate-to-heavy system use was chosen as a reasonable guideline.

Educational Computer System (ECS) Configuration

The original system design called for implementation in two phases. The first phase would be a trial or feasibility study and the second would be the full-blown scale system that would be expected perpetually to meet the above-specified needs of the College of Dental Medicine. The first system was a PDP 11/20 computer system with 28K words of core memory. Primary storage for the ECS was two 1.2-million-word disk cartridges. The initial system had five CRTs which ran at 2400 bits per second and which served as both data entry and retrieval devices. A 60-line-per-minute printer, a 30-character-per-second printer, and an industry-compatible magnetic tape unit completed this system. The 5 CRTs are permanently located in carrels in the College of Dental Medicine's Learning Center where they are readily available, along with other learning aids, to all students, faculty, and staff.

One of the primary motivations for selecting the Digital Equipment Corporation system was the availability of the powerful operating system, Resource Sharing Timesharing Systems (RSTS). RSTS is a single-language system which uses BASIC-PLUS, an extension of Dartmouth BASIC. The primary virtues of this extension are its capability for handling strings and files. This is essential for CAI and for dynamic data entry and retrieval. Further, the RSTS operating system allows extended-precision calculations and matrix manipulations and permits the use of a hardware floating point processor. It is exceedingly fortunate that this system was conceived as part of a feasibility plan rather than as the ultimate system because we very rapidly ran out of disk storage space due to system storage allocation schemes. Furthermore, we found that adding a second interactive user to the system downgraded terminal response time so severely that the system was virtually unusable for interactive applications. This occurred in the complete absence of computer-bound jobs on the system.

The second installation, which is presently in operation at the college, is an upgrade of the PDP-11 to a model 40. Additional enhancements are a 40-million-word moveable head disk system, a 132-line-per-minute printer, and 16 additional CRT terminals for the dental school clinics. Before system acceptance, a benchmark was run which required that 10 simultaneous interactive users would have at worst a 2-second response time. An additional requirement was that all terminals could be driven at the rate of 1200 bits per second. The operating system for the upgrade is an extension of the RSTS system already in use here, RSTS-E. The decision to upgrade to another DEC PDP-11 system rather than to change vendors or operating systems was based on the fact that the new system won in a competitive bid. The hardware for both the trial and permanent systems is listed in Table 1. It should be noted that the transition to the larger system was very smoothly made.

Initial Implementation

While administrative endorsement, adequate funding and staff, and acceptable hardware and software are certainly essential to the initiation of a CAI effort, certainly no less important are the issues of user acceptance. We were demanding considerable interaction with our users because of the selected methods of data

Table 1. Trial CAI System

1 PDP 11/20-CA	System[a]
1 LA30	DEC writer
2 MM11-L	8K words of core memory
1 MM11-E	4K words of core memory
1 KW11-L	Real-time clock
1 BM792-YB	Bulk storage bootstrap loader
1 RK11	DEC pack disk controller
2 RK05	1.2 mil word DEC pack disk
5 VT05	CRT display
1 TM11-A	MAG tape controller
1 TV11-EA	9-Track master transport
1 KE11-A	Extended arithemetic element[a]
1 Centronics 101	60-LPM line printer
Permanent system additions	
1 PDP 11/40-BK	System
1 KE11-E	Extended instruction set
1 KT11-D	Memory management
1 MM11-UP	16K words of parity memory
1 LP11-VA	132-LPM printer
1 RP11-CE	Control and disk drive
16 Hazeltine 1200	CRT display

[a]Deleted for upgrade.

entry, editing, and report generation; therefore, their cooperation and enthusiasm were essential to even initial success of our operation. In the purely educational area, we felt that there must be incentive for the faculty to develop instructional materials. There is no basic reason for a faculty member to spend many hours developing a rather crude instructional program that may or may not be liked by the students and that would most certainly detract from the teacher's responsibilities. In addition, if we wanted to generate hard data showing the value of CAI, it was essential that our students feel no more antipathetic toward the computer as an instructional medium than they would feel toward any other medium, such as tapes or textbooks or even lectures. So, although our overriding mission was to produce computer software and courseware that would be of genuine service to the educational process and to the administration of the college, it was certainly essential to educate our faculty, staff, and students in the benefits of computer usage and to have a high profile of accomplishment early in our endeavor. Accordingly, for the students, we immediately made available a set of old National Board questions for review. These questions can be ordered from the American Dental Students Association for $7.00 a set; however, apparently it was much more rewarding for the student to review through interaction with the computer than to order the sets. We made available to the students some 700 questions in 14 different disciplines, 7 basic and 7 clinical. At the end of each session with the computer, a simple scoring mechanism is used to display scores for the students. This program of National Board questions, which has no feedback other than the evaluation at the end, has served as the backbone of our attempts to interest and educate people in the direct educational use of the computer. The National Board Review is used in all student orientations and at demonstrations throughout the country. This program is available for all students to use at any time the Learning Center is open.

Concurrently with the development of the Boards program, a program to register patients in the clinic was developed. Now, certainly in a minicomputer system concerned with educational management, nothing is more useless than the address of a patient. However, the registration program, with all of its retrieval, editing, and report-generation features, certainly illustrates very graphically to the faculty, and in a manner to which they can easily relate, just what sorts of data could in fact be stored, recombined, and retrieved by the computer. This program has been used at a faculty retreat and several workshops to demonstrate computer service.

It was and is our belief that staff who will be required to use the computer should come to view it as harmless, helpful, and easy to use, rather than as an added chore. Accordingly the registration program, along with the National Board Review and other dummy programs, has been made available to the staff in the clinics. This has helped create a low-pressure atmosphere for orientation and indoctrination in computer use.

In addition to direct computer use, a variety of other instruction was used. For example, each entering student was assigned a computer password, and the freshman class was oriented in small groups to the use of the computer for CAI using

National Board Review. A seminar course entitled "Computers and Society" and a Special Projects course involving problem solving and programming were also offered. For faculty and staff, a series of workshops, demonstrations, and discussions were held. The workshops dealt variously with computer-assisted-managed instruction, computers in dental education, and computers for problem solving. All of these activities continue along with an increasing use of our capability for statistical analysis and research data base management.

Ongoing Implementation

In the next sections, a discussion of our CAI projects will be followed by a presentation of our unique use of the computer-managed instruction concept and other educational applications.

Computer-Assisted Instruction (CAI)

It was our intention to pursue actively only that CAI which would be innovative and exciting. We believe that worthwhile CAI should offer genuine enhancements to dental education. This can be accomplished in many ways, including simulation exercises that allow students to learn how to make and to practice making judgments for real clinical situations. Other enhancements might be the management of a complex learning resource environment or the replacement of a tutor when one-to-one instruction is needed. Since dentistry is in large part a manual art and science, we wanted to try to teach dental students a practical manual skill using the computer. The idea behind this is that manual skills now have to be taught on a tutorial basis in the laboratory. It seems reasonable that students might miss learning important skills because the instructor cannot observe every student through every step of the procedure. In order for a manual skill to be amenable to instruction by computer, it is necessary to have a mechanism of eliciting data from the student for the computer that can be evaluated and serve as a measure of success of the student's procedure. This means, for example, that presently a student cannot be taught how to fill a cavity using CAI, because there is no mechanism by which the courseware can determine a successful performance.

The selected program that met the criteria set forth in the previous paragraph was arch-length analysis, which is taught during the student's second year Pedodontic course.* The students are given an instructional guide, a set of models of a child's dental arch to be analyzed, and a Boley gauge for measuring tooth width. Because of the high correlation between a child's present primary tooth size and the eventual dental arch space for permanent teeth, it is possible to measure the primary teeth and to predict whether or not there will be sufficient space in the

---

*This program and the pedodontic simulations were developed by Dr. Frank Farrington, Department of Pedodontics, and the staff of the Office of Computer Resources.

dental arch. This allows assessment of whether or not the child will need ortho-
dontia in the future. If the student is measuring teeth properly, making the appropriate calculations, and entering these values in the computer, then it is apparent
that the student is executing the technique successfully. Sample dialogue is shown
in Figure 2. It is seen that measurements are noted, and the student is given immediate feedback which coaches him or her on how to correct the measuring technique. An exciting feature of this type of program that is not possible using a
paper-and-pencil programmed-instruction method is that the computer can automatically allow a tolerance for the student's measurements. This program has been
in routine use for several classes.

Our other major CAI effort is in the area of clinical simulations. To date,
students are able to exercise their diagnostic skills with three pedodontic cases,
one physical diagnosis problem, one oral pathology problem, and one prosthodontics case. A case requiring the handling of a medical emergency in the dentist's
office is presently under development. It is in the area of dental simulations that we
hope to put most of our future efforts in CAI. Because we are using a minicomputer
system and we believe that a 2-second response is the maximum tolerable for
clinic personnel and student interactions, it is not feasible for us to utilize extensive
text analysis in the simulation exercises. Nonetheless, a variety of interactive styles
are still available for incorporation in simulation courseware.

```
C  ENTER TOOTH NUMBER
S    23
C  ENTER TOOTH WIDTH TO NEAREST TENTH OF MILLIMETER
S    5.4
C  ENTER ANOTHER TOOTH NUMBER
S    23
C  YOU HAVE ALREADY MEASURED THIS TOOTH.  PLEASE MEASURE ANOTHER ONE.
   ENTER ANOTHER TOOTH NUMBER
S    24
C  ENTER TOOTH WIDTH TO NEAREST TENTH OF MILLIMETER
S    5.0
C  YOUR MEASUREMENT IS MORE THAN .1MM LOW
   PLEASE RE-MEASURE TOOTH NUMBER 24
   ENTER TOOTH WIDTH TO NEAREST TENTH OF MILLIMETER
S    5.1
C  YOUR MEASUREMENT IS MORE THAN .1MM LOW
   BE SURE THAT YOU ARE POSITIONING THE POINTS OF THE BOLEY GAUGE AT THE
   WIDEST PART OF EACH TOOTH.  THIS IS CRUCIAL WHEN DEALING WITH THE DESIRED
   DEGREE OF ACCURACY.  IF YOU ARE UNABLE TO MEASURE THE TOOTH FROM ABOVE
   BE SURE THAT THE BOLEY GAUGE IS PERPENDICULAR TO THE MESIAL AND DISTAL
   MARGINS WHEN TAKING YOUR MEASUREMENTS.  PERHAPS YOUR ERROR STEMS FROM
   INCORRECTLY READING THE BOLEY GAUGE.  REFER TO THE PAGES OF INSTRUCTION
   ON THE USE OF THE BOLEY GAUGE INCLUDED IN YOUR PACKET OF MATERIALS.
C  PLEASE RE-MEASURE TOOTH NUMBER 24
   ENTER TOOTH WIDTH TO NEAREST TENTH OF MILLIMETER
S    5.2
C  ENTER ANOTHER TOOTH NUMBER
     27
```

Figure 2. Arch-length analysis dialogue.

C BOBBY'S TREATMENT WAS COMPLETED YESTERDAY. THIS MORNING HIS MOTHER
   CALLS SAYING HE WAS JUST SENT HOME FROM SCHOOL WITH A SEVERE TOOTHACHE.
   AT THIS POINT YOU WOULD:
   1. CALL DR. KEALL
   2. SEE BOBBY IMMEDIATELY
   ITEM #?
S   2
C BOBBY PRESENTS TO YOUR OFFICE IN EXTREME DISCOMFORT. EXAMINATION
   REVEALS MARKED TENDERNESS OVER AREA OF MAXILLARY LEFT CENTRAL INCISOR
   WITH INCREASED MOBILITY OVER THE PREVIOUS DAY. OTHER FINDINGS ARE
   ESSENTIALLY THE SAME AS BEFORE.
   AT THIS TIME YOU WOULD:
   1. CONTINUE WITH CLINICAL EXAM
   2. INITIATE FURTHER TREATMENT
   3. CONSULT LIBRARY
   ITEM #?
S   2
C YOUR PULP TREATMENT WILL CONSIST OF: (CHOOSE ONE)
   1. PULP CAP
   2. PULPOTOMY
   3. STIMULATION OF APEX FORMATION (FRANK'S TECHNIC)
   4. CONVENTIONAL PULPECTOMY AND ENDODONTIC THERAPY
   5. CONSULT LIBRARY
   ITEM #?
S   3
C PULP TREATMENT COMPLETED
   BECAUSE THE ROOT OF THE AFFECTED TOOTH IS FULLY DEVELOPED AND THE APEX
   IS CLOSED, CONVENTIONAL ENDODONTIC THERAPY CAN BE INITIATED AT THIS
   TIME.

Figure 3. Simulated treatment choices.

In most of our programs of this type, the student is presented with a menu of choices, as shown in Figure 3. Where it might be appropriate for the student to query the computer for information, as in history-taking or in obtaining lab values, standard phrases are provided among which the student may choose. Figure 4 illustrates yet another mode of teaching information collection. Here, the student selects relevant questions by number. Some attempts have been made to score the student's clinical decision-making ability by subtracting points for poor decisions and returning some of these points for proper recovery from an error.

Another type of decision making that is especially important in dentistry is that of treatment planning. In medicine, treatment planning is often dynamic, with succeeding treatment depending on the outcome of a previous treatment. Further, in medicine, patients' problems are usually dealt with singly as they are presented by the patient. Unlike medicine, however, dental treatment begins with developing a coordinated plan for restoring the patient's oral health, so learning treatment planning is an important part of the dental curriculum. A student using the computer can leisurely study models, X-rays, charts, history, and clinical findings to derive a plan. As the plan is entered at the CRT terminal, the courseware can give step-by-step feedback to the student in tutorial form and can provide as well a comprehensive evaluation at the end of the session. A model program of this concept is being tested at the College of Dental Medicine, and sample dialogue is

12. Have you ever been told Bobby needed braces?

13. Does Bobby have any history of heart disease?

14. Any history of allergies?

15. Any history of serious illness in the family?

16. Is your water fluoridated?

17. What childhood diseases has Bobby had?

18. Is Bobby covered by insurance?

19. When was Bobby's last tetanus booster?

20. Is Bobby in pain now?

21. Does his tooth hurt when he chews?

Figure 4. Preformatted simulation questions.

shown in Figure 5. Treatment planning exercises could be used for teaching or testing and could thus provide a new modality for dental board exams.

In other activities, the previously mentioned Office of Education of the College has completely mediated a 2-quarter course on pain control for dental students. In winter of 1976, this course was managed by computer to the extent of providing student self-evaluation and weekly progress reports to the instructor. For the second quarter of the course, computer management was extended to provide test—retest and remedial feedback suggestions for the students. It is further important to note that CAI development has been dependent on faculty enthusiasm. Although no release time is granted for development of CAI courseware, college promotion guidelines do give credit for courseware development. However, since the University Promotions Committee does not recognize these achievements, faculty participation has been voluntary and sporadic.

```
C  ARE THERE ANY ORAL HABITS?
S  NO
C  IN DESCRIBING ORAL HABITS IT IS IMPORTANT TO DETERMINE THE
   FREQUENCY, INTENSITY, AND DURATION OF THE HABIT.
   IN THIS PARTICULAR CASE WE THINK THERE IS A POSSIBLE
   FINGER HABIT, BUT WE CANNOT ACCURATELY DETERMINE THIS FROM THE
   DATA AVAILABLE.
   IS THERE ANY EVIDENCE OF SPACE LOSS OR ARCH LENGTH DEFICIENCY?
   ENTER YES OR NO.
S  NO
C  RIGHT!!
   TO PROPERLY ASSESS SPACE LOSS, IT IS NECESSARY TO HAVE ADEQUATE
   RECORDS.  THIS USUALLY CONSISTS OF DIAGNOSTIC MODELS, AN ARCH
   LENGTH ANALYSIS, AND COMPLETE RADIOGRAPHIC SERIES.
   ARE ANY SPECIAL PRECAUTIONS NECESSARY?  ENTER YES OR NO
S  NO
C  GOOD!  WE FEEL THAT NO SPECIAL PRECAUTIONS ARE NECESSARY.
```

Figure 5. Simulated treatment planning feedback.

Clinical Instruction Management

This system was targeted for initial use on January 1, 1976. The phases of the system are appointments, student requirement status, patient treatment progress, and clinic utilization reports. As was described earlier, the concept being implemented is that the patient's problem can be viewed as an instructional unit. The utilization of this learning resource (i.e., treating the patient) can be scheduled by computer for each student as to place and time (operatory, procedure, day, and hour). This information is seen to be immediately useful to clinic personnel in the college's 14 clinics. If the dental assistant can obtain timely information of this sort, operatories can be properly equipped and staffed for patient visits.

Figure 6 shows a simplified flow diagram of the *appointments* phase of the system. The dynamic data base updated in this example consists of the student's record, and patient's record, and the clinic utilization file. Appointment information is entered at the appointment center, and relevant information is displayed on a CRT terminal in each clinic prior to and during each clinic period. The outcome of each student–patient visit is entered by CRT terminal in the clinic also. This elaborate system must allow for the fact that the instructional units (patient problems) are human and do not always show up and that often several appointments may be required to complete a dental procedure to the point of grading. In addition, students are responsible for all their patients' dental problems, whether or not the student needs credit for the necessary treatment. So there are no-credit appointments that must still be recorded to keep the patient record and clinic utilization file updated.

The system complexity is increased further by the fact that patient records are categorized by *problem*, but student records are categorized by *procedure*, and procedures used to remedy a problem may vary considerably. Presently,

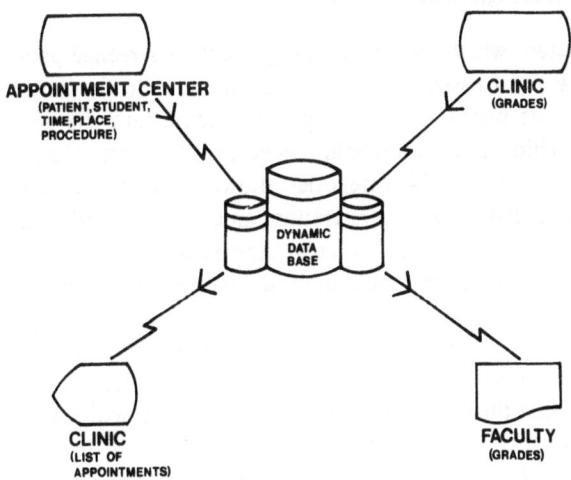

Figure 6. Appointments flowchart.

patient problems are classed into 24 different categories, and patients are assigned to students on the basis of these categories. However, student requirements are described by a large number of different procedures each of which the student must accomplish a certain number of times before graduation. An equivalence table between problem and procedure is being used initially for record update.

All other phases of the Clinical Instruction Management System are made possible by the first, or appointments, phase. It is apparent that regular update of the dynamic date base by clinic personnel as to the outcome of the day's appointments is essential. Student Requirement Status Reports will be generated on demand at the department chairman or clinic director level comparing each student's progress to his or her requirements. Grades for each part of a procedure will be kept only on a department-by-department basis. The reason for this is that many departments have highly specialized grading schemes appropriate only for their procedures. Further, day-by-day grades are not of general interest to the administration of the college, so no attempt will be made to develop an overall automated grading system, other than in summary form. This is a more realistic goal for a minicomputer system.

The *patient treatment progress* phase will update patient records by altering information in the 24 treatment categories to reflect work in progress or work completed, in addition to treatment needed. The basis for this phase of updating patient records is in routine use at the college, and this application, called Student— Patient Assignment, is described in detail in the next section. In the computer-managed instruction analogy, student—patient assignment is equivalent to providing the student with a set of learning resources. Clinic Utilization Reports are of course analogous to utilization studies of any learning resource center.

Student—Patient Assignment

This is a system which aids in the assignment of screened patients to the dental students, and is most easily described with reference to the flow chart in Figure 7. First, it should be noted that when patients come into the dental clinic and are accepted as teaching cases, a screening sheet is made up and the patient's diagnostic plan is developed in the 24 categories shown in Figure 8. Through a terminal located in the oral-diagnosis—registration area, the patient's diagnostic plan and the registration date are entered on a real-time basis.

As the dental student is required to see patients with given problems and to solve these problems and treat them, it is apparent that the appropriate selection of patients to be assigned to students is very important. Even when a patient with specific problems that match the requirements of a particular student is identified, it is important that the patient not have other problems which the student is unable to handle. It is also critical that patients not be assigned to students who will be graduating before there is time to complete their total dental treatment plan.

In order to meet the needs of the student, even for a student body of only 156

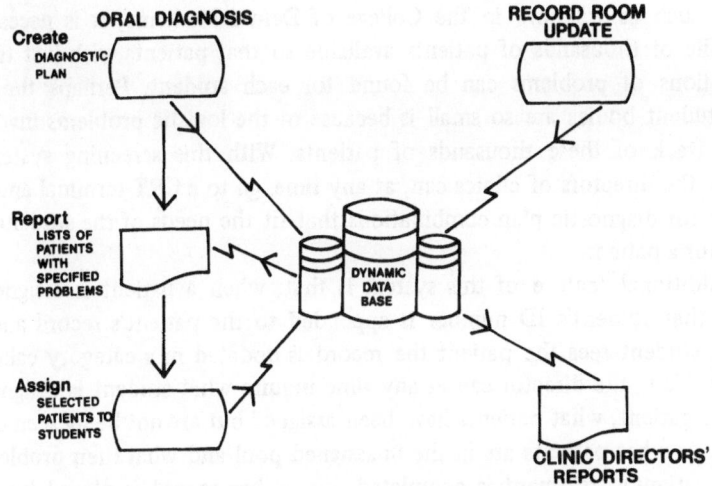

Figure 7. Student–patient assignment flowchart.

(ENTER "Y" INSTEAD OF CHECK MARKS, EXCEPT WHERE NUMBERS ARE REQUESTED)

DIAGNOSTIC PLAN:

Periodontia: 1. localized problems_____
                      2. generalized problems_____
                      3. occlusal equilibration_____

Endodontia: 4. anterior_____
(enter   5. bicuspid_____
numbers)   6. molar_____

Operative: 7. amalgam_____
(enter   8. resins_____
approximate   9. inlay_____
numbers)   10. foil_____

Crown & Bridge: 11. anterior crown_____
(enter   12. anterior bridge_____
Numbers)   13. posterior crown_____
                     14. posterior bridge_____

Surgery: 15. anterior extraction_____
(enter   16. posterior extraction_____
numbers)   17. impaction_____
                     18. alveoloplasty_____

Prosthodontics: 19. partial mandibular_____
                     20. partial maxillary_____
                     21. complete dentures_____
                     22. maxillary complete denture_____
                     23. denture reline_____

24. Orthodontics_____
     Pedodontics_____
     Oral Pathology_____

Figure 8. Patient's diagnostic plan.

students such as we have in the College of Dental Medicine, it is necessary to keep a file of thousands of patients available so that patients with just the right combinations of problems can be found for each student. Perhaps the reason dental student bodies are so small is because of the logistic problems involved in keeping track of these thousands of patients. With this screening system now available, the directors of clinics can, at any time, go to a CRT terminal and search the bank for diagnostic plan combinations that fit the needs of the student who is looking for a patient.

An additional feature of this system is that, when a patient is assigned to a student, that student's ID number is appended to the patient's record and every time the student sees the patient the record is updated in a category called *date last seen*. Now, the director can at any time inquire what student is assigned to a particular patient, what patients have been assigned but are not being seen by their students, or what patients are in the unassigned pool and what their problems are. When a patient's treatment is completed, his or her record is placed by record-room personnel in a completed file for periodic recall. If a patient's record is turned in uncompleted because of graduation or other good reason, the record is reentered as unassigned in the patient file. The screening plan is updated to reflect only the amount of work left to be done so the patient can be appropriately reassigned. Another feature of this system is that it is possible for the clinic director to ascertain at any time the diagnosis profile of the entire patient file. This information allows the director to close registration to patients with problems of a kind of which the college has an excess and to recruit actively in deficient areas. A similar screening program is being carried out separately in Pedodontics, since this department registers its own patients.

Didactic Grade System

This system functions only for the didactic portion of the student's curriculum, but it does include both basic science and clinical didactic work. At present, the level of detail recorded in this system is the students' final grades in each course for each quarter. The motivation for keeping grades automatically came from the fact that there is already an automated grade-keeping system available to the dental school but the summary grade reports are not available to the promotions committee until about 3 weeks after the end of the quarter. Since students often do not complete their requirements for graduation until virtually the day before graduation, it is essential that these reports be considerably more timely. Accordingly the objective of developing the grade-keeping system was to provide the promotions committee with grade summaries for the immediate past quarter for each course and student, summarized by course or presented by course or by student. This includes the student's grade point average and quality points for the past quarter and the cumulative grade point average and quality points for his entire school career. Also available is an indication of whether each student was in some way special (e.g., whether or not a course was taken in the normal sequence of the curriculum or was repeated). Grades are calculated by various standards depending on whether or not the student had been required to repeat a course or only a portion of a course. Different standards are also used for calculating class standings. The grade-keeping system is somewhat unusual in that it is almost completely on-line as well as being real-time. There are many grade-keeping systems that are real-time because of the need for timely grade reporting. But on-line grade entry and report generation is another matter. Figure 9 illustrates the flow of the system for this design. Note that the system is built as three sets of programs. The first set is used for building master files of student name and ID and the general course files of the school. Naturally, each new class of students is entered once a year in the student file. The course file may be modified in any way at any time to reflect changes in course credit, etc., for quarterly data entry and report generation. The most important feature of this system is that data entry and report generation are accomplished completely by the Office of Admissions. There is a CRT terminal in the Office of Admissions, and all quarterly grades are entered in any order at any time that it is convenient for that office. This is not merely a data entry function, since the personnel in that office have considerable flexibility in file editing. When all grade entry has been accomplished, the Admissions personnel initiate a program that computes all relevant grade

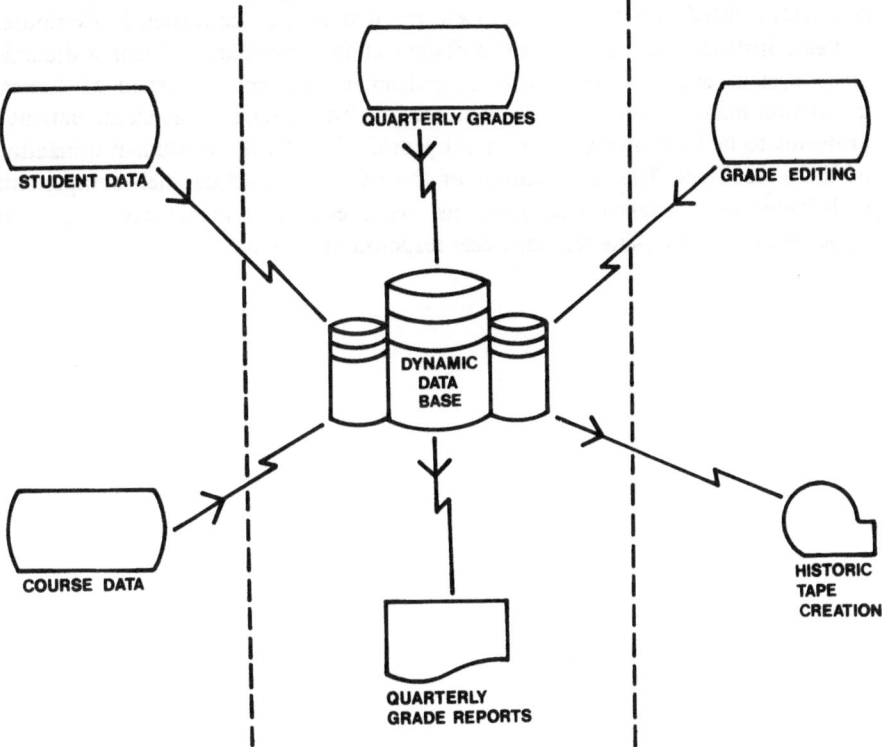

Figure 9. Didactic grade system.

points, quality points, and class standings. The Admissions Office may then initiate a printout of a wide variety of reports from the CRT terminal. At the present time, the printers are located in the machine room because location elsewhere is not warranted by volume of use. However, when the clinic areas or an administrative area of the school has sufficient output to justify it, a small printer can be placed in those areas. The third set of programs in the grade-keeping system have to do with historic records. Each quarter, there are always grades that are turned in late or that have to be modified. This is done for the records of the previous quarter at the discretion of the Admissions Office in the first few weeks of the new quarter. When the Admissions Office notifies the computer group that, in fact, the quarter's grades are complete, the sole responsibility of computer personnel is to dump the previous quarter's records to a tape. The system is now ready for grades for the new quarter. At present, no use is being made of these historic grade records; however, it is hoped that faculty with expertise in educational testing will see fit to use these reports for analyses in the future.

Summary

The College of Dental Medicine has an ongoing program of development in computer-assisted instruction courseware within its Educational Computer System. Instructional management software in full operation includes a didactic grade system and a student—patient assignment system. A system of clinical instruction management is near implementation. This system considers the patient's problems to be learning resources, and it provides logistically for student utilization of these resources. The key features of the ECS are its off-the-shelf components with tailor-made applications programs, its integrated dynamic data base, fast response time, and on-line real-time user responsibility for data.

5

Computer-Assisted Instruction in Health Professions Education: Guidelines for Utilization

John Casbergue

Introduction

The demands for health care and health manpower are outstripping the ability of educational institutions to meet these demands with traditional educational approaches and methods (Keller, 1965). These demands, coupled with the changing roles of the health professions, and the varied learning styles of students, are creating a growing sense of the need for better educational methods. Medical education is being challenged as never before (Stewart, 1968). Educators are seeking to modify their approaches to instruction in order to improve the effectiveness of teaching and learning systems. Jason (1968, p. 37) states:

> Patterns and techniques of instruction which had been hallowed by decades of use are being modified and even jettisoned and the search is on for new instructional modalities which hold the promise of getting more done in less time.

Thus, the need to educate and to provide continuing education for the large numbers of people in the specialized disciplines required for the delivery of modern health services mandate the development and use of newer instructional techniques (Herskovitz and Skolnick, 1972, p. 85). Health professions educators and administrators should be aware of the capabilities of the computer and the potential of computer-assisted instruction (CAI) when seeking new techniques for improving their educational programs. The computer is becoming an increasingly significant and available tool for instruction and research.

In the health professions educational programs, progress toward improving instructional effectiveness through the use of the computer and CAI is just beginning. In a survey of 561 health sciences institutions (Brigham *et al.*, 1973), over one third stated that they were using or planning to use computerized instruction in their curriculum.

John Casbergue • Office of Medical Education Research and Development, Michigan State University, East Lansing, Michigan.

In most cases, however, this represented a small experimental teaching unit (developed by an enthusiastic faculty member) and used in a few courses. Of all the reported computerized teaching material developed in medicine, 44% was developed at a single institution and 74% of the total comes from only three institutions (Brigham *et al.*, 1973, p. 186).

The apparent lack of acceptance of CAI as an educational tool in health professions education, in spite of its potential, is usually attributed to several factors. The factors most often cited are the high investment cost of CAI instructional systems, institutional resistance to change, and the lack of available CAI course material. Though factors, such as the above, are alluded to in the literature, a careful literature search reveals a lack of empirically based evidence concerning the influence of these and other factors on the development and use of CAI in health professions education. Greater knowledge of the interaction of these factors on the development process would enable educators and administrators to plan more effectively for, and make sounder educational decisions regarding the use of CAI as an instructional medium (Anastasio and Morgan, 1972, p. 1). Such decisions might include (1) the consideration of CAI, (2) the development and implementation of a CAI system, or (3) the utilization of CAI materials and/or systems developed at other institutions.

Related Research

Though the focus of this book and this chapter is on computers in medical and health professions education, there are several studies in related areas, in addition to those dealing with medical education, that provide important insights into the human aspects of introducing CAI. It is therefore appropriate to review briefly a portion of the literature published since 1968 in the following three areas:

1. Studies of factors facilitating the development of CAI in general education
2. Studies of factors inhibiting the development of CAI in general education
3. Studies of applications of CAI and of factors influencing the development of CAI in health professions education

Studies of Factors Facilitating the Development of CAI in General Education

Tuttle (1970) conducted an extensive descriptive study of the historical development of computer capabilities as an educational medium from 1958 to 1968. Among his conclusions are two that are seen as potentially influencing the acceptance of CAI. They are:

1. The teacher's role shifts "from purveyor of information and record-keeping to specialist in educational management, diagnostics, prescriptive procedure, etc." (p. 380)
2. The student's role shifts from passive to active involvement in the educative

process, and toward increasing control of teaching-learning activities. (p. 381)

Although Tuttle assigned no positive or negative value to his findings, he recommended these areas be studied further to identify the effects on roles and their relationships to student learning. Further, he recommended that studies be made to identify the problems that are encountered when CAI is implemented for purposes of guiding administrators in their decision making.

Christopher (1969) found from his literature review three obstacles that commonly occur in the use of computers in instruction:

1. The fledgling state of the art of computer-assisted instruction
2. The necessary financial commitment required by the medium
3. The resistant attitudes among professional educators toward the use of mechanically controlled instruction. (1969, p. 2)

He described most programs as being in developmental stages and attributed the lack of progress both to the inadequacy or absences of sufficient compatible and tested software and to the reluctance of educators to commit their resources to CAI systems that may soon be modified. But despite the decrease in the cost of utilizing computers as technology, Christopher felt that incompatability of hardware and software as well as competition among manufacturers were delaying the willingness for educators to make the investment required by CAI.

Christopher also stated that resistant attitudes of educators were more likely due to the magnitude of changes that CAI may cause than to the computer itself; and he referred to the fear, apprehension, and attitudes among educators that prohibit the "intelligent investigation" of the capabilities of CAI.

As part of the same study, Christopher conducted an empirical investigation to determine if school administrators' attitudes could be affected by "an acceptable computer assisted instruction experience." He found that (1) a structured experience with CAI did cause attitudes to become more favorable toward CAI, (2) the experience caused a decreased apprehension toward CAI among school administrators, and (3) administrators who were knowledgeable about computer applications in education possessed a more favorable attitude toward CAI.

Another of the studies examining factors influencing the development of CAI was conducted by Robardey (1971). He examined the relationships among attitude, knowledge, and other variables regarding CAI among 256 teachers and principals in one Michigan county. After an extensive survey directed at determining attitudes toward CAI, he suggested that "exposure to the computer and computer assisted instruction tends to foster a positive attitude toward this mode of instruction" (p. 34). On the basis of survey results, he concluded that there is a positive, statistically significant, relationship between knowledge and attitude with respect to CAI.

The third of the studies included here was by Hess and Tenezakis (1973) who sought to examine the long-term effects of CAI on educational institutions and particularly on the role of the teacher and the attitudes of students toward CAI.

This was accomplished by comparing attitudes of 189 seventh- to ninth-grade students toward CAI and other learning modes, such as classroom lecture and reading. Hess and Tenezakis reported that in the eyes of both CAI and non-CAI students the computer had a more favorable image than the teacher or textbooks. It appeared that these favorable student attitudes were related to some predicted role changes of teachers and opportunities for more personal and creative instructional contact with students.

In summary, there is some evidence to support the position that knowledge of CAI and a positive experience with it will cause administrators, students, and teachers to have a more positive attitude toward CAI as an instructional medium. The studies by Christopher and Robardey suggest that educational leaders within an institution who are contemplating the use of CAI should initially plan to acquaint administrators, faculty, and students with CAI through various activities, such as internal or external educational workshops, and provide experiences with CAI. Hess and Tenezakis's study demonstrates further the need to recognize the implications of technological developments upon individuals and educational institutions, as does Tuttle's work.

Studies of Factors Inhibiting the Development of CAI in General Education

Two empirical studies, one by Luskin (1970) and the other by Anastasio and Morgan (1972) identified the factors that inhibit or negatively influence the development of CAI. As evidenced in the studies reported in the previous section, attitudes are a significant factor to consider in planning the CAI. Awareness of other obstacles to the introduction of an educational innovation is likewise helpful to educational planners.

Luskin (1970) sought to identify and to examine the obstacles to development of CAI in junior colleges. It should be noted that Luskin included all instructional uses of computers in his definition of CAI. The study data were derived from 127 individual interviews. Twenty-two obstacles to CAI were identified which Luskin then included in a survey instrument. The survey instrument was administered to 75 of the personnel already interviewed. The personnel included educators with expertise in CAI, junior college administrators, and representatives of hardware/software companies active in CAI. The purposes of the survey were: (1) to classify the 22 factors (obstacles) obtained from the interviews as critical inhibitors, considerable inhibitors, or minor inhibitors and (2) to determine when in the future, if at all, these obstacles would be resolved. Of the 22 obstacles to CAI development, 7 emerged as critical inhibitors. These were:

> (1) Availability of individuals with appropriate component skills, (2) sufficient local funds, (3) sufficient funds for research and development, (4) attitude of faculty, (5) lack of incentives to stimulate preparation of educational software, (6) poor documentation of educational software, and (7) the existence of a communication gap between educators and representatives of industry.

Ten obstacles were reported as considerable inhibitors:

(1) High costs; (2) lack of definition of required skills, (3) lack of definition of appropriate personnel combinations, (4) inability to share developed software, (5) poor distribution mechanisms, (6) the traditional nature of education, (7) inadequate copyright laws, (8) attitude of administrators, (9) general availability of audio-visual devices, and (10) general availability of appropriate terminal devices.

Five obstacles were reported as minor:

(1) Ability to choose between instructional strategies, (2) attitude of the public, (3) lack of sufficiently powerful author languages, (4) ability to measure educational effectiveness, and (5) attitude of students (p. xiv).

Luskin concluded, "The shortage of individuals with appropriate component skills is the most critical obstacle appearing in the findings of the study" (p. xiv). He also concluded that CAI may eventually win acceptance in education but that acceptance may come as late as 1988 (p. xv).

A more recent study done by Anastasio and Morgan (1972) was undertaken to identify the obstacles to the widespread use of computers in the instructional process and to outline strategies for overcoming the difficulties. Anastasio and Morgan defined CAI to include all aspects of computer use in an instructional context. The study methodology utilized the Delphi technique with 30 participants from the areas of curriculum development, educational research, educational administration, law, computer science, and computer hardware and software production. The study classified the inhibiting factors derived from the Delphi questionnaires as having the following dimensions:

1. The lack of "good readily available" CAI materials was cited as the most critical inhibiting factor.
2. The lack of demonstration capability of "high quality use" and economic feasibility of CAI.
3. The failure to recognize that CAI requires an extensive reorganization of course materials and pedagogy in order to be utilized effectively. (p. 31)
4. CAI requires a high capital investment even when good cost effectiveness can be achieved in the long run. (p. 41)
5. The use of CAI will require a change in the established patterns of instruction and a restructuring of the traditional role of the teacher. (p. 35)
6. The design of more appropriate hardware and software systems is moderately inhibiting in the development of CAI.

In summary, the Luskin and the Anastasio and Morgan studies emphasize the problems inherent in introducing and developing applications of CAI in general education. They provide comprehensive, empirically derived lists of obstacles to the development of CAI. As such, the studies are useful to educational planners as they consider CAI. Yet, it is not clear that the above findings can be generalized to health professions education. In the next section, the research literature on factors influencing the development of CAI in health professions education will be reviewed.

Studies of Applications of CAI and of Factors Influencing the Development of CAI in Health Professions Education

In 1967, four publications directly relating CAI to health professions education appeared in the literature (Stolurow, 1967; Stolurow *et al.*, 1970; Geertsma, 1967; Fonkalsrud *et al.*, 1967; Starkweather *et al.*, 1967). Stolurow states:

> The health sciences and professions seemed an excellent place to start, not only because of the cost of instruction and the critical personnel shortages, but also because of the problems attendant upon the education and training of the various members of this community of specialists. (1970, p. 3)

In contrast, Skolnick states:

> This concept (CAI) has always been and still is full of promise, but the promise has been very slow to be fulfilled. The difficulties have not primarily related to hardware. ... The problem instead has been one of software, of the instructional materials and the computer program to control the new medium. (Skolnick and Jolly, 1972, p. 43)

A number of references have recently appeared in the literature that provide a more optimistic perspective on the state of the art of CAI in the education of health professionals. In the earliest of these, Griesen (1971) attributed the growth and positive acceptance of CAI in medical education at The Ohio State University to the fact that faculty were involved in developing concepts about CAI and its use in teaching and learning rather than just being involved in the details of computer coding. The involvement of students in education and medicine in the planning stages was another factor that contributed to the favorable response to CAI (p. 54).

Griesen also examined medical student preferences and performance in an independent study mode (in which CAI was a significant medium of instruction) versus traditional group instruction. He reported:

1. Students who elect independent study and enroll in such a curriculum display more positive reactions to their school environment at the completion of their programs than do students who complete a group instruction curriculum. (p. 154)
2. Students who enroll in an independent study curriculum possess certain personality characteristics that differ from those choosing a group instruction curriculum. (p. 153)

Brigham *et al.* (1973), in a *Guide to Computer Assisted Instruction in the Health Sciences*, provide a listing of specific current applications of CAI and a comprehensive bibliography of the CAI literature directly related to health sciences education. This study lists each of the 362 courses offered in 109 of the 561 schools responding to the survey. It should be noted that many of these institutions offer only one or two courses while some offer a large number. For example, The Ohio State University has 81 CAI courses in the College of Medicine, University of Kansas School of Medicine has 20, and Harvard Medical School has 38. But the number of institutions employing CAI is increasing rapidly. Of the 561 institutions reporting, 78 reported they were using CAI as an instructional medium, 116 anticipate using CAI, and 367 do not anticipate using CAI. Furthermore, the Health Education Network (formerly the Lister Hill Biomedical Communications Center CAI Experimental Network) now offers CAI to health professions educational institutions without CAI capability through a national network.

The rapidly increasing number of CAI users and the appearance of several articles regarding CAI in health professions education indicates CAI is an increasingly integral part of many health professions educational programs (Ingersoll, 1974; Meyer and Beaton, 1974; Brigham and Kamp, 1974; Kamp, 1975; Virgo and Hody, 1976; Goroll *et al.*, 1977). Furthermore, a general of the literature indicates that questions regarding the adoption of CAI are more of "when" and "how" rather than "if" (Hickey, 1968, p. 7).

Finally, a recent study (Rubin *et al.*, 1975) provides a comprehensive look at the Lister Hill Experimental CAI Network on the use and impact of computers in medical education. (The Network is further described in Chapter 8 of this volume) The Rubin study reports that 95 institutions had participated in the Network experiment as of October, 1974. The report states that administrative support at user institutions was lacking and that, though administrators were impressed with CAI, they were not convinced that the "add-on" costs could be justified. They sought proof of the learning benefits of CAI at a time when CAI was still very much in the evolutionary stage.

Bitzer and Bitzer (1973), in an experimental study in nursing education, utilized CAI to present simulated patients with commonly encountered problems to student nurses and found that students taught by CAI learned the same materials as well as or better than a control group taught by conventional classroom methods and that they learned the material in one-third to one-half the time. Bitzer and Bitzer also stressed that CAI must be accepted by both students and instructors if it is to be of practical use. This finding is supportive of Robardey's observation that acceptance of CAI is influenced by the way it is introduced and by teachers' and students' preconceived attitudes (pp. 6–7). Bitzer and Bitzer's attitudinal studies revealed that 54% of the nursing students initially had difficulty concentrating on the lesson because attention needed to be given to operating the terminal equipment. However, shifts in attitude toward acceptance of CAI in the learning of difficult material occurred as students became familiar with the terminal operation. Thus, Bitzer and Bitzer stated:

> By the end of their courses, over 50 percent of students typically rate PLATO (the CAI system) as the "best," "easiest," and "most preferred" medium over lecture, textbook or movie; while from 0 to 15 percent rate PLATO as "worst" or "hardest" to learn from. Instructor evaluation of the material was almost uniformly favorable. (p. 201)

Gaston's (1972) study related students' attitudes toward CAI and their achievement in dental school tests and on the Dental National Board Examinations. He found that students who were favorably disposed toward CAI (1) achieved higher grades in the courses when CAI was used as adjunct material and (2) received higher grades overall in the first two years of dental school. However, Gaston also reported that the favorably disposed students who scored higher during the last two years of dental school had a lower entering grade point average than did other students. Thus, CAI was perceived by the faculty as a helpful learning resource to these less promising students.

In summary, the literature on CAI in the health professions consists mainly of reports on surveys, specific institutional experiences with CAI, and the viewpoints of educational leaders. The empirical studies are more recent. Rubin, Stolurow, and others have described the appropriateness of recognizing and exploiting the potential of CAI in meeting health and educational needs. CAI's feasibility for increasing rates of learning is now being demonstrated. Yet, the literature is incomplete as a guide to health professions administrators or faculty in planning for the development and utilization of CAI as an instructional medium. However, projection of CAI's future role in university-based and continuing-education programs for health professionals indicates exciting opportunities.

Generalizations from the Review of the Literature

The following generalizations have emerged from this review of the literature:

1. Technological developments such as CAI have implications for changes in roles and relationships of teachers and students as well as instructional design.

2. The acceptance of CAI by teachers and school administrators is strongly related to their knowledge of how CAI can be utilized in instruction.

3. Educational planners must recognize that there are cognitive and noncognitive variables that impinge on individuals' achievement in and attitude toward independent study modes such as CAI.

4. CAI is a feasible instructional medium to consider in health professions education in terms of learning effectiveness, increasing numbers of students that can be served, and the limited numbers of faculty and educational programs presently available.

5. There is a limited amount of empirical evidence defining the factors inhibiting the development of CAI in general education, but no empirically based studies were found that sought to identify factors that facilitate the development of CAI.

This review of the literature reveals a lack of widespread knowledge of important considerations and factors among educators. To assess the need for greater knowledge of factors impacting on the developing or utilizing CAI in health professions education, the author surveyed deans and directors of health professions educational programs to determine whether as not identification of factors influencing the development of CAI would be helpful to educators and administrators in health professions programs. All responded in the affirmative to the questionnaire.

The author therefore felt that this response further indicated there was need for more research. A study designed to examine the factors that influence the development and utilization of computers in health professions education was then undertaken.

The goals of the study were (1) to identify the critical factors that facilitate or inhibit the development and utilization of CAI in health professions education as perceived by current, experienced users of CAI in medical education and (2) to develop a set of guidelines for health professions administrators and faculty to use in planning for the utilization of CAI as an instructional medium. The guidelines for planning as well as the understanding of the crucial factors associated with effective planning and utilization of CAI which come from the study data may provide educators with the confidence needed to consider objectively CAI as an instructional medium. Thus, the guidelines developed in this study and presented at the end of the chapter should be helpful in facilitating planning and increasing effectiveness in the utilization of CAI in health professions education through better informed administrators and faculty. Such guidelines should also aid in reducing the negative effects of a poorly planned or improperly introduced innovation.

Method of Conducting the Study

A methodology was utilized in which critical factors influencing the development of CAI were identified by CAI-experienced personnel in three medical education (ME) programs. The extent to which these factors play a crucial role was then determined for both CAI-experienced and CAI-inexperienced health professions personnel. The data thus derived were then used in preparation of a set of guidelines to aid health professions educators in the development and utilization of CAI.

The first phase of the study consisted of the identification and prioritization of the critical factors influencing the development of CAI as perceived by CAI-experienced administrators, faculty, and technical staff in three medical education programs (Massachusetts General Hospital, The Ohio State University, and The University of Illinois). The nominal group process was the methodology used (Delbecq and Van de Ven, 1971). (Further information on the research methodology can be found in Casbergue, 1974.)

The second phase of the study consisted of a mail survey to members of the American Society of Allied Health Professions (ASAHP). The survey was designed to determine the perceived importance of each of the factors obtained in the Phase I study.

The third phase of the study was directed at preparing a set of guidelines for utilization in planning CAI. The guidelines were derived from data gathered in the first and second phases.

Results of the Study

The facilitating and inhibiting factors influencing the development and utilization of CAI which were identified by personnel at the three CAI-experienced medical education institutions and the rating of those factors are here presented and discussed. This section concludes with a comparison of the findings of this study with the findings of other related studies.

The first-phase, nominal-group process meetings identified the most critical factors (those facilitating and those inhibiting) influencing the development and utilization of CAI in medical education at the three institutions providing CAI programs to the Lister Hill Network. Over 200 factors influencing the development of CAI were generated by the three groups. The lists of the ten highest priority facilitating factors and ten highest priority inhibiting factors from each group are presented in Tables 1, 2, and 3.

It is interesting to note that there are some high-priority factors that are listed by all three CAI-experienced institutions and several that are listed by only one such institution. For example, "high costs of CAI" appears as a critical inhibiting factor among all three institutions but "funding for CAI based on task analysis" is mentioned by only one CAI-experienced institution. This suggests that there may be factors that can be generalized across institutions but that some may be institution-specific. This is an area of inquiry suggested for further research.

Table 1. *University of Illinois Medical Center, Critical Factors in the Development of CAI*

Rank	Facilitating factors	Rank	Inhibiting factors
1	Top administrative support	1	Administrative structure restricted promotion of CAI
2.5[a]	Top-level health professions administrator is liaison between CAI staff and faculty	2	No ongoing faculty−CAI-staff organization exists
2.5[a]	Operational computer facility available	3	CAI programs do not relate to existing curricula of users
4	Funding for CAI based on task analysis	4	High costs with little documented results
5	Joint faculty and CAI staff production and evaluation of software	5	Incompatibility of CAI material with educational goals
6	CAI is an integral part of the curriculum	6.5[a]	Lack of understanding of CAI by faculty and students
7.5[a]	Easy student access to terminals	6.5[a]	Central computer facility is not a part of total educational program
7.5[a]	Direction of CAI defined by the curricula	8	High operational costs
9	Continuous production and evaluation of CAI materials	9	Competition between CAI groups to promote own brand of programs
10	Establishment of written priorities and objectives	10	Cost for development of software in terms of time and resources

[a]Ties in ranking

Table 2. Massachusetts General Hospital with Harvard University, Critical Factors in the Development of CAI

Rank	Facilitating factors	Rank	Inhibiting factors
1	Adequate funds for personnel, hardware, and software	1	High initial investment
2	Validated, documented CAI programs available	2	Lack of institutional framework
3.5[a]	Competent faculty and technical staff available	3	Lack of perceived need by faculty
3.5[a]	Availability of CAI network	4	Inadequate evaluation mechanism for cost–benefit and cost analysis
5	Commitment to CAI as an educational tool	5	Transmission problems
6	Reliable CAI network with guaranteed access to users	6	Lack of money to develop content
7	Availability of support personnel	7	Lack of validation of CAI program
8	CAI terminals in institutions are highly accessible to users	8	Nontransferability of CAI program
9	Appropriate educational orientation to faculty and others	9	Lack of faculty commitment to schedule students for CAI
10	Trial use of CAI system before institutional commitment	10	Lack of clearly defined objectives for CAI programs

[a]Ties in ranking

Thirteen questionnaires were received from participants (the same number participating in the nominal group meetings). Ninety-five percent of the questionnaires sent to the ASAHP member schools were returned, of which 83% were usable and included in the analysis of the data from the CAI-inexperienced group.

Table 3. The Ohio State University, Critical Factors in the Development of CAI

Rank	Facilitating factors	Rank	Inhibiting factors
1	Top-level administrative support	1	High investment costs
2.5[a]	Adequate budget for implementation and development	2	Time investment for planning and development period
2.5[a]	Qualified director of CAI	3	Lack of administrative support
4	Stable and reliable computer facility available	4	Faculty do not perceive proper use of CAI
5	Independent study curriculum in progress	5	Lack of adequate software
6	Qualified technical staff available	6	Cost benefits unknown
7	Students' interest and support of use of CAI	7	Unknown effectiveness of CAI instruction
8	Abundance of courseware	8	Inadequate computer compatibility
9	Time saving for faculty	9	Requires large support staff
10	Authoring recognized as a publishing endeavor	10	Lack of recognition and reward system for faculty

[a]Ties in ranking

Preparation of Guidelines

The guidelines presented at the end of this chapter were prepared based on an analysis of the ratings done by the CAI-experienced and CAI-inexperienced groups of the facilitating and inhibiting factors. The mean ratings for each item were converted to a rank-ordered listing. These data are summarized in Tables 4 and 5.

While preparing guidelines, considerable variation was noted in the rankings of the inhibiting factors by the CAI-experienced group compared to the CAI-inexperienced group. For example, in Table 5 the CAI-experienced group lists "cost benefits are unknown" as the least crucial of the 12 inhibiting factors rated, while the CAI-inexperienced group rates this as the third most crucial factor.

These observed differences led to an analysis of the items using the Spearman rank-order correlation coefficient (Seigel, 1956, p. 204). The following correlations between the CAI-experienced and the CAI-inexperienced group were found:

$$\text{Facilitating factors} \qquad r_s = 0.8213$$
$$\text{Inhibiting factors} \qquad r_s = 0.0909$$

The large positive correlation indicates that both groups tend to rate the facilitating factors in the same way. However, there is relatively little agreement on the inhibiting factors that have a rank-order correlation which is close to zero (0.0909 is not statistically different from zero at the .01 level).

Table 4. Crucial Facilitating Factors Rated in the Study

Facilitating factors	CAI-experienced group	CAI-inexperienced group
Reliable computer facility available	1	2
Adequate funds available	2	1
Availability of large number of appropriate CAI programs	3	6
Top-level administrative support	4	5
Establishment of central office to lead, coordinate, and develop CAI materials	5	8
Faculty commitment to CAI	6	3
CAI is an integral part of curriculum	7	13
Faculty and CAI staff work together in planning and development of materials	8	4
Highly qualified director of CAI available	9	7
Funding for CAI based on task analysis	10.5	10
Students committed to and support CAI	10.5	12
Individualized learning is an accepted learning mode	13	9
Competent faculty and technical staff available	13	11
Existence of a national CAI network in health professions education	13	16
Top level health professions educator is liaison between CAI staff and faculty	15	15
Faculty perceive CAI as means of saving time	16	14

Table 5. Crucial Inhibiting Factors Rated in the Study

Inhibiting factors	CAI-experienced group	CAI-inexperienced group
High initial investment for people, time, and hardware	1	1
Lack of institutional framework for development of CAI	2	12
Faculty do not recognize how to utilize CAI as an integral part of curriculum	3	4
Lack of perceived need for CAI by faculty	4.5	6
No ongoing faculty and staff organization exists	4.5	9
Lack of top-level administrative support	6.5	7.5
Lack of adequate software	6.5	2
Transmission problems cause frustration and loss of interest	8	11
Available CAI programs do not relate to curricula of multitude of health professions education programs	9.5	7.5
Inadequate evaluation mechanisms for cost-benefit and cost-effectiveness analyses	9.5	5
Faculty do not recognize alternative forms of CAI (tutorial, problem solving, simulation, etc.)	11	10
Cost benefits are unknown	12	3

In the development of guidelines, it becomes important to emphasize both those factors that are prioritized differently between the groups and those that are ranked similarly by the two groups. The reason for this is not to lose sight of important, or highly crucial factors for CAI development merely because they do not differ between the two groups. For example, in Table 5 both groups rated "high initial investment for people, time, and hardware" as the most crucial inhibiting factor in the study. This underscores the important nature of this factor. Therefore, not to include it or comment on it in the discussion would be a serious error, because any list of recommendations for the development of CAI guidelines must include this factor.

It is equally important to note that prioritizing *within* each group can lead to a misinterpretation of the data. It should be stressed that all the factors, facilitating and inhibiting (Tables 5 and 6), are important by virtue of how these factors were originally determined (i.e., they are high-priority concerns of CAI-experienced faculty and staff). Therefore, the reader should view each factor in the guidelines as important, and further research can indicate which subset of these factors, if any, are both necessary and sufficient for adopting CAI.

A final point of discussion refers back to the high correlation of perceptions of facilitating factors and the low correlation on inhibiting factors. It could be suggested that, since the CAI-inexperienced group perceived the facilitating factors in the same way as the CAI-experienced groups, guidelines for naive health professions educators need only address the inhibiting factors where reported perceptions differ. Thus, why bother the administrator with something he already "knows"? It must be noted that the crucial factors were identified by the CAI-experienced groups and then the factors were presented in an instrument to the inexperienced group for a review and rating. The naive raters had the opportunity to consider a factor *presented* to them; they were not asked to derive the factors and then rate them. Thus, one cannot say with certainty that the high correlation on facilitating factors means that the inexperienced group would perceive or even generate these same facilitating factors if they were not suggested to them. Indeed, the low correlation on the inhibiting factors suggests the inexperienced administrators may put the emphasis on the wrong factors and not deal with the more critical factors as specified by the experienced people. This point supports, in the author's view, the need for guidelines incorporating both facilitating and inhibiting factors. This was further supported during the guideline validation process. The inexperienced health professions educators who reviewed the prototype guidelines included such comments as: "Yes, very helpful; [the guidelines] raise questions we should attend to and identify the necessary support," and "Yes, particularly [useful] in communicating these CAI considerations to other faculty and administrators."

The guidelines themselves are presented later in this chapter.

Discussion of Critical Factors

The facilitating and inhibiting factors identified in this study that form the basis for the guidelines fall into seven logical categories: (1) attitudes (includes recognition and reward), (2) economics, (3) learning and instruction, (4) organization and administration, (5) personnel, (6) software, and (7) technology.

Attitudes

Factors identified in this category include the need for faculty and student commitment to CAI and a system of recognition and reward for motivating faculty to undertake the necessary development effort. Over 94% of the raters stated that faculty commitment to CAI was among the most crucial factors in the development of CAI. Such commitment is a critical element in (1) the objective consideration of CAI as an instructional medium, (2) the appropriate use of the medium, and (3) student acceptance of CAI as an effective learning medium. For, as described in the literature by Tuttle (1970), CAI will not only change most faculty members' way of teaching, it will affect their way of relating to students, their relationship with peers, and their work setting. Therefore, plans to consider and diffuse an innovation such as CAI should include careful consideration to the factor of faculty commitment and how this might be accomplished.

Further, during their discussions, the CAI-experienced groups indicated that this aspect of attitude and commitment to diffusion of CAI is a factor that must be considered and dealt with at the earliest stages. Gaining commitment does not require capital investment for hardware or technical staff, the most critical inhibitor reported. But it does require a planned approach to involving faculty, including selection of faculty CAI planners on the basis of openness, status, and leadership (as change agents or opinion leaders). Considering the state of the art of CAI in health profession education and the presently limited amount of software, the educational preparation of administrators and faculty is likely to be the most promising opportunity to increase objective consideration of CAI or other technologically based instructional media.

The aspects of recognition and reward were reported as important factors in maintaining a positive attitude and commitment toward CAI. Recognition within the institution as well as monetary and professional recognition were referred to in both written comments on the survey instrument and verbal comments during the meetings of the CAI-experienced groups. Financial incentives were reported as desirable, but faculty release time for development was also reported as important. By and large, institutions do not yet recognize the knowledge and time commitment required for CAI materials' development. Recognition of CAI development efforts by a faculty member's peers both within and external to the institution was also found to be crucial by the CAI-experienced institutions as was the need to consider the authoring of CAI materials as a publishing endeavor – an historical source of evidence of academic achievement.

In summary, the commitment of faculty and students to value and support CAI is considered a critical element in its development. This study indicated that passive acceptance of CAI will not lead to its effective utilization as an integral part of the instructional systems even with financial support. In addition, there must be systems for recognition and reward of development efforts. Financial support and reward systems are needed, but internal and external professional recognition of faculty as authors and developers of CAI will increase the likelihood of continued faculty commitment to CAI.

Economics

The primary concern of both experienced and potential users of CAI was the high initial investment costs. From the perspective of CAI-experienced respondents, cost effectiveness was not as critical an issue as attitudes but was still important because the investment costs are significant, particularly when coupled with other activities competing for funds. Likewise, the present study revealed that experienced medical education CAI users did not rate the inadequacies of cost-effectiveness measures and the fact that the cost-benefit ratio is unknown as critical to the development decision as did the CAI-inexperienced group. Verbal comments at the meetings of the CAI-experienced users suggested that increased motivation and effectiveness and increased learning rates of students were factors that had to be considered in establishing cost effectiveness. This perspective on cost effectiveness and learning effectiveness is particularly relevant to health professions educational programs because, as described earlier, increasing demands for health manpower, an increasing number of students, and a limited number of faculty and educational programs are emphasizing the need for improved effectiveness. When weighing the relative advantages of CAI, the health professions administrator must recognize the economic as well as social-organizational implications. However, due to rapid changes in technology and in computer-related costs, administrators should not disregard CAI as an instructional medium because of present costs. Again, the author found that "cost benefits are unknown" was the least inhibiting factor of those rated by the CAI-experienced groups. But systematic analyses of the cost and learning effectiveness of present instructional methods, projections of the impact of CAI and other innovations on the educational program, and related development activities should still be a part of any effort to develop or utilize CAI on a wide-scale basis.

Learning and Instruction

The lack of integration of CAI into the health professions educational programs and the lack of understanding of the alternative forms of CAI were reported (by over 65% of the raters) as crucial factors that are directly related to the faculty's understanding of and commitment to CAI as a medium of instruction. These and related factors indicate the need for faculty education and understanding of CAI as an instructional medium rather than merely a technological innovation. This would 'rclude an understanding of the need for an instructional system to be redesigned and restructured if CAI is to be used effectively. There must also be a movement from teaching-oriented pedagogy to learning-oriented approaches. In this respect, the acceptance of individualized instruction as a learning mode was rated by over 80% of both groups as a critical factor or one of considerable importance in the development of CAI.

There was also agreement among the groups that CAI would be most effective as an integral part of curricula (70% rated this critical or of considerable importance). However, verbal and written comments also support the value of CAI for remedial learning and as an optional resource for students. The somewhat limited number and types of CAI courses available suggest this has been a feasible and widely used alternative.

In summary, both faculty knowledge of the instructional alternatives provided by CAI and an understanding of how to integrate CAI with other instructional modalities remain as crucial factors in the development of CAI. Again, the need is demonstrated for educational planners to provide educational opportunities including demonstration as a means of interesting faculty in learning about and "trying-out" CAI as an instructional medium before a long-range development effort is undertaken.

Organization and Administration

In the perception of over 91% of both groups, the development and implementation of CAI on more than an experimental basis will require top-level administrative commitment to CAI in order to provide the necessary support and organizational structure. (The factor was reported as lacking in the Rubin *et al.* [1975] study.) Crucial factors were the establishment of a central office to lead, coordinate, and facilitate the development of CAI materials and the establishment of an organizational mechanism whereby faculty and CAI technical staff can work together in the development of these materials. Discussion within the CAI-experienced groups suggested that this need for faculty and CAI technical staff to work together is apparently more important as CAI is being planned than as it is being implemented. Once faculty and staff understand their responsibilities, there is a decreased need for joint efforts in developing CAI programs. But continuing joint efforts were suggested for long-range planning, review of new developments, and formative and summative evaluation. Also, joint efforts were seen as helpful in keeping CAI available primarily for instructional purposes rather than solely for research and/or administrative purposes.

In summary, top-level administrative support of and commitment to CAI is necessary for its development and implementation. Cost factors and developments in CAI technology will influence administrative decision-making; but once there is a decision to develop and implement CAI, support must be provided for computer-system capabilities and for educational programs for faculty, for leadership, and for instructional and technical staff.

Personnel

Among CAI-experienced groups, four personnel categories emerged as crucial for the development of CAI. There must be available (1) a highly qualified director of CAI, (2) a top-level health professions educator to serve as liaison between CAI staff and faculty, and (3) faculty knowledgeable in computers and health care and (4) an experienced CAI technical staff.

There was agreement that the recruitment of a competent staff is an important element for effective diffusion of CAI. The CAI-experienced groups reported most success in developing and utilizing CAI materials when the faculty did not have to become experts in the technical aspects of CAI but could restrict their role to that of content experts. Even in those schools where CAI is made available through a network, the availability of a technically competent person to assist faculty and students in using hardware or software was reported in discussions as highly desirable in overcoming the frustration that can occur with errors in input (or output), unanticipated disconnections, or systems failures.

Software

The availability of a large number of appropriately documented and validated CAI programs is ranked third as a facilitating factor by the CAI-experienced groups. However, problems of program adequacy were also cited as inhibiting factors, including

(1) a lack of adequate software and (2) the fact that available CAI programs do not relate to the curricula of most health professions educational programs.

The lack of adequate software is ranked seventh as an inhibiting factor by the CAI-experienced group and second by the CAI-inexperienced group. It cannot be stated with any high degree of certainty, but this may be partly a dissemination problem as well as an actual lack of courses. The literature revealed that there are approximately 85 courses available through the Health Education Network. The discussions indicated that though these may be primarily for physician education, many of the programs are in the basic sciences (i.e., histology, gross anatomy, physiological chemistry, and physiology). At least part of these are potentially adaptable for health professions educational programs, such as dietetics, nursing, occupational or physical therapy, or other programs. Moreover, the available programs are presented using a variety of instructional strategies. This capability would be most helpful for demonstration or experimental applications by potential users of CAI.

The factors related to software reflect the fact that CAI is in its adolescence. The past difficulties attributed to weakness and/or complexity of programming languages are less important due to strengthening of programming capability and the use of CAI personnel to carry out the technical programming of faculty-designed CAI courses. However, the lack of programs *per se* will remain a problem until there is an expanded number of faculty or other content specialists involved in program design and development for the varied needs of the health professions educational programs.

Technology

The availability of a reliable computer, on-premises or by network, is ranked as the first or second most critical facilitating factor by the CAI-experienced and CAI-inexperienced groups, respectively. The existence of a national CAI network was perceived as slightly less crucial. The only inhibiting factor in this category was "transmission problems cause frustration and loss of interest."

Access to a CAI system is, of course, a requisite for the operational and instructional use of CAI. The development of a computer system, *de nova*, can be a time-consuming and often discouraging activity. The developing technology is reducing the difficulties, but the technical difficulties in setting up any computer system are still a cause for concern to potential users. Experienced CAI users stressed the need for "tolerance" and "patience." One "law" often referred to in this respect was "Things take longer than they do."

The inhibiting factor of frustration due to system failure or transmission problems is a serious one that cannot be negated simply by alluding to the early state of the art. However, experienced users emphasized that faculty and students could accept occasional problems and delays if there were an adequate orientation to this aspect of CAI and if users were to understand the kinds of problems that occur as well as the reasons for their occurrence.

Summary and Conclusions

This study had two goals; (1) to identify the critical factors that facilitate or inhibit the development of CAI in health professions educational programs and (2) to develop guidelines for health professions administrators and faculty to use in planning for the utilization of CAI. The health professions educational program populations included in the study were (1) the three medical educational institutions providing CAI programs nationally through the Lister Hill Biomedical Communications Center CAI Experimental Network and (2) the 108 institutions in the American Society of Allied Health Professions.

Using the nominal group process, the CAI-experienced medical education groups provided a prioritized list of the crucial factors influencing the development and implementation of CAI. Utilizing this list of crucial factors, a questionnaire was developed (1) to identify the current state of adoption of CAI in allied health educational programs and (2) to determine the perceptions of the relative importance of factors which influence adoption of CAI. The perceptions of the three CAI-experienced medical education programs and the ASAHP (CAI-inexperienced) institutions were elicited. The ASAHP group reported that they (71% of those responding) expect to be utilizing CAI as an integral part of their educational program within 5 years, and 94% agreed that CAI is an appropriate instructional strategy to consider in the education of health professionals.

Conclusions

There are two sets of conclusions in this study. The first relates to the critical factors that facilitate or inhibit the development or utilization of CAI in health professions education — the first goal of this study. These conclusions were useful in deriving the guidelines for the utilization of CAI in health professions education — the second goal of the study. These guidelines, presented in the last section of this chapter, were drawn from an examination of the critical factors influencing the development of CAI. These conclusions provide insight into differing perceptions depending on (1) the level of CAI experience of the health professions educator and (2) the field of health professions education of the respondents.

Conclusions Regarding Crucial Factors

1. *The high financial investment required for the development of CAI is a primary inhibiting factor to those considering the use of CAI.* These costs and the lack of evidence of documented cost effectiveness are seen by some allied health professions educators as so prohibitive that they will not consider CAI.

2. *A reliable computer system must be available or accessible for the consideration or development of CAI.* Further, there is a need for continued development of relevant CAI software that meet the needs of the multitude of health professions curricula.

3. *There must be an institutional commitment to the development and utilization of CAI.* In addition, an institutional framework or organizational structure that supports such utilization must be established. This includes recruitment and/or development of a competent team of faculty and technical staff that can plan, coordinate, and assist in evaluating any development or utilization efforts. These are critical organizational factors for any health professions educational programs contemplating the utilization of CAI.

4. *There must be educational programs for faculty, administrators, and technical personnel.* Educational planners must recognize the need for faculty and administrators' awareness, knowledge, and interest prior to introducing an innovation such as CAI.

5. *Faculty must understand how to integrate CAI with other instructional modalities.* Furthermore, they should be aware of the various instructional strategies available through CAI. Faculty experience with learner-oriented pedagogy was found to be a facilitating factor in the acceptance of CAI as a part of health professions curricula.

Conclusions Regarding Differing Perceptions of Factors Influencing the Development of CAI

1. There is only partial overlap in both the highest priority facilitating and inhibiting factors cited by the three medical education institutions with CAI experience. This leads the author to conclude that there are some institution-specific factors influencing the development of CAI.

2. CAI-experienced and inexperienced health professions educators tend to agree on perceptions of crucial facilitating factors and fail to agree on several crucial inhibiting factors.

3. The most critical inhibiting factors identified in this study are different, in part, than those reported by Anastasio and Morgan (1972) and Luskin (1970). The "lack of institutional framework for development of CAI" (rank of second most critical factor by the CAI-experienced education groups) and lack of reference to the need for "top-level administrative support" and commitment to CAI as an instructional medium are two examples. The CAI-experienced medical educators view these as highly critical yet these factors are only alluded to indirectly by Luskin and not reported by those who participated in the Anastasio and Morgan study. (Rubin *et al.* [1975] does report on the need for administrative support.) Thus, there are particular factors that are perceived differently in health professions educational institutions than those reported in studies of inhibiting factors in general education.

Guidelines for the Utilization of CAI in Health Professions Educational Programs

This section presents a set of guidelines for administrators in health professions educational programs who are considering the use of computer-assisted instruction. The guidelines can be looked upon as actions necessary for the utilization of CAI.

The items listed under each guideline are specific factors or considerations that elaborate on the action(s) stated in the guideline. These guidelines should be helpful in assisting the educational administrator in posing the question: Is this institution ready to commit its resources to the development or utilization of CAI?

GUIDELINE I. *The high initial investment costs of CAI must be weighed against the potential gains in learning effectiveness, rate of learning, and overall cost effectiveness of the total curriculum.*

A. Studies have reported increased learning effectiveness and reductions of time for learning via CAI, when compared to traditional methods of instruction.

B. The costs of development of health professions instructional materials can be reduced through shared network systems. However, top-level decision-makers in using institutions must be involved as a means of insuring top-level support for long-term network support.

C. Instructional programs (software) can be developed for multiple purpose use with advance planning, thereby reducing overall development costs.

D. When high initial investment costs are amortized over large numbers of students and/or long periods of time, the cost per unit of instruction compares favorably with other modes of instruction in health professions curricula.

E. The availability of the Health Education Network provides an opportunity for many health professions educational programs to utilize CAI without significant investment.

GUIDELINE II. *Reliable computer facilities and services must be made available.*

A. Access to reliable institutional facilities or access to computer facilities by telephone network (where several institutions share CAI materials) is a requisite. The crucial factor is the reliability of the system. Frequent breakdowns, delays or limited access are frustrating to users.

B. There must be a recognition by faculty and students that CAI is in its technological adolescence and that there will be occasional system delays or failures. Recognition and acceptance of the state of the art will help facilitate satisfaction in spite of occasional interruptions.

C. The availability of mini-computers and computer networks are altering requirements for hardware, software, and staff. The Health Education Network provides an established base of CAI materials and opportunities for further development to many health professions educational programs.

GUIDELINE III. *The institution must make a commitment to the development and utilization of CAI.*

A. Top-level administrative support and commitment to CAI as an instructional medium are required for continued development, utilization, and effective evaluation. Such support and commitment must be clearly communicated to other administrators and faculty.

B. Support by the institution must include facilities, space, and staff as well as recognition and reward systems for faculty. Further, support must be provided for faculty to attend educational workshops or programs and to purchase appropriate reference materials. Access to resource personnel is also an effective means of demonstrating institutional commitment to CAI development. Release time is also necessary for the faculty to author materials.

C. There must be an institutionalized system of professional reward and recognition of faculty involved in CAI development. The present reward structure of many colleges and universities may actually discourage such efforts as CAI development or authoring.

D. Consideration should be given to cooperative work among institutions and faculty in the development of materials.

GUIDELINE IV.   *The faculty must make a commitment to use of CAI.*

A. There must be at least part of the faculty who value and are committed to the use of CAI as an instructional medium. This may initially be one or two faculty innovators or opinion leaders who can demonstrate to others the utility and potential for CAI in health professions education.

B. Faculty members who are part of the ongoing instructional program must be actively involved in the planning and development of CAI.

C. CAI has been successfully developed and integrated into curricula where the faculty were given educational orientation to individualized learning and CAI. Educational workshops and other educational support must be provided and/or supported by the institution.

D. CAI can be more readily integrated into curricula which already utilize individualized instructional modes. There are specific examples through which computer-based simulations and problem-solving exercises have also proven excellent for group instruction. In this context, CAI can respond to the needs of an individual even though in a group setting.

E. The availability of a CAI demonstration unit is a crucial element in developing awareness and interest in CAI. Faculty members and administrators need opportunities to test the capabilities of CAI and its relative advantage over other instructional media for various instructional problems.

F. Student acceptance of CAI is dependent on acceptance and valuing by the faculty. CAI materials which have been identified as major components of a course are perceived as more valuable by students than any "optional course materials."

GUIDELINE V.   *The utilization of CAI is facilitated by development of collaborative efforts between faculty and CAI technical staff.*

A. Traditionally, faculty work as individuals in the development of instructional materials. In developing CAI programs, however, few faculty possess the technical knowledge and skills required for computerization. The production of CAI materials is best accomplished when technical staff participate in the design and development of programs – a collaborative relationship. The faculty prescribes the context, sets the objectives, and designs the instructional strategy; the technical staff works with the faculty member in these activities and then takes over the technical aspects of preparing and testing the CAI programs.

B Rational growth and objective evaluation are facilitated by (1) a central office or committee composed of faculty knowledgeable of computers in education, and (2) a technical staff knowledgeable in CAI to guide and coordinate development.

C. Educational institutions developing CAI should consider utilizing internal resources such as faculty or staff from the areas of educational psychology, evaluation, instructional development and computer science. Long-term team development relationships are necessary in addition to the occasional support and guidance provided by external consultants.

GUIDELINE VI. *CAI must be made an integral part of the health professions curriculum.*

A. CAI is more than the use of computer-based materials to augment conventional instruction. CAI is best utilized when integrated into the total curriculum. This will require an analysis of the alternative modes of instruction for established objectives, and if CAI is appropriate, it is most effective if integrated with other instructional activities.

B. To assure proper use of CAI, the faculty must recognize the alternative modes of instruction provided by CAI. These are: tutorial, drill-and-practice, problem solving, and simulation.

C. Utilization of CAI is best when designed to meet the instructional objectives for a given course or curriculum. However, for demonstration purposes and experimental use, CAI materials developed for other courses may be utilized.

GUIDELINE VII. *Educational workshops, programs and processes must be provided to prepare faculty, students, and staff for change due to the utilization of CAI.*

A. Educational planners must recognize that the development of CAI will affect roles, relationships, and settings of teachers and students.

B. When various modes of individualized instruction and independent learning are provided, the primary contact between teachers and students may be shifted to an individual or small-group basis to resolve problems or discuss materials rather than in a lecture environment oriented toward presentation of content. The implications of such shifts in roles and relationships should be well considered in light of the knowledge of the roles of attitudes and the historical resistance to change.

C. The change in roles, relationships, and settings has implications for organizational structure as well as physical design of teaching and learning facilities to accommodate such changes.

References

Anastasio, E. J., and Morgan, J. S., 1972. *Factors Inhibiting the Use of Computers in Instruction*, EDUCOM, Interuniversity Communications Council, Inc., Princeton, New Jersey.

Bitzer, M. D., and Bitzer, D. L., 1973. Teaching nursing by computers: An evaluative study, *Comput. Biol. Med.* 3(3): 187–204.

Brigham, C. R., 1973. Editorial, *Comput. Biol. Med.* 3(3): 337–342.

Brigham, C. R., and Kamp, M., 1974. The current status of computer-assisted instruction in the health sciences, *J. Med. Educ.* 49(3): 278–279.

Brigham, C. R., Kamp, M., and Cross, R. J. (Eds.), 1978. *A Guide to Computer Assisted Instruction in the Health Sciences*, Rutgers Medical School, New Brunswick, N.J., and the University of California, San Francisco (December, 1972). Available from National Technical Information Service, U.S. Dept. Commerce, Springfield, Va., as PB 214 351 for 9.00.

Casbergue, J. P., 1974. Computer Assisted Instruction in Health Professions Education: Guidelines for Utilization. Unpublished doctoral dissertation, Michigan State University.

Christopher, G. R., 1969. The Influence of a Computer Assisted Instruction Experience Upon the Attitudes of School Administrators. Unpublished doctoral dissertation, The Ohio State University.

Delbecq, A. L., and Van de Ven, A. H., 1971. A group process model for problem identification and program planning. *J. Appl. Behav. Sci.* 7(4): 466–492.

Fonkalsrud, E. W., Hammidi, I. B., and Maloney, J. V., Jr., 1967. Computer assisted instruction in undergraduate surgical education, *Surgery* 62: 141–147.

Gaston, G. W., 1972. Dental Students Attitudes Toward Computer Assisted Instruction. Unpublished doctoral dissertation, The Ohio State University.

Geertsma, R. A., 1967. A student oriented learning center in the biomedical sciences, *J. Med. Educ.* 42: 681–686.

Goroll, A. H., Barnett, G. O., Bowie, J., Prather, P., 1977. Teaching differential diagnosis by computer: A pathophysiological approach, *J. Med. Educ.* 52(2): 153–154.

Griesen, J. V., 1971. Independent Study Versus Group Instruction in Medical Education: A Study of Non-Cognitive Factors Relating to Curricular Preferences and Academic Achievement. Unpublished doctoral dissertation, The Ohio State University.

Herskovitz, A., and Skolnick, M., 1972. Instructional technology *in* E. J. McTernan and R. O. Hawkins, Jr. (Eds.), *Educating Personnel for the Allied Health Professions*, C. V. Mosby, St. Louis.

Hess, R. D., and Tenezakis, M. D., 1973. The computer as a socializing agent: Some socio-affective outcomes of CAI, *AV Communication Review* 21(3): 31–325.

Hickey, A., 1968. *Computer Assisted Instruction: A Survey of the Literature*, 3rd ed., Entelek, Inc., Newburyport, Mass.

Ingersoll, R. W., 1974. The computer in the health services center, *J. Med. Educ.* 49(3): 298–299.

Jason, H., 1968. Computers in undergraduate medical education, *in* Proceedings of the Conference on the Use of Computers in Medical Education, University of Oklahoma Medical Center, Oklahoma City, Ok. (April 3, 4, 5).

Kamp, M., 1975. *Index to Computerized Teaching in the Health Sciences*, University of California, San Francisco.

Keller, M. D., 1965. *In* J. P. Casbergue (Ed.), *Proceedings of the First Conference on Computer Applications in Nutrition and Food Service Management*, The Ohio State University. Available from Clearinghouse, U.S. Dept. of Commerce, Springfield, Va. 22151.

Kerlinger, F. N., 1973. *Foundations of Behavioral Research*, Holt, Rinehart, and Winston, New York.

Luskin, B. J., 1970. An Identification and Examination of Obstacles to the Development of Computer Assisted Instruction. Unpublished doctoral dissertation, University of California.

Meyer, J. H. F., and Beaton, G. R., 1974. An evaluation of computer-assisted teaching in physiology, *J. Med. Educ.* 49(3): 295–297.

Robardey, C. P., 1971. A Study of Selected Michigan Elementary and Secondary Teachers' and Principals' Attitudes Toward Computer Assisted Instruction. Unpublished doctoral dissertation, Michigan State University.

Rubin, M. L., Hunter, B., and Knetsch, M., 1975. Evaluation of the Experimental CAI Network (1973–1975) of the Lister Hill National Center for Biomedical Communications, National Library of Medicine, Final Report No. LHNCBC 75–03, Human Resources Research Organization, Alexandria, Va.

Seigel, S., 1956. *Non-Parametric Statistics for the Behavioral Sciences*, McGraw-Hill, New York.

Skolnick, M., and Jolly, H. P., 1972. Electronic data processing, *in* E. J. McTernan and R. O. Hawkins, (Eds.), *Educating Personnel for the Allied Health Professions and Services*, C. V. Mosby, St. Louis.

Starkweather, J. A., Kamp, M., and Monto, A., 1967. Psychiatric interview simulation by computer, *Methods Inf. Med.* 6: 1523.

Stewart, W. H., 1968. Statement of the Surgeon General, *in: Proceedings of the Conference on the Use of Computers in Medical Education in Oklahoma*, University of Oklahoma Medical Center, Oklahoma City, Ok. (April).

Stolurow, L. M., 1967. Computer-Assisted Instruction (CAI), Technical Report No. 2., Harvard Computing Center, Cambridge, Mass.

Stolurow, L. M., Peterson, T. I., and Cunningham, A. C., 1970. *Computer Assisted Instruction in the Health Professions*, Entelek, Inc., Newburyport, Mass.

Testerman, J. D., and Jackson, J., 1973. A comprehensive annotated bibliography on computer-assisted instruction, *Comput. Rev.* 1973: 483–553.

Tuttle, J. G., 1970. The Historical Development of Computer Capabilities Which Permitted the Use of the Computer as an Educational Medium in the United States from 1958 to 1968, with Implications of Trends. Unpublished doctoral dissertation, New York University.

Virgo, J. A., and Hody, G. L., 1976. Computer-based instruction and the health sciences library, *J. Med. Educ.* 51(8): 644–647.

6

Planning for Educational Communication Networks

Richard F. Walters

Introduction

After a relatively disappointing start during the decade of the 1960s, computers have finally begun to play an important role in education in many disciplines. Networks have been important in encouraging the use of computers. Single-host configurations, such as the Dartmouth and PLATO systems, have served local and sometimes even remote users. Groups of colleges and universities have combined resources in several local or regional networks, such as the New England Computer Network, the Triangle University Computer Center (North Carolina), and the California State Universities and Colleges. In medical education, the National Library of Medicine had almost too much success in sponsoring such a network on a national scale to link medical institutions with the computers at the University of Illinois Medical College, Ohio State University, and Massachusetts General Hospital. As a result, and due to the keen interest generated by this experiment, the Health Education Network was formed; it is described in Chapters 7 and 11 of this book.

Networks have thus far played a role that has allowed users in remote locations to access programs available from one or perhaps a few centers of development. In the future, however, networks will play an expanded role, one whose character will depend on many factors, some of them technical and others relating to educational methodology. In order to plan for the future, it is necessary to understand these factors both in terms of their historical development and the trends that appear to be emerging for the future.

In this chapter, we will consider the background factors associated with computer network applications to medical education, and we will then propose a plan for future growth and development on the basis of this information.

Background

Education networks are influenced by the educational objectives and strategies employed by developers and users of such networks, by the computer hardware

Richard F. Walters · Medical Learning Resources, School of Medicine, University of California, Davis, California.

and software available to support such uses, and by the communications technology which is used to collect, switch, and disburse information. Each of these three major fields can be characterized by rapid growth and development. Each also appears to be likely to continue to evolve rapidly over the next several years. In order to place in perspective the future role of networks, it is necessary to examine briefly each of these contributing elements in the light of their potential effect on the design of networks for the future.

One of the factors leading to the disappointing performance of computers in education during the 1960s was the failure to understand the appropriate educational strategies that might be applied to technology-mediated instruction. (Anastasio and Morgan, 1972; Carnegie Commission, 1972). The success in medical education's use of computers in recent years has come in part from the realization that certain methodologies are indeed suitable for computer-based learning, and those institutions whose contributions are the most outstanding represent an interesting combination of successful strategies, as reported in this book. The trend will continue for these institutions to provide the majority of instructional materials, as one might expect. Despite the availability of learning materials to other institutions through national networks, the gap between the sophisticated development centers and the newer user schools appears to be growing rather than shrinking, at least up to the present. This cumulative growth effect will probably continue for some years, although it is equally true that, as a result of a broader base of awareness, many other institutions will also become originators of learning materials.

In the context of educational methodology, networks serve two roles, first as disseminators of basic material and second as indirect training vehicles for new user institutions. The natural consequence of this process is that new institutions will want to become developers of materials, sometimes requiring consultation with more advanced centers, sometimes independently, and sometimes serving to introduce still other new users to materials that they have developed. It is important that the role of networks be re-examined in this evolving process.

Computer hardware has evolved at a blinding and accelerating rate over the past decade, profoundly influencing the character and potential of networks as they exist today and as they will be designed for the future. One of the most obvious factors is cost effectiveness of computing. The computer industry has achieved remarkable progress in reducing costs of computation in absolute as well as relative terms. These economies have been accomplished by orders-of-magnitude improvements in speed of central processors, costs of production and maintenance, and size of computer components. Modular design of computers and peripherals make it possible to configure almost any sized system to meet a particular application, and then to expand its capabilities as the need dictates.

The development of smaller and cheaper computers has given rise, first to minicomputers and then to microprocessors, some of which are small and inexpensive enough to be housed directly in interactive terminals, resulting in an "intelligent terminal" capable of performing many functions in a stand-alone mode. This capability offers potential for computer-assisted instruction (CAI) that has already been effectively used in medical education (Kamp and Starkweather, 1973).

The effect of these trends has been to increase the instructional strategies available for the designer of a computer-supported learning exercise. No longer is it required that a large, time-shared computer be available in-house before even considering implementation of such material. In terms of networks, one might assume that this increased flexibility would result in a decreased dependence on communications, since low-cost computing is more readily available. However, the reverse may well be true. Increasing the options for implementing learning modules also increases the requirement for communication between developers, as will be shown later.

An additional subtle element must be taken into account in light of the accelerating rate of computer hardware development. At the same time that more and cheaper options for hardware will be available, the degrees of freedom and the resulting choices that must be made between such systems will become more complex, and the decisions made by various educators will differ, thus adding greatly to the needs for coordination and, most likely, for communication links to provide a means for compatibility between otherwise nonstandard systems.

Just as hardware has rapidly evolved in recent years, so too has the area of software technology. New and more powerful CAI languages have been developed, better adapted to modern concepts in the use of computers for instruction. Operating systems capable of supporting responsive timeshare systems are becoming available on many large systems. As a result, educators are finding more attractive systems, ones that are better received by students and hence permit increasingly successful application programs to be written. The successes in MUMPS (Bleich, 1971), COURSEWRITER (Griesen, 1973), and other languages attest to these significant improvements.

However, as in the areas discussed above, the improvements in software have themselves led to increased diversity, and, in many cases, incompatibility. PLATO, a system with a large library of educational programs (some of them medically oriented), is not readily capable of being implemented on systems departing from the particular configuration used at the University of Illinois. The TICCIT approach is specific to that hardware, and other languages also suffer from varying degrees of incompatibility. Some languages, such as BASIC, are ostensibly available on several machines, but in fact the languages are sufficiently dissimilar that major conversion efforts are required to transfer a program from one system to another even though the languages and machine are both "standard."

There have been efforts at standardization. MUMPS, a language originally implemented on minicomputers of one manufacturer, has now been made available on many different systems of varying sizes, and a Standard MUMPS language has been adopted, bringing together a whole host of dialects that developed from the original version during the past few years. Use of general purpose high level languages (such as FORTRAN) has aided in transferability of educational programs. A parallel software development, one that is still in its infancy but that offers promise for future benefits is in the general area of automatic translator systems; that is, programs that can be used to generate source code in more than one language from a conceptual definition of the solution to a particular problem. These systems may well become increasingly important in years to come. They have already been used in the creation of at least one medically oriented education system (Wilcox, 1974).

Still another trend that offers promise in compatibility is that of using a hybrid form of programming called "firmware" to emulate one machine on another. This process, involving the use of microprogrammed instruction sets that can make one hardware system capable of simulating one or more other systems, is already in use to permit small computers to serve useful educational functions without recreating a whole library of software for the new system.

The impact of all of these developments on networks is complex. One of the principal trends visible through this maze of rapidly changing capabilities is the concept of "distributed computing," in which different machines will serve different functions in the learning process. In such a networked system, large machines may play a role in storage, dissemination, and execution of certain levels or types of programs, whereas smaller systems might undertake to provide independent functions for less-demanding learning tasks. The logistics necessary for such a system are indeed complicated, but the capability is technically on hand for their implementation. As compatibility is achieved between several sizes and configurations of computers, then networks must be designed to support the communication links to tie these components together at speeds appropriate for their applications.

The spectrum of devices and capabilities associated with data communications networks has expanded just as dramatically as have the fields described above. Since many people involved in computer applications are not familiar with the basic concepts of communication networks, the following paragraphs set forth some of the most fundamental elements of such systems, so that the reader may be able to understand their effect on the design of educational systems for the future.

Communication between a terminal and a computer may be accomplished by directly wiring the terminal into the computer (Figure 1); this type of link is characteristic of many minicomputer systems. In fact, in the case of intelligent terminals, the "computer" is embedded in the terminal itself. If several terminals are linked to a single computer, it may become advisable to share the communications link into the computer, particularly since the average interactive user only uses the communications link a fraction of the time that he sits before the terminal. In order to accomplish this common use of a single communications channel, it is necessary to have a "multiplexer" (Figure 2), a device that distinguishes between the different terminals and sorts messages to and from the computer so that each

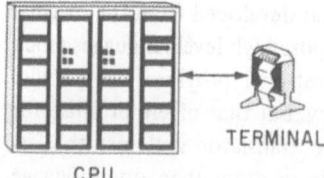

CPU   TERMINAL

Figure 1. Single terminal directly linked to central processor.

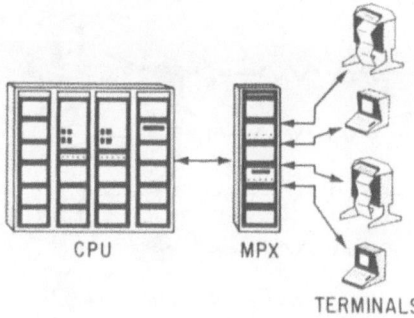

Figure 2. Groups of terminals connected to central processor via multiplexer.

TERMINALS

user will have his messages identified as belonging to him and will receive from the computer only those messages intended for him. Multiplexers can be designed to handle several terminals; characteristically they will "concentrate" from 4 to 16 such devices over a single channel.

If the terminals are located some distance from the computer, it may become necessary to use long-distance lines to link them with the computer. Telephone lines ordinarily transmit voice sounds, but digital signals can be converted to travel on telephone lines if they are "modulated" at the sending end to convert the digital information to a frequency code and later "demodulated" back into the appropriate digital signal at the receiving end. Devices that perform these modulation and demodulation functions are called "modems" (Figure 3). The rates at which modems send information are measured in terms of bits or characters per second (sometimes the term "baud" is used to express a more precise definition of the bits per second which include coded signals other than the basic character transmitted). Rates typical of today's modems are 10 to 30 characters per second for printing (110–300 bps) and low-speed cathode ray tube terminals, ranging up to 9600 bits per second for some devices. Normal telephone lines ("unconditioned") can be relied on to transmit up to 240 characters per second in many environments; higher speeds require varying degrees of special treatment or "conditioning" to overcome difficulties in the switched telephone system.

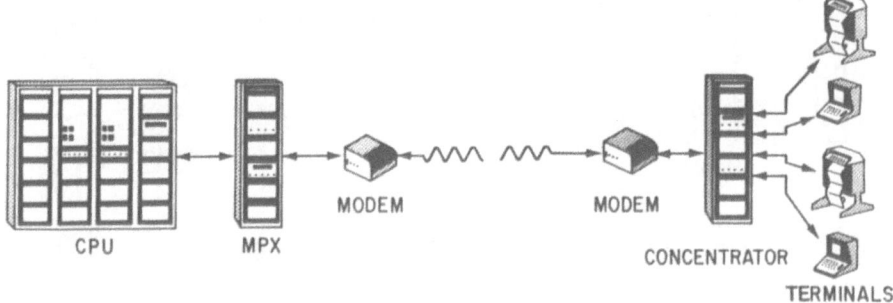

Figure 3. Groups of terminals connected through modems for remote connection to central processor.

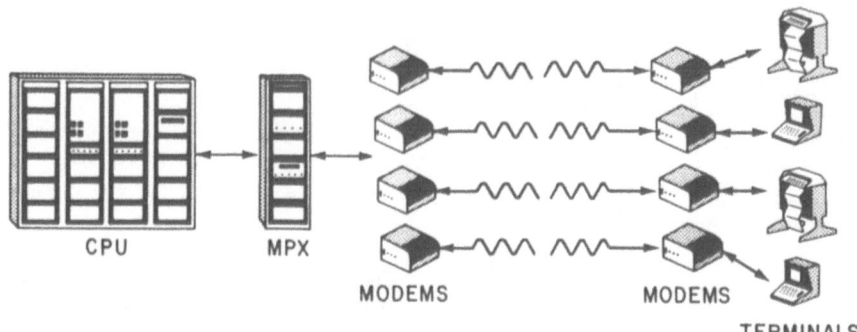

Figure 4. Use of a concentrator to transmit multiple terminal messages on a single line.

Putting these pieces together, it is possible to have a multiplexer at a remote site which concentrates messages from several terminals, codes them by a modem and reads them through a communications channel (we will stick with the telephone line for the present), where at the other end a second modem and multiplexer perform the opposite functions for the computer (Figure 4).

If a large number of terminals are connected to a single computer, the task of sorting out the messages, decoding them, and interpreting them so as to act on each, becomes a fairly time-consuming task which may interfere with the other duties of the central processor. In order to increase the efficient use of the central processor, therefore, many computers have "front-end processors," whose function is to take the chore of data communications away from the main central processor, allowing it to act on messages that have been preprocessed and are ready for handling (Figure 5). This front-end processor is itself a computer, sometimes a rather powerful one, but its function is secondary to the main processor, and it has no general-purpose responsibilities. Such a front-end processor is positioned in the network described above between the multplexer and the central processor. Because

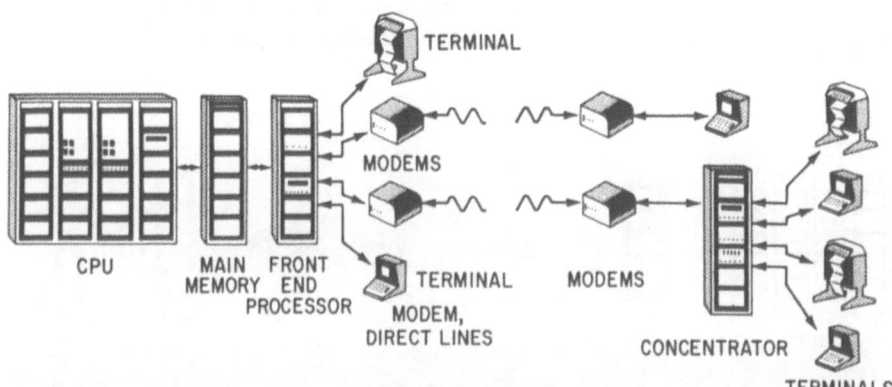

Figure 5. Separation of communications processor activity from central processor. Front-end processor handles messages and communicates with central processor via main memory.

of its power, such a front-end processor can usually handle several multiplexers, thereby enlarging the number of terminals that can be accommodated by a single computer system.

In many networks, a user may wish to access more than one computer, although not at the same time. In order to allow for this flexibility, it is necessary to have a communications controller that can switch messages to the appropriate computer, depending on the user's request (Figure 6). Such communications controllers can be inserted at several places in a communications network: they may be at single computer sites, they may serve as a front-end processor for two or more adjacent computers, or they may belong to a regional or national network, switching messages to the appropriate channel in order to reach the proper computer.

In such a system, therefore, several "computers" may be involved in transmission of a single message. A communications controller within a network may be programmed not only to switch and transmit messages, but also to monitor the entire system, reporting troubles encountered in data transmission to the systems monitors or engineers so that they can take corrective measures. It can also collect usage statistics and therefore facilitate the design of optimal configurations for the particular usage.

A primer on communications networks is incomplete without a brief discussion of the carrier media available. In this discussion we have so far considered terminals which are either directly wired or telephone-system wiring. There are, however, other options. Microwave links can be used for electronic communications, including data; these networks are capable of transmitting several million bits per second, or multiplexing data signals along the same beam that simultaneously

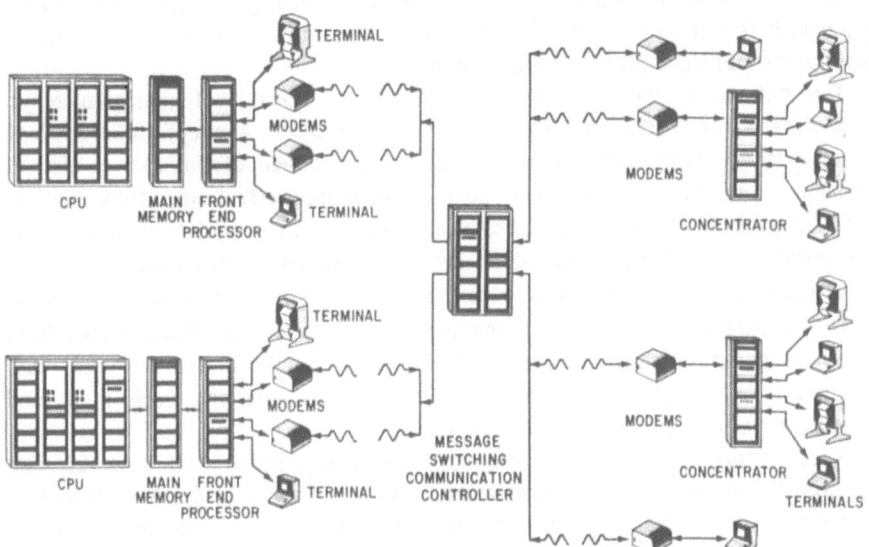

Figure 6. Multiple central processors accessed through switched network.

carries a television signal and its associated audio channels. Several such microwave links are in use for data communications, and the telephone company uses many microwave links as part of their network. Television networks, because of their relatively large communications capabilities, offer potential for incorporation of the lower-volume data signals. Hence, community coaxial cables systems loom as important future carriers of data into private homes, and campuses with television networks may well wish to explore the use of these networks for simultaneous data communications (perhaps even for combined computer and television camera-generated signals on the same screen).

Earth satellite transmission, used for telephone and television, is also being used for data communications (the University of Hawaii uses such links). The use of satellites in such an application is dictated primarily by economics; when it is economical to lease such channels or perhaps even to put up a data communications satellite, it will not require any new developments in technology to put such a system to use.

Another communications medium in use for short distances is the laser. Because of its capability for carrying large volumes of information, it offers potential for computer-to-computer line-of-sight transmission, using wavelengths that are relatively unaffected by fog and other atmospheric complications. Such systems are not generally designed for distance over a mile or two at present, but their carrying distance may increase with time. "Light pipes," cables designed to transmit optical information for longer distances, are now under development.

This section should serve to confirm the fact that the technology of communications has indeed come a long way. When one adds to this hardware-oriented discussion the complexities of error detection and correction, modes for packaging the data to be sent, and other techniques that improve the efficiency and reliability of such systems, it is fair to say that the art of data communications is evolving just as rapidly as other elements in computer design.

Two national networks serve to illustrate the range and potential of such systems. One is the ARPA net (Advanced Research Projects Agency), linking several major research computers across the nation. The design of this system aims at efficient communication between such large computers, transmitting data in 1000-bit packets at rates of 50,000 bits per second with appropriate error detection and correction strategies. The second system is offered by TYMSHARE, Inc., as a commercial service. This network, covering most major cities in the nation, assumes communication between numerous relatively slow-speed terminals and a few (about 40) host computers. The system is designed to provide interactive users with maximum reliability through alternate pathways connecting each node and constant monitoring of the network for malfunctions.

Recent years have brought increased interest in regional or local networks, such as those linking several computers within a single hospital or group of hospitals, providing hierarchical connections between different-sized systems, including terminals within a single campus or state, and other configurations designed for various mixes of dedicated and general-purpose systems.

The remarkable success of the Lister Hill Biomedical Communication Center in sponsoring data networks for medical education and research is documented in Chapters 7 and 11 of this volume. These successes point first to the benefits provided by such networks, and at the same time they raise the question as to effective long-term goals for such systems. Clearly, large data bases such as those maintained in the MEDLINE and ERIC bibliographic files need to remain on national networks, but a question arises as to whether the costs of duplicate storage of smaller data bases in different locations will at any time, present or future, offset the costs of long-distance communication. Since there is no simple answer to this question, it is necessary to formulate plans in which these variables remain as flexible as possible, in order to take advantage of current and changing factors in communication storage.

Minimum Basic Assumptions for Planning Educational Communication Networks

Analysis of the admittedly scanty overview provided in the previous section will reveal several factors that make planning difficult. None of the basic components involved in educational uses of computers is static; each is changing, and at a different rate. Even the acceptance of computers as valid resources in education is changing, hopefully for the better after a negative reaction to early failures. In the face of these uncertainties, it might seem foolhardy even to attempt to plan for the future. Yet, as amply documented in Toffler's *Future Shock*, survival in time of change characterizes our lives in today's world, and the planner must learn to adapt to these conditions.

What follows is an attempt to create some stability within the sifting sands of change — a frame of reference that will permit orderly development while at the same time incorporating new improvements as they arise. This is no easy task, and the author pleads for understanding and tolerance if, some few short years hence, his structure will require substantial revision.

A broad spectrum of expertise is required to develop effective computer-based learning. Not only must there be faculty competent in this unique approach to learning; there must also be technical experts to design and implement systems responsive to the pedagogical requirements, education experts available to adapt new concepts in learning to the task at hand, an administration ready to fund such efforts and provide proper incentive and reward mechanisms for the several contributors (both faculty and students) who can participate actively in the painstaking task of program review, revision, and refinement. Although federal or foundation support may be available for new institutions wishing to enter this field, the number of institutions successful in the overall effort will probably remain a small fraction of those making use of such programs.

Most successful CAI programs have matured through a process of successive revisions before they were considered stable. The Lister Hill Center for Biomedical Communications support and distribution of the Massachusetts General Hospital programs, for example, provides for feedback from students in many institutions, and this feedback is still used extensively in the revision of programs that have been in use for some time at the parent institutions. The important role of the network in this process is twofold, providing program access for students in many institutions and also collecting helpful comments for the authors' use in program revision. The network also offers a vehicle for remote authoring and thus for accelerated development of learning materials. In this context a network serves to augment program review and hence to improve program quality.

Technology will continue to develop at a rapid pace for the foreseeable future on all three fronts of hardware, communications, and software. This assumption has been stressed earlier in this chapter. However, it should not be taken to imply that the current state of the art or of equipment at any one time will become obsolete by virtue of new resources developed in the interim. Rather, it will require that designers of computer-based media must provide for a state of flexibility that can accommodate existing resources while leaving open the doorway to new improvements that are sure to evolve.

Some of the critical elements essential for compatibility and transferability will have to be defined and developed by research institutions, not by manufacturers of equipment. This assumption is based on the observation that the type of compatibility required for flexible future growth necessarily requires independence from specific equipment. Development of machine-independent languages, operating systems, and supporting communications is of value to a specific manufacturer only if his product is likely to benefit by greater sales. Successful manufacturers, particularly of large systems, will not be anxious to develop the means whereby materials operating on their system will run on other systems. The smaller manufacturers will have only limited interest in the same product, since they will not stand to gain a long-term advantage over similar-sized manufacturers in such an environment. Since a considerable investment in time and resources will be necessary for the development of such a complex of languages, operating systems, and communications, the justification for corporate investment in this effort appears to be minimal. Federal or other grant funds may be essential in this area.

Network Requirements Resulting from these Assumptions

If one accepts the premises listed above, then one can attempt to outline the broad framework of a network that would be designed to operate within those boundaries and still to provide for growth and development in the future. Such a network must be defined not only in terms of the communications, but of the nodes that are linked by the network, since an understanding of the nodes is essential to an appreciation of the communications requirements.

One way for computer-assisted learning to grow will be through increased exposure of the medical community to successful programs. Novice users must be offered the means to experiment with learning materials proven elsewhere and a mechanism must exist whereby they can commit themselves gradually to increased use of these materials as the level of acceptance increases. This need will continue, initially involving medical and other health professions schools, then moving gradually to smaller hosptials. It may well be that continuing education will extend to physician's offices and even patient's homes, maintaining the supply of novice users for the foreseeable future.

The network design must provide for the identification and technical and educational growth of centers of development. These centers may be single institutions or loose consortia of several institutions. It seems certain, however, that growth from user to developer status will occur in many places. An education network should encourage this growth and provide adequate recognition for those institutions that achieve program-origination status. Implicit in this process is a wide variety in the interests and competencies of different institutions and students, so that varying qualifications for acceptance to development status must be defined.

The need for a network to disseminate resource materials is obvious. Perhaps less obvious is the continuing need for a return communication link whereby the learning modules are continuously evaluated and/or updated on the basis of user reaction.The nature of such as a communications link, or links, is not restrictive. Mail service may be sufficient under certain circumstances to fulfill the communication requirements. In other situations an on-line system with instantaneous response across the nation may be required. Nor are these two extremes mutually exclusive; in all probability provision will be made for a continuum of communications extending from mail, phone, travel, and other human-mediated forms of communication to sophisticated systems connecting two or more machines.

Network systems of the future should support research necessary for development of machine-independent learning resources.

Current technology permits development of machine-independent language capable of executing on microprocessors as well as large central systems, for creation of hierarchical operating systems that encompass distributed computing on different systems and different sizes of systems, and for establishing communications links whose role includes dynamic transfer of learning materials, user responses, and even programs. However, it does not appear that these systems will become commonplace without a coordinated effort to encourage their growth. One essential element in such a system is the availability of a grant-supported experimental communications network through which such a system may be defined, tested, and implemented.

Components and Responsibilities of an Educational Communication Network

Throughout this chapter, the contribution of hardware, software and communications technology has been linked with the human factors responsible for development of existing or proposed education systems. In this section we will attempt to define the general opportunities and limitations in potential or responsibility for each of these components.

Human Resources

The most important component of any education network is the human resource factor. Any plan for development of a system must first include a viable plan for the involvement of individuals who will be responsible for the generation, maintenance, use, and evaluation of such a system. There are several vital components of this porttion of the design. There must be adequate opportunities to develop and train specialists in each of the disciplines necessary for such a system, as defined earlier: computer technicians, education experts, content experts, communications experts – all must be encouraged to enter into this field and to bring with them their experience in related application or development areas. Faculty and students interested in the health sciences must also be aware of the educational methodology that will serve them if they are to participate effectively in planning for its future. There must also be adequate mechanisms for these individuals to communicate with each other in the constant process of program definition, creation, revision, and certification (improved techniques in human communications such as telecommunications conferences may be developed to facilitate this process). Even when programs are in use, it will be important for users to provide feedback to originators. Some network systems may provide both human and machine communications. No network system will be complete, however, if it fails to take into account the human element in design, revision, and acceptance.

Hardware

It appears likely that minicomputers and microprocessors will play an increasingly important role in computer-supported learning over the next several years. There is no reason to counteract this trend, since it is likely to result in low-cost entry into this mode of learning by groups and individuals for whom startup costs were previously prohibitive. Two basic design characteristics should, however, be included in plans for incorporation of small systems into the learning process. First, such devices should be capable of exchanging machine-readable information with other devices. This criterion may call for on-line communications (a characteristic that increases flexibility) or it may call for physically removable storage systems such as cassettes, disks, or other media which can be read or prepared by other systems.

The design of a hierarchy of computers of different sizes and capabilities should permit the inclusion of other technologies. One promising new development is the videodisk, capable of storing large volumes of pictorial or digital information at very low costs. A second concept, offering potential as yet unrealized, would be that of holographic memory devices capable of performing complex pattern recognition through optical computation. Although this technology has not and may never be developed, it is indicative of the unknown potential that may become vital to tomorrow's educational resources.

If these simple guidelines are followed — communications capability and receptiveness to the incorporation of new media and technology — it appears that a reasonable configuration of hardware could be designed involving components available today. With appropriate attention to other components of the networking plans, devices available today will be capable of serving a useful purpose for an extended period into the future, supplementing new concepts and equipment as they become available.

Software

It is unlikely that any language currently available will represent the ultimate answer in educational methodology even for the short-term future. This premise is by no means a source of discouragement; new developments will lead to new capabilities that can be translated into new languages for the learning process. However, in terms of planning for the future, it is important that language developments take place in a coordinated effort of the medical education community. The model provided by the MUMPS Development Committee is important in this regard from several standpoints. First, it represents a cooperative effort by a community of researchers to arrive at a common language definition that will serve the entire group, provide for exchange of applications software, and pave the way for future language modifications and improvements. Second, the standardization effort includes generation of a package of routines that provide the semiautomatic translation of existing dialects into the newly defined standard MUMPS. If this model can be followed by others in the development or evaluation of CAI languages, the potential for transferability will be immeasurably increased.

The development of new concepts in software, operating systems for hierarchical, distributed computer configurations, and metacompilers for machine-independent program development and maintenance are goals to be sought with enthusiasm, even if initial results prove disappointing. Recognizing that our understanding of these concepts is incomplete at present, it nevertheless seems likely that educators will have more at stake in the creation of such systems than most other groups. For this reason, the impetus for development of new concepts in software support will have to come from within this group, medical education appears to have the opportunity to provide a leadership role in educational software development over the next 5 to 10 years. Because such systems are by nature heterogeneous, they will probably require for their development several research groups interested in testing the new concepts as applied to intra- or interinstitutional learning projects.

Communications Systems

Development of effective computer-mediated instruction will call for the continued dependence on communications ranging from human, face-to-face conversations to long-distance transmission of information between computers. Several factors will be important in the design of these systems.

The designer of a communication link for education purposes must keep in mind the real (not imagined or hoped for) time requirements of his application. It is pointless and wasteful, to build an on-line coast-to-coast communications link to transfer information that can be as readily mailed from an origination to a recipient site. Costs will become increasingly important as new systems capable of providing stand-alone service are brought into the educational process. On the other hand, some guarantees of two-way communication must be preserved even in mailed distribution, so that a system requiring return of a previous data set in order to receive a newer one may be desirable to ensure effective slower-speed information exchanges.

Communications links will rapidly become just as important at the local level as they are on regional or national scales. Links will be needed between hospital mini-computers and microprocessors to provide for shared education systems, for intra-campus links to classroom and study carrel facilities, or between video systems accessed by computer control for local CATV or intracampus distribution of pertinent images. To date most attention has been focused on larger networks, neglecting the equally important local links. It would further appear likely that experience gained on a local network configuration may well provide the models whereby regional or national hierarchical networks may be designed.

Communications designs must include provision for communication between people as well as between machines. In the medical education setting, this means conferences to arrive at definition of program areas requiring support, review and demonstration of new programs, concepts or technologies, and specification of new support systems made feasible by new educational or technological advances. Indeed, human communication links may well continue to be the most important factor in the evolution of computer-supported education.

The bandwidth of data communication links is at present an uncertain element. If hierarchical systems are developed capable of supporting dynamically allocated resources, it may be necessary to transmit large volumes of information (programs and data bases) from central to distributed sites; on the other hand, mail trans-mission of large-volume items supplemented by on-line return of usage statistics and pertinent feedback information may prove to be adequate in many learning situations.

No mention has been made in this section about preferred communications media or message disciplines. Although some forms of standardization will be necessary in the selection of these elements, their importance is considered secon-dary to the overall architecture of an education-communications network. It would appear reasonable to assume that the physical links will be available either through common carriers or by other privately or regionally owned systems, and the educational requirements outlined in this chapter should not present an excessive technical burden on such links, available or under development at present.

Summary

This chapter has outlined briefly the factors associated with development of educational communication networks. The concept of continuing change looms as the single most consistent characteristic of the technical and methodological factors associated with such a system. The architecture of the future will have to take into account the potential for change without losing sight of the fact that successful educational programs are already available within the medical domain and that these programs could continue to exist side-by-side with new concepts and learning materials for some time to come. Potential for new developments remain largely undeveloped owing in part to lack of sufficient stimulus; other concepts are already at hand awaiting application to the educational domain.

The architecture of future systems will have to take into account first, the complex technical base required for effective design and implementation of such systems, and second, the probable hierarchical structure of an education network that links small and large systems as well as user groups into a coherent structure. The system will have to maintain an additional degree of freedom as the small systems develop increasing capability to handle more sophisticated tasks. Such a system can be envisaged within the body of knowledge available today. What remains as the prime requisite is that medical educators of good faith join to plan for such a system.

References

Alper, D., and Bitzer, D. L., 1970. Advances in computer-based education, *Science* 167: 1582–1590.

Anastasio, E. J., and Morgan, J. S., 1972. *Factors Inhibiting the Use of Computers in Instruction.* EDUCOM Interuniversity Communications Council, Inc., Princeton, N.J.

Baker, L. H., 1974. Hierarchical networking in higher education, *in North American Perspective* (Proceedings of EDUCOM Fall Conference), pp. 159–165.

Bleich, H., 1971. The computer as a consultant, *N. Engl. J. Med.* 284(3): 141–147.

Carnegie Commission on Higher Education, 1972. *The Fourth Revolution: Instructional Technology in Higher Education*, McGraw-Hill, New York.

Cornew, R. W., and Morse, P. M., 1975. Distributive computer networking: Making it work on a regional basis, *Science* 189: 523–531.

Denk, J., 1974. The fear is gone: A study of the adoption of computer-based curricula in North Carolina's Institute for Undergraduate Curriculum Reform, *Proceedings of 1974 EDUCOM Fall Conference*, pp. 129–140.

Greenburger, M., Arnofsky, J., McKenney, J., and Massey, W. F., 1974. *Networks for Research and Education*, MIT Press, Cambridge, Mass.

Griesen, J. V., Beran, R. L., Folk, R. L., and Prior, J. A., 1971. A pilot study program of independent study in medical education, presented at the 5th Rochester Conference on Self-Instruction in Medical Education, April 1–3, 1971.

Kamp, M., 1975. *Index to Computerized Teaching in the Health Sciences*, University of California, San Francisco.

Kamp, M., and Starkweather, J. A., 1973. A return to a dedicated machine for computer assisted instruction, *Computers in Biology and Medicine*, 3, 293.

Kimbleton, S. R., and Schneider, G. N., 1975. Computer communications networks: Approaches, objectives and performance considerations, *ACM Computing Surveys* 7(3): 129–173 (September).

O'Neill, J. T. (Ed.), 1976. *MUMPS Language Standard*, Handbook 118, National Bureau of Standards, Washington, D.C.

Parker, L. Jr., and Denk, J., 1974. A network model for delivering computer power and curriculum enhancement for higher education: The North Carolina Educational Computing Service, *EDUCOM* 9(1): 24–30.

Toffler, A., 1970. *Future Shock*, Random House, New York.

Wilcox, J. C., 1974. MUMPS on large computers, continued progress, *Proceedings 1973 MUMPS Users' Group Meeting*, St. Louis, Mo., pp. 147–150.

7

Sharing Computer-Based Simulations for Clinical Education

Barbara B. Farquhar, Kathleen T. Famiglietti,
Craig J. Richardson, Edward P. Hoffer, and G. Octo Barnett

Introduction: Costs to Develop Simulations

During the past decade, Massachusetts General Hospital has written and distributed a series of computer-based simulations designed to supplement other instruction in the process of clinical problem-solving. Sharing educational resources is a commonly accepted academic responsibility, and sharing the end products of federally sponsored research and development is implicit in grants and contracts. Sharing computer-based materials can be accomplished in a variety of ways. The purposes of this chapter are (1) to describe three modes of sharing (program transfer, remote authoring, and networking), (2) to consider the costs and benefits of each mode from the points of view of both the originating and receiving institutions, and (3) to describe the evolution of a community of medical educators whose goal it is to enhance sharing of educational resources among institutions. This chapter is an overview of the issues and concerns associated with sharing computer-based educational materials, and it is written from the perspective of an originating or host institution.

One reason to share computer-based simulations is that they are costly to develop. Cost to develop a simulation varies and depends primarily on the time of personnel to design, implement, refine, and evaluate the simulation (Chapter 21, this volume). If an experienced author uses an established, straightforward instructional strategy (a "driver") and provides the medical content and logic for that

---

Barbara B. Farquhar • Educational Computer Group, Digital Equipment Corporation, Marlboro, Massachusetts. *Craig J. Richardson* • Digital Equipment Corporation, Marlboro, Massachusetts. *Kathleen T. Famiglietti* • Laboratory of Computer Science, Massachusetts General Hospital, Boston, Massachusetts. *Edward P. Hoffer* and *G. Octo Barnett* • Massachusetts General Hospital and Harvard Medical School, Boston, Massachusetts.
Development of the MUMPS language and the simulations was supported in part by Grant No. 5 R01 HS 00240 from the National Center for Health Services Research and Development. Development of the simulations was supported by the National Fund for Medical Education. Distribution of programs was supported initially by Contract No. N01-LM-2-4716 from the National Library of Medicine.

driver, it might take as little as 16 hours to prepare a rough draft of several cases for a simulation. An inexperienced author would likely require 40 hours to write the same cases in the same driver because the inexperienced author must first learn the format in which to put his data. At the other extreme, it has taken authors a year to design a new instructional strategy and to have that implemented in MUMPS, tested and evaluated.

Medical content experts who use a driver require far less assistance from a MUMPS programmer than those who wish to specify a new means of presenting and collecting information from students. If an author who is using a driver wishes to deviate slightly from the logic of the driver, he may ask a programmer to insert MUMPS routines into the program logic to allow for his modification. This is usually a simple procedure and takes little time from a MUMPS programmer. When a medical content expert "starts from scratch," he must demonstrate first no existing driver meets his needs, design and specify a new instructional strategy, and then either program it himself in MUMPS or transmit the strategy to a MUMPS programmer who can implement it for him. Such development of a new instructional strategy may require 4 to 18 months of programming support.

The library of programs available from Massachusetts General Hospital has been developed and tested over the past decade. The library consists of 30 different simulations, and there are multiple cases within each simulation. The cost to develop the library is difficult to estimate precisely, but it is well over $300,000. Development of the simulations was possible because they were created in a facility where there were other ongoing projects related to patient care. The development costs cited are merely the incremental costs to support staff engaged in the production and developmental testing of the programs.

Program Transfer

Program transfer usually includes transmission of computer program code, program documentation, and user documentation from the originator to the recipient. In concept, providing copies of computer programs at "cost of reproduction" is reasonable. In practice, however, requirements for successful program transfer exceed merely copying and mailing existing materials (Chapter 26, this volume). The true costs of program transfer include expenses incurred by the originating institution in (1) developing extensive program and user documentation that are not usually necessary for in-house development or maintenance, (2) providing each recipient with individualized consultation to make programs operational at each institution, and (3) establishing and maintaining some mechanism of communication between the originator and recipients for updating programs. These costs are substantial, and they generally are not included in grants or contracts.

A major problem in program transfer is overcoming language differences between the originating and the receiving institution. When programs have to be rewritten in another computer language or adapted to different equipment, requirements of time, effort, documentation, and consultation on the parts of originators and recipients increase by an order of magnitude.

Prerequisites for Program Transfer

Several conditions must exist at both originating and receiving institutions for successful program transfer to take place. The receiving institution must have the appropriate computer hardware, computer software, technical and instructional staff, and an institutional commitment to support and maintain the transfer. Similarly, the originating institution must have the technical capabilities to produce materials for transfer, funds to support personnel involved in the initial transfer and follow-up activities, and a strong desire to support program transfer. If any of these components is lacking, successful transfer is not likely.

Benefits of Program Transfer to Recipients

Transfer of programs written at another institution may provide the critical mass necessary to make computer-based educational materials a useful part of the curriculum. In most cases, the receiving institution will wish to modify or expand the program content to meet its peculiar institutional requirements. Faculty who modify or write programs are generally more enthusiastic about including them in the curriculum. Perceived control over program content is also important for user acceptance. Users place demands on computer-based educational materials that they do not require of other media, and local control of program content permits users to make the modifications which will make programs acceptable.

Another potential benefit is stimulation of awareness among faculty members who might otherwise show no interest in creating computer-based educational materials. Modifying an existing program is a much less awesome task than creating something completely new. Medical faculty rarely want to learn a programming language, but modifying program content introduces them to the potentials and limitations of the technique, and permits them either to communicate with instructional programmers or to write programs themselves in a formatted, near-English language (driver).

Costs of Program Transfer to Recipients

Costs of program transfer to the receiving institutions will be relatively high if they reimburse the originating institution for the costs of additional documentation, consultation, and updating. Recipients will have to bear the costs of local computers, technical and instructional support staff, and faculty time to modify or create programs.

When comparing the costs of renting programs (as in networking) vs. buying programs (as in program transfer), it is important to look beyond the hourly charge for connection to computer. This cost is usually less when programs are transferred and terminals are connected to local computers; however, the real cost incurred during the actual transfer process (for documentation materials, consulting fees, etc.) and the often "hidden" costs incurred after transfer (for off-line storage, data analysis, etc.) may make renting programs the more attractive option.

Benefits and Costs of Program Transfer to Originator

For the originating institution, costs to prepare programs for transfer are high, and these costs are not usually completely reimbursed by recipients. Each recipient is slightly different and requires individualized support and consultation from the originator. No mechanism exists for orderly updating of material, and original authors may resist having colleagues modify their creations. Benefits of program transfer to the originating institution are small, especially if there is a more attractive means to fulfill the obligations of sharing.

Massachusetts General Hospital's Experiences with Program Transfer

Massachusetts General Hospital has experience with three forms of programs, and for purposes of discussing transfer, each will be considered separately.

The first type of program is a driver, which does not contain medical content, but consists of a set of utility programs that are designed to perform a repetitive task independent of the medical content. The driver can be considered the instructional strategy; it includes options, format, branching, and the structure of the program. The driver and its associated on-line editor elicit the medical content and logic from the author, check syntax, and verify that the medical content and logic are consistent with the structure of the driver.

Massachusetts General Hospital has prepared and documented two drivers in Standard MUMPS. This work was supported by the Lister Hill National Center for Biomedical Communications. DIALOG is a branching, multiple-choice driver. POSER is a free text, narrative driver; GROPER is the author-input editor associated with it. Transfer of these drivers has proven to be difficult and costly primarily because of lack of a standard MUMPS language and standard MUMPS system. Progress in developing the language and systems should facilitate transferability and minimize the level of personnel support required from Massachusetts General Hospital. Of the three types of programs, driver programs are least costly to transfer and are potentially of greatest benefit because they provide the structure for recipients to create their own materials. Drivers are less likely to require modification than the medical content associated with them, and the possible consequences of an error in a driver are much less serious than either an error or lack of update in the medical content.

Secondly, a program can be considered the medical content and logic that are contained within the structure of a driver. The transfer of a simulation written in a driver is usually relatively simple if the driver has been transferred successfully.

Problems that arise with transfer of medical content and logic are associated with authorship, ownership, copyright, medical liability, updating, the locus of control and responsibility, and rights for distribution and redistribution. These problems have not been resolved and remain an impediment to transfer of medical content.

Copyright of computer programs is not very effective. There have been instances in which a computer programmer has translated a program from one computer language to another and claimed credit for the program. In other cases, a programmer or medical content expert has changed a few lines of code and considered the results to be his version of the program. Most program authors receive little or no pay for writing programs. The only compensation many program authors receive is acknowledgment of their work. It takes as long to write a good simulation as it does to write a chapter for a book or a good journal article, yet the academic recognition for writing simulations is almost nonexistent. The issues of academic honesty and incentives for authors are exacerbated by program transfer. Standards, procedures, and funding mechanisms to support orderly, systematic, and responsible transfer and update of programs are needed. Groups qualified to develop such standards and mechanisms are the Health Education Network, the MUMPS Users' Group, the Association of American Medical Colleges, and the National Library of Medicine.

The third type of simulation is one that is programmed directly in MUMPS (a computer language) without benefit of a driver. Before these programs become candidates for transfer, they will probably have to be rewritten in Standard MUMPS and in driver format. The most useful documentation that could be provided on these programs at this time would be independent of any computer language and consist of logic diagrams, formulas, and written descriptions of how the programs operate.

Indications for Program Transfer

Despite the difficulties involved, program transfer is indicated when both the originator and recipient agree in advance on the form and terms of the transfer, the programs are stable and well-documented, and there is no liability associated with the transfer. Expense to the originator to prepare programs for transplant must be reimbursed by some mechanism. The recipient may be willing to underwrite these expenses and the follow-up costs associated with updating and maintenance. If it is cheaper for the recipient to pay for documentation, consultation, and updating than it is to develop the programs himself, program transfer will probably be his choice.

Remote Authoring

For faculty at institutions in which there is not a strong or rich computer-based educational environment, remote authoring might provide many of the same capabilities they would enjoy if they were at such centers. Faculty would have the opportunity to construct the logic and content of programs to meet their needs precisely. In addition, they could be given feedback on their programs, including records of student performance and the comments of all those who have used the programs. Feedback is essential in the development and improvement of computer-based simulations, and faculty at remote institutions could be provided feedback so that they could modify programs and answer comments while they were improving program content and logic.

Remote authoring could provide faculty local control over programs they prescribe for their students. Just as it is likely that a faculty member will recommend or require a textbook that he or one of his colleagues has written, faculty would probably behave in much the same way with regard to computer-based educational materials. With remote authoring, an institution that does not have a computer facility dedicated to computer-based education would not need to make the large investment in the hardware and personnel required to support such a facility.

Faculty at many institutions have expressed an interest in authoring new programs on the Massachusetts General Hospital system. Others have asked to modify existing programs to meet the needs of their home institutions. Drivers shared via the Health Education Network (Chapter 11, this volume) could provide the facilities for faculty at remote institutions to write new clinical case simulations, and also create modified versions of existing programs to be stored on the Massachusetts General Hospital system for use at their particular institutions.

Requirements for Remote Authoring

Remote authoring is feasible technically and may be desirable educationally, but requirements are costly in terms of personnel and hardware resources. Institutions wishing to pursue a remote-authoring project must be willing to commit substantial resources for content development, evaluation, and program maintenance. Simulations proposed by remote institutions should correspond with the objectives of the host's clinical curriculum. The cost to the host institution to support remote authors is high, and funding mechanisms will have to be found to meet those costs before remote authoring will be feasible financially.

Review and Appraisal of Materials

Remote authoring brings into focus questions about review, appraisal, and evaluation of programs, and it demands answers to these questions with greater urgency than has been felt heretofore. The Health Education Network has a task force working to develop criteria for evaluation, methods for disciplinary review of programs, and means for disseminating information to medical educators on programs that have been reviewed. The Association of American Medical Colleges and the National Library of Medicine are collaborating to develop criteria for appraising computer-based medical educational materials. Massachusetts General Hospital and other institutions who have produced large numbers of programs have internal procedures and policies which they use to review a program before it is released to other institutions through the Health Education Network (Chapter 21, this volume).

The processes of review and updating programs are continuous. New programs may undergo almost daily change while older, more stable programs require less frequent modification. New medical knowledge or a major change in accepted medical practice may require program modification. This may be as trivial as adding a new reference to the reference list or as major as rewriting a majority of the content. For example, the cardiopulmonary resuscitation program developed at MGH was reviewed by the American Heart Association's Committee on CPR when it was first written several years ago. After the standards for CPR were revised and the computer program was modified to reflect changes in CPR standards, the AHA's Committee on CPR reviewed the program again to insure that it conforms to national standards. Computer simulations, unlike most texts, are dynamic.

Review and updating are simplified when a program is shared through a vehicle like the Health Education Network because only one version of the program exists. As soon as the author updates the master copy of the program, all subsequent presentations of that program through the Network will be the most current version.

With remote authoring, the original author or his designee must provide the content of the program and must also continue to have responsibility for updating it. However, without an established review and evaluation process, there is no guarentee that the content and logic of the program meet some minimal standards of acceptability for release via transfer or networking. Such standards need to be developed and authors need to demonstrate that their programs meet these standards.

Networking

An alternative to program transfer is networking. In networking, the program resides on the computer at the originating institution, and recipients are provided access to the programs through a telecommunications network. The originators maintain and update one copy of the program, and they supply recipients with extensive documentation on the *use* of each program. User documentation, as opposed to program documentation, changes less frequently and does not need to be modified extensively for each recipient. Recipients share the cost of program distribution. A small staff at an originating or host institution can maintain and update an entire library of programs and make these available to a wide audience. Networking appears preferable to program transfer when programs are changed frequently and the resources at either the originating or receiving institutions are very limited. The costs to both the host and recipient are frequently less for networking than for program transfer for an equivalent end product.

Benefits to Originators of Networking

There are several advantages to the host in networking. By providing access to programs through a network, the host fulfills his obligation for sharing the end products of research and development responsibly and economically. Networking accelerates the development and refinement of programs because many more people use and comment on programs than they would if programs were restricted to use in-house. Authors have extra incentive to keep programs up-to-date and non-parochial when they know their materials are used nationwide by an audience of students and peers. Documentation required for in-house maintenance of programs is relatively simple. A small staff at a host institution can maintain a library of programs and provide access to that library at a reasonable cost.

Cost to Originators of Networking

Network host costs are for computer resources, communications services, and personnel. Costs for computer resources may be fixed if a portion of a computer is dedicated to networking, or costs may vary with usage if the computer is capable of serving others when not being accessed by a user of the network. Similarly, communications services may be at a fixed rate with unlimited usage of fixed number of lines, or they may vary with the locations of users, number of characters transmitted, or total amount of usage (measured in time). Personnel are required at the host institution to maintain computer programs and systems, develop and up-date documentation, respond to users' questions, and handle billing. Personnel costs to perform maintenance functions are relatively low. Personnel costs to provide net-work users with the technical, educational, and faculty development support could be very high if the host provided users with all the services from which users could benefit. There are economies of scale; in general, the higher the level of usage, the lower the unit cost to the host.

Benefits of Networking to Recipients

Network users enjoy many benefits. Accessing programs through a network permits people who have an interest in trying computer-based educational materials to do so without a large capital investment. The programs they receive are the most current available, and the recipients need not be concerned about transforming them for local computer requirements. Network users do not require a local computer installation, technical staff, operations staff, or faculty commitment to update programs. Users share the resources of a complex facility such as Massachu-setts General Hospital, and they have access to both the programs and the people responsible for them. Networking also allows the potential for fostering remote authoring of simulations.

Costs of Networking to Recipients

Two disadvantages some users attribute to networking are cost and control. Renting programs is often perceived as more costly than running programs on a local computer system. Cost considerations tend to be deceptive because users usually consider and compare costs assuming that program transfer has taken place. Costs of transferring and updating may well be greater than those for networking. Then, too, users do not always compare costs of equivalent end products. Massachusetts General Hospital has redundant computer systems, can guarentee access through a reservation system, has a full-time operations staff with personnel on call for educational and technical assistance, and faculty who respond daily to users' comments and revise programs. Providing equal services at a remote site can be extremely costly, especially if the sole use of the computer were for computer-based educational materials.

The other disadvantage to networking that some users perceive is lack of absolute control over program content. Control is exerted on program content by external sources such as nationally accepted standards, generally accepted medical practice, and comments from users. Complete control over program content could be exercised by each using institution if we permitted remote authoring and allowed each institution to tailor and store a copy of each program. Currently, MGH avoids writing procedurally oriented programs and controversial material which tend to have little general applicability over a range of institutions.

Initial and ongoing costs to network users include charges for computer terminals, local and long-distance communications, computer usage at the host institution, documentation, other supplementary materials, and assistance from host personnel. A computer terminal must be compatible with the network to which it connects; not all computer terminals will work on all networks. Some sophisticated terminals with capabilities to handle graphics, color, microfiche, film, slides, and sound must be purchased and cost over $10,000. Basic alphanumeric terminals can be purchased for under $2000 and rent for as little as $50 per month. Communications charges may be as high as a long-distance call to the host on a specially conditioned telephone line or as low as a local phone call to a network node on a regular phone line. Charges for use of the host computer may be based on the time that the user is connected to the host's system or they may be figured on the amount of central processing unit used, characters transmitted, or storage required. Documentation and supplementary materials, such as slides or tapes to be used in conjunction with programs, may be provided to users or available at a fee. The host usually makes staff available for on-call assistance from his site to answer users' questions. If the host provides special services for individual users, there may be additional charges for these services.

The costs to recipients for networking with Massachusetts General Hospital are limited and under the user's control. Prices for accessing the programs range from $10 per connect hour to $4 per connect hour; rates depend on the user's minimum monthly commitment for usage and the time of the day or night he uses the system. Users provide their own terminals, which rent for as little as $50 per month, and pay local telephone charges between their sites and the nearest TYMNET nodes. Users have limited liability and may change their levels of service or terminate service on 60 days' notice.

Evolution of the Health Education Network

In 1971, the Council of Academic Societies of the Association of American Medical Colleges (AAMC) developed a plan for the National Library of Medicine's Lister Hill National Center for Biomedical Communications (LHNCBC) (Stead *et al.*, 1971). One of its recommendations was that the LHNCBC establish a biomedical communications network to support interinsitutional sharing of expensive or scarce resources. The LHNCBC implemented an Experimental CAI Network in July of 1972 (Chapter 8, this volume), and Massachusetts General Hospital was the first operational host (provider of programs by access to its computers) on the Experimental CAI Network. During the next 35 months the Lister Hill Center supported distribution of programs through the Network. Ohio State University (Chapter 15, this volume) and the University of Illionois Medical College (Chapter 19, this volume) were other hosts on the Experimental CAI Network.

After 18 months of operating the Network, the LHNCBC announced (Schoolman, 1974) that it had achieved its research objectives and would be forced to terminate support after an additional 17 months; it had demonstrated that the Network was feasible technically and that programs developed at one institution could be used successfully at other institutions. Both the hosts and medical institutions using the Experimental CAI Network asked the Lister Hill Center to provide transitional support (beyond May, 1975) for the Network which would enable it to survive, grow in an orderly fashion, and develop mechanisms for central coordination. Lister Hill replied that its mandate is for research rather than support of an operational service or development of materials for networking, and they terminated support of the Experimental CAI Network in May of 1975.

Lister Hill's Experimental CAI Network made computer-based educational materials available to at least a hundred institutions and thousands of users a decade earlier than would have been possible otherwise. It gave faculty a new tool to supplement other modes of instruction. The Experimental CAI Network gave students an opportunity to use technology with which many of them were already familiar in ways they found useful in their clinical education. Acceptance of clinical simulations by the students for whom they were designed is the ultimate test. Many of the next generation of medical school faculty will have had experience with clinical simulations, and they may be the first generation of clinical faculty to teach others with techniques other than the traditional exclusive clerkship. Perhaps the greatest legacy of the Experimental CAI Network was that it helped to identify the people who would form the core of innovative medical educators throughout the country. Lister Hill maintains an interest in computer-based educational materials and has a learning resource center at the Lister Hill Center.

When users of the network learned that federal funding would be withdrawn they formed the Health Education Network to facilitate, maintain, and preserve economical nationwide access to computer-based materials for health education. The Health Education Network began in June of 1975 and is user-directed and user-supported. It is the first fully operational national network for health sciences. It provides users 20-hour/day access to the largest instructional medical data base in the world, and that data base is growing. Hosts are seeking to develop mechanisms for remote authoring so that faculty throughout the nation will have the capability to develop instructional programs at their home institutions.

Goals of the Health Education Network are:

1. To maintain and enhance medical education through interinstitutional sharing of computer-based instructional materials
2. To investigate academic and professional aspects of computer-based education aids such as faculty development, curriculum development, authorship, evaluation, and peer review
3. To investigate technical and functional aspects such as networking alternatives, program transfer, documentation, distribution, and cost-effectiveness
4. To develop computer-based education materials into a disciplined literature
5. To communicate with users and with medical educators in general on the status, availability, and effectiveness of computer-based educational materials
6. To provide means through which health professionals can engage in self-assessment and continuing education

The Health Education Network (Chapter 11, this volume) became incorporated in 1975. It had its organizational meeting, adopted by-laws, and elected its Board of Directors and Officers in 1976. Nine directors were elected by the members, and each host appointed one member to the board. Officers are Dr. Robert G. Votaw, President, University of Connecticut Health Center; Barbara B. Farquhar, Secretary, Digital Equipment Corporation; Dr. Charles S. Tidball, Treasurer, George Washington University Medical Center.

The Health Education Network exists because users of the Experimental CAI Network organized and took the initiative to develop a structure and mechanisms to insure its survival. The Health Education Network Users' Group of the Association for the Development of Computer-based Instructional Systems was a vital organization in the formation of the Health Education Network, Inc., and it is a continuing forum for the users.

Operation of the Network

Programs from host institutions are available to remote users through the Health Education Network. For example, certain ports on the Massachusetts General Hospital computers are allocated exclusively to the Health Education Network. The hospital has a contract with TYMNET, a commercial time-sharing company, to provide communications services to Network users. The communications network has 86 nodes or local access points located in major cities throughout the United States. Users dial the phone number of the nearest node and gain direct access to simulations on the Massachusetts General Hospital computer system. Use of the system is simple, and no technical expertise is required at remote sites. Massachusetts General Hospital provides documentation on how to use the programs and on-call assistance for technical or educational services.

Use of the Massachusetts General Hospital Programs

During the past 6 years, more than 150 institutions in more than 40 states have used approximately 80,000 hours of time on the Massachusetts General Hospital system for medical education by accessing programs through the Network. Major users are medical students (68%) and practicing physicians (18%); the remaining usage (14%) is by nurses, dentists, and allied health personnel. Institutions who have access to the programs consist of medical schools (68%), hospitals (16%), national medical organizations (11%), and physician groups (5%). Medical students in their clinical training use the programs to practice clinical decision-making. Practicing physicians use the programs for self-assessment and for continuing education. Many of the programs have been reviewed and approved by the Harvard Department of Continuing Education for Category I credits toward the American Medical Association's Physician's Recognition Award. Potential uses of computer-based materials for licensure, certification, and recertification are great.

Conclusion

Many institutions have asked to share the computer-based simulations developed at the Massachusetts General Hospital. Sharing educational resources is an academic responsibility, and an originating institution must judge the ways in which it can maximize that responsibility with the resources it possesses. Sharing responsibly means that an originating institution should provide (either through program transfer or networking), the best, most up-to-date programs available to the most recipients at the lowest cost possible. Transferring programs to another institution requires extraordinary personnel time, and the time involved is allocated for a limited number of recipients. Each program transfer to a different institution requires additional staff time. There are no mechanisms for orderly transfer and maintenance, and there are apparently insufficient funds to pay for the high costs of program transfer. To date, Massachusetts General Hospital has found networking the most responsible and economical means of sharing programs with colleagues.

ACKNOWLEDGMENTS

The authors wish to acknowledge the editorial assistance of Mrs. Rita D. Zielstorff, R.N.

References

Schoolman, H., 1974. Address to the Association for the Development of Computer-Based Instructional Systems, Washington, D.C.

Stead, E.A., Smythe, C. McC., Gunn, C. G., and Littlemeyer, M. H., 1971. Educational technology for medicine: Roles for the Lister Hill Center, J. Med. Educ. **46**: Part 2 (July).

8

The LHNCBC Experimental CAI Network, 1971–1975: An Administrative History

Harold Wooster

From July, 1972 through May, 1975, the Lister Hill National Center for Biomedical Communications (LHNCBC) of the National Library of Medicine (NLM) operated an experimental biomedical computer-assisted instruction network. This network, perhaps the first of its kind, connected three university data bases through a commercial time-sharing network to as many as 100 institutional users providing, at its peak, up to 3000 terminal connect hours per month. Information from and about the network has appeared in the literature: four papers by LHNCBC staff members (Lewis and Wooster, 1973; Wooster, 1973; Wooster and Lewis, 1973, 1974); two outside evaluations published as technical reports (Wakefield *et al.*, 1973; Rubin *et al.*, 1975), and as a journal article (Wakefield, 1973); and four special reports (Brigham, 1973a, b; Brigham *et al.*, 1972; Kronick and Robinson, 1974). This paper attempts to fill a remaining lacuna — an administrative history of the network.

Dates are the skeleton of history. The key dates in the history of the network are these:

August, 1968	Lister Hill Center established
March, 1971	"The Stead Report" (Stead *et al.*, 1971)
February, 1972	First NLM contract with TYMSHARE
July, 1972	Massachusetts General Hospital connected to network
September, 1972	Ohio State University College of Medicine connected
January, 1973	University of Illinois Medical Center, Chicago connected
February, 1974	Network users charged $2.50 per connect hour, communication costs
March, 1974	University of Illinois withdraws from network
May, 1974	Portion of Illinois data base transferred to Ohio State computer

Harold Wooster · Special Assistant for Program Development, Lister Hill National Center for Biomedical Communications, National Library of Medicine, National Institutes of Health, Public Health Service, Department of Health, Education, and Welfare, Bethesda, Maryland.

| July, 1974 | Network users charged $5 per connect hour communication costs |
| May, 1975 | NLM support of network terminates |

Preamble

The formal "Statement of Organization and Functions and Delegations of Authority," dated November 8, 1968, charged the Lister Hill National Center for Biomedical Communications, in part, with designing, developing, implementing and managing a biomedical communications network; assisting the biomedical community in identifying and developing products and services for dissemination through the network, and developing networks and information systems to improve health education, medical research, and the delivery of health services.

In the fall of 1968, the Lister Hill Center started a continuing relationship with the Council of Academic Societies of the Association of American Medical Colleges (AAMC) to discuss ways in which the academic medical community might become actively involved in the planning of services to be rendered by the Lister Hill Center to the medical schools. These conversations led to a conference, "Potential Educational Services from a National Biomedical Communications Network," held at the National Library of Medicine in February, 1969 (Smythe, 1969). The conferees concluded that:

1. There is a need for a nationally based biomedical communications network.
2. There is a great range of educational services such a network might provide.

This conference led to another contract with the AAMC to provide more specific recommendations in the areas of content development for a biomedical communications network, as well as to suggest steps that might be taken in furthering relations between the National Library of Medicine and the academic medical community. A Steering Committee was appointed, chaired by Dr. Eugene A. Stead, Jr., Professor of Medicine, Duke University. The Steering Committee consulted or interviewed some 100 individuals in site visits to 10 medical schools. The committee report (Stead *et al.*, 1971) was issued as a technical documentary report in March, 1971, and reprinted as a supplement to the *Journal of Medical Education* in June of that year.

"The Stead Report," to use its familiar eponymn, became an instant classic. Like other classics, the wealth and prolixity of its recommendations — some 53 all told — made it easier to quote than to summarize. The task of rank-ordering these recommendations was assigned to a Priorities Review Committee. This committee finished its task in October, 1971, presenting four recommendations to the November 22–23, 1971 meeting of the Board of Regents. As adopted unanimously by the

Regents, the second of these recommendations reads:

> 2. The committee advocates the organization of a biomedical communications network fundamentally conceived as providing the mechanism by means of which inter-institutional cooperation and sharing of resources will be used to meet some of the needs of medical education and medical practice.

Translating Theory into Practice

The major ancestor of the LHNCBC Experimental CAI Network was the National Library of Medicine's involvement with on-line bibliographic search services (McCarn and Leiter, 1973). Davis B. McCarn, then Deputy Director of the Center, and the first Director of the Center, Dr. Ruth M. Davis, began early in 1970 to develop an on-line search system. Their system needed, just as the future CAI network would need, a base of computer-stored data and efficient economical communication lines to that computer. Unlike the CAI network, the data base they chose was provided by a NLM product already in machine-readable form — the computer tapes used to photocompose *Abridged Index Medicus* (AIM). AIM, a sub-set of the full *Index Medicus* data base limited to citations from 100, English-language, clinically oriented journals, began publication in January, 1970. The communication lines to be used were those of the Teletypewriter Exchange Network (TWX), inasmuch as some 500 medical institutions already had TWX terminals.

LHNCBC planned and contracted for an experimental service, AIM-TWX, which was provided from an IBM 360/67 Computer at the System Development Corporation in Santa Monica, California. That computer was the first to be connected without special arrangements to the TWX network. The system became operational in June, 1970. Users of the system had to make long-distance telephone calls, either to Santa Monica or to an East Coast multiplexer. These costs were averaging over $6.00 per search. (As explained later in this chapter, MEDLINE was the successor to this system as of December, 1971.)

In February, 1971, LHNCBC, with the assistance of the National Bureau of Standards, began looking at alternative communications networks. The Phase 1 network which resulted provided local telephone access to the NLM computer for the regional libraries and MEDLARS centers in the NLM's regional medical library network. Access was provided by Western Union Datacom service, supplemented by leased telephone lines. The Phase 2 network went into operation in February, 1972. It largely replaced the Western Union Datacom and leased telephone lines with a commercial, time-sharing, value-added network operated by TYMSHARE, Inc. The NLM computer was the first "alien" computer to be added to the TYMSHARE network.

Changes at the Lister Hill Center

Dr. Ruth M. Davis became Director of the Center for Computer Sciences and Technology of the National Bureau of Standards in November, 1970. Her successor,

Albert Feiner, became Director of LHNCBC in May, 1971. (Davis B. McCarn was Acting Director of the Center during the interregnum. He left in January, 1972, to continue MEDLINE development as head of the Office of Computer and Communications Systems, another Division of the National Library of Medicine.)

As a dynamic, aerospace executive, Feiner was eager to start new projects of his own; as a "communicator" he was quick to see the possibilities of the AIM-TWX pattern of using commercial wire-lines to connect remote users to central computer data bases.

A number of leads were explored during the spring and summer of 1971. By August 19, 1971, there was enough information compiled to send the following memorandum to Mr. Feiner:

August 19, 1971

Subject: *Biomedical data communications network*

In about 5 months LHNCBC/NLM is to start leasing services from a large commercial time-sharing computer network. The purpose of this lease is to afford better and less costly communications service to, eventually, 500 AIM-TWX/ MEDLINE user terminals to be connected to the NLM computer through this communications network. The purpose of work under this project is to determine what other on-line biomedical computing services can be offered to our terminal users through this same network.

During the preceding 10 years many on-line, interactive computer programs for undergraduate and continuing medical education have been developed at such centers as Ohio State University, Massachusetts General Hospital, the University of Illionois, the University of California School of Medicine, the University of California at Davis and at Irvine, the San Francisco Medical Center, and the University of Washington. All of these can be accessed on-line at their home computers; some are telephone-accessible from anywhere in the country. To the best of our knowledge, no attempt has been made to tie these services together through a common communications network. A major problem is that these programs have been written in a wide variety of languages for an heterogeneous assortment of computers; each of them requires the user to learn its own keyboard conventions to call-up, log in, and interact...

Programs selected for inclusion in this experiment must be accessible through the terminals planned for the AIM-TWX/MEDLINE network. They must not require the use of cathode ray tube displays, nor accompanying audiovisual material, nor the creation by the user of permanent data files. (Important though they are, we are not concerned with hospital records or patient billing systems.) They will fall into general category of computer-aided instruction for undergraduate and continuing medical education.

The following tasks are envisaged during the coming year:

1. Setting up a demonstration on-line carrel at LHNCBC. This would consist of one of our terminals plus user's instruction sheets for each available program. This would use existing services, in their existing formats, on their home computers.

2. An inventory of existing, on-line biomedical computing programs, described in precise detail, to be considered for inclusion in the network. Publication of this survey would be a useful project in itself.

3. Establishing standard interface conventions and format for programs on their home computers, to be called up through the network, or to transfer them to a compatible computer already on the network.

4. Choosing four of the programs for inclusion in the network and determining the cost of rewriting them in the standard format.
5. Rewriting these programs in standard format. (N.B. This is *not* writing new programs; it may involve translating programs from one programming language to another.)
6. There are many desirable and useful programs which may not be suitable for inclusion in the network, but which should be made more widely available. Some of these, for example, require accompanying audiovisual materials, which could be made available through NMAC. The feasibility of establishing a clearinghouse for biomedical computer programs, as suggested in the AAMC report, should be explored. Such a clearinghouse would maintain an inventory of de-bugged computer programs and upon request would copy them in a desired format and send them to requestors to use on their own computers. This service should be performed on a cost reimbursable basis.
7. By the end of the first year the following items should have been accomplished:
   A. Demonstration carrel at LHNCBC.
   B. Survey of available biomedical computing programs completed and in process of publication.
   C. A small number of programs made available to AIM-TWX/MEDLINE and other users through the biomedical data communications network.

Item A came to pass, in a very informal way, as soon as we had a network, a terminal, and an articulate demonstrator. It was the anlage of the LHNCBC Learning Resource Center, to be discussed in another chapter by Mr. Goldstein. Item B became Chris Brigham's *A Guide to Computer-Assisted Instruction in the Health Sciences* (Brigham *et al.*, 1972). The steps taken to accomplish item C are the subject of this paper.

The Overtures Begin

September 2, 1971 is the key date in the history of the network. On that day, the Lister Hill Center brought together, at the Center: William G. Harless, Ph.D., Chief of Instructional Systems, University of Illinois Medical Center, Chicago; G. Octo Barnett, M.D., Director, Laboratory for Computer Sciences, Massachusetts General Hospital, Boston; James V. Griesen, Ph.D., Director, Division of Research and Evaluation in Medical Education, College of Medicine, Ohio State University, Columbus; and Stephen Yarnell, M.D., University of Washington Medical School, Seattle. Their travel orders read: "To participate in a meeting ... to discuss programs available for networking through the AIM-TWX system."

The Lister Hill Center entered this meeting with the assumption that it would be possible to acquire a sample collection of good CAI programs from their developers, transfer them to a central computer, and make them available to what we came to call "trial" users on a demonstration basis.

Our visitors made it quite clear that they were not interested in letting go of their proprietary programs. If we wanted to use their programs we would use them on their home computers, and pay for the privilege. Although they were willing to tolerate trial users, emphasis and priorities were to be placed on "operational" users who would (a) attempt to integrate the CAI materials into their curricula, and (b) enlist faculty cooperation in writing additional units of instruction. The Lister Hill Center wanted to make the proposed services as widely available as possible; the visitors were interested in working more intensively with a smaller number of users.

This approach postponed – it certainly did not eliminate – the problems of standardization, compatibility, translation and portability of CAI programs. It added the problems of networking three computer centers. AIM-TWX and eventually MEDLINE had an established potential library/librarian clientele; we were being asked to develop a faculty/curriculum clientele from scratch.

The second meeting on October 2, 1971 with Griesen, Harless, and Yarnell (Barnett was weather-bound) reached the following conclusions:

1. The TYMSHARE network would be used.
2. Programs would be left on their home computers.
3. Computers must be connected to the TYMSHARE network through a Varian 620 at each site. Basic cost to LHNCBC for the Varians would be $2000 per month each.
4. Users would be operational and "demonstration." Demonstration users were to be limited to a fairly short time, say, 2 weeks.
5. Tying Dr. Yarnell's programs, resident on a Boeing computer, into the TYMSHARE network would be impractical.

1972, the Year of Decision(s)

Negotiations in 1972 proceeded, almost simultaneously, with the potential contractors, with the potential users, and with our management. Working with the NLM Contract Management Office, the contractors and we had to translate vague feelings of mutual goodwill into specific contractual documents, with price tags attached – price tags that were within the funds we had set aside for the network long before we had talked prices. Management needed to be convinced that we could manage the planned network and that we were not asking for funds to provide a service that nobody would use. With the users, we had a Catch-22 situation. We could not get users until we had a network, and on our bleaker days, it looked as if we could not get a network until we had users.

The Contractors

Requests for proposals were sent to the contractors on March 28, 1972, with a deadline of April 14, 1972 for return of the proposal. About a week after the deadline, Dr. Harless called us to say that he was leaving the University of Illinois Medical Center by the end of August. Illinois was at first reluctant to submit a proposal until a replacement for Harless had been selected.

Table 1. *Cost of University CAI Contracts*

Contractor	Duration of contract	Months of contract	Total cost	Cost per contract month
Ohio State	6/28/72–5/31/75	33	$281,391	$8,527
Massachusetts General	6/28/72–5/31/75	33	314,408	9,527
University of Illinois	10/1/72–2/18/74	16	81,695	5,105
		82	$677,494	$8,262

The proposal they finally did submit came in too late to be processed before the July 1 start of a new fiscal year. The Illinois contract was eventually awarded on October 1, 1972 and, what with one thing and another, Illinois did not go on the network until January of 1973.

Our major discussion with the potential contractors during this period was over the price of the services they would provide and the basis on which they would calculate their costs. We wanted to be charged per connect hour used, plus a base charge for the computer and a minimum number of hours a month. Hourly charges would have made it a lot easier to monitor usage of the system and, thereby, expenditures at any time. We also assumed that the universities' charges to NLM for personal contact and training of the users would be held to a necessary minimum inasmuch as the operational users, on whom the universities had insisted, would be contributing additional units of instruction to the universities' data bases.

We based our estimates of costs on commercial time-sharing fee schedules published by "profit-making" vendors operating similar computers, and assumed a computer base cost of $1300 per month, with an additional $8.00 per hour terminal connect charge. The funds we had programmed would, we thought, provide approximately 2750 terminal connect hours* from each university for the first 10 months.

At commercial rates, then, the university contracts would have cost $3500 per month for computer services, with an additional $1050 per month added for developing evaluation plans and reviewing the new material to be provided by the operational users, giving an average contract cost of $4550 per university month.

We were to find that we did not really understand university pricing systems. The universities, in submitting their cost sheets, ignored the "incremental cost" understanding, and pro-rated their "total service cost" to the number of ports into their computers. Their proposals were priced on numbers of ports to be made available, rather than connect hours. On top of that, they added estimated costs for reprogramming, supplies, staff assistance to the users, evaluation of service and, needless to say, overhead. The effect was to almost double our original cost estimates. Table 1 gives a summary of our costs by university. The average works out to $8262 per university contract month.

---

* We based our estimate of usage on the only data we had, the AIM-TWX figures. The final, operating network logged as high as 3000 hours a month!

A typical university contract would provide five ports at $600 per port month; The difference between the $3000 per month port cost and the average cost of $8000 per month went for the "hand-holding" that the universities and, eventually, the Lister Hill Center, realized was necessary, at that time, to make sure that these new users would be able to use this method of instruction effectively.

The Users

We were reasonably sure, and time has borne us out, that the "turnpike effect" (a new road almost always attracts more automobiles than it was originally designed for) would take over once the CAI network was started, but how to get started? Each of the contractors had its own list of contacts — not infrequently potential users who had been scared off by connect costs. But this was to be a Lister Hill/ NLM network, not an OSU, MGH, nor a UI network. (All three contractors had had some experience in providing their services over telephone lines to off-campus sites.)

The only direct mail announcement we made was to the members of the Health Sciences Interest Group of the Association for the Development of Computer-Based Instructional Systems (ADCIS). A letter was sent early in May, and reprinted in the May, 1972 issue of the *ADCIS Newsletter*.

This letter was the Lister Hill Center's first direct contact with the computer-assisted instruction community, as represented by ADCIS. We sent out 26 letters; 12 of the institutions addressed eventually became users of the network. Perhaps most importantly of all, we had started a relationship with an organization that was to form a users organization, the Health Education Network Users Group, (HENUG) and eventually to take over operation of the network.

Management

The LHNCBC Experimental CAI Network's problems began when we took the first steps needed to spend real money, $159,000, on it. Our first draft of a Request for Proposals was prepared on February 14, 1972. The final RFP was issued on March 28, with a deadline of April 14 for receipt of proposals. The contracts with Massachusetts General Hospital and Ohio State University were signed on June 28, 1972, two days before the end of the fiscal year. It should not be surprising that the paper work took this long. LHNCBC was seeking approval for the expenditure of federal funds to offer an untried service for which there was no predictable demand. Approval, in principle, was granted early in 1972, but there were a lot of details to be worked out before the final contracts were signed.

The first of these was the "Data Communication Service Management Plan," formally approved on March 16, 1972. This document treated the CAI network as a subset of the functions of the Data Communications Service — the branch of LHNCBC primarily concerned with the contracts with communication contractors involved with AIM-TWX and MEDLINE. The Data Communications Service Manager was responsible for defining the requirements for becoming "operational" or "trial" users of the "service" (sic), and to act as Project Officer on all contract operations affecting the service. There were to be two advisory groups, a contractors group, and two staff "functions," a user services and evaluation function and a communication and network operations function.

This document also defined for the first time the two classes of users, operational and trial. Trial users were to have access to the network for limited period of time, such as 2 months (an increase from the 2 weeks originally to be allotted to demonstration users). Emphasis during the start-up phase of the network was to be placed on selecting and working in close cooperation with a limited number of operational users, who must be endorsed by one or more of the participating contractors. These operational users, in a pattern that would later be published in our Memorandum of Understanding, were to make a serious effort to integrate the programs offered through the network into their curricula, to assist in the development of new content material, and to participate in the evaluation of the material used.

For the first but not the last time, we listed prospective operational users, from lists of contacts supplied by the three potential contractors. At the suggestion of G. Burroughs Mider, M.D., then Deputy Director, NLM, we starred those located at network nodes and presumably therefore able to use the network without paying long-distance bills. The following eleven institutions were listed as being in node cities:

Baylor University College of Medicine, Houston
Boston University
Columbia University
George Washington University
Medical College of Wisconsin, Milwaukee
Stanford University
Tufts
University of California, Los Angeles
University of California, San Francisco
University of Colorado
University of Texas, Houston

Only two of these institutions did *not* eventually become network users.
On June 19 we received permission to proceed, in the following memorandum:

June 19, 1972

Subject: Proposed Obligation of $145,000 for the Support of Biomedical Data Network Regarding CAI

1. Your request for obligation of $145,000* is approved, contingent upon the provision of information supporting the assumption of adequate numbers of anticipated users of the network.

2. It is understood that this project is clearly an experiment in which the committment is specifically limited to the duration of the experiment, and no further

---

* This was the amount for the two university contracts. The difference between this and the $159,000 mentioned earlier was for communication costs.

commitment is implied at this time. It is understood that this point will be
made absolutely clear to all prospective users, as well as to the contractors.

3. You will provide, within the next 30 days, the following:

   A. An explicit statement of the objectives of this experiment

   B. The data required for you to make a decision regarding each of those objectives

   C. The basis upon which a decision will be made regarding further developments in this area

   D. A description, including scope and management, of the ultimate organization of this material as you now visualize it

4. It is understood that the data requirements for the judgments indicated will be incorporated into the implementation of these contracts, and that the data necessary will be accumulated with the funds obligated. If this is not the case, no funds should be obligated until projections are presented indicating the additional time and money which will be required to reach this point.

Predictions of Possible Users

The first paragraph of the above memorandum asked for the evidence on which we based our assumption that the network would have enough users to make it worth funding. We had two sorts of evidence on which to base our reply. The direct evidence was the Center's correspondence with prospective users; the indirect evidence was the contacts the prospective contractors had made in their own right. In the reply which went back the same day we listed our best guesses in a ranked list of potential users. That list, prepared in June, 1972, is given in Table 2, together with the use these institutions actually made of the network.

We also named eight more institutions as probable users. Seven of these institutions: University of California, Davis; SUNY, Stony Brook; University of Texas, Houston; Wayne State College of Medicine; Baylor University School of Medicine;

Table 2. Projected and Actual Ranking of Network Usage by Institution

Projected rank[a]	Institution	Time used[b]		Mean hours/ month usage	Actual rank[c]
		Months	Hours		
1	Univ. of Pennsylvania	22	2583.7	117.5	1
2	Univ. of Michigan School of Dentistry	4	23.1	5.8	7
3	Univ. of Kentucky College of Dentistry	16	29.8	1.9	5
4	Rutgers Univ.	4	27.7	6.9	6
5	Northwestern Univ.	15	573.3	38.2	2
6	New England Deaconess	22	146.7	6.7	4
7	Univ. of Alabama	22	483.9	22.0	3
Total		105	3868.2		

[a] Based on subjective impressions from correspondence with prospects.
[b] Rubin *et al.* (1975). Time is logged through August, 1974.
[c] On basis of total hours used.

University of Texas, Dallas; and Michigan State University did become users, totaling 1556 hours of usage.

Ohio State University nominated four candidate institutions; University of Washington, Seattle; University of Wisconsin, Madison; SUNY, Stony Brook; and the University of Michigan. All four of their candidates became users, totaling almost 4000 hours. (Although it must be admitted that one of these schools accounted for 3662 hours and another only 4!)

Massachusetts General Hospital offered a list of 21 institutions. Five of these institutions never joined the network, 2 more used only token amounts (1–3 hours); their remaining 14 institutions, however, logged a total of 8324 hours.

June 20, 1972 was our first attempt to estimate transaction costs over the network. We were unhampered by any practical experience, but did have cost estimates from TYMSHARE and knew the costs of the OSU and MGH contracts. At "normal" usage of 8 hours/port for 22 days a month, the estimate worked out to be $13.00/hour for OSU and $14.44 for MGH.

Massachusetts General Hospital connected a PDP-9 computer to the TYMSHARE network at 8:00 A.M. EDST on July 1, 1972.* The LHNCBC Experimental CAI network was in being, and would continue, in various configurations, from then till 5:00 P.M. PDST on May 30, 1975.

Meanwhile, we were writing the Memorandum of Understanding to be signed by us and by prospective users, outlining the commitments and obligations of both NLM and the using institution. Our draft of August 2, 1972 contained, as the second paragraph on the first page, the following statement:

> It is understood that the Educational Component of the Data-Communication Service is an experimental service, and that the NLM makes no assurance, either explicit or implicit, that this service will be permanent or continuing. This experiment is a planned two/three year effort, but the NLM reserves the right to terminate the service to any participating institution by giving a ninety (90) day written notice.

This statement was, presumably, read by all who signed this document.

Two other events occurred in August, 1972. I broke my left arm in a bicycling accident on August 19, 1972 and was effectively *hors de course* for some 6 weeks. Jinnet Fowles Lewis started work with the Lister Hill Center that same month, after a year of postgraduate training at NLM as a Library Associate. Ms. Lewis found herself with a network to run and a crippled boss – strangers both. She coped.

By October of 1972 we had sent out almost 100 "User's Packages" to prospective users. This was a formidable document as evidenced by the Table of Contents:

A. Introduction to the Experiment
B. Educational Material Developed by the Massachusetts General Hospital

---

* This is the "official" start-up time. Rumor has it that Massachusetts General Hospital, following a venerable New England tradition that permits engaged couples certain liberties, had, in fact, coupled with the TYMSHARE network on June 24, 1972.

C. Educational Material Developed by the Ohio State University
D. Educational Material Developed by the University of Illinois
E. Communications and Terminals
    E.1 Data on Terminals
    E.2 Current Nodal Cities
    E.3 IBM 2741 Users
F. Requirements for Participation – the Memorandum of Understanding
G. Network Personnel Directory

In November, 1972, we tackled a housekeeping problem. Massachusetts General Hospital, with our enthusiastic approval, had been adding trial users *ad libitum*. We knew who they were. They did not necessarily know who the Lister Hill Center was. We needed signed pieces of paper from these users for our files. The full ritual User's Package and Memorandum of Agreement represented administrative overkill for these kittle cattle. Our new Trial User's Package reduced the pieces of paper to be signed and returned to two, a Trial Users Letter of Intent and a Background Data Sheet. This form was designed to meet the immediate MGH users crisis. It turned out to be increasingly useful as the years went by and the emphasis changed from operational to trial users.

Our contract with the University of Illinois became effective on October 1, 1972, although it would be January, 1973 before the problems of connecting their IBM computer to the TYMSHARE network were, at least temporarily, solved.

1973 – The First (and Only) Year of Full Network Operation

Network Status and Objectives

On January 4, 1973, we sent forward a Request for Proposals to continue the OSU and MGH contracts, which were due to terminate on the 30th of April. In response to a request for supporting information, we reported on February 21 that we now had 45 operational and trial users, and that we had received Material Use and Evaluation Plans from the following 15 institutions:

    The Medical Center, the University of Alabama in Birmingham
    American Heart Association – Boston Hospital for Women
    CAPO Project – Bolt Beranek and Newman
    Case Western Reserve University
    Michigan State University
    The School of Medicine, University of Pennsylvania
    The University of Texas, Dallas
    Stanford University School of Medicine
    State University of New York – Downstate Medical Center
    University of Texas Medical Branch, Galveston
    College of Medicine, University of Utah

Medical College of Virginia
University of Washington
Medical College of Wisconsin

We then went on to state the objectives of the CAI experiment:

1. To determine the best way to foster interinstitutional sharing of resources
2. To establish the foundations for a network that will ultimately be managed and supported by its users
3. To design the functions and procedures for an optimal CAI network
4. In conjunction with the Network Plans and Management Branch, to define the most cost-effective network

The question, "What data are required for you to make a decision regarding each of these objectives?" was answered by providing a series of questions which we hoped to have answered from network operating experience (my current answers to each of these are given in parentheses after each question).

1. If CAI services are made available over a time-sharing communications network, will people be willing to use them? (Yes, enthusiastically.)
2. Can the material offered over the network be integrated in a meaningful and useful way into existing curricula? (Scattered successes, but not proven.)
3. Can it produce measurable benefits? (In a few instances, yes.)
4. What is the mechanism whereby material may be generated most efficiently and cost effectively? (Still unknown. The barter system proposed did not work out in practice.)
5. What is the best mechanism for reviewing and updating material placed on the network to assure quality? (Not answered during lifetime of network.)
6. What is the mechanism whereby gaps in the data base are identified and filled? (Not answered during lifetime of network.)
7. How should the system be organized and managed? (We did not, but the Health Education Network Users Group, q.v., did answer this question.)
8. What is the most cost effective distribution (networking) mechanism? (Still unanswered, but our Computer Technology Branch is working on it.)
9. Can the network be made economically viable, i.e., be placed on at least a partially self-sustaining basis? (Unanswered during the duration of the network, but the Health Education Network will answer this question.)

The concluding paragraph to our February 21, 1973 Memorandum reads:

It is our belief that the full, three-computer network will have to be in operation for the equivalent of 3 semesters before the necessary information for decision making can be obtained.* The fall semester was largely spent in start-up, both for two of the three computers, and in gaining necessary faculty involvement and participation. The coming semester will see extensive trial use for all three...

---

* In fact, the full three-computer network was in existence for almost three semesters.

FY 74 funds are required to renew all three network contracts to continue through June, 1974, in order to gather the information required to make decisions or to modify approaches

Revised Management Plan

In February, 1973 we issued a new management plan for the CAI network. The previous plan of March, 1972, Data Communication Service Management Plan, treated what was then called the Educational Component Service as an integral part of the Data Communications Service. Experience with actually operating the CAI network showed the desirability of separating these two functions. Responsibility for operating the network was assigned to the then chief of the then Research and Development Branch, with the CAI network becoming a subscriber/user to the Data Communications Service. This new plan is important for two reasons: the CAI network received the name which it was to carry to its grave, the LHNCBC Experimental CAI Network, and this plan also stated where we expected to be in 1975:

> The demand for CAI services will have increased past the point where NLM can afford to pay the full operating costs of the CAI network. Users of network services will pay an increasing portion of the costs, either to the communications and CAI contractors directly, or to a consortium established to run the network. Major institutions may find it desirable to transfer certain CAI programs to their own computers. The network will have made it possible for them to experiment with CAI without first making a substantial capital investment. Smaller institutions will continue to require an external supplier of on-line CAI programs, and will represent a continuing market for such services.

First (and Only) Meeting with Operational Users

On May 18, 1973 the network contractors and operational users were brought together for the first time. The meeting was held in Billings Auditorium of the National Library of Medicine and moderated by Gary E. Striker, M.D., Assistant Dean for Curriculum, University of Washington School of Medicine. Most of the operational users, as requested, brought along at least one medical student – a population which added a certain tang to the proceedings. My summary of the meeting reads, in part as:

> The general mood was one of enthusiasm, tempered with network communication difficulties and busy signals at the home computers. Massachusetts General Hospital reported that 60% of their seven ports were busy from 10:00 A.M. to 10:00 P.M. EDST. It is now necessary to reserve ports for specific high-priority purposes, such as demonstrating CAI to a dean. Plans are under way to set aside specific blocks of time for specified periods at each of the contractor's locations.
>
> The users reported, almost unanimously, that the network had made it possible for them to use computer-assisted instruction for the first time.
>
> Uses ranged from familiarizing medical students with computer terminals through remedial tutoring. In the latter case, a gross anatomy sequence, the use of CAI raised the grades of 15 failing students to the class average. It was considered a major use of this form of teaching.

The University of Washington acknowledged that if the Ohio State University data base had not been available for modification to their specific needs, their Independent Study Program would never have gotten off the ground.

Several users reported that introduction of this new technology is raising fundamental questions in the evaluation of medical education, especially when the same modality is used for teaching and testing.

Questions were raised about continuing National Library of Medicine support of the CAI network, especially at this early state. Fears were expressed that NLM would withdraw support just as they were making progress toward convincing their faculties of its usefulness. The need for eventual support by the users was recognized, but the consensus seemed to be that the benefits and costs still have to be more carefully evaluated through continued experience. Many expressed the view that they had no doubt that cost sharing will be acceptable, but that it was too early at this time to make this determination.

Midyear Status Report

In June, 1973, we issued a progress report for the Board of Regents which stated:

Organizing the CAI network was the Center's first encounter in depth with computer-assisted instruction. The Library has had extensive experience with mechanized information-retrieval systems where it is relatively easy to transfer retrieval program and data bases from one computer to another. CAI programs are not so easily tranferred. The programs at present are treated as experimental prototypes, which need to live in a laboratory atmosphere. The contractors as well as we did not want them to be treated as interesting toys, but rather to be integrated into the curricula of the using institutions in a meaningful way. Two of the three contractors wanted faculty members of using institutions to learn to write additional units of instruction and contribute them to the common pool; the third wanted primarily to provide access to a wider body of students.

We have many more trial than operational users. At the moment, that ratio is 4:1, with 47 trial users and 11 operational users. The programs are used for three general purposes (some institutions use them for more than one purpose):

Demonstration – 31
Teaching – 32
Writing new units of instruction – 8

As of the latest reporting period (February 15 to March 15, 1973) the network computers showed the following usage pattern:

Massachusetts General Hospital	1408 hours
University of Illinois Medical Center	438 hours
Ohio State University	559 hours
	2405

We average 2.5 encounters per hour, which gives us 6000 encounters a month. It probably represents at least twice that number of users; some of our users report that the students cluster five deep around the terminals, with decisions reached by group consensus. Approximately 5% of current usage is by physicians; 70% by medical students. The remainder of the time is used by nurses, dental students, allied health personnel and nonmedical personnel.

An ideal communications network should be transparent to its users; that is, it should have no impact on the procedures, language, or any other aspects of the users' mode of operation. Our users report that the network is at best translucent and frequently opaque. The chief problem with our CAI network is its success; from 11:00 A.M. to 5:00 P.M. on most days, all ports of all computers are saturated. We have added two ports to the computer at Massachusetts General Hospital; the University of Illinois has given us five additional ports.

Our contractors and we have been surprised by the amount of hand-holding our users require. Neither they nor we had much experience with off-campus operations. Naive users need to be told what sort of terminal to buy, and how to turn it on; sophisticated users demand increasing amounts of feedback from the contractors in terms of detailed individual test results. Preparation of adequate manuals for remote users of the systems has been another necessary, but unexpectedly high expense.

Contractors and the National Library of Medicine staff are reviewing the basis of user charges to defray communication expenses. Although the MEDLINE rate schedule and approach has been proposed as a guide, a time frame for implementation has not yet been established.

The User Charge Problem

At least as early as February, 1973, the problem of recouping at least part of the costs of operating the LHNCBC Experimental CAI Network from its users had been raised. There were at least two precedents for user charges.

One was Bureau of the Budget Circular No. A-25, dated September 23, 1959 with the subject: User Charges. This circular established the following, as "General Policy": "A reasonable charge, as defined below, should be made to each identifiable recipient for a measurable unit or amount of Government service or property from which he derives a special benefit."

The other, closer to home, was the Library's experience with AIM-TWX and its successor, MEDLINE. AIM-TWX started in June, 1970; MEDLINE, December, 1971. Creating and maintaining the MEDLINE data base, references to approximately half a million citations from 3000 biomedical journals, was regarded as a logical extension of the National Library of Medicine's functions, as specified in Public Law 941 of the 84th Congress (August 3, 1956).* The cost of the telecommunications necessary to access this data base was not regarded as a cost the Library should bear. MEDLINE user charges, at $6.00 per connect hour, were inaugurated August 20, 1973.

It was obvious to Lister Hill that the network users would eventually have to pay

---

*This law specified that the Surgeon General, PHS, through the Library, shall:

"Acquire and preserve books, periodicals, prints, films, recordings and other library materials pertinent to medicine.

Organize the materials specified by appropriate cataloging, indexing and bibliographic listing.

Publish and make available the catalogs, indexes and bibliographies referred to.

Provide reference and research assistance; and

Engage in such other activities in furtherance of the purpose of this part as he deems appropriate and the Library resources permit."

a portion of their communication costs. Discussions of when, and how much, occupied at least the last 5 months of 1973.

Formal announcement of the pending user charges was made by Ms. Lewis and me at the August 10, 1973 meeting of the network users group held in conjunction with the Ann Arbor meeting of the Association for the Development of Computer-Based Instructional Systems. We announced that network users would be expected to share a portion of the communication costs from January 1, 1974, and to assume a greater portion of these communication costs after July 1, 1974.

This statement was followed by a letter, on September 5, 1973 mailed to all network users of record. This letter also became a part of the "package" sent to all new and/or prospective users of the network. It said in part:

> The user population must assume a larger and larger share of the management and financial support (of the network) with time. At the present, the network is averaging over 2000 hours of use a month. Network costs are of two sorts, fixed and variable. The fixed costs reflect costs which are not a function of the number of users. At a constant monthly expenditure, the actual hourly rates vary inversely with the amount of message traffic. At 2000 hours of use a month, the costs amount to $14.275 per hour:

University contractors (MGH, OSU, UIMC), per month	$22,050
3 TYMCOMS (interface minicomputers), per month	6,500
	$28,550

> Fixed cost per hour, @ 2000 hours/month = $14.275
>
> The rates for variable costs are $4.50 per hour:

2.5 log-ins/hour @ .40	$1.00
Connect hour cost	.80
Transmission (6 characters/second)	2.70
Connect hour cost	$4.50

> This gives a total hourly connect cost at present levels of *$18.775 per hour.*
>
> At present this total cost has been underwritten by NLM. Beginning in this fiscal year the users must begin to assume appropriate fiscal responsibility. We are therefore proposing a graduated payment scale, which will begin to underwrite the cost of accessing the system. This is a temporary minimal expedient until we can develop an appropriate distribution of responsiblity and derive from that more inclusive rates to become effective in beginning of FY 75...
>
> Details of our FY 75 pricing policy are yet to be developed. It can be safely assumed that they will be proportional to the hours of use, and that we will expect to recover the variable costs. There is also the possibility of a fixed billing cost added to these hourly rates. It would probably be safe to assume, for tentative budgeting purposes, connect cost of $5.00 to $8.00 an hour after July 1, 1974.

Background of Charges

By December, 1973 the eventual rates of $2.50 and $5.00 per hour had been chosen. Some, but not all, of the reasons for this decision are set forth in a memorandum of that period:

The plans for the CAI network have historically included the provision for users assuming part, if not all, of the program's costs. The timing for this cost transfer was not laid out in the initial plan, although it was assumed that a period of subsidization would be required.

The communications budget for FY 74 was $145,000. If utilization were to continue at its Spring, 1973 rate (approximately 2000 hours/month) the experiment would run out of communications funds in March, 1974.

In June of 1973, it was stated verbally that no funds would be committed for CAI communications in the FY 75 budget.

In July, 1973 plans were begun to develop a charging system for CAI users. The rate structure was to be administered in two phases, the first to recover our deficit from January, 1974–June, 1974 and introduce user charges; the second to recover communications costs after July 1, 1974. At this time communications costs were defined as those costs exclusive of TYMCOM charges, incurred with TYMSHARE, Inc. TYMCOM charges are considered part of the computer costs. Because the first phase of charges was introduced on short notice (within the fiscal year), it was decided not to pass on the full communication charges as that time. Instead, a graduated rate structure was developed in which the user would pay for the entire 6-month period according to the category in which his anticipated use fell. (See September 5 letter.) At this time (August, 1973) there had been no experience with MEDLINE charges although their charge system had been designed. It was anticipated that the CAI charge schedule would avoid dependence on TYMSHARE statistics (unreliable at that time) and also elimate the dependence on the contractors' three unequal sets of statistics.

When the supplementary statement to the TYMSHARE contract was written (November, 1973) it was felt that the legality of the proposed system would be questioned and that it would be more expedient to charge an hourly rate as MEDLINE had begun to do. The rate was set at $2.50/hour, more than the most favorable case in the previous charging structure, but less than the $5.00/hour total communications cost. It is still hoped that this charge can be instituted in January.

After July 1, 1974, users will be charged $5.00/connect hour. Studies are now underway to determine the impact of this charging schedule. If the result is to decrease the number of users below critical mass, it will be difficult to justify the expense of maintaining the data bases. A preliminary telephone survey indicates that the majority of users contacted to date find the $5.00 charge reasonable.

A Contractor Problem

One of our crises occurred when Dr. William Harless left the University of Illinois for the College of the Pacific. The pattern seemed to be recurring in July of 1973, when we heard that our two co-principal investigators at Ohio State University, J. Griesen and A. Weinberg, were leaving: Griesen on November 1 to go to the University of Michigan; Weinberg on August 1 to go to Ohio Osteopathic Hospital. The Lister Hill Center felt strongly that assurance of an adequate replacement was critical; otherwise the thing to do would be to let the OSU contract terminate on October 31, 1973.

Ohio State University reacted strongly to this suggestion. On August 16, 1973, Dr. Henry Cramblett, new Dean of OSU Medical School, and Jerry Huddleston, Dean for Fiscal Affairs, met with us. Also present were Dr. Robert Beran and

Dr. Robert Folk, whom OSU proposed as the new co-principal investigators. What had threatened to be Armageddon turned into agape, particularly after Dr. Cramblett made a ringing affirmation of his faith in computer-assisted instruction, even to the point of putting some of his budget in it.

1974–1975, The Beginning of the End

My letter anouncing user charges of $2.50 per hour, starting February 1, through June 30, 1974, was mailed to all users of record on January 4, 1974. It contained the following paragraph:

> Continuation of the network after July 1 will depend on the number of users who wish to continue to use the services of the $5.00 per hour connect charge in effect after that date. The decision to renew the CAI contracts for FY 75 will be made in April; it would not be cost-effective if only a few institutions could or would pay this increased connection charge. It is urgent that I hear, as soon as possible, of your institution's intentions in this regard. Are you interested in continuing to use the network's services after the first of July?

Our users, a remarkably resilient group, took the user charges in stride. The first month of charging shook out a few users, mostly in the token group that used 0–10 hours per month, but actually increased both the net number of users and the number of connect hours per month used.

By mid-March, we had received almost 50 signed contracts from users, most of whom indicated their intentions to use the network after July 1, when the $5.00 per hour charge would apply. My management had been pessimistic about the impact of user charges, expressing concern that they would reduce the number of users to a point where it would no longer be cost effective to pay for maintaining the data bases. As a result of this user response, funds were released to fund the computer/contractor cost of the network through May 31, 1975. As Figure 1 shows, the number of users continued to increase through the lifetime of the network.

As Dr. George Miller of the Center for Educational Development, University of Illinois, had announced at our December, 1973 Contractor's Meeting, the University of Illinois withdrew from the network on February 28, 1974. Illinois released their CASE programs to Ohio State University. CASE became operational there on May 28, 1974 and has flourished happily in its new environment ever since.

On May 10, 1974, the Lister Hill National Center for Biomedical Communications was reorganized. All four branches, including the Research and Development Branch which had been responsible for the CAI network, were abolished. Three new branches were established in their stead: Communications Engineering; Computer Technology; and, soon to be transferred, Educational Technology. I became Special Assistant for Program Development, but continued to run my existing programs including the CAI network until May 31, 1975. The Computer

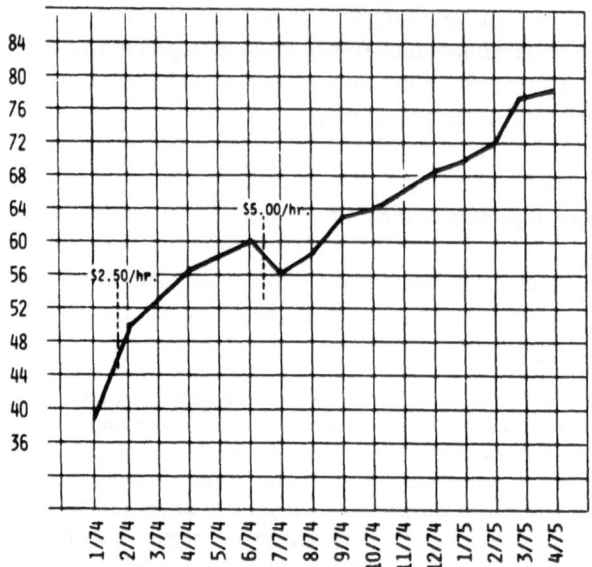

Figure 1. Number of users on the LHC Experimental CAI Network.

Technology Branch under its new Chief, Charles Goldstein, who came on board in September, 1974, was to take care of CAI-Future. Albert Feiner, who had been Director of LHNCBC since May, 1971, left later in May. His replacement as Director, Dr. Robert M. Bird, did not start work until September, 1974. Operation of the Center during the lull between Mr. Feiner and Dr. Bird was the responsibility of Dr. Harold M. Schoolman, Assistant Deputy Director of NLM. Jinnet Fowles (Lewis) left for graduate studies on June 28, 1974. Her successor, Becky J. Lyon, assumed responsibility for operating the network on July 1, 1974.

On July 1, 1974, $5.00/hour communication costs were charged against the using institutions. Of the 59 institutional users in June, 1974, 55 signed to continue at the increased rate. In addition, 8 new institutions were added bringing the total of using institutions up to 63.

Table 3, prepared in September, 1974, shows the impact of user charges on hours of use.

The period March, 1974–June, 1974 ($2.50/hour) reflects only a 4.7% decrease in overall hours used. The July and August figures, however, show a decrease of 7.9% overall.

With funding firm through May 31, 1975, we were left with two problems.

One was to operate the network efficiently during the remaining 10 months of existence; the other was to prepare our users for the day when NLM support of the network would cease. Strictly speaking both of these subjects are out of the scope of history; the first because it was uneventful, the second because most of the key events occurred outside our walls, and certainly out of our control.

Table 3. CAI Experimental Network Usage

	Hours per month, 1973 (no charge)	Hours per month, 1974 (charge instituted)	Change in number of hours used
March	1686	2290	+604
April	1893	1830[a]	– 63
May	2806	2287[a]	–519
June	1806	1393[a]	–413
July	1570	1407[b]	–163
August	1294	1228[b]	– 66

[a] Hours used after $2.50/hour charge instituted.
[b] Hours used after $5.00/hour charge instituted.

As Figure 1 shows, the network grew steadily. We allowed, although we certainly did not encourage, users to join through April, 1975. As user charges increased, we relaxed the distinction between operational and trial users, and loosened our reporting requirements, seeking instead to expose the greatest number of users to the greatest number of contact hours.

Dealing with the users was another problem. Fortunately, Dr. Robert M. Bird started work, as Director Designate, on September 3, 1974, just as the storm broke. As a former medical school dean (University of Oklahoma), he was accustomed to saying "No"; as a Virginian born and bred, he said "No" politely. He was to need both of these skills in the coming months. Dr. Bird had inherited the network; he had also inherited the decision to terminate the network on May 31. Both of these were facts. A lot of people would have been saved a lot of counter-productive effort if they had realized that the decision in April, 1973 to fund the network terminally was final.

Our major source of outside pressure came from the Health Education Network users. This group had its start with a letter from Robert G. Votaw, Ph.D., of the University of Connecticut School of Medicine inviting representatives of some 30 institutions from New England, New York, Pennsylvania, New Jersey, District of Columbia and Virginia to attend a meeting at the University of Connecticut Health Center on May 30–31, 1974. The letter said, in part:

> A number of users feel that we should form a CAI Network Users Group to foster communication among medical CAI users, to support the development of a cost-effective alternative to the existing network, to consider problems related to inter-institutional sharing and to impress upon the LHC the necessity of support during this period of transition.

The meeting was attended by representatives of 14 network user institutions, as well as by representatives of the Lister Hill Center, AAMC, and the Health Sciences Interest Group of ADCIS. The meeting agreed, as reported by Votaw in a letter of July 1, 1974 that (1) the network should be continued, and (2) a national Users Group should be formed.

At the Lister Hill User's Pre-Session to the ADCIS meeting in Bellingham, Washington on August 3, 1974, the New England group expanded to include all users of the network, elected a chairperson (Dr. Votaw), outlined their basic purposes and petitioned to become a Special Interest Group under the auspices of ADCIS. At that meeting they voted to recommend that Lister Hill continue the support of the network for 3 years past 1975 "to allow for the development of an alternative to the network."

The Health Education Network Users Group's (HENUG) first formal contact with LHNCBC occurred on October 1, 1974 in the form of a 6-page letter from Dr. Votaw as Chairman of the Steering Committee, HENUG, ADCIS, to Dr. Robert M. Bird. HENUG asked the Center to:

1. Convene a meeting to consider network continuation.
2. Reconsider the LHC position on support of the network.

The gist of the paper was a table outlining four possible network models: (1) *the network as is*, with all users paying $5.00 per connect hour; (2) *the network as is*, with operational user costs set at $8.00 per connect hour; (3) NLM guarantees a 600-hour-per-month minimum for OSU, and provides a $1.10-per-hour subsidy through TYMSHARE. Contractors provide "bare port" service, with no hand-holding. NLM subsidizes new users and holds user costs to $8 per hour; (4) the HENUG fall-back position, a model without NLM subsidy of costs over $8.

November must have been a busy month for HENUG. They ran a booth at the AAMC meeting in Chicago, prepared a brochure, circularized their constituents for firm estimates of network use for the year beginnning June 1, 1975, and prepared a proposal for presentation to the NLM at a meeting held on December 3. This meeting was attended by representatives from HENUG, OSU, MGH, and the AAMC. My notes on the meeting contain the following comments:

1. HENUG represents a potentially valuable organization for expressing user interests. It does not now (Dec., 1974) have legal status, except through ADCIS, necessary to be a recipient of federal funds.
2. Ohio State University, as a state university, is very properly concerned with maintenance of financial control over state funds. They can only enter into contractual relations with established, financially sound institutions.
3. MGH and OSU should be encouraged to set up their own distribution networks, either directly or through HENUG. If, in the future, LHNCBC should desire to use either MGH or OSU CAI material in educational experiments, it should expect to pay an equitable price for the materials used.

HENUG now understood the LHNCBC position. Votaw, in a circular letter of January 8, 1975 reported to HENUG members that:

> LHC has answers that they are satisfied with to their research questions vis a vis the existing network, and LHC *will not* provide *further dollar support to operate* [emphasis in original] the network. LHC will probably respond to requests to help that involve no dollar outlay.
>
> Our need to buy time to organize and to implement a self-supporting and user-directed network is unmet. It is clear we must plan for network continuation,

starting 1 June 1975, without LHC dollar support...We must rely on OSU and MGH for leadership in the next few months. ...We now recognize the inadequacy of the networking model embodied in the LHC effort. With what do we replace it?

Votaw's letter of February 7, 1975 to his colleagues reported that MGH and OSU had reached an agreement with TYMSHARE, and that the new network would "look" like this:

1. Users will access the network much as they do at present.
2. Each user/institution will have a memorandum of understanding with OSU and a memorandum of understanding with MGH, to replace the memorandum of understanding now in force with the Lister Hill Center. Each user will be billed bimonthly according to usage by the appropriate courseware contractor(s).
3. Costs will be:
   A. Ohio State University, $10.15 per connect hour and no minimum charge.
   B. Massachusetts General Hospital, $8.00 per connect hour and a minimum charge of $100 per 2-month billing.

In April, 1975 the Lister Hill Center, in fulfillment of a commitment to provide administrative support, provided $16,000 via a supplement to our contract with MGH to pay for a "network coordinator" for 10 months, who would report to us on the progress of the network.

On May 30, 1975, at 5:00 P.M. PDST, the LHNCBC network entered the pages of these, and we hope other, histories.

On February 21, 1973 we had stated as an objective of the Lister Hill CAI experiment: "To establish the foundations for a network that will eventually be managed and supported by its users."

On June 1, 1975, the Health Education Network, financed and managed by its users, started to operate. It now has almost 60 institutional users.

References

Brigham, C. R., 1973a. Programming Languages Used for Health Sciences Computer-Assisted Instruction. Massachusetts General Hospital. Available from National Technical Information Service, U.S. Dept. Commerce, Springfield, Va., as PB 224 421 A/S for $3.50.

Brigham, C. R., 1973b. Minicomputers in Health Sciences Instruction. Massachusetts General Hospital, Boston. Available from National Technical Information Service, U.S. Dept. Commerce, Springfield, Va., as PB 224 397 A/S for $3.00.

Brigham, C. R., Kamp, M., and Cross, K. J., 1972. A Guide to Computer-Assisted Instruction in the Health Sciences. Rutgers Medical School, New Brunswick, N.J., and the University of California, San Francisco. (December, 1972). Available from National Technical Information Service, U.S. Dept. Commerce, Springfield, Va., as PB 214 351 for $9.00.

Kronick, D. A., and Robinson, C. K., 1974. Remote Access Computer Assisted Instruction: User's Guide to the LHNCBC (National Library of Medicine) Computer Assisted Instruction Experimental Network. The University of Texas Health Science Center at San Antonio.

Lewis, J. F., and Wooster, H., 1973. Utilization of the Lister Hill Center Computer-Assisted Instruction (CAI) Network, *Computer Medicine* Unpaged special report, September (1973).

McCarn, D. B., and Leiter, J., 1973. On-line services in medicine and beyond, *Science* 181: 318–324.

National Library of Medicine News, 1973. (January).

Rubin, M. L., Hunter, B., and Knetsch, M., 1975. Evaluation of the Experimental CAI Network (1973–1975) of the Lister Hill National Center for Biomedical Communications, National Library of Medicine. Human Resources Research Organization, Alexandria, Va., (January, 1975). Available from National Technical Information Service, U.S. Dept. Commerce, Springfield, Va., as PB 239 358 for $4.75.

Smythe, C. McC., 1969. Potential Educational Services from a National Biomedical Communications Network. Association of American Medical Colleges, Washington, D.C.

Stead, E. A., Jr., Smythe, C. McC., Gunn, C. G., and Littlemeyer, M. H., 1971. Educational technology for medicine: Roles for the Lister Hill Center, *J. Med. Educ.*, 46(7): Part. 2 (July), 97p.

Wakefield, J., 1973. CAI: Report on the NLM network, *Biomed. Commun.* 2: 18, 32, 35, 36.

Wakefield, J. S., Minner, D. E., Oszustowicz, R. J., and Miller, D. E., 1973. CAI Network Evaluation and Methodology. Medical Computer Services Association (MCSA), Seattle, Wa. Available from National Technical Information Service, U.S. Dept. Commerce, Springfield, Va., as PB 226 484 A/S for $6.25.

Wooster, H., 1973. The Lister Hill CAI Network – A progress report, *The Physiologist* 16: 626–630.

Wooster, H., and Lewis, J. F., 1973. Distribution of computer-assisted instruction materials in biomedicine through the Lister Hill Center Experimental Network, *Comput. Biol. Med.* 3: 319–323.

Wooster, H., and Lewis, J. F., 1974. The utility of computer-assisted instruction – An experimental network, *in* P. L. Zunde (Ed.), *Information Utilities – Proceedings of the 37th ASIS Annual Meeting, 1974*, pp. 213–217, American Society for Information Science, Washington, D.C.

9

The PLATO System:
An Evaluative Description

G. L. Hody and R. A. Avner

Introduction

PLATO is a fast, flexible, and responsive system designed expressly to present inter-active instructional lessons attractively and economically. From initial research data collected on three predecessor systems over a period of 15 years, PLATO developers concluded that they would have to make extensive modifications in existing computer equipment before it would be suitable for delivering the kind of individualized instruction they wanted. They also found that they had to depart from the traditional architecture of computer systems and to develop a new author language. These tasks were necessary because available computer systems had been optimized for scientific and business applications with requirements that were very different from those of the instructional setting.

Although PLATO is probably best known for the resulting unorthodox approach to equipment and systems design, it is really the underlying philosophy that is its most distinguishing feature:

> ... [that] education is an extraordinarily difficult human enterprise ... [which] requires a flexible and powerful medium. (Bitzer *et al.*, 1973)

Thus, while PLATO, like other computer-assisted instructional (CAI) systems, can relieve instructors from tedious repetitive facets of teaching, it is intended more to expand the spectrum of possible educational approaches than to reduce the role of the human teacher. In order to encourage the full range of teaching techniques within the reach of computer technology, PLATO does not require specific educational strategies or formats. Instead, it strives to maximize for each category of user the accessibility of the features most needed for their specific tasks. This goal is sought by careful attention to the user–system interface. For example, speed of response, full graphics displays, touch input, and an extensive group of author

G. L. Hody · School of Basic Medical Sciences, University of Illinois College of Medicine, Urbana, Illinois and *R. A. Avner* · Computer-Based Education Laboratory, University of Illinois, Urbana, Illinois. The PLATO system has been supported by the State of Illinois, the National Science Foundation, The Control Data Corporation, and the Advanced Research Projects Agency (ARPA) of the Department of Defense. This work was supported, in part, by Contract number NO1–PE–34068 between the University of Illinois College of Medicine and the Health Resources Administration, Department of Health, Education, and Welfare.

and student aids built deeply into the system software are important interface features. The intent of this design is to intrude minimally upon the user during the preparation as well as the use of instructional materials.

PLATO developers were also sensitive to the need for ultimate low-cost, high-volume operation. Fortunately, careful analysis of the way computer resources are used in the course of instruction revealed that economy could be consistent with good performance if the systems design were tailored from the start for the educational user.

It is very difficult for a prospective new user to get an accurate picture of a computer-based educational system from a written description. Long lists of technical specifications are of little use to nonspecialists, and written examples of "typical interactions" are apt to be misleading because they involve experienced users who are attuned to the idiosyncrasies of the system and can make it behave well, even where a typical student might have a great deal of trouble. Cost and performance claims that originate with the developers rather than with objective evaluators should be scrutinized for overoptimism – the host of interactions involved in the design and the complexity of the systems often result in unforeseen limitations that do not become evident until they are revealed by users outside of the design group. The authors, a physician–educator and an evaluator, have no ego-involvement with the design of the PLATO system and have had extensive experience with other time-sharing computer applications so that their views should be relatively unbiased. Nevertheless, readers who want an accurate impression of the capabilities and limitations of CAI systems should realize that there is no substitute for extensive personal experience and painstaking quantitative analysis of the specifications, performance, and cost data.

This chapter describes the PLATO system in use at the University of Illinois in 1976. Care has been taken to differentiate claims of future performance from objective data on current characteristics – a particularly important precaution for a system that is as rapidly growing and changing as PLATO. Instead of the traditional hardware–software–lessonware characterization, an orientation to applications will be used to structure the information for readers with specific interests outside of the computer sciences.

The authors believe that there is room for many approaches to computer-based education in health sciences and that innovative methods should be enthusiastically supported. For each new system, it is critically important to set specific objectives and to evaluate carefully how well these are met. As an initial suggestion for a framework from which to view the question of evaluation, the following questions should be considered by the reader when studying the systems described in this book:

1. *Accessibility*. How easy is it for users to make use of the major system capabilities? How much training is needed before students can make efficient use of the system? Does the system give adequate support to authors as well? Can non-computer specialists learn to write effective lessons?

2. *Availability*. Does the system perform with adequate speed and without "busy" signals? To what extent is the system "up" and available for use, and what is the relationship between operating costs and reliability?

3. *Flexibility*. Does the system permit a wide variety of educational approaches and methods? What features promote or inhibit the creation of innovative course materials? Can the capabilities be extended to change and grow in response to past experience and user needs?

4. *Experience*. Has the system been used in its present form by enough people and institutions for enough time to obtain valid information about its performance in a variety of settings? Are objective data being collected and evaluated on a regular basis?

5. *Costs*. What are the true costs of operating the system? How do these costs change when the system expands from a small-scale prototype to high-volume "production" operations? What is the cost basis to the user? Does the pricing structure encourage efficient use of available resources?

The aim of this chapter is to provide as much of the above information as is currently available so that the reader will be able to decide if the PLATO system is suitable for the delivery of high-quality health sciences education.

General Description

PLATO is an acronym for **P**rogrammed **L**ogic for **A**utomated **T**eaching **O**perations. The name is associated with a wide variety of equipment and methods developed mainly at the Computer-based Education Laboratory (CERL) of the University of Illinois. The original concept and overall direction of the project since its inception are the work of Dr. Donald Bitzer, a professor of electronics engineering, and the director of CERL.

This chapter describes specifically the time-shared teaching system in operation by the University of Illinois. This system, committed to research, is also used to present accredited instruction in a variety of academic settings during at least 80 hours of the typical work week. Its main facility in east-central Illinois communicates with about 950 terminals, many of which are located at long distances. Full PLATO service at present requires a special terminal – teletypewriters and conventional CRT terminals will not work with PLATO. The processing power resides in a specially modified Control Data 6000-Cyber series computer, generally considered to be a "large" machine. The size of the central processor, its speed, and special additional equipment let each user access a large resource of information and lesson material and perform massive computations rapidly.

The User–Machine Interface

PLATO interactions are carefully made as flexible and natural as possible. The concern for the comfort and speed of the system–user interface is reflected both in the design of the terminal equipment and in PLATO's systems software that operates "behind the scenes" to cue, prompt, correct and otherwise assist both student and author users. These built-in aids come into play whenever errors are made or information is requested and are designed to anticipate a large variety of difficulties that are known to occur frequently in the creation or delivery of CAI. Not specific to any particular subject content area, the messages are delivered in plain language and conversational style.

Because even extensive written descriptions and cross-references will often fail to solve a problem, PLATO encourages direct interpersonal communications by allowing the use of the terminal as a combined electronic mail and teletype service. These highly humanizing features are automatically available to authors and students alike without the need for special programmer attention.

Any terminal on the PLATO system may be used for all functions – to study instructional materials, design curricula, write new materials, or perform systems programming. At the time of sign-on, the system identifies each user, on the basis of previously entered information, as a student, instructor, author, programming consultant, or system programmer. On the basis of this identification, the system allocates appropriate resources and capabilities. The services provided to students may be considered the basic level available to all categories of users. Others have the same capabilities as students plus additional features necessary for their tasks. The way in which the system interacts with students will be described first.

The Machine-to-Student Interface Part 1: The Display

The major sensory pathway for learning by computer-based instruction is visual, which makes the terminal display device extremely important. In contrast to the industrial user who typically looks at computer displays infrequently and for short periods, the student may use the terminal for several hours continuously. Under these conditions, the display must be sharp, absolutely steady, and of ideal brightness and contrast. Unfortunately, the usual computer terminal displays are deficient in one or more of these desired features: CRTs often distort straight lines, particularly at the edges; the vector method of generating graphics causes disturbing flickers when graphics become complex or dense; many storage tubes fade out with prolonged viewing unless refreshed and have generally poor contrast. To remedy these problems, Bitzer and his associates designed a new display panel for PLATO, the "plasma matrix" display (Bitzer and Slottow, 1968; Stifle, 1970; Johnson *et al.*, 1971). Figure 1 shows a typical PLATO terminal.

The PLATO terminal display is a 22 × 22 centimeter screen (about 8.5 inches square or about the same dimensions as the typical textbook page). It contains a little over a quarter of a million points arranged in a matrix of 511 positions in the vertical and horizontal directions. By ionization of a noble gas (roughly similar in principle to the neon lamp), any point can be independently illuminated. Once "lit," the addressed point glows bright orange on a black background and remains bright until specifically extinguished by a computer command. In practice, the

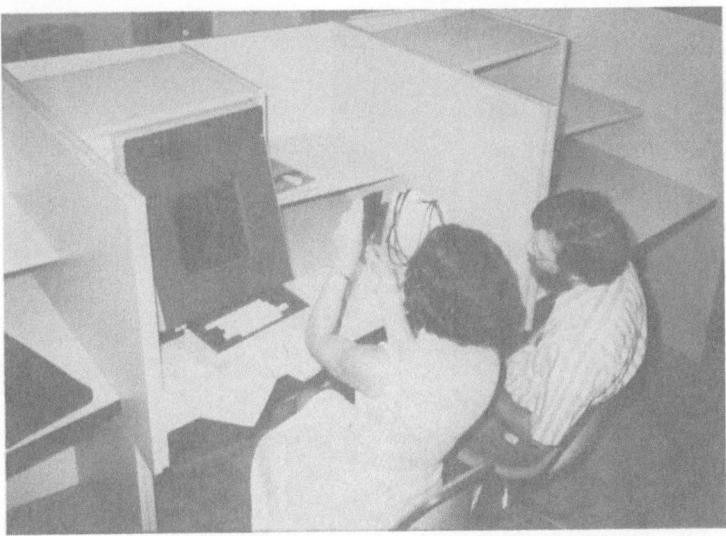

Figure 1(A). The PLATO terminal is a versatile multimedia device, slightly larger than conventional CRT terminals. It is most conveniently installed in custom-designed carrels, such as this example from the language laboratory of the University of Illinois at Urbana.

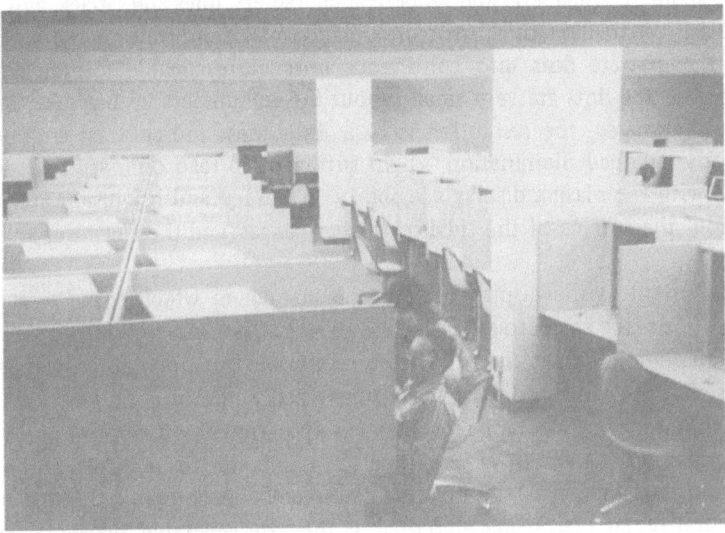

Figure 1(B). The language laboratory of the University of Illinois at Urbana includes 64 PLATO student consoles in an air-conditioned, properly illuminated environment – the classic "classroom cluster" envisioned in the original PLATO designs.

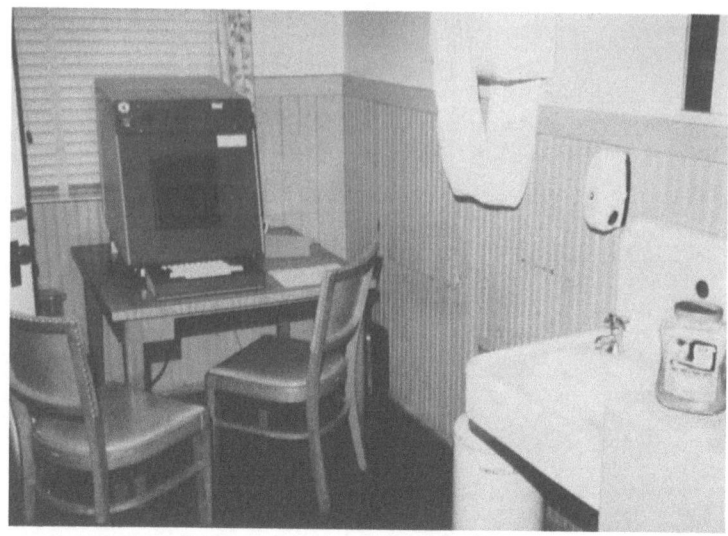

Figure 1(C). Some PLATO installations are more Spartan than others, and this terminal appears to thrive in unusual surroundings as well – (with a sign on the door: "The quality of the product is not implied by the location of the terminal").

computer does not frequently address individual dots on the panel but rather sends simple commands to the terminal which contains enough internal circuitry to generate standard alphabetic and numerical characters, lines and circles, and a group of "special" characters that are stored in a small solid-state memory. The eye merges the discrete dots into continuous lines at reasonable reading distances, and, because the dots are very small (about 0.4 millimeters in diameter) and very accurately arranged, the resolution is high. Brightness and contrast are optimized for slightly subdued illumination – light sufficient to read ordinary text does not interfere with the plasma display's legibility. Accuracy and resolution are uniform throughout the surface of the tube to the very edges, and there is never any flicker or fading.

As important as the display itself is the manner in which each "screenful" is generated. Looking ahead to extensive use of PLATO for interaction and simulation, a page-orientation, rather than the more traditional line-orientation, was selected. Displays that are written one line at a time usually do not permit backspacing or returns to lines already completed. They rarely permit selective printing or erasing of any point on the screen at any time. If graphs are to be displayed on a line-oriented device, they must be built up completely in computer storage prior to presentation rather than being presented as they are generated, because everything appearing on a given screen line must be printed at the same time (when the line in question is generated).

On the PLATO terminal, there are no discrete lines, pages, or frames as such – rather, the display can be altered at will – from a complete erasure of the panel to repositioning of a single dot. Interactive displays and simulations can be structured in any desired temporal sequence, irrespective of where the result is to appear on the screen — an essential requirement for "real-time" simulations. Further, the alteration of small sections of displays is almost instantaneous; if small pieces of a display are sequentially and rapidly written, erased, and rewritten in a slightly different location, a primitive but effective animation effect results.

Pictorial aids are an essential part of the teaching style of many if not most classroom educators and are even more essential in a system intended mainly for self-paced instruction. Although these are not available on most current computer-based systems,* they are richly supported on PLATO. With the help of information stored permanently in the terminal, computer commands create straight and circular line segments at very high speeds (typically 60 lines per second for straight segments). The terminal also contains the patterns for the standard alphanumeric character set in a read-only memory. Another memory within the terminal has the capability of storing up to 126 author-designed special characters. These are normally "loaded" from the computer into the terminal under program control at the start of a lesson (a 20-second operation). Special characters are used for symbols such as chemical formulas and structures, foreign language text, and even, in combinations, for realistic pictorial illustrations.

Elaborate graphics would be useless if they were slow — speed is so essential to computer-based education, given normal human impatience, that its importance is hard to overemphasize. PLATO characters, both standard and special, plot at 180 per second. Standard text is thus presented at a rate corresponding to a reading speed of about 2000 words per minute. The time required to generate a complete display varies widely, mainly as a function of the complexity of the display. A typical amount of text, accompanied by simple graphics can plot in about 5 seconds, while a really full picture made up of complex line drawings might require as much as 15 to 30 seconds to complete. For most readers, text appears sufficiently fast that writing speed is not a significant limitation to the learning process and display generation is perceived as essentially instantaneous. Figure 2 gives an example of PLATO graphics display.

The major limitations of the PLATO display are that it cannot reproduce colors and that displays which are both large and highly complex require appreciable time and computer resources to create. Attempting to solve both of these problems at once, PLATO provides a microfiche projector within the terminal. With this option, color photos, copied from slide originals, are projected on the same display screen as the computer-generated graphics and text. This superposition enables the lesson program to use the slides much like a human instructor — by pointing to desired portions (see Figure 3). The color slides are arranged 256 slides to a single 4 X 6 inch microfiche card. The card is loaded into the terminal by the user. Under computer control, any slide can be accessed within 0.2 seconds, using energy

---

*The TICCIT system (Mitre Corporation, 1974) and the physics computer development project at the University of California (Irvine) (Bork, 1975) are two CAI projects other than PLATO that emphasize graphics.

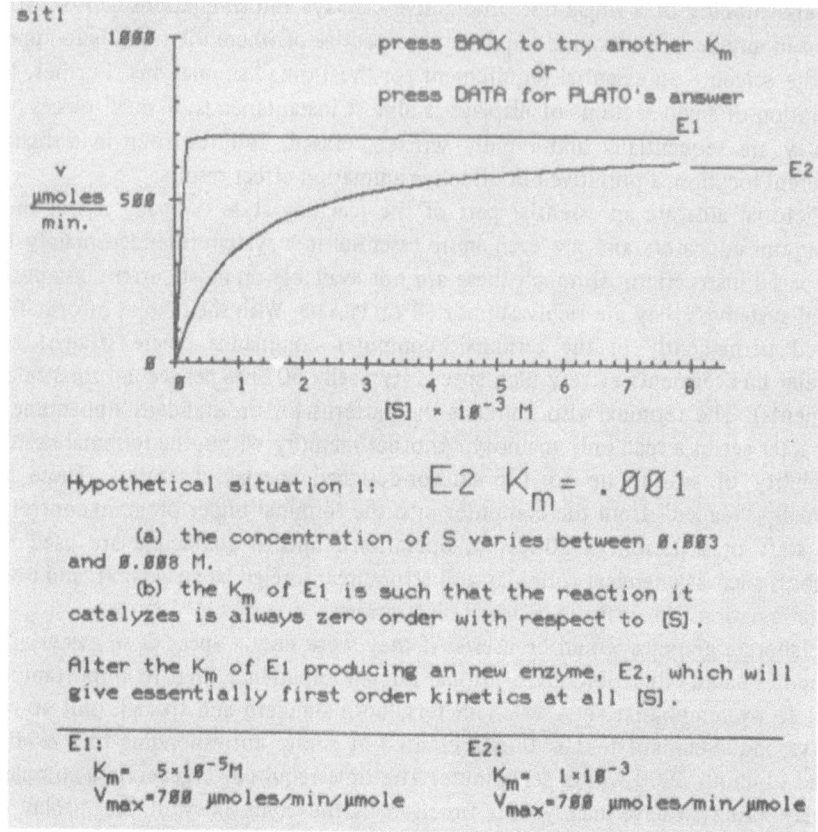

Figure 2. The PLATO display can easily write sub- and superscripts so that chemical formulas appear in their usual manner. Writing of larger than standard size is used to set off important items. The use of the graphics features, including the automated drawing of coordinate axes, is richly supported by TUTOR commands. This figure also illustrates the rapid computing that can be performed for each student – in this case, curves are drawn from parameters entered *ad lib* by the student. In a sense, this represents a minisimulation embedded within a lesson whose format is basically tutorial. (This is a photograph of an actual display from a lesson in biochemistry – series by C. Agee, T. Ahasic, and J. Baxter.)

supplied by any small compressed air supply (about 15 psi). Unfortunately for the health science user for whom it would be an ideal feature, microfiche is still in the research prototype stage and is supported with varying degrees of enthusiasm by CERL. Although the fiche is suitable for many applications, its resolution, color fidelity, and contrast control are not as good as one would want for demanding uses, such as the reproduction of histological, microbiological, or radiographic images. Because the format is nonstandard, the fiche is also expensive to produce. Hopefully these deficiencies will be solved rapidly because the concept of superimposed computer graphics over program-selected random-access slides is an excellent one.

For applications that require sound, PLATO provides a random-access device

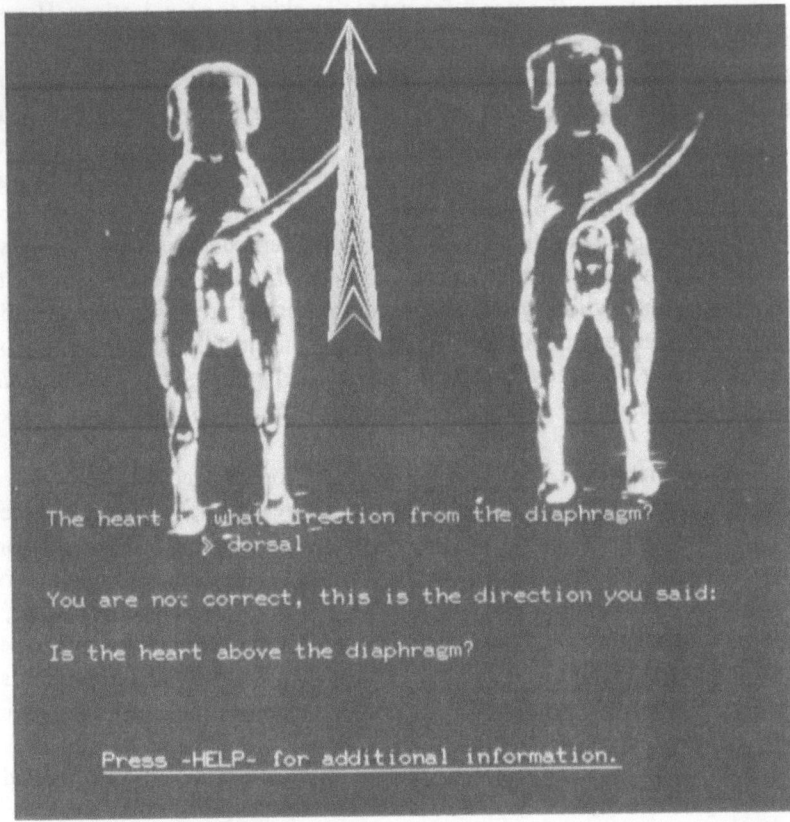

Figure 3. Superposition of computer-generated graphics over microfiche images gives the computer the ability to present full color pictures. In this illustration, the problem is presented to the student using both the microfiche (for the illustration) and the computer graphics (for the question). After the student has responded (in this case, incorrectly), feedback is given by more computer output — an arrow and text based on the nature of the student's error. All three actions are presented at once on the same frame to illustrate the point compactly, but the reader should realize that the text and graphics appear sequentially in response to student input. (From a lesson on the anatomy of the dog from the Department of Veterinary Medicine of the University of Illinois, Urbana; G. Grimes, Project Director.)

that handles audio much like the microfiche projector provides visual images. Lesson programs are able to access segments of sound tracks recorded on a custom-made magnetic disk that is played on an auxiliary instrument connected to the terminal. Segments can be as brief as 0.3 seconds and up to 4096 can be combined smoothly for a total time of about 17 minutes.

Student-to-Machine Interface

A fast and comfortable way of entering information into the system is as critical as a good display. PLATO uses a rather unremarkable keyboard and a somewhat more unusual touch-sensitive panel for user to machine communications. However, it is what happens to input which is the most important aspect of this interface.

When a key is pressed (or a touchpanel input is made), the terminal immediately transmits the information to the central processor. Rapid but complex interpretation of the input is then carried out and, in general, the system takes some specific action. In the simplest case, PLATO "echoes" the key pressed back to the display — if for example the student pressed the key "a," PLATO writes an "a" on the screen. Echoing of this type is traditionally handled by the terminal itself, and PLATO's use of the central processor for the purpose has been criticized as inefficient. In fact, the PLATO communication system that links the central processor to the terminals is designed for frequent exchange of information and handles the echoing process very economically. The advantages of letting user input go through the entire system without delay are essential to the proper operation of PLATO (Sherwood and Stifle, 1975).

Because key presses are processed within a fraction of a second in all cases, it is possible to do without the traditional "enter" or "return" key. Single key presses can cause rapid changes in the display, move figures around on the screen, or, in combination provide teletype-like, rapid communication between two users at different terminals. Because key information is sent to the central processor, the entire keyboard may be redefined to produce, for example, Greek letters or special symbols rather than ordinary alphanumerics. Finally, essential PLATO options, such as the use of superscripts and subscripts, keys to control branching, and selective erasure and backspacing, all require this feature.

The PLATO keyset is basically a typewriter keyboard to which have been added numerical operators ($+$, $-$, $\times$, $\div$) and a small group of special-function keys. The function keys are useful for student-control of branching within a lesson as well as to create subscripts and superscripts and to shift the terminal into alternate fonts. The ERASE, EDIT, and COPY key are used mainly to correct typing errors as explained below.

Most PLATO terminals are equipped with a touch-sensitive panel which overlays the display screen (Figure 4). Along each side of the touchpanel are transmitters and receivers for beams of infrared (thermal) energy — 16 in the vertical and 16 in the horizontal directions, respectively. When a student touches the screen, a unique combination of one horizontal beam and one vertical beam is interrupted, indicating to the system where (within a half-inch resolution) the screen has been touched.* As in the case of microfiche, system support for the touchpanel is not as elaborate as that accorded to most other features. Nevertheless, touch is a useful feature where typing skills can be expected to be poor — as with grammar school children and postgraduate physicians, to cite a couple of examples.

Machine-to-Student Interface Part 2: Response to Student Input

Whenever a student has progressed in a PLATO instructional lesson to the point where the author has specified that a response is needed from the student, an "arrow"

---

*A quarter-inch resolution prototype is already available.

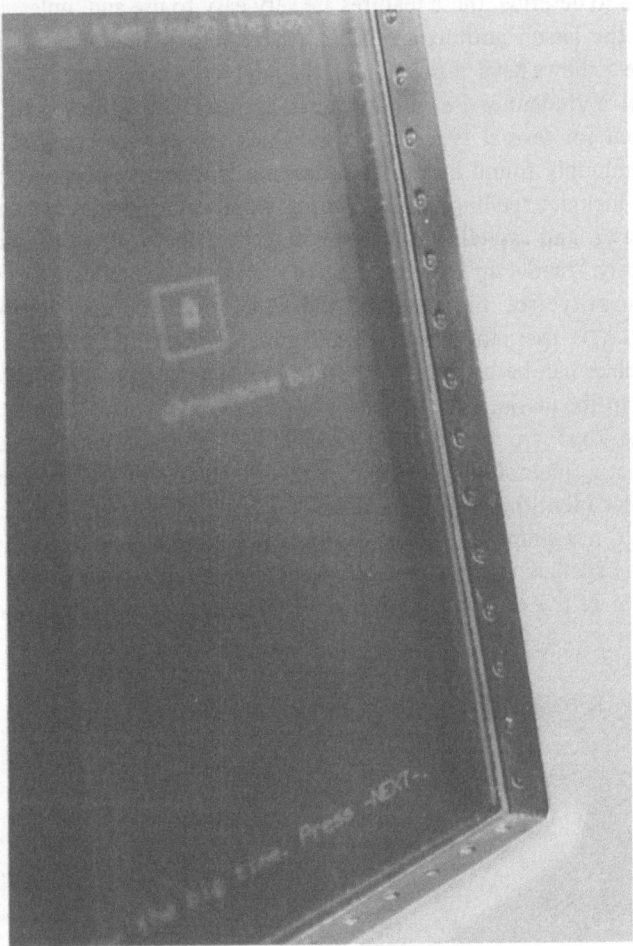

Figure 4. The touch-sensitive panel is really an invisible grid of infrared beams originating from light-emitting diodes located at half-inch intervals around the periphery of the display screen (small vertical and horizontal circles around the edges of the display). This panel is a very popular feature with physicians who dislike typing. Many lessons can be programmed so that either the panel or the keyset can be used to respond – at the option of the user.

symbol appears on the display. In general, the student's typed response appears at the arrow, and a number of features are automatically activated. The first group of these is intended to permit rapid correction of typing errors. By pressing the ERASE key, the student can delete single characters from his or her response (corresponding erasure of the displayed response accompanies the action). A SHIFT-ERASE will delete entire words rather than single characters – the system automatically recognizes word boundaries. Pressing the EDIT key stores the student response in a temporary storage space and blanks the display of the response which can then be recalled (for possible correction by the ERASE key) one character or an entire word at a time by successive presses of appropriate function keys.

Burdensome to describe, these features are very easy to use and, unless intentionally deleted by the lesson author, are made available each time the arrow symbol is used. Figure 5 shows keys in position on the keyboard.

Whenever a student writes an answer in an instructional lesson, it is automatically checked for several types of errors which are of such a general nature that they are commonly found in almost all lessons, irrespective of the subject matter. The checks include: spelling, missing words, words out of order, extraneous words, broken phrases, and capitalization. Upon detecting one of these errors, the system simultaneously "marks up" the response and sets the value of a system variable to a specified quantity (see Figure 6). If the student can be assumed to be an experienced PLATO user, the markup itself gives sufficient information. If not, the system variables can be used by the author to select an appropriate error comment to supplement the markup.

Error markups are particularly valuable in scientific lessons. Suppose, for example, that a microbiology student had worked through a complicated exercise to the correct identification of an unknown but had misspelled the answer. The system would not simply reject the response but would, most probably, recognize and mark the spelling error, potentially saving the student a great deal of time and the repetition of the exercise. Note that the system need not accept the misspelled

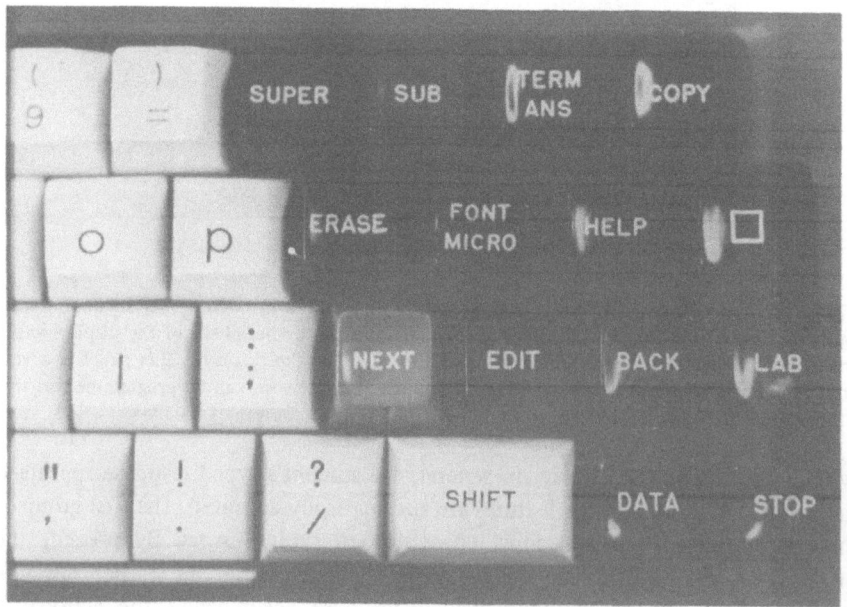

Figure 5. The PLATO keyset is like a standard typewriter keyboard except for numerical operators and the "function" keys that allow for student-controlled branching and very rapid alteration of incorrect entries. The SUPER and SUB keys are used to create super and subscripts while the FONT MICRO, and □ keys assist in using alternate fonts and special characters.

```
From which side does the superior rectus approach
the eyeball?

> laterraly
  ========
```

```
PLATO thinks that you may have misspelled the
underlined word.  Try typing it in again.
```

Figure 6. An implicit feature of the TUTOR language is the markup of many commonly made student errors – those, such as misspellings and words out of order, that are generally independent of the nature of the content material of the lesson. In this example, the author has used a system-reserved variable to identify the spelling error and to provide additional feedback. This requires some programmer attention while the markup (double underline in this case) itself is automatic. (From a lesson in the anatomy of the extraocular muscles – an original lesson written in ATS by W. Hagamen of Cornell University Medical College, TUTOR conversion by P. Cohen, edited by R. McCormick and G. Hody.)

response (though it can if the lesson designer so specifies). The student may be required to correct misspellings before being allowed to proceed. The algorithms that allow the computer to recognize a student response as a misspelled or incorrectly ordered version of what has been specified as the correct response are an integral part of the PLATO software. Thus, the lesson designer need not provide a list of all possible student errors in order to recognize departures from expected answers. Once the anticipated responses and the particular options desired are specified by the designer, the PLATO system itself can take over the judging of "near misses" (Tenczar and Golden, 1972). These options can also be disabled by the lesson author if desired, for example, in a spelling quiz.

Most students learn to use the terminal with the aid of a brief written "handout" and one of several introductory computer-based lessons available on the system. The choice of which lesson to use depends on the age and experience of the student. The typical user, whether in grammar school or postdoctoral training, becomes comfortable with the terminal and keyset within a few hours.

Machine to Student Interface Part 3: Access to Instructional Materials

Just finding a desired lesson to study is a common barrier in the customary CAI system. PLATO students need not be involved with cryptic code numbers or computer "file" names. Instead, they are identified by name and "course"* at sign-on time, and on the basis of this identification, they may be sent directly to specified lesson materials. If desired, they can be taken instead to an index display that lists the titles of all lessons which they can access. This computer-based lesson index may be customized to any necessary degree because it is written, like most other PLATO programs, in the standard PLATO language – TUTOR. If an instructor wishes, a unique curriculum can be designed for a single student, or a complex, multipage, branching index, a bit like the index of a sizeable textbook, can be assembled. Such an index would normally be used by a whole class. The instructional designer has the option of using either a system-provided routing routine for which it is only necessary to provide a "menu" of instructional programs or may design his or her own routine to suit needs unique to particular students. An example of such a special routine is an index that uses the language-processing capabilities of the PLATO system to permit conversational indexing of materials. This option is under experimental development by the Health Science Network. Finding one's way within an instructional module or segment can also be elusive. PLATO's speed and the judicious use of intuitively labeled function keys, such as NEXT and BACK, can be used to let the student leaf through instructional material more easily (Figure 7). After an interrupted session, students can be returned to the approximate place where they were previously working; however, this feature is not automatic – it requires the insertion of a few extra commands into the lesson program.

The Interpersonal Interface

The same technical features that allow for a variety of instructional lesson formats also encourage highly effective communications options for use by students, lesson authors, and classroom instructors. There are three ways that students can use the PLATO system to get help or information directly from human rather than computer resources. The most obvious is the "electronic mailbox." This entity, dubbed a "notefile," permits students to write notes, one page at a time. The notes may be "public" in which case they can be read and responded to by other PLATO users, or they can be designated "personal" in which case they must be addressed to an individual. In the case of personal notes, both originals and the automatically routed replies are private.

The second option is for students to enter comments while using an instructional lesson. Recently, PLATO announced a plan to make this option a standard system-supported feature of all lessons that would be available automatically without specific programming. At the moment, it requires the use of a special program segment that can be added to the lesson program with a few simple commands (Cohen, 1975). The comment feature is especially attractive because remarks can be

---

*PLATO "courses" designate groups of users for identification and data collection. Instructional modules often called "courses" on other systems are referred to as "lessons" on PLATO.

```
                          INDEX


  →  1.   Introduction to the nervous system

  →  2.   Anatomical differences between pns and sns

   **3.   Location of neurotransmitters

     4.   sns actions / α and β receptors in review

     5.   Review of organ innervation (sns)

     6.   pns actions

     7.   A diagram of the nervous system with
          a short quiz on transmitter location

     >

        (→  indicates completion of a section)
        (** indicates the last section studied)

  Please choose a number or press ███ alone to
  proceed in sequence through the lesson.
```

Figure 7. PLATO students select lessons from index displays rather than by mnemonic names and use additional indexing within lessons to overcome the problem of disorientation within programs. This illustration is a lesson index from a sequence in central nervous system pharmacology. (From a lesson written by the Kansas Medical Center Department of Pharmacology originally in COURSEWRITER III, converted to TUTOR by B. Cohen, series edited by R. Stull, G. Hody, and J. Woods.)

addressed from student to author without deletion of the display under study (the messages are written on the bottom two lines of the display screen – lines purposely left unused in lessons which permit comments). When the author reads back the student comments, each such note identifies the student, date on which the remarks were entered, and a mnemonic word keyed to the display that was on the screen at the time the comment was composed. These features as well as a sorting program for the comments are available without extra programming effort. Authors can reply to student comments by either private or public notes and they may choose to modify their lessons to incorporate new suggestions (a step which must be taken with caution due to the dangers of creating errors in programs already in frequent use).

The third communication method provides for monitoring of students by establishing an electronic link between the student and instructor or author displays so that both become the same. The monitor and monitoree can communicate about the lesson by typing on the bottom two lines of the screen and by using a cross-hair (cursor), they can point to items on the display if needed to illustrate their discussion. To prevent possible invasion of privacy, all monitoring is accompanied by an automatically generated message on the left-lower corner of the display that warns of the monitoring and identifies the monitor by name.

PLATO students in the health sciences are instructed regarding the PLATO communications features and are encouraged to use the human resources and the computer system in proportions that suit their individual needs.

Summary of Interface Features

The net result of speed, page orientation, rapid entry and correction of responses, full graphics capability, and high legibility of displays is a facility that is pleasant to use – even for extended periods. This means that instead of simple multiple choice entries, it is comfortable for students to respond in phrases, or by moving a cursor, or by pointing to something. Even more important, it is not necessary for explanatory text and diagrams to be the sparse, abbreviated output that many believe is the only way that computer-based systems can deal with humans. It is now possible to use almost the same range of visual expression on the system as is available in the classroom.

Authoring PLATO Lessons

PLATO programs, like most other computer-based educational materials, are groups of computer instructions. All PLATO lessons are written in TUTOR. The TUTOR commands for a given instructional segment, usually enough to occupy a typical student for between a few minutes and an hour, are contained in a TUTOR "file" that has a mnemonic name.*

Using the mnemonic name for a lesson, authors can choose either to "execute" the program, meaning to run it as a student would, or they can "edit" the file – make additions, deletions, or other changes to the computer instructions. In general, no security codes are needed to execute lessons but, of course, a lesson security code must be entered to see or change a lesson program.

To edit a file, an author types the name of the lesson on the entry display and presses the NEXT key. If the security codes match, the system provides, at the

---

*As previously noted, students do not need to know mnemonic names and can only access lessons from a predetermined index.

same time, access to both the contents of the requested lesson file and the system-editor routines. The process is far faster than reading this simple description of it.

The editor programs take full advantage of the system's speed and page orientation. Authors are able to write or modify the computer instructions with a broad choice of powerful editing options. Simple directives allow the user to locate desired segments, copy pieces of lesson programs electronically, or alter the contents of the programs by inserting, deleting, or changing anywhere from a single character to an entire line with a single keypress. Descriptions of the directives are always immediately available by pressing the HELP key while editing. The editor, as well as the HELP sequences, takes advantages of the instant key echoing of key presses and rapid processing of inputs that have been described under the options available to students.

Given the broad range of possible graphics that are instructionally useful on PLATO, the system must facilitate the design of drawings as much as possible. All PLATO graphics can be specified from the outset by TUTOR instructions. However, most authors find it vastly more convenient to use a versatile group of interactive drawing options available to all.* Using the interactive options, an author can create graphics with the help of a cursor controlled from the keyboard or touchpanel. Critical parts of the desired display (centers and diameters of circles, end points of lines, and position of text for example) are designated by single key presses. As in the editor, the HELP key supplies complete instructions at any time. The resulting designs can combine text, special characters, straight and curved line segments, single dots, and rotated, enlarged, or reduced combinations of the above into figures that are seen in the editor exactly as they will later be reproduced for the student. When the display appears satisfactory, a press of the function key, BACK, activates a rapid conversion that creates TUTOR instructions for the display in a few seconds and places the resultant commands and tags into the appropriate location of the lesson program.

Small but intricate figures can be drawn with "special" or "lineset" characters. Authors can either choose to create new illustrations with an interactive generator much like the one described above, or an existing set can be copied from a large and well documented library. As with display-editing options, an author does not need to manipulate TUTOR instructions to create or display special characters and linesets.

Testing PLATO Lessons

Once a lesson segment has been completed by the author, it can be tested immediately. Within a few seconds, the TUTOR instructions are prepared for execution by a routine called the "condensor,"† a routine initiated by a single keypress.

---

*The most useful of these were designed and produced by Richard Blomme, David Frankel, and Marshall Midden of the PLATO software staff.

†Technically, PLATO'S "condensor" is mainly a compiling routine that converts "source code" (human-readable instructions) into "binaries" (machine-executable instructions). Binaries are stored between sessions so, in general, re-condensing is done only if changes have been made in the lesson (or in the operating system).

After "condensing" the lesson, the author can experience all the displays and inter-actions that a student taking that lesson would. At any time, the author can, with a single keypress, return to the PLATO editor to make further changes to the lesson program.

Documentation "On-Line" and Author AIDS

Comprehensive and frequently updated documentation of the author language is available on line in a program called "AIDS."* AIDS contains descriptions of all TUTOR commands and words, explanations of the workings of the system, and includes suggestions for instructional design. It also provides a guide to the system's libraries of subroutines for computation and display materials and illustrative, inter-active examples of how the TUTOR options described therein actually work. Sections of AIDS are accessed by a detailed conventional index and, in addition, with the help of a recognition routine that can identify any one of over 1400 forms of natural-language requests for about 700 different information presentations.

Based on data from over 1700 requests per day over a period of 128 days, it has been found that 93.3% of requests are handled without problems by this technique. Another 2.6% are identified as possible misspellings of recognized concepts and, as would be done by a human, are routed to the information that is thought to be needed. For the small balance of unsatisfied requests, the author can normally obtain an answer from colleagues, system notefiles, "on-line" consultants, off-line documents, or by experimenting a bit.

AIDS is fast: for over $\frac{2}{3}$ of the requests, by actual measurement, the information is provided in less than half a second, while the average delay for the balance is 3 seconds (Kraatz, 1976).

One of the advantages of large or linked CAI systems is the fact that a "critical mass" of experienced users is accessible via public notes with very short turnaround time. This means that the experience commonly represented by "interest groups" for most CAI systems can be communicated in a matter of hours rather than the weeks that are necessary when such groups must resort to printed communication and the mail.

In cases where an extremely fast response is needed (or where problems are too minor to bother other users), the author can "page" a consultant. Communicating on the bottom two lines of the screen, the author and consultant can discuss the problem and either one can show their screen display to the other to illustrate their discussion. Consultants are usually available during the normal workday and often work at other times as well.

A potential disadvantage of the communications features of a large system like PLATO is the risk of information overload. The proliferation of notefiles, comment files, and other options for exchange of opinions and data becomes difficult to

---

*Developed jointly by James Ghesquiere and members of the consulting and software staffs of CERL.

keep up with and can take an inordinate amount of time from the work schedule of conscientious authors. One method of ameliorating this difficulty is logical indexing and classification of the notefiles. This problem with reference to "computer-based conferencing" has been discussed by Vallee (1975).

When PLATO detects an error — either incorrect use of the TUTOR language or attempts to perform in some manner outside of the permissible range of options — lesson execution is interrupted by a special error display. If this occurs to a student (and such occurrences should be extremely rare with well-tested lessons), the display asks students to copy the information and relay it to an instructor. Authors who encounter error displays during lesson testing can return to "edit mode" at the precise program statement that is causing the problem. Alternatively, they can request an expanded and detailed computer-assisted analysis and explanation of the error and, if the matter is still obscure after that, can opt to see the specific section of AIDS that describes the problematical command or feature. All of this is done within seconds and without leaving the system or losing one's place in the work. All error comments are in plain language and contain a minimum of abbreviations and codes.

The TUTOR Language

All PLATO instructional material is written in TUTOR; however, it is not always necessary to learn any TUTOR to write PLATO lessons (alternatives will be elaborated further below). TUTOR is analogous to "high level" languages used for science and business programs in that it has a "command and tag" structure and allows the user direct access to computer functions and storage spaces. It is totally different from the traditional languages in its capabilities. Included in TUTOR are features that handle both graphics and text, accept and respond to student input, and store student-response data for later analysis.

Features of the Language

TUTOR contains built-in inferences about the way in which computer—human communications should be handled in the instructional setting; commands used to accept and/or store student input and responses are an excellent example of this. These "judging commands," in recognition of the difficulty of anticipating human responses in dialogues, make it simple for the author to specify the synonymity of words or concept phrases that, once entered, remain in effect for the duration of the program unless revoked. The ability of the system to make assumptions about the handling of student inputs is further illustrated by the way it detects and indicates spelling and other errors as has been described previously. The system also handles automatically many other tasks that would normally have to be constantly reprogrammed by the author of instructional materials. For example, when a student receives a feedback comment after an erroneous response, the comment is automatically erased by the system at the time the student attempts a new answer. All TUTOR features for the inferential handling of human—machine interaction are readily inhibitable by lesson authors, but the automatic availability of the features is both a timesaver for authors and a major factor that improves the quality of lessons delivered to the students. A basic style suggestion proposed for all basic medical science authors is therefore: "Never inhibit built-in TUTOR options unless you are sure of precisely why you are doing so!" Such advice can be given only because these automatic features are the result of many years of evolutionary experience in presenting a wide range of instructional materials in an equally wide range of teaching approaches.

TUTOR files are called "lessons" on PLATO — even if they are not instructional in function. PLATO employs a 60-bit computer word of which a PLATO file designed for instructional use can hold a maximum of 13,375. Because a single character consists of 6 bits of information, one TUTOR file can hold a maximum of 133,750 characters, which is equivalent to about 50 double-spaced typewritten pages of text. Of course, computer instructions and text are not all that comparable in any practical sense, but the figures are useful for giving an idea — albeit very rough — of the amount of information in a file.

The internal organization of lessons is entirely up to the author; however, in many cases, it is convenient to arrange instructional material in such a way that all necessary components of an instructional sequence will be in one file. TUTOR lessons can be linked readily so students can "jumpout" from one to another, either under program control or by making a voluntary selection from an index display. Thus, the capacity of a single file is not an absolute limit on the potential length or complexity of a PLATO lesson. Nevertheless, frequent "jumpouts" from file-to-file increase the rate of use of computer resources and are discouraged in some cases, particularly during high load periods. This means that a single TUTOR file normally covers a specific, rather narrow, single-topic area rather than several hours of instruction.

Within a TUTOR file, commands and tags are organized into "units," addressable sequences of computer instructions that are usually relatively brief. Units can contain the instructions for displays, accepting student responses, calculating, and branching to other units, or any combination of these. Any TUTOR unit in a program may be "called" by any other unit in the program and may be rapidly repeated as often as desired without having to be rewritten. Thus, the language inherently structures the programs into easily readable subroutines. The use of units also decreases redundancy, because pieces of programs that must be repeated during execution need be written and stored only once.

It is often assumed that sophisticated computational capabilities are not needed in instructional computer systems. Experience over the past 10 years with the PLATO system has shown this to be a self-limiting view. In order to provide instruction that requires mathematics and in the physical sciences as well as to provide the high-level simulations that can uniquely be done by computer in all subject-matter areas, powerful computational capabilities are a necessity (Smith and Sherwood, 1976).

TUTOR has an extensive group of calculational commands that are reduced essentially to direct machine-level instructions at "condense" time (when a lesson is made executable). These give the system an efficient way to compute rapidly — a capability that is used not only to facilitate the student's work but also to take over a good bit of the labor of structuring displays, creating animations, and taking data. PLATO is gradually being supplied with increasingly advanced facilities for the manipulation of arrays and matrices although, for some time, these will remain modest in maximum size to conserve memory space and processing time. The system has built-in standard mathematical functions, such as the trigonometric and logarithmic ones, and a powerful calculator may be called into play from any PLATO display unless inhibited (as in an arithmetic lesson) by an author.

TUTOR display commands are nearly plain English. They are supplemented by a group of commands expressly for the construction of coordinate graphs. These can use either Cartesian or polar axes and can plot points, author-designed symbols, curves, or vectors. The commands rapidly create dimension and label axes — all by interactive computation. Many other TUTOR commands are available to provide for sequencing of operations, conversational interaction with the students, and a whole armamentarium of specialized technical functions.*

Learning TUTCR or Avoiding it

In 1967, disgusted with the amount of extraneous labor necessary to program computer-based lessons in existing languages, Paul Tenczar, then a zoology graduate student, created TUTOR to provide a simpler way for good teachers to prepare instructional materials. It was originally intended to be a language in which authors could be quickly trained and for whose use they would not need to know much about programming methods and computers. As the PLATO community increased in size, commands and features were added to TUTOR in response both to user requests and to data from student and author interactions. The resulting language is now rather complex and difficult to master completely. While it is still simple to use TUTOR to create uncomplicated lessons, there is general confusion, outside of the PLATO community, about just how difficult it is to get started authoring on PLATO. Perhaps Nelson (1974) sums it up most accurately:

> To learn the first steps in TUTOR — how to set up drill and practice lessons for instance — is unusually easy. To do anything complex, however, requires you to learn the bulk of the TUTOR language.

Early data from the PLATO evaluation team support the estimate that an experienced teacher who has never used a computer before (Figure 8) will have to work on PLATO for about 3 months on the basis of half-time release to begin to write acceptable programs in TUTOR (Avner *et al.*, 1972). This lag period can be

---

*For example, there is a TUTOR command that causes the terminal to write from right to left for Hebrew and Persian lessons.

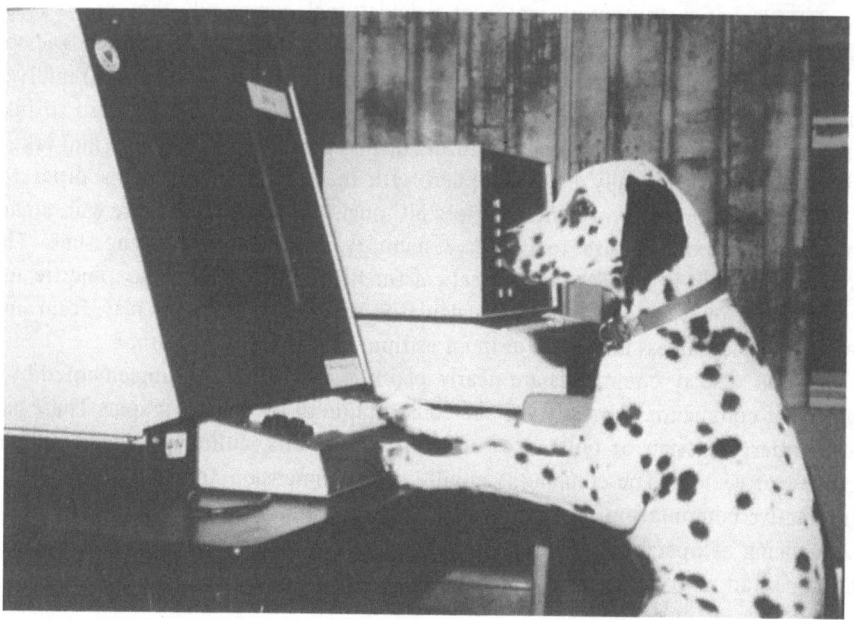

Figure 8. While PLATO can be used by almost any student with very little instruction, authors require time and practice with TUTOR in direct proportion to the sophistication of the materials they expect to produce. In fact, this user, whose name is Embers, was probably not studying at all but, rather, was enjoying one of the many PLATO recreational lessons — in this case, probably "Dogfight."

dramatically shortened by the use of prepared formats that allow the creation of lessons without any knowledge of the TUTOR language.

A team approach in which a programmer codes the computer instructions for a content specialist is used by many PLATO author groups in frank departure from the original philosophy of the system. Often this method yields poor results, mainly due to communications problems and the difficulty of understanding the system's capabilities in the absence of significant experience with it. The use of "driver" programs that accept author input in *student mode* is another compromise. Many such special programs are available on PLATO including a group of them specialized for the generation and scoring of examinations. Perhaps the most elaborate such routine is used instead to create complex computer-based lessons. It is called QWRITER (Stull *et al.*, 1976).

QWRITER, created by the Basic Science Author Group at the University of Illinois, queries the author for questions, text, answers, and help sequences and then generates all of the TUTOR code necessary for the lesson. QWRITER includes sufficient prompting and error interception that it takes only a 3 to 5 day workshop session (or a few days of self-paced experimentation) to learn its use — even without any previous similar experience. A brief intervention by a PLATO programmer is needed to make the QWRITER module operational at the start and again at the end of the authoring period (this takes less than 5 minutes). The resulting program calls on run-time subroutines already established by QWRITER insuring error-free program execution, consistent standards of programming quality, built-in data collection, and a student comment facility. While QWRITER does not at present generate graphics, it may be modified to do so in the future and, in any case, the system permits programmers to edit and modify further already activated QWRITER lessons. While QWRITER rather limits the format of the resulting instructional module to a predetermined and essentially linear structure, it gives new authors an early start toward improved productivity and has resulted in some excellent health science lessons.

It strikes the authors as ironic that many computer systems that are used heavily for teaching cannot teach their own programming language and methods. This is increasingly less true of PLATO, on which many lessons that teach the TUTOR language by interactive experimentation and testing are becoming available. The PLATO Service Organization (PSO) and the Military Training Centers Project (MTC) have been particularly attentive to the need for these types of instructional lessons.

Excellent off-line documentation of the TUTOR language and a clear and easy to read how-to-do-it textbook on TUTOR are now available (Avner, 1975; Sherwood, 1974). AIDS includes some suggestions for programming standards and instructional design, and these helpful sections for new authors will hopefully continue to be extended.

Data Collection

One of the more attractive features of many computer-based educational systems is that they can collect objective data that can be used to improve the lesson materials. It is important to select with care the nature and quantity of the data and to analyze and organize the information in a manageable manner. The PLATO system has had a unique advantage in data-collection procedures because of its evolutionary development from the PLATO III system, which preceded the curent version in the mid 1960s. One PLATO III project used PLATO's generous computational and storage capability to collect complete data on selected lessons and student groups (Easley, 1966). These data were so detailed that they permitted the experimenters to "play back" and simulate the interaction of an entire class! Thus, an instructor or researcher could stroll about the PLATO classroom and observe the same activity at each terminal that had earlier occurred while the students were present. The advantage of this rather heroic experiment with exhaustive data collection was that helpful items could be identified by the process of eliminating nonessential information rather than by the inverse method of sequentially testing selected items of data hypothesized to be of value. This project also produced some very useful new analytical software that was able to identify patterns of student interaction with instructional materials. One of the surprising outcomes of the study was that most instructional designers used only the most basic sort of collected information. The most often-requested items were unanticipated student responses and unsuccessful attempts to perform branching. Despite the availability of much more quantitative and statistical information, few instructor/authors made use of the routines. At the same time, limiting data-collection options on PLATO to the very basic information alone proved to be unsatisfactory, because a small but significant proportion of the authors needed additional information that was unique to special instructional techniques they were using. It was also noted that under production pressures authors who did not have rapid and easy access to data tended to minimize its use in making revisions of material — often with the result that large numbers of students were exposed to materials of dubious quality before necessary revisions were made.

A compromise approach, used in the current system, incorporates into the TUTOR language special commands that give lesson designers total access to virtually all possible student interactions with the instructional material. Thus, experienced authors can design in TUTOR their own data-collection and processing routines explicitly suited to their special instructional approach. At the same time, the most often-requested items of information are provided by standard system features that do not require explicit instructions from authors. Thus, an instructional designer may specify with a very few commands that, for all or a subset of students using a given lesson, all unanticipated responses should be stored (for later analysis for content by system-provided search, selection, and display routines). This example does not require writing of new TUTOR routines by the author. An author who, on the other hand, wants to introduce special measures of redundancy in a problem-solving simulation would have to write a special program to collect that highly specific and unusual information. Summaries of commonly used administrative data, such as the amount of time spent in a lesson, the percentage of questions answered on the first attempt, and similar data, are collected and summarized automatically by the system.

System Reliability

Although a user of a CAI system can generally adapt to limitations in its design, it is seldom the case that one can get used to unreliability. Loss of time due to system unreliability works a particular hardship in medical education where resource costs are high and time itself is at a special premium. Unfortunately, estimation of system reliability for a CAI system is often a very difficult matter. Many systems are in a constant state of modification or expansion. The state of the art of hardware is changing rapidly, and cost considerations frequently dictate the use of components for which no complete history of reliability is available. Even well-seasoned components may be used under conditions for which no adequate reliability experience exists. In the case of the PLATO system, these factors are further affected by the fact that a substantial number of the components have been designed specifically for the system and, hence, are in a near-prototype rather than production form. Against these considerations is the fact that the PLATO system has been subjected, in the course of well over two-million terminal-hours of use, to a wide variety of physical environments and system-wide reliability data have been continually kept. In order to insure validity of data, any user having "author" or higher privileges has access to an on-line program that identifies all current sources of system unreliability and summarizes past experience. Thus, "customers" are able to verify that a report of a terminal or communication problem has been recorded or to read a description of the time, cause, and duration of system-wide problems that have happened in the recent past during "prime time" (the hours from 7:40 A.M. to 10 P.M. on weekdays and 8 A.M. to 12 P.M. on Saturdays when the PLATO IV system attempts to provide service of highest reliability).

From the viewpoint of the user, the three major causes of unreliability of service are the central computer complex, the communications channels, and the individual terminal. Communications problems are largely a function of the distance of the user from the central computer. Once established, short local links cause few problems. Unfortunately, the same is not the case for long links that rely on services of several commercial common carriers. Although virtually all telephone services in the continental United States offer communications lines that ostensibly meet standards of quality required for data transfer, many local services do not yet, in fact, have the experience required to these standards. The most common effect of such communications problems for PLATO users at distances of hundreds or thousands of miles from the Urbana computer is degraded service. High error rates in communication cause perceptible delays when the automatic error-correction devices in the PLATO terminal and at the computer require several retransmissions of data before data meeting internal consistency checks are received. At very high error rates, it becomes possible for parity checks of data to be met by chance alone, and the terminal or computer will accept isolated items of "noise" as legitimate data. In a sense, the automatic error correction built into the PLATO system can lead to acceptance by the user of poor service, because it can compensate (with resulting loss in response time) for communications links that are substantially below the standards specified by the common carrier.

The balance of reliability problems is about equally divided (in terms of total lost time) between the terminal and the central computer complex. Terminal problems of remote sites generally have more serious impact simply because of the delays in transportation of required service personnel or replacement parts from a central location. Thus, although "remote" terminals (those outside the Urbana and Chicago areas) actually have a somewhat lower frequency of problems because of less severe use, they tend to remain out of service for a substantially longer period of time.

For the first 5 months of 1976 the mean time to failure for a PLATO terminal or its auxiliary equipment was 10.96 weeks. On a system-wide basis, a terminal reported "down" was back in operation in an average of 1.36 days (this figure includes night, weekend, and holiday time when terminal maintenance service is not normally available). For "remote" terminals alone the average delay in return to operation was over twice as long. Such differences are basically a matter of economics. The Chicago metropolitan area, while physically "remote" from Urbana, has a sufficient number of terminals to justify support of a local maintenance staff. Though terminals in the Chicago area are widely dispersed, the mean down time can be kept close to the system average of 1.36 days.

Mean time to failure for the central PLATO system during the first 5 months of 1976 ranged from a catastrophic 4.99 hours during December (resulting from the trauma of installation of a new computer) to 26.40 hours during a more settled March with an average of 18.45 hours for the entire period. The combined effects of central system, terminal, and communications reliability resulted in an average availability of 95.4% of scheduled hours during the period. In addition, approximately 90% of nonscheduled hours were available to users willing to be interrupted for brief periods by system tests of experimental software. Test versions of software are commonly evaluated during nonscheduled hours of operation. Such a procedure has been found to be of mutual benefit to users (usually authors preparing new instructional materials) who are able to have added access to the system, and to the system staff, which is able to test new system software under realistic conditions.

Basic Principles of PLATO Design and Operation

The most essential aspects of PLATO design, seen from a user perspective, are speed and potentially very low operating costs. Under the constraints of traditionally designed data-processing systems, speed and economy are considered to be tradeoffs – they are mutually exclusive properties. PLATO provides both by redistributing the pattern of use that is normally seen in data processing – from a basically intermittent function to an essentially continuous one.

There are two components to this novel approach. The first is philosophical and financial in nature – services are billed to users on an *annual basis* – the charges are completely independent of the amount of time the user is on the system, the amount of processing that is done, or the size of the memory space that is used. This promotes increased and efficient use of PLATO's relatively costly terminal equipment and frees users from budgetary worries while using the terminal. Billed "by the hour," a computer-based education system could be affordable only if it had a modest number of hours of use. By contrast, PLATO depends for economy on a very high utilization rate. The more it is used, the less the hourly cost.

The second component of the PLATO approach to data processing is mainly technical. It includes the use of special processing, memory, and communications equipment designed for education, and the management of these key resources by monitoring programs that insure equitable distribution of computer service to all users. The important "hardware factors" are (1) a powerful processor, (2) extremely rapid information access and transfer between the computer's processor and the short-term "working memory," and (3) a communications system that never impedes data flow from the system to the terminals.

The PLATO system consists fundamentally of about 950 terminals connected mostly by dedicated telephone lines to a central processing facility. The equipment in Urbana includes a controlling and formatting device for communications (the network interface unit or NIU); magnetic disks for long-term storage of massive amounts of lessonware and data, the central processing unit (CPU), and the high-speed memory system (CDC "extended core storage" or "ECS"). Figure 9 provides a schematic overview of the system. From the user point of view, the resources that are allocated by the management software are the high-speed memory (ECS), processing power (CPU), disk access rates, and the use of the condensor (compiler program). The communication system is available at all times at the same high transmission rate (it is not "managed"). This is crucial for rapid response and will be explained further.

PLATO communications are mediated through a network of special-purpose mini-computers — the network interface unit (NIU). The NIU combines the output data for all terminals and formats it for transmission on a standard television channel. The system is designed to serve "classroom clusters" of 32 terminals. Each cluster is equipped with a device called the "site controller" that recovers the data from the TV channel and transmits it to the appropriate terminal. The terminals need not be physically near the site controller — they can be connected to it with ordinary voice-grade telephone lines (up to 4 terminals may be multiplexed on one phone line).*

The speed of the computer processing would be wasted if there were "hangups" in the transmission system. By leaving the communications job to a series of mini-computer "peripheral processors," and by the use of an unusual data transmission format (which structures the data in a time-divided multiplexed fashion), the system maintains what its developers describe as an "open pipeline" that can provide data to each terminal at a continuous (not average) guaranteed rate of around 1200 bits per second (baud) (Sherwood and Stifle, 1975). This insures that output will be developed smoothly with time — or more precisely that the system will not be "input/output bound" with respect to speed. An integral component of the communications apparatus checks for line errors and retransmits data that might have been scrambled.

In most cases, then, response speed is a function of available computing power. This is a major reason for the use of a large computer for PLATO. In many time-sharing systems used for CAI, the system permits individual users to monopolize the computing power for appreciable periods. PLATO, on the other hand, permits users very high peak computing rates for *very* short periods. The average rate of use for each user is frequently measured and closely controlled. If the system is under a heavy load, users who exceed an average of 2000 machine operations per second during a given session are "stopped" by a TUTOR feature, called autobreak, that is designed to interrupt program execution at points where no data will be lost. When autobreak occurs, the result is a brief hesitation in program execution —

---

*A new multiplexer that will couple 8 PLATO terminals to 1 voice-grade phone line is in a prototype development stage at CERL.

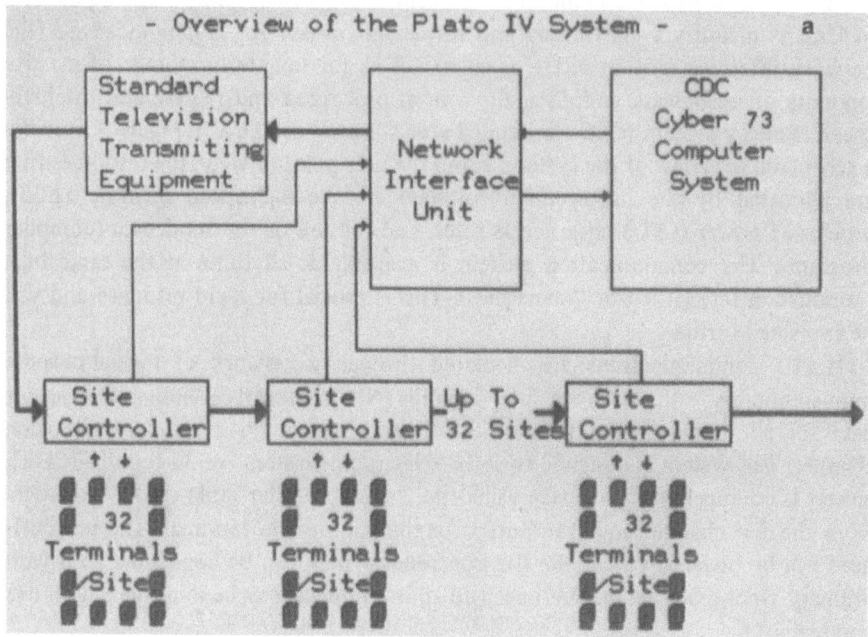

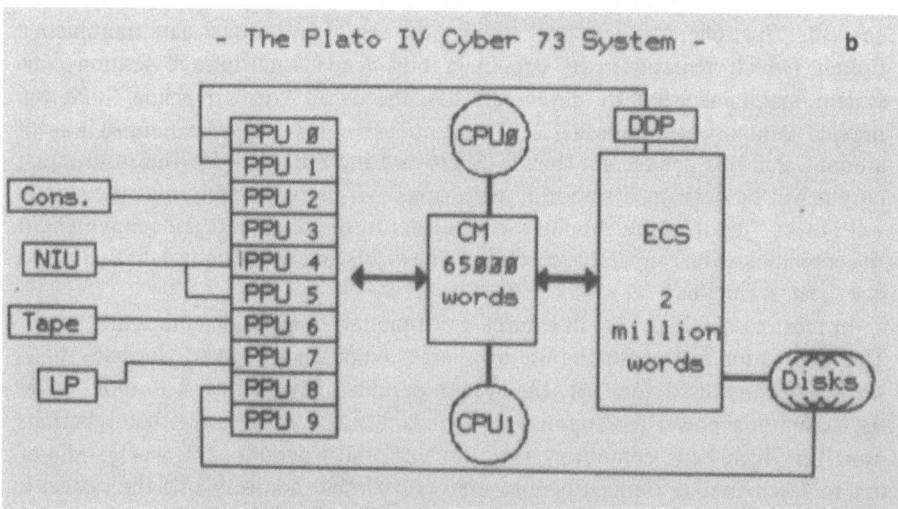

Figure 9. The PLATO system is possible because of special equipment for communication between the terminal and the computer system as well as special organization and design of the components within the processing center. These features are discussed in the text and explained in more detail in the referenced articles.

rarely more than a few seconds. Well designed lessons never autobreak when executed under normal circumstances by students, since peak demands for computations or simulations will be balanced by periods of low load when the student is thinking or responding. Autobreaks generally occur either because the author has assumed that extra computing power will be available (lessons designed expressly for "off-peak" periods) or because the executor of the lesson is familiar with the materials and is running through the program at a much higher rate than would the primary audience for which it is designed.

Fast access to stored data, as important as processing speed, requires electronic memory. Electromechanical devices, such as disk and tape, are fine for long-term lesson storage but hopelessly slow for giving access to active lessons. On the other hand, extension of computer-fast central memory to accommodate the lesson materials for an appreciable number of students would be extremely costly. The solution selected for PLATO was ECS (extended core storage). Because ECS is easily available only on Control Data computers, PLATO, as a system, is currently designed to be run on machines made by that manufacturer. A typical PLATO lesson occupies between 4000 and 6000 words of ECS; thus, even the 2,000,000 words of ECS available on PLATO* are insufficient to give each of 950 terminals a unique lesson program to run. A partial solution is to separate the lesson program from each user's status information for that program. As many users as desired can then "share" an existing copy of a lesson program in ECS, each new entrant adding only a 400-word-long "status bank" to the drain on ECS. Even with this feature, the current PLATO system can support fewer lessons than there are terminals. Either lessons must be "shared" or fewer than 950 terminals must be in use.†

PLATO lessons are stored for the long term on large disks. The current disks each have a capacity of approximately 2.5 million words of storage or about 500 typical PLATO lessons. By adding more disks, capacity can be expanded almost indefinitely. Because the system is under continuing evolution, all of its information is kept on disk in dynamically alterable form. Thus, when evolutionary changes are made in the operating system, they can be immediately reflected in all the courseware — a condition that could not be met if the materials were stored as paper tape or cards and distributed to the individual authors.

System Resource Management

> If the system does not respond for more than five minutes, you can assume it is down and you should telephone a systems programmer. (From a sign on the wall of an anonymous laboratory in computer-based education)

---

*Approximately 20% of the ECS is required for the PLATO operating software including TUTOR and author aids of various types — this is considered operating "overhead."

†Between 200 and 400 simultaneous *different* lessons can be supported by the current system without exceeding ECS supplies. Other considerations discussed elsewhere in the chapter also influence the number of possible simultaneous users.

That sign would never be found in a PLATO facility. The feeling of responsiveness that is characteristic of the system is due to the short time allowed to elapse between the time of a user input and the time at which the system *first* starts to respond. For terminals within a 35-mile radius, this interval is guaranteed to be less than 0.2 seconds, for "remote" sites, it may be up to 0.1 second longer. For simple operations, such as the echoing of key presses, it is *completely independent of system load* from 0 to over 400 simultaneous users (Tenczar, 1975). To accomodate a large number of users, many of whom may have unusual requirements, the system has an elaborate "real-time" dynamic software management program that allocates resources to users in such a way as (a) to guarantee absolutely all users a minimum level of service at all times; (b) to permit very high rates of peak resource use for any given user — provided average rates of use are within prescribed limits; and (c) to apportion unused "overflow" resources (if any) equitably among all users.

As a result of allocating unused resources on demand, the general expectation of level of service is higher among users than can be supported under conditions of maximum system load. Thus, satisfaction with service is very high for all classes of users when less than about 350 terminals are in use on the University of Illinois system. With from 350 to 400 running at once, satisfaction is slightly less, especially for nonstudent types of operations such as editing files (response time is still superior to most other systems and tolerable for PLATO). Over 500 users are rarely seen, mostly because, in a group of 1000 terminals, many are bound to be unused as a result of individual scheduling considerations but also because, at that point, surplus resources have diminished to the stage where experienced PLATO users begin to find it increasingly unpleasant to work — ECS becomes hard to find, processing slows, and authors get very unhappy. Students, in many cases, can continue contentedly with 400 to 500 simultaneous users. Although it would be easily possible to limit all users at all times to the service available at peak load conditions, such a policy would limit applications to those that fit a preconceived notion of how CAI should work. The present policy (based on a conscious evolutionary viewpoint) allows testing of styles of instruction that, admittedly, cannot currently be supported on a guaranteed basis. The cost for this exploration is an apparant degradation in the level of service for users who have become accustomed to using PLATO during off-peak hours and find they must suddenly share it with a larger group.

Cost

Although cost is one of the most important factors in the selection of a CBE system, it is difficult to determine it. The diversity of fund sources and the multiplicity of services supplied by CBE systems do make accounting and reporting tedious, and systems still in the research and development phases can validly claim that they have too little data to make firm cost estimates. However, the majority of institutions and vendors alike are so reticent to cite cost estimates in public that they appear to harbor paranoid fears of what might be done with that information! Perhaps what happened to PLATO in this respect has taught them a lesson. During the planning phases for the current version, CERL was a picture of candor regarding projected costs. The best example of this open policy was a scholarly analysis, appearing in *Science*, that placed the maximum cost estimate for PLATO service at $0.75 per student contact hour (Alpert and Bitzer, 1970). Unfortunately, the original estimates proved wide of the mark and were roundly ridiculed by the educational computing community. Perhaps, as a result, PLATO is now extremely reluctant to issue cost information. The most recent article about PLATO in *Science* has only a short section on costs — one that can best be characterized as delicately evasive (Smith and Sherwood, 1976).

In the absence of official data, the authors have elected to compute their own estimates. After making a few reasonable assumptions, this is not difficult to do with a good chance of "ball-park accuracy." It is particularly important, however, for the reader to understand the nature of the assumptions behind the numbers and, armed with this understanding, to be able to correct the figures for hypothetical cases in which some of the basic parameters may differ.

The first assumption concerns the number of hours a year terminals are used (see Figure 10). Normally, the cost of computer-based instruction in the health sciences is expressed per student contact hour. For such systems as PLATO that charge per terminal per year, irrespective of how much a terminal is used, the hourly rate is obtained by taking the annual charge and dividing it by the number of terminal contact hours per year. By actual measurement, PLATO terminals on the Illinois system are used for an average of 1300 hours a year (Smith and Sherwood, 1976). Many health science users get higher rates than that, and it is not unreasonable to assume that a CBE facility successfully embedded in an enthusiastic health science school setting could amass 2000 hours a year per terminal — this would mean only 40 hours a week for 50 weeks a year, for example.

The second conjecture concerns the cost of student terminals. Since the current price is about $10,000 in single lots, a figure of $7500 seems reasonable for the 1000-lot purchase hypothesized for this estimate.* Taking similarly conservative estimates for the costs of rather lush supportive services and overhead, one arrives at the figures in Table 1 — an annual cost of $6400 per year per terminal or $4.92 per student contact hour based on the 1300-hour-a-year estimate, and $3.20 per contact hour if a 2000-hour-a-year rate is realized. No doubt a more Spartan, yet still acceptable, facility could be acquired for considerably less.

Two sources of highly tentative information are available to test these estimates. First, CERL has recently announced that its NSF contracts will terminate soon and that thereafter it will offer PLATO service to current users outside of the university on a cost-recovery basis. The unofficial figure that is often heard for this cost is about $2400 a year for users with their own terminals. If one adds the estimated pro-rata annual fee of $1500 for the terminal and a little extra for local

---

*The PLATO terminals now owned by the University of Illinois were, in fact, purchased 1000 at a time at a unit cost of slightly under $6000 (Smith and Sherwood, 1976).

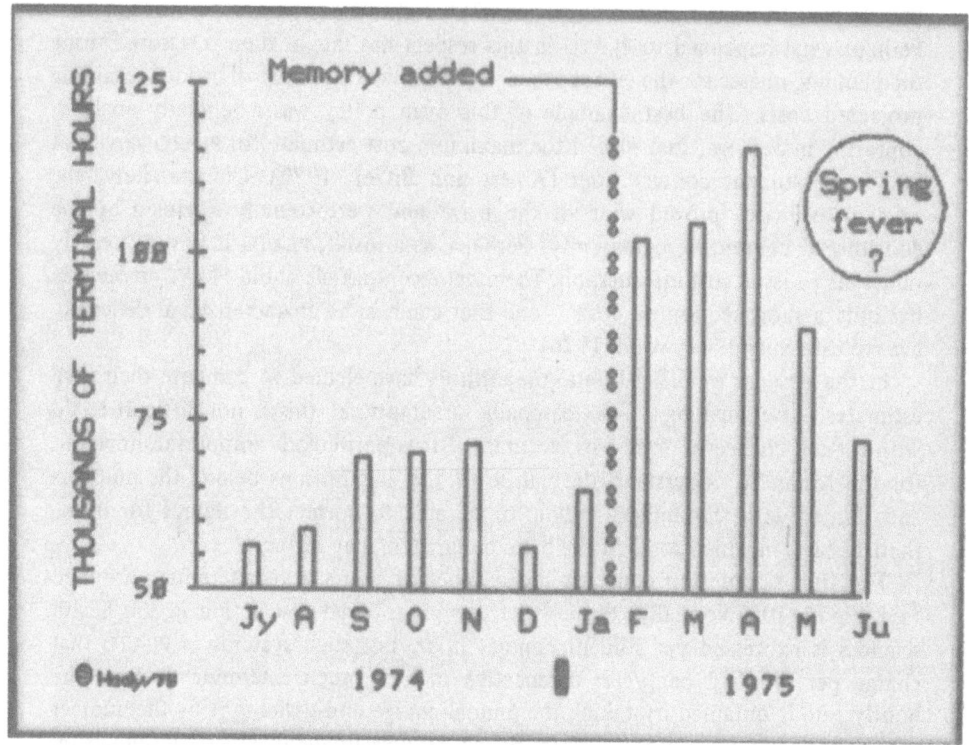

Figure 10. The economy of the PLATO system depends upon a high volume of use and the system's ability to sustain a rapid response in the face of heavy use. A hundred thousand hours of student and author contact per month (as much as 5000 student contact hours per day) are not unusual. This graph, generated by PLATO, illustrates a typical rate of use for a period of a year and a half, subdivided by months. In January, 1975, new active memory (ECS) was added and the effect of this new resource on the user population is seen in the use rate figures. Data are from the PLATO Educational Evaluation and Research (PEER) Group.

Table 1. The Estimated Cost of PLATO Service

Item	Annual Cost ($)[a]	
	Total	Per student terminal
Terminals	1,500,000	1,500
Computer facility	2,300,000	2,300
Staff and related overhead	1,400,000	1,400
Communications and miscellaneous supplies	1,200,000	1,200
Total	$6,400,000	6,400

[a]Rental or amortization of purchase cost over 5 years.

communications, the result is not too far from the postulated $6400 annual rate. The second piece of supporting information comes from recent announcements by Control Data Corporation, which plans to market PLATO services. Including the terminals, on a 2-year contract, the cost is expected to be about $8000 a year per terminal – within a reasonable distance of the estimate above (Pantages, 1976).

Finally, if one corrects the original Alpert and Bitzer data for the decrease in the numbers of connected student terminals from their postulated 4096 to the actual 1000 and then multiplies by a factor of 1.5 for inflation since 1969, the result, $4.50 per hour, also supports the current estimate. In conclusion, it appears that, for the next few years, PLATO services will cost somewhere between $3.50 and $5.00 per student-contact hour* and should decrease thereafter.

Future Developments

The future plans for PLATO include expansion, commercial marketing, and serious attempts to maintain communications and compatibility between the various systems expected to be established. The Control Data Corporation (CDC) has completed contractual negotiations with the University of Illinois as the result of which it will be able to market not only the PLATO terminal and other special equipment but also the TUTOR language and agreed-upon portions of the course materials. CDC has announced plans to form at least five regional PLATO centers in the United States with a combined total of 2000 terminals by the end of 1977 (Pantages, 1976).

The Florida State University has the first private institutional PLATO system outside of Illinois and will be expanding its facilities.

Technical developments, some of which are already in prototype stages, include plasma display terminals equipped with built-in microprocessors that can take over some of the display tasks as well as adapt themselves to the parameters of non-PLATO computers (in particular those that use the ASCII conventions) (see Figure 11). A multiplexer that can couple as many as eight PLATO terminals to a single telephone line is said to be under development to cut the communications costs at long distances. Finally, a number of PLATO features, including the use of the TUTOR language and the PLATO display, may be available in whole or in part on other systems including some "mini" and "midi" computers as the result of work performed by Schuyler, Chen, and others (Schuyler, 1974; T. Chen, personal communication). Hopefully, the technologists will cooperate with the educators to insure that all PLATO and PLATO-like systems that are designed in the future will remain compatible so that course materials can be interchanged for sharing between systems with a minimum of effort.

---

*The cost of lesson materials, not included in this estimate, may add from $0.10 to $0.50 per hour additional, in author royalties (a current, rough, "best guess").

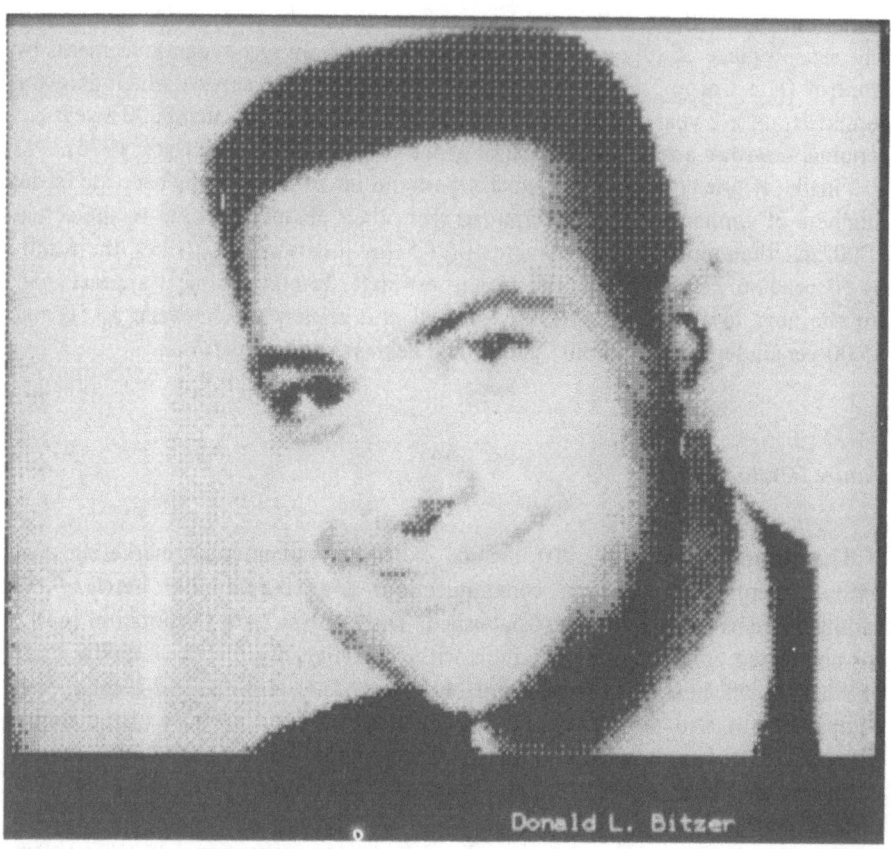

Donald L. Bitzer

Figure 11. The present PLATO system allows testing of special features that use computer resources at a high rate, provided this is done when there are modest demands on the system. An example of such a feature is the computer-generation of high-quality, full-screen, halftone images, such as this photo of PLATO's originator and director, Dr. Donald L. Bitzer. The use of microprocessor terminals and other future developments are expected to make such illustrations, now requiring excessively long plotting times and memory allocations for prime time use, practical for unrestricted access. Halftone illustrations of this type, restricted to a smaller portion of the display and limited to a few examples per lesson, are successfully used.

ACKNOWLEDGMENTS

Additional information about the PLATO system may be obtained from the Director, Computer-based Education Laboratory, University of Illinois, Urbana, Illinois 61801. Inquiries about health science applications should be addressed to the Director, Medical Information Science Department, School of Basic Medical Sciences, University of Illinois, Urbana, Illinois 61801. The commercial version of PLATO is available from the Control Data Corporation, P.O. Box 0, Minneapolis, Minnesota 55440.

References

Alpert, D. and Bitzer, D. L., 1970. Advances in computer-based education, *Science* 167: 1582–1590 (March 20).

Avner, E., 1975. PLATO user's memo (A summary of TUTOR commands and system variables), No. 2, 2nd ed. (June) CERL, University of Illinios, Urbana.*

Avner, A. *et al.*, 1972. Planning estimates for production of TUTOR lessons, *PLATO Evaulation Report*, No. 3 (November), CERL, University of Illinois, Urbana.*

Bitzer, D. L., and Slottow, H. G., 1968. The plasma display panel – A new device for direct display of graphics, *in* D. Secrest and J. Nievergelf (Eds.), *Emerging Concepts in Computer Graphics*, W. A. Benjamin, New York, pp. 2–28.

Bitzer, D. L., Sherwood, B. A., and Tenczar, P., 1973. Computer-based science education, CERL Report X-37 (May). Originally a paper presented to the conference on Utilization of Education Technology in the Improvement of Science Education, UNESCO, Paris (September 13–16, 1972).

Bork, A. M., 1975. Effective computer use in physics education, *Am. J. Phys.* 43(1).

Cohen, P., 1975. PLATO lesson "cmode," personal communication.

Easley, J. A., Jr. 1966. First annual report for Project SIRA, SIRA report to the U.S. Department of Health, Education, and Welfare, Office of Education (October 1965–September 1966).

Johnson, R. L., Bitzer, D. L., and Slottow, H. G., 1971. The device characteristics of the plasma display element, *IEEE Transactions on Electron Devices* 18(9): 642–649 (September).

Kraatz, J. 1976, personal communication.

Mitre Corporation, 1974. An overview of the TICCIT program, No. M74-1 (January) (available from Mitre Corp., 1820 Dolly Madison Blvd., McLean, Va. 22101).

Nelson, T., 1974. Is it better to toot? *in Dream Machines* (No. DM-27), Hugo's Book Service, Chicago.

Pantages, A., 1976. Control Data's education offering: Plato would have enjoyed PLATO, *Datamation* 22: 183 (May).

Schuyler, J., 1974. The complete guide to HYPERTUTOR, (June) (available from Computers and Teachings, Northwestern University, 2003 Sheridan Road, Evanston, Illinois 60201).

Sherwood, B. A., 1974. The TUTOR language, CERL, University of Illinois, Urbana.*

Sherwood, B. A., and Stifle, J., 1975. The PLATO IV communications system, *CERL Report* X-44, University of Illinois, Urbana.*

Smith, S. G., and Sherwood, B. A., 1976. Educational uses of the PLATO system, *Science* 192: 344–352 (April 23).

Stifle, J., 1970. A plasma display terminal, *CERL Report* X-15 (March). (Revised March, 1971) (revised February, 1972, and appears as The PLATO IV student terminal.) University of Illinois, Urbana.*

Stull, P. E., Cohen, B., and Hody, G. L., 1976. QWRITER: An automatic lesson programmer, presented at the Summer Conference of the Association for the Development of Computer-based Instruction (ADCIS), Minneapolis, August, 1976.

Tenczar, P., The evolutionary design of CAI software (in press). Presented at the 1975 annual meeting of the American Educational Research Association, Washington, D.C., April 1975.*

Tenczar, P., and Golden, W., 1972. Spelling, word and concept recognition, *CERL Report* X-35 (October), University of Illinois, Urbana.*

Vallee, J., Lipinski, H., Johausen, R., Wilson, T., 1975. Computer conferencing, *Science* 188: 203 (April 18).

*All PLATO reports and manuals may be ordered from CERL, University of Illinois, Urbana, Illinois 61801.

CAIREN: A Network for Sharing Health Care Learning Resources with Ohio Health Care Facilities and Educational Institutions

Mark H. Forman, Ruann E. Pengov, and Jeanne L. Burson

Introduction

The availability of quality learning resources to complement basic and continuing education activities is, at best, sporadic in most disciplines. The supply many times fails to meet the demand, forcing educators or training coordinators to make do with tried but true resources that have long since been shown to be something less than totally effective.

The problem is most evident in the health sciences, where basic education for the training of health professionals continues to spread to ever-increasing numbers of students. Responsibility for providing this educational support is also growing to include not only large universities and teaching hospitals but also vocational–technical colleges and small community hospitals.

The problem also manifests itself in the area of continuing education, a concept that is linked to a number of issues, such as malpractice, peer review, relicensure, continued competency, and professional concern for optimum patient care. Members of the health care team are under fire to mandate continuing education activity – and yet, where are the resources to support such activity?

Given its history of involvement in computer-assisted instruction (CAI), The Ohio State University College of Medicine recognized the potential for using computers in the development of quality learning resources. This chapter will focus on a specific example of an operational network designed to facilitate the sharing of such materials in support of basic and continuing health education throughout the state of Ohio.

The choice of computerized interactive learning experiences as a potentially efficient means of helping to meet the continuing education needs of health professionals is summarized in the following quote by a previous network administrator:

Mark H. Forman, Ruann E. Pengov, and *Jeanne L. Burson* · Division of Computing Services for Medical Education and Research, Ohio State University, Columbus, Ohio.

The health professional, in order to function at maximum, has found it necessary to continue year after year to add to his knowledge and skills. However, the work schedule of the professional makes it almost impossible to attend programs presented at set times and scattered sites throughout the country. Therefore, the expressed need is for *accessible, relevant* and short *specific* programs that deal with the important, reinforcing and innovative principles that confront the individual.

Moreover, the mode of learning should be adaptable to the personalities and past experiences of *individuals* who vary in the rate, comprehension and retention of what is learned. A method of continuing education, therefore, should relate to the needs of the individual, so that what needs to be learned can be learned *when needed* and can instill within the individual the ability to *apply* this knowledge in reality.

Many of the expressed needs suggest individualized – even independent study programs. Individualized independent study cannot replace actual clinical laboratory instruction, but coupled with *other media* this instructional combination can offer much as a learning activity in health care education. Therefore, it will become necessary to develop more effective and efficient means of teaching knowledge. While knowledge itself may give no assurance that the care of patients will be improved, knowledge is the first step upon which both ability and motivation to use information rests.

One innovative method, which relates to these views, seems to have eluded effective utilization by the health-related professions. This is computer assisted instruction. CAI emphasizes the active involvement and appropriate responses provided the user by the computer system. (Burson, 1972)

CAI affords accessibility at the health care students' or practitioners' site of work, is available according to the user's time schedule, and is adaptable to the personalities, past experiences, and needs of the individual. In addition, programs dealing with a specific subject area are constructed with multiple pathways to meet the differing educational needs of a wide variety of audiences from students to practicing health professionals in the medical, nursing, and allied health areas. Individual program modifications may also be implemented to accommodate varying institutional procedures, norms, and practices.

Such are the variables that help to explain the birth of a statewide CAI network for sharing learning resources of The Ohio State University College of Medicine* with Ohio health care facilities and educational institutions. Having survived an exciting yet unstable infancy, the Computer Assisted Instruction Regional Education Network (CAIREN) now exists as a self-supporting educational outreach of the college. As it approaches adulthood, this network has taken an expanded and flexible view of the type of computerized educational and service programs that can and should be offered by a central facility. The history, growth, and current operation of CAIREN will now be examined in detail.

---

*The Ohio State University College of Medicine includes the School of Nursing and the School of Allied Medical Professions.

History

In July of 1967, the Ohio State Regional Medical Program funded a 2-year planning and development phase of a project to investigate both the usefulness of CAI in meeting information needs of local health practitioners and the practicality of networking such materials from The Ohio State University College of Medicine to community hospitals throughout Ohio (HEW, 1968). Then, as now, the network functions on the premise that "the quality of patient care and health care services is contingent on the knowledge and skills of health professionals. Therefore, the maintenance and expansion of current knowledge and skills are of vital importance to health practitioners" (Burson, 1972).

The CAI Project Staff later admitted that their initial objectives were overly optimistic. As one administrator put it, "We proposed to develop a network for CAI, to develop the software necessary to support CAI on this network, to develop coursework which properly utilized this new medium, to establish administrative relationships with the affiliated communities, to assess the needs for continuing education, to conduct research regarding behavioral change affected by utilization of our network, and in short, to solve all of the problems of continuing education" (Report of The Ohio State Regional Medical Program Computer Assisting Instruction Conference, 1970). Fortunately, the project staff prioritized the assessment of the feasibility of the medium and the delivery system that supported it.

During the first 2 years of the project, a small number of CAI courses were written, evaluation was begun, and equipment was installed and tested. In the summer of 1969, the project began the testing of equipment and the utilization of CAI programs at four remote community hospitals. Equipment and processes were debugged, additional programs were written, personnel changes were made to insure continued development, data were gathered for evaluation, and hospital personnel became involved in the examination of utilization and future potential of the CAI system.

Much of the initial project staff time was involved in the development of community relations. It was chiefly a matter of getting out into the community and finding hospitals that were interested in this type of involvement with Ohio State. One interesting aspect of this effort was noted by a member of the project staff:

> Assessing continuing education needs and designing evaluation studies proved somewhat difficult in certain communities. As representatives of a federally funded program, we were sometimes viewed by the practicing health professionals with a certain amount of apprehension. . . . We had to spend great amounts of time just developing good relations with these health practitioners. We did this by involving them in the development of the project, by building their confidence in our ability to be of help, and by convincing them that our motivations were genuine, and that we were not really "federal spies" (Report of The Ohio State Regional Medical Program Computer Assisted Instruction Conference, 1970).

Operating under a second continuation grant funded in 1969, the network membership was extended to include 10 hospitals. By July of 1972, there were 15 institutional members; the 5-year funding was extended for 10 months; and the consortium of users had become the Computer Assisted Instruction Regional Education Network (CAIREN). In July of 1973, outside funding support terminated and CAIREN was incorporated into ongoing College of Medicine efforts to utilize computer technology in the advancement of medical education and research.

As is the case with any resource, the success in incorporating the CAI learning materials into existing hospital programs and educational efforts is dependent upon a number of institution-controlled variables. Therefore, the network membership fluctuated according to the educational needs and program coordination of each member institution. Institutional memberships have ranged from 1 year to 7 years in length; from small community hospitals of less than 300 beds to large teaching hospitals of nearly 1000 beds; from mental health institutions to health-related educational institutions and technical schools offering nursing and allied training programs. Figure 1 summarizes the membership profile by institutional type during the course of CAIREN'S 7-year history.

The significance of the evolvement of CAIREN as a part of the larger whole (the College of Medicine CAI System) manifests itself in two very important ways:

1. The program library of CAI programs and instructional materials is created by users from all components of the College of Medicine CAI System. Thus, programs developed for College of Medicine student usage are made available to CAIREN, just as programs developed specifically for CAIREN are made available to college users. This sharing of the CAI program libarary has provided a larger quantity and a higher quality of CAI courseware for all audiences.

2. The central support costs (hardware, software, and personnel) for operation of the CAI system are not borne by any one user group but are borne jointly by CAIREN, the college, and other users of the system.

The evolvement of the College of Medicine CAI System and subcomponents of that system are discussed in other chapters of this book. Suffice it to say, that as

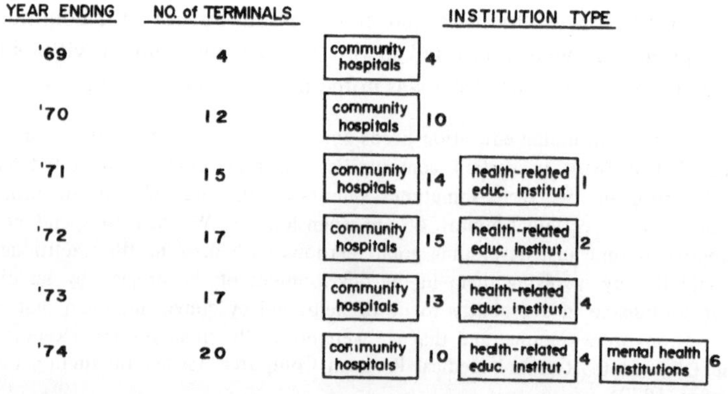

Figure 1. CAIREN membership profile. Copyright 1975, The Ohio State University College of Medicine.

the CAIREN effort was evolving, so too was the utilization of CAI in the curriculums of the School of Allied Medical Professions, the School of Nursing, and in the M.D. and Ph.D. curriculums within the College of Medicine. In summary, it is important to note that in its short 7-year history, CAIREN has evolved (a) from a federally-supported network to a self-supporting network, and (b) from an experimental network to a fully operational network.

The CAI Program Library

Complete indexing and description of the CAI program library is available in *The Ohio State University College of Medicine's User's Guide to Computer Assisted Instruction.* A total of approximately 100 programs offers over 350 interactive terminal hours of instruction to CAIREN users. Audiences include patients and their families, clerical support personnel, and, of course, students and practicing professionals in allied health, nursing, and medicine.

During the first 5 years of the network, the Regional Medical Program funding enabled the project staff to develop materials specifically for continuing education purposes. Hospital continuing education committees helped in identifying subject areas where program development was needed. Courses developed included A Basic Review of Nursing in Coronary Care, Stroke Rehabilitation, Oral Cancer Recognition, and Juvenile Diabetes. Initial thrusts in programs designed specifically for practicing physicians and nursing personnel were later augmented by materials developed by the College of Medicine for its students. It became apparent that the practicing nurse was much more receptive an audience than the physician.

A majority of the CAI materials are constructed for self-evaluation and are individualized by participant response. However, some programs include formal evaluation such as pre-, interim and/or posttesting. All programs are simulation — task simulation or tutorial presentation. A task-simulation program allows a participant to interact in a situation closely resembling the actual experience. A tutorial presentation, as the name implies, is a simulation of a tutorial session between the instructor and the learner.

Programs are written for primary or adjunct instruction, overview, and/or review. The programs include several types of learning activities — question and answer, dialogue, drill-and-practice, case study, minisimulation, and problem solving. Audiovisuals of various forms are employed when essential for objective achievement. The capabilities of the computer and the author language, coupled with branching, coaching, and feedback mechanisms, allow the learner to acquire or reinforce knowledge at his own level of competence.

One motivating item in utilization is the code name assigned to each specific program. Aside from being "catchy," the code name is descriptive of the content and/or purpose (e.g., "aciba," Acid—Base Balance; "bugout," Hospital Infection Control; "cvterm," Cardiovascular Terminology; and "obtox," Toxemia of Pregnancy).

It is critical to note that professional societies are moving toward continuing education requirements for their members. CAIREN has a vested interest in this area given CAI's suitability as a vehicle for providing materials that will meet these requirements. Users have expressed a keen interest in accessing accredited continuing education materials via CAIREN. In response to this need, all CAI programs are viewed and evaluated to determine if they will meet the requirements of the societies. Based on this review, selected programs are then submitted to the appropriate society for accreditation consideration. For each approved program, a computer-generated statement is available to the participant who completes the program. Information regarding usage is also available, upon request, to the institution or accrediting society. The following societies have granted continuing education activity approval to selected CAI programs (Progress Report, 1976):

	Hours approved for credit
American Dietetic Association	108
American Medical Association	70
American Osteopathic Association	All programs eligible for category II-A credit
Ohio Nurses Association	6
State of Ohio Board of Pharmacy	106

CAI Usage

CAIREN members currently account for approximately 30% of the total College of Medicine CAI System usage. Again, the impact of cost and data base sharing (in that 70% of the central system support costs are borne by other users) is significant in accounting for the cost effectiveness of the state network.

Figure 2 offers a detailed perspective of the utilization by CAIREN institutions. It shows the average usage per institution per month for each time period and gives the total number of interactive sessions during the same period.*

The year-to-year variances in total network usage are for the most part attributable to the number of institutions terminating or initiating membership in *CAIREN*. The increased monthly usage from 1971 to 1973 was related to the growth and development of the CAI project itself. The decrease in that figure from 1973 to 1975 is most probably the result of several variables:

1. Given the absence of federal funding, the amount of field support from central staff to individual institutions is considerably reduced. Those institutions that do not lend personnel support to this activity and that do not, in general, prioritize continuing education activity, find the maintenance of high levels of usage difficult.

---

*A student interactive session is based upon the average student time at the terminal (30 minutes); therefore, each usage hour accounts for two student interactive sessions.

TIME PERIOD	TOTAL HRS. USAGE	AVER. USAGE / INSTIT. /MO.	TOTAL STUDENT INTERACTIVE SESSIONS
JUNE – DEC. 1971	3217	41.3 HR.	6434
1972	8536	50.4	17072
1973	13300	60.2	26600
1974	11374	50.6	22748
1975	8430	40.4	16860
TOTALS	44875	48.6	89714

Figure 2. CAIREN utilization statistics. Copyright 1975, The Ohio State University College of Medicine, Division of Computing Services for Medical Education and Research.

2. In the absence of federal funds, little support is available for the development of programs designed specifically for continuing education activity. Although institutional input is still solicited for program development, it is only useful insofar as it meshes with the priorities for program development efforts within the College of Medicine.

3. The withdrawal of federal funding found some institutions unable to continue usage, so the size of the user population decreased.

Present usage is now on the increase after 2 years of decrease. Some of the factors that account for this trend reversal include:

1. The CAI materials are increasingly applicable to the basic educational programs (i.e., nursing) offered by several CAIREN institutions (Forman and Mourad, 1976). The programs are also attractive learning resources for students who are gaining clinical experience in the community hospitals.

2. Continuing education activity is being mandated by several professional societies. Nursing and allied health professionals, in particular, appear to be utilizing CAI resources in greater numbers.

3. The transition from a federally subsidized network to self-sufficiency is complete. During this period, the organization and availability of central staff resources required several iterations of refinement before network operations were stabilized.

4. Physicians are becoming acquainted with CAI via a variety of professional society projects. This formalized acquaintance with the medium will hopefully accent its attractiveness as a continuing education resource tool. The American Board of Internal Medicines' MERIT (Model for Examination and Recertification through Individualized Testing Project) (Harless *et al.*, 1975) is one such project that links competency-based individualized examinations with recertification. The Ohio State University Medical School renders the computer support for this effort.

It is interesting to note that the average usage hours per month linked with the fixed costs each institution incurs provides the administrator with accessible monthly data for cost–benefit analysis – he can easily calculate a cost per hour of instruction utilized. Since each CAIREN institution is afforded "round-the-clock" access to the CAI materials, the extrapolated cost per hour, if all available hours were used, is approximately $1.00 per hour.*

Although Figure 2 demonstrates that the average usage does not begin to approach maximum usage, it is nonetheless important to note that the institution, through a number of mechanisms, actually influences the cost per hour of instruction. Scheduling of the facility, effective utilization of the medium, promotion of the materials available, and monitoring of the system are mechanisms that ultimately influence the cost effectiveness of CAI as a learning resource.

Operation of the Network

User Access

The hardware network for CAIREN is a star formation linking the central computer site with each institutional member via General Services Administration TELPAK, State TELPAK, and/or local telephone company facilities. No multiplexing or shared-line facilities are used at this point, although such configurations are possible if the usage and institutional locale dictate. Figure 3 offers a conceptual view of the star-form network structure of CAIREN.

The user at each individual institution encounters CAI in a learning-resource carrel located in a library or other centrally accessible room. In this carrel, he finds a computer terminal, slide projector, and associated learning resources (slides, tapes, etc.) necessary for his utilization of the CAI programs. In each institution, a monitor is assigned to assist new users with the first encounter at the CAI terminal and to help users with any ongoing access problems. The computer terminal is a high-speed thermal typewriter that provides hard copy output as the student interaction proceeds. The slide projector is self-controlled by the student and is used when called for in the learning sequence. Figure 4 depicts schematically the on-line linkage pattern from the student terminal via data sets, telephone lines, communications controllers, and minicomputers to the central computer site.

Given the above configuration involving terminal, communications hardware, and computer hardware rental from several different vendors, it becomes crucial that support staff be available to troubleshoot, monitor, and continually upgrade the quality of the hardware support network. Without stability and reliability of both hardware and software operation, CAI cannot succeed. The Ohio State University system reliability is high with "up time" sometimes exceeding 100%† and always exceeding 95%. A full series of reports provide data to help insure the continued stability and reliability of network operation.

---

*The system is generally accessible at least 20 hours per day, 7 days a week, providing a potential of 600 hours of monthly usage to each institution.
†This access of greater than 100% can occur when the system is up longer than guaranteed.

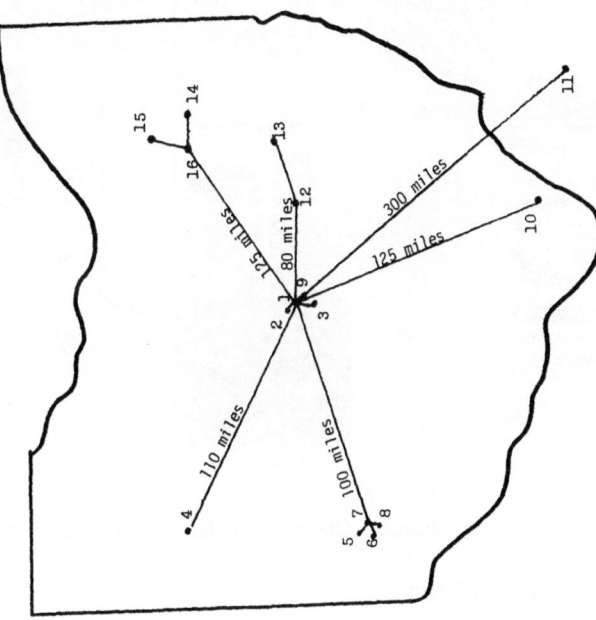

1. CAIREN Headquarters - Division of Computing Services For Medical Education and Research
   The Ohio State University College of Medicine, Columbus, Ohio

2. The Ohio State University Hospitals, Columbus, Ohio

3. Columbus State Hospital, Columbus, Ohio

4. Lima Technical College, Lima, Ohio

5. Grandview Osteopathic Hospital, Dayton, Ohio

6. St. Elizabeth Medical Center, Dayton, Ohio

7. Dayton Mental Health Center, Dayton, Ohio

8. Kettering Medical Center, Kettering, Ohio

9. Columbus Technical Institute, Columbus, Ohio

10. Holzer Medical Center, Gallipolis, Ohio

11. University of Virginia, Charlottesville, Virginia

12. Good Samaritan Medical Center, Zanesville, Ohio

13. Cambridge State Hospital, Cambridge, Ohio

14. Aultman Hospital, Canton, Ohio

15. Akron City Hospital, Akron, Ohio

16. Massillon State Hospital, Massillon, Ohio

Figure 3. The star-form network structure of CAIREN.

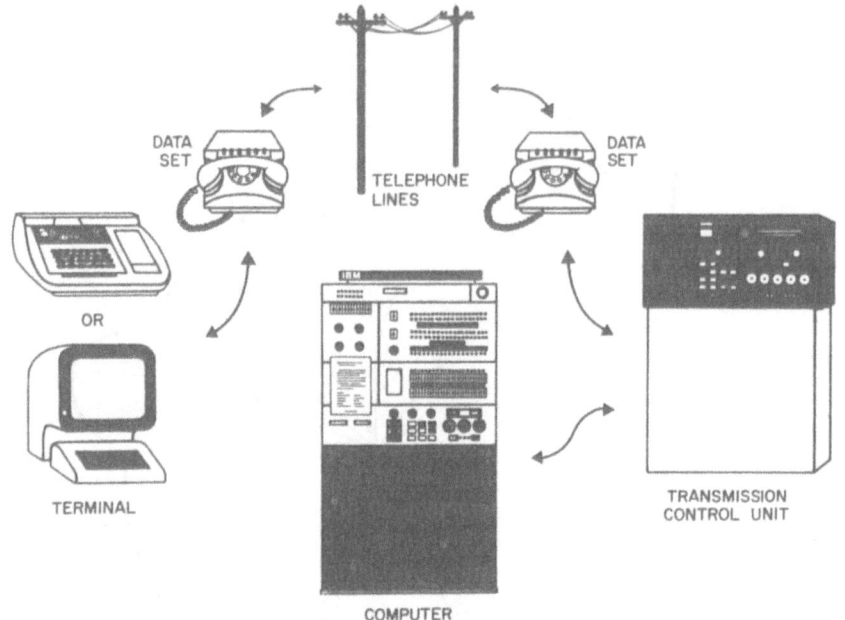

Figure 4. On-line computer configuration.

The Central Support Team

As essential as the computer network to the continued operation, reliability, and stability of CAIREN is the personnel support provided by the central CAI staff in the College of Medicine's Division of Computing Services for Medical Education and Research. The Division's CAI User Services Unit provides administrative and operational support for the network. This support embraces producing and disseminating materials describing the numerous CAI programs, maintaining and updating program catalogues, providing system troubleshooting, implementing and coordinating communications mechanisms, providing user information regarding the access and use of the resource materials, and promoting a general awareness of the full capabilities that exist in the CAI system.

The User Services Unit includes $2\frac{1}{2}$ full-time staff who are responsible for the provision of the above services to all users of the CAI system. It should be stressed that CAIREN institutions receive a unique set of field services not afforded to other users, which are discussed later in this chapter.

The Division also contains a unit that is responsible for the development and maintenance of the CAI programs. Appropriate mechanisms have been employed to assure that this unit receives input from CAIREN users regarding the value and content accuracy of existing materials as well as the critical areas where new materials need to be developed.

Here again, the cost effectiveness of a central support team in servicing all audiences allows for amortization of costs to user groups. The maintenance of a full CAI support team for the CAI Regional Education Network alone would require a significant increase in the monthly cost to CAIREN users.

The CAIREN Communications Model

At the heart of effective interface between the central CAI support team and the individual user is the CAIREN Coordinator, as shown in the CAIREN communications model (Figure 5). The CAIREN Coordinator interfaces continually with the institutional monitor and the institutional CAI Committee. This triangular communications mechanism is critical to the success of CAI in any CAIREN institution. Figure 5 delineates major responsibilities of the institutional CAI Monitor and CAI Committee.

The CAIREN Monitor, as the primary contact person responsible for the day-to-day operation of the terminal, must be an individual who is dependable, relatively constant in physical location, and able to respond quickly to user problems. More often than not, in-service education coordinators or medical librarians serve this function, subsequently training additional staff members to provide support when necessary.

The CAI Committee is formulated by an institutional administrator and usually includes representatives from all appropriate areas of the hospital. Many times an existing committee on in-service education and training is charged with these tasks. Generally, the institutional CAI Committee works with the Monitor and the CAIREN Coordinator to set up priorities for usage, new course development, and strategy within the institution. The CAIREN Coordinator, as a staff member of the

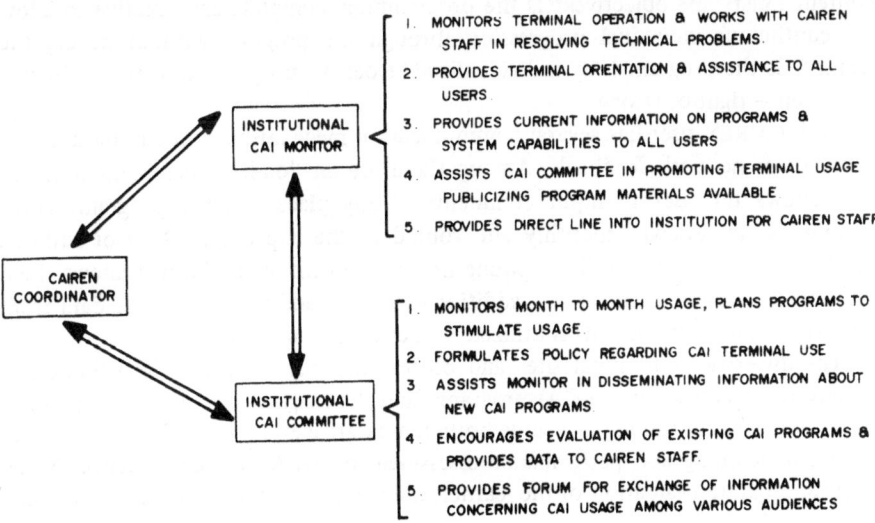

Figure 5. CAIREN communications model. Copyright 1975, The Ohio State University College of Medicine.

Division of Computing Services for Medical Education and Research, continually interfaces with the appropriate support personnel in the Division.

To promote the network, CAI and CAIREN literature is distributed at demonstrations, meetings, and workshops and in response to written inquiries. To augment the actions of the coordinated CAI committees, assistance is given to individual member institutions as requested, and field trips are made regularly by CAIREN staff to member sites. A comprehensive descriptive *User's Guide to CAI* is made available at each terminal location. Descriptive flyers, promotional material, and *User's Guide* updates are sent to all member institutions as releases and changes are made. Usage reports are sent monthly to the CAI Monitor and administrative personnel at each institution. In addition, workshops and demonstrations are planned to offer the opportunity for users to increase their knowledge and understanding of CAI and its potential and application as a learning activity.

The importance of the CAIREN Coordinator in providing a personal interface between the central support group and the user institution is crucial, given the innovative nature of CAI and the requirements for user education in the potential use of CAI and the specifics of the CAI programs available in the existing library at Ohio State University.

Evaluation

Since the individual objectives of the CAIREN participants vary greatly, it is difficult to evaluate the amount of knowledge "transferred." Therefore, evaluation is, for the most part, limited to individual program appraisal. Attempts are made to answer such questions as: Is the program content correct? Does the program content satisfy the objectives? Is the programming complete and creative to allow for continuous individual progression through the program without boring the learner? Is the program truly individualized? Does the program allow for difference of option — right or wrong?

Each CAIREN user has several communication mechanisms that can be used for program or network feedback. Among these are an "on-line" comment function that allows the user to input comments at any place within a program. These comments are reviewed monthly and routed to the appropriate staff or authors. CAIREN users also have a direct phone line to the central staff which allows them unlimited communication at no additional cost. In addition, computer data from student terminal interactions is utilized for periodic program evaluation.

The diversity of terminal sites and professional participation, the volume and variety of objectives of the CAI programs, and the usage at various stages of education (basic and continuing) preclude both comparative evaluation of CAI with other modes of learning and performance assessment of participant competence. Nonetheless, separate evaluation of the learner, the media, and the network has not been overlooked.

Printout review by instructors or supervisors is the major means of learner management. CAIREN utilizes anonymous identification numbers for "bookmarks" only.

Participant reaction to CAI as an instructional methodology is obtained through voluntary response to a semantic differential survey form. Although these informal surveys seem to express a high degree of favorability toward CAI, additional effort needs to be expended in more formally evaluating user attitudes. Any comprehensive evaluation of CAIREN would have to embrace many of the aforementioned areas.

Costs

One of the more interesting aspects of the envolvement of the Computer Assisted Instruction Regional Education Network has been its movement from a totally federally supported endeavor* to an endeavor supported by institution user fees.

As is shown in Figure 6, the transition from federal money support to institutional support was a gradual one that began in 1971 and was fully effected in 1974. Again, it must be stressed that cost-effective institutional support of the endeavor is possible only in light of the larger system of which CAIREN is a part and with which it shares the central operational and support costs. Figure 7 evaluates the total cost on an institution (or computer terminal) basis and shows the average monthly dollar costs per terminal dropping from an initial $5000 per terminal per month† in 1969 to the current $600 per terminal per month. Also shown in Figure 7 is the drop in federal dollar support and the gradual increase in institutional dollar support during the evolution of the network.

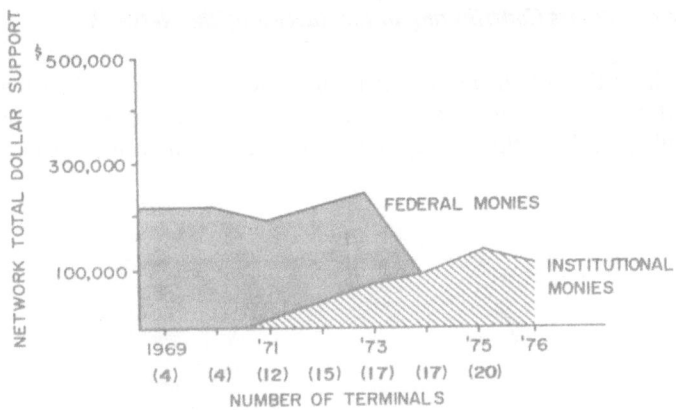

Figure 6. CAIREN financial support of network. Copyright 1975, The Ohio State University College of Medicine, Division of Computing Services for Medical Education and Research.

---

*Approximately $1,000,000 in funds from the Ohio State Regional Medical Program was invested in the initial development and operation of CAIREN.

†The high initial cost per terminal is due to the experimental nature of the first project effort. Development, evaluation, the initial design and testing costs are included in the first year of the project, whereas current total dollar support covers operation only.

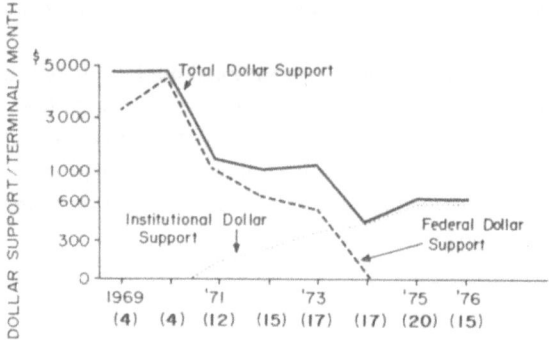

Figure 7. CAIREN terminal dollar support. Copyright 1975, The Ohio State University College of Medicine, Division of Computing Services for Medical Education and Research.

From another perspective, Figure 8 shows the distribution of the user dollar expenditure in terms of the service provided. The largest percentage of each user dollar (48%) goes to communication linkage between the user site and the central computing facility. Thirty-one percent is used to purchase computing power, 13% is for terminal rental fees, and a minimal 8% is spent for network administration which includes items such as terminal insurance, terminal paper, field services, staff travel, office supplies, a marginal portion of program development, and visual material updates, etc.

Discussion of Factors Contributing to the Success of the Network

A full discussion of all the factors influencing the success and current viability of CAIREN would constitute another full chapter. For the sake of brevity, the authors will note here the major factors that have been significant in the success

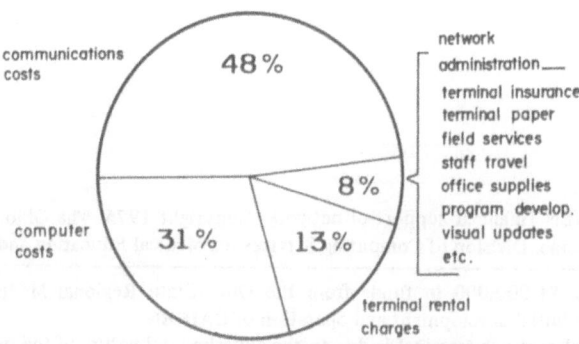

Figure 8. CAIREN average user dollar expenditures. Copyright 1975, The Ohio State University College of Medicine.

of the CAIREN network. These are by no means the only factors involved but have been chosen due to their potential generalizability to other similar endeavors.

1. The CAI materials provided on the network are generally of high quality and have been proven effective for the education of health professionals. The educational strategy, the quality of content, and the curriculum application of CAI materials hold priority over elegant hardware and/or computer systems. In brief, the network has a good product that is being distributed to the user institutions. It offers variety of content and variety of educational strategies of the CAI medium. Many of the materials are independently paced, allowing for user entry based upon his background, experience, and knowledge level. Materials are regularly reviewed and updated. New programs are constantly being developed and added to the library.

2. User access to the materials is well maintained via (a) The technical network of hardware and software necessary for an operational system with reliable and stable provision of services and user access to the services; (b) the facilitating network of central support staff using the CAIREN/Communications model (this network assures effective user interface with the hardware network and the CAI program library; and (c) the management network with responsibility for marketing, administration, and general management of the technical and facilitating networks. Longevity of College experience with all three networks allows CAIREN to operate in an environment of cumulative knowledge and shared expertise.

3. The use of CAI on an individual institution basis has proven to be a cost-effective resource for the institution. This factor must be linked to the college's ability to amortize the central support costs among various user groups. User willingness to pay the monthly fee for access is the first indicator of the value of CAIREN to the institution. Comparatively, the monthly fee could be equated to much less than the salary of one full-time equivalent medical educator. Via CAIREN, a variety of already developed and tested learning materials covering the full spectrum of health professions education is available.

Implications for the Future

CAIREN as an exemplary network for the use of computer-assisted instruction in facilitating basic and continuing medical education has an exciting future. Several specific developments in the area of continuing health education enhance the potential of CAI as a tool:

1. Some professional associations require continuing education credits for membership in their associations.
2. Recent legislation, such as that in the state of Ohio, will require continuing education credits for relicensure of physicians.
3. The Area Health Education Center Plan makes colleges of medicine responsible for health education at the community level. This effort works hand-

in-hand with items 1 and 2 above to underline the increasing importance of continuing education of health professionals and the vital role that medical centers play in this outreach.

4. The Professional Standard Review Organization (PSRO) concepts calls for in-house review, control, and improvement of the quality of patient care delivered. The key here is that, once a deficiency is noted, the organization must also identify means of corrective action for the deficiency shown.

5. Several professional societies are investigating the use of computer-based materials as a part of the recertification process. One example was that used to facilitate a pilot test of the American Board of Internal Medicine's MERIT Project.

In summary, the Computer Assisted Instruction Regional Education Network has evolved as an operational and self-supporting network serving a viable role in facilitating the sharing of health care learning resources with students and practitioners.

References

Burson, J., 1972, Effects of a Terminal Context Summary (TCS) in a Multi-Media Individualized Instructional Approach to Statistics for Quality Control (QUCOST), Dissertation, The Ohio State University, Columbus, Ohio.

The Computer Assisted Instruction Regional Education Network (CAIREN): A Report Prepared for the Committee on Educational Applications of the Computer, The Ohio State University College of Medicine, 1974.

Division of Computing Services for Medical Education and Research, 1973. *The User's Guide to Computer Assisted Instruction (CAI).* The Ohio State University College of Medicine, Columbus, Ohio.

Forman, M. H., and Mourad, L. A., 1976, The Role of Computer Assisted Instruction in the Nursing Program at The Ohio State University, Columbus, Ohio.

Harless, W., Farr, N. A., Gamble, J. R., and Zier, M. A., 1975, MERIT–A Model for Evaluation and Recertification Through Individualized Testing, *Proceedings of the Fourteenth Annual Conference on Research in Medical Education.*

HEW, 1968, Proposed Planning for the Use of CAI in Meeting Information Needs of Local Community Health Practitioners, Division of Regional Medical Programs 1 C03 RM 00070 01, Public Health Service, Department of Health, Education and Welfare, Washington, D.C.

Progress Report, January 1974–December 1975, 1976, Division of Computing Services for Medical Education and Research, The Ohio State University College of Medicine.

11

Health Education Network

Charles S. Tidball

Introduction

The Health Education Network, Inc., is an outgrowth of the Experimental CAI Network sponsored by the Lister Hill National Center for Biomedical Communications (LHNCBC) of the National Library of Medicine described in Chapter 8. Convinced of the utility of sharing of health-related courseware and the inherent advantages of networking, a group of former users of the Experimental CAI Network have taken steps to preserve nationwide access to the libraries of CAI programs (data bases) available at The Massachusetts General Hospital (MGH) and The Ohio State University (OSU). The purpose of this new support structure is to facilitate, maintain, and preserve economical, nationwide access to computer-assisted instructional materials for health education (Health Education Network, 1975).

During the last decade, the development of computer-assisted instruction (CAI) has occurred with increasing momentum at various levels of the total educational effort. The status of implementation for this technology was assessed in the fall of 1975 for the schools of medicine in North America (Lefever and Johnson, 1976). Eighty institutions provided data on their involvement. Fifty-eight of these schools generated original programs at their own institutions. Fifty-four accessed other institutions' programs via networking or time-sharing arrangements. Forty-three had permanent facilities for computerized instruction. Thirty-seven exchanged programs with other institutions. More importantly, for this total group, as shown in Figure 1, the number of courses involving CAI increased from 1 in 1965 to 351 in 1975 (Tidball, 1976). The clear-cut, exponential growth in this activity establishes that the long-awaited CAI revolution has arrived, at least in the area of health sciences education.

It is against this background of expanding activity in devising and testing new instructional strategies, as well as incorporating additional content areas into an ever-widening data base, that the Health Education Network Inc., has come into being. This chapter will examine four topics: Rationale for Networking, Current Capabilities, The Birth of a User-Directed Network, and Challenges for the Future.

Charles S. Tidball · Computer Assisted Education and Services, George Washington University Medical Center, Washington, D.C.

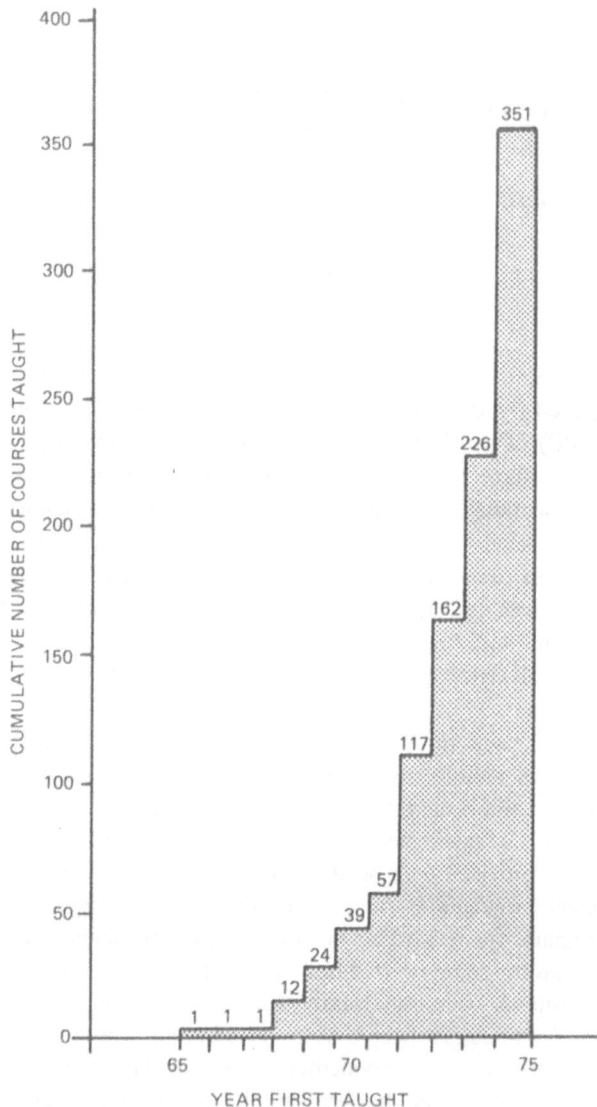

Figure 1. Cumulative number of courses involving CAI vs. the year in which they were first taught (Tidball, 1976).

Rationale for Networking

The development effort summarized above is being made on a broad variety of computer hardware and in more than a dozen computer languages that run under different computer operating systems (Kamp, 1975). Networking can provide compatibility across this tangle of individual differences without requiring cooperating institutions to alter computer hardware or software. For example, in my own institution, students and faculty employ the same computer terminals to communicate with a variety of networks, with a number of computers in the Washington area, and with several different internal mainframes.

The second advantage of networking is that items of courseware remain on the computers where they were originally developed and where there is the greatest responsibility and interest in updating and improving the unit as learner feedback becomes available.

Third, networking is of value because a larger number of learners can be exposed to a newly developed item of courseware in a shorter period of time than can ordinarily be accomplished at the developing institution alone. Given responsiveness to user comments that are collected on the computer system (see chapter 9) and prompt action on the part of courseware authors, a more rapid enhancement of the courseware can occur. Thus, it is brought to a higher level of acceptability, from both the faculty and the student point of view, than would be achieved if its use were restricted to a single institution.

A fourth advantage of networking obtains for institutions that have no CAI capability. Their costs in becoming involved in this innovative educational technology consist of acquiring a standard computer terminal and paying network access fees including, where necessary, telephone costs to the nearest node city of the communications carrier (see Figure 2); such costs are considerably less than those involved in developing an equivalent, full-scale CAI environment locally, even if this is done on low-cost minicomputer equipment.

Fifth, a network is based on several computer mainframes. Thus, a network generally provides a greater degree of reliability since alternate courseware delivery equipment is accessible at such times when a given system may become temporarily unavailable.

Sixth, a properly designed network distributes the costs of CAI development across several institutions while making available the fruits of this development on a broad scale. In so doing, networking contributes to economical distribution of what can otherwise be an expensive feature of the educational environment. By being affiliated with a network, a user is also under less pressure to expand the data base available on an internal courseware delivery system.

Seventh, membership in a network creates opportunities for interaction with colleagues at other institutions who desire to use information technology in support of health science education. Involvement in such a community of users increases the likelihood of appropriate and economical use of the advancing technology.

Finally, it should be acknowledged that networking provides access to a larger data base than can probably be created or maintained by any single institution. It seems likely that a combination of network access to a broad, general-purpose data base and internal access to a somewhat more specialized data base will provide the best solution for most academic medical centers interested in this mode of education.

Arizona	Hawaii	New York
Phoenix	Honolulu	Buffalo
California	*Illinois*	New York
Cupertino	Chicago	Rochester
El Segundo	Freeport	Syracuse
Los Angeles	*Iowa*	*Ohio*
Mountain View	Des Moines	Akron
Newport Beach	*Kansas*	Cincinnati
Oakland	Wichita	Cleveland
Oxnard		Columbus
Palo Alto	*Louisiana*	*Oklahoma*
Riverside	Baton Rouge	Oklahoma City
Sacramento	New Orleans	*Oregon*
San Diego	*Maryland*	Portland
San Francisco	Baltimore	*Pennsylvania*
San Jose	*Massachusetts*	Philadelphia
Canada	Boston	Pittsburgh
Calgary	Cambridge	Valley Forge
Edmonton	*Michigan*	*Texas*
Toronto	Ann Arbor	Austin
Vancouver	Detroit	Dallas
Colorado	Kalamazoo	El Paso
Denver	*Minnesota*	Houston
Connecticut	Minneapolis	Midland
Darien	*Missouri*	San Antonio
Hartford	Kansas City	*Utah*
District of Columbia	St. Louis	Salt Lake City
Washington	*North Carolina*	*Washington*
Florida	Durham	Seattle
Miami	*New Jersey*	*Wisconsin*
St. Petersburg	Englewood Cliffs	Madison
Tampa	Union	Milwaukee
Georgia	Wayne	
Atlanta		

Figure 2. Node cities for access to TYMNET (data as of June, 1976).

Current Operation and Capabilities

The Health Education Network, Inc. (Network), like its predecessor, is composed of four basic elements: (1) institutions with well-developed health-related CAI materials on their own computers, (2) a communications carrier with a nationwide network, (3) institutions desirous of accessing the courseware items made available, and (4) a management structure to preserve and enhance the interinstitutional sharing.

The formalities for becoming involved are not extensive. It is merely necessary to execute an agreement with one or both of the data-base hosts (MGH and OSU).

Membership in the Network is not required, although participation in its gatherings is desirable in order to meet colleagues from other institutions using these services and to influence decisions related to future operations of the Network. All ASCII (teletype-compatible) terminals and some IBM terminals are currently compatible with the TYMNET,* the international, commercial network currently being utilized by the Health Education Network to enable access to the courseware available at MGH and OSU.

The cost to the user for accessing the Network during its support by the LHNCBC varied between no charges and $5.00 per hour that a computer terminal was connected to the Network. In the transitional year just passed, fixed fees per terminal connect hour were assessed of $9.00 from OSU and $8.00 from MGH (the latter was also subject to a minimum billing of $100.00 per 2-month billing period). Since July 1, 1976 the charges have been reduced! Now charges are based on three factors: (a) the time when the terminal connection takes place (i.e., there is a reduction for non-prime-time use), (b) the total amount of use per month (i.e., there is a reduction for high-volume use), and (c) the magnitude of the committed monthly minimum (i.e., there is a reduction for a higher monthly minimum). Items (b) and (c) are interlocked with the terms of the Letter of Agreement and can be varied with adequate notice to the data-base hosts. For example, by committing a monthly minimum of $375.00, an institution can reduce the prime time rate to $7.50 per hour and the non-prime-time rate to $5.50 per hour on both hosts. Other levels of commitment provide different rates; there are five possible levels at MGH and six at OSU. The net outcome of these new reduced rates is that actual terminal connect charges can vary from $10.00 all the way to $4.00 per connect hour.

Logging-in to the Network

In Figure 3 is shown a typical dialogue between the user and the various computers that establish the legitimacy of an access attempt and create the communication link for the courseware desired. The interaction depicted is for access to MGH; that for OSU is similar except that the intial response requests a student number and a six-character code name for the "course" desired. A standard Health Education user student number is provided for those institutions not wishing to assign student numbers for persons making use of that system.

Documentation of Courseware Items

For both data-base hosts, the particulars on the available courseware items can be found in user manuals that are distributed to each user institution after acknowledgment of the Letter of Agreement. An index of the topics can be found in Table 1. The User's Manual from MGH comprises approximately 200 pages.

---

*TYMNET is a registered trademark of the TYMSHARE Corporation of Cupertino, California.

please note your terminal identifier E (Note 1)

-1022-15-- (Note 2)

please log in: GWU222M; (Note 3)

password: GWUMEDU; (Note 4)

INTERACTION 025646 (Note 2)

MGH LINE 23 PORT 1 04/30/76 12:45 PM

ARE YOU USING A CRT (TERMINAL WITH TV SCREEN)? N (Note 5)

DO YOU NEED INSTRUCTIONS ON USE OF TERMINAL? N

TYPE YOUR INITIALS (FIRST, MIDDLE IF ANY, AND LAST): CST

I ASSUME YOUR NAME IS CHARLIE TIDBALL
IS THIS CORRECT? Y

WELCOME BACK, CHARLIE

TYPE 3 LETTER CODE OF THE PROGRAM YOU WANT TO TRY, OR TYPE ? IF YOU
NEED A LIST OF PROGRAMS AND CODES.
PROGRAM:

Key

lower case: originated by TYMCOM computer at node city and printed by terminal

upper case and underlined: typed by user at local terminal and printed by terminal

upper case and underlined twice: typed by user at local terminal but not printed by terminal

upper case and not underlined: originated by courseware delivery system at desired remote site
and printed by terminal

Note

1. The letter E is used to signify an ASCII terminal operating at a speed of 30 characters per
second (300 baud). Other letters are used for terminals with different characteristics.
2. An identification number used by TYMSHARE and/or MGH in troubleshooting hardware
and software difficulties.
3. These eight characters represent six characters of account code (GWU222), a letter to indicate the desired remote computer (M=MGH in Boston, Massachusetts), and a semicolon to
close the field. This response is terminated by pressing the key, of ten labeled RETURN,
which sends the message to the computer.
4. These eight characters represent seven characters of password (GWUMEDU) and a semicolon
to close the field. Since passwords are considered confidential by the computer system,
they are not printed by the terminal. The semicolon is printed only after the account code/
password combination has been accepted by the computer supervising the TYMNET system.
5. For users of CRT terminals which often have restrictions in the amount of text which can
be displayed, a different format for the courseware items is made available.

Figure 3. Typical sequence for logging-in to the Network.

In addition to directions on accessing the system and the interpretation of system
messages, there is a specific section for each of the 30 courseware topics available
from this host. Each topic is designed in such a fashion that students who engage
the program on subsequent occasions are exposed to new and different patient
material. All visuals are contained in this source and no other supplementary
material is needed for MGH programs. All these specific sections include a typical
interaction between a user and the program.

Table 1. Index of Topics Available on the Network[a]

Abbreviations, medical	Drug use in renal failure
Abdomen, anatomy of	Duodenum
Abdominal pain	Electrocardiography
Acetone, testing for	Electrolytes
Acid–base balance	Endocarditis
Alimentary tract	Endocrinology
Anatomy	Endometrium
Anesthetics	Endotracheal intubation
Anticoagulant simulator	Enzymes
Appendix, diseases of	Esophagus
Arrhythmias	Experimental trauma case
Atrial	Family medicine
Heart block	Fluid and electrolyte balance
Ventricular	Gastrointestinal system
Arterial blood gases	Genetics
Arteriosclerotic heart disease	GI bleeding
Basic patient care	Growth and development
Biliary tree	Hematology
Biochemistry	Histology
Biometrics	Human biology
Biostatistics	Human sexuality
Bleeding disorders	Hypertension diagnosis
Blood pressure	Hypertensive emergencies
CAI, general introduction	Hypertension management
Cardiac simulation	Idiopathic RDS in the newborn
Cardiopulmonary resuscitation	Ileum
Cardiovascular system	Immunohematology
Cell function	Immunology
Cell structure	Infectious diseases
Central nervous system	Infection control
Clinical nuclear medicine	Inflammation
Closed drainage systems	Internal medicine
Coagulation and bleeding disorders	Jaundice
Colon	Jejunum
Coma	Joint pain
Congenital disease	Juvenile diabetes
Congestive heart failure	Kidney
Connective tissue	Lab test simulator
Contrast media reactions	Leadership and management
Degenerative processes	Learning and motivation
Dental pharmacology	Liver
Dentistry	Lymphoreticular diseases
Developmental disorders	Malabsorption
Diabetes	Maldigestion
Diabetic ketoacidosis	Male genital tract disorders
Diagnostic tests	Math
Digestive system	Medical records
Digitalis	Medicine
Digoxin dosage adviser	Medicine, nuclear
Diseases of infants	Medicine, social
Drugs	Metabolic system

Table 1 (continued)

Microbiologic mechanisms	Psychosocial development
Musculoskeletal system	Pulse
Muscles	Radiation therapy
Myopericardial diseases	Radiology
Neontology	Renal excretory system
Neoplasms	Renal vascular disease
Nervous system	Reproductive system
Central	Respiratory distress syndrome
Muscular and peripheral	Respiratory simulation
Neurology	Respiratory system
Neuroscience	Respirations
Newborns	Shock
Nuclear medicine	Skeletal system
Nutrition	Skin
Obstetrics/Gynecology	Social medicine
Breech delivery	Statistics
Oral contraceptives	Stomach
Opthalmology	Surgery
Optometry	Temperature
Oral cancer	Terminology
Oral contraceptives	Basic perceptual concepts
Orthopmedics	Cardiovascular
Pancreas	Medical
Pathologic mechanisms	Medical abbreviations
Pediatric cough and fever	Obstetric
Pediatrics	Thromboembolic disorders
Peripheral nervous system	Toothache
Pharmacology	Trauma
Physics, nuclear	Urinalysis
Physiological chemistry	Urology
Physiology	Veins
Pregnancy	Virology
Preventive medicine	Vital signs
Psychiatry	
Psychology	

*a*Over 600 hours of terminal interactions are offered.

The CAI User's Guide from OSU is a compilation that contains over 150 pages. It too has general instructions and the courseware topics (200 as of this writing) are presented not only alphabetically by name but also by 90 subject classifications and by 17 projected audiences. The individual listings are generally restricted to a single page and call attention to the number and kinds of supplementary materials (hard copy visuals or 35-mm slides) required but do not actually provide them. The latter may be obtained from OSU for each specific courseware item at nominal cost. Both user manuals are kept up-to-date by addition and/or substitution of pages at regular intervals.

Other Services Provided

Each data-base host maintains an inquiry service for users encountering difficulties. Most of this troubleshooting can be done by telephone. As an institution becomes more familiar with utilising the Network, less reliance on this service is needed. This is true, in part, because internal personnel know how the interaction should proceed and also because local problems associated with the terminal or the communication carrier are more readily diagnosed and referred to the appropriate level rather than to the data-base host.

Both data-base hosts make available a reservation system whereby there is a guarantee that an access port will be available at a predetermined time for a specified period. The latter is particularly useful for demonstrations of system capabilities to decision makers and for scheduling access to the Network as a part of a class or laboratory exercise.

Remote authoring is available on the OSU system by using the same terminal that a student would use to engage the courseware. The latter can be accomplished by the author learning the computer language COURSEWRITER or by interacting with the CAI support personnel at OSU. This institution has developed extensive authoring aids that are available as a hard copy manual (see Chapter 15) and also provides consultation services to bring new courseware items to a high level of performance. An automated patient generator for the program CASE (Harless *et al.*, 1971) enables clinicians to create new patients for this program in an average of from 6 to 8 hours.

At the moment, only limited experience with remote authoring has occurred on the MGH system. It is possible to send courseware copy in English to Boston and have it entered into the system by MGH personnel. There are also two recently developed interactive authoring aids available on their system, DIALOG and POSER these programs make it possible for the content expert to answer queries from the computer; then the driver program generates the appropriate data base without further author intervention. To what extent this new development will impact program production remains to be determined. At MGH, there is a large reservoir of experience available in the design and implementation of sophisticated computer simulations of clinical situations (see Chapter 21).

The Birth of a User-Directed Network

In May of 1974, Dr. Robert G. Votaw, then Director of Multidiscipline Laboratories of the University of Connecticut Health Center called a meeting of the Experimental CAI Network users residing in the northeast region of the United States. It was known at that time that support for the Experimental CAI Network from the LHNCBC was scheduled to be discontinued on May 31 1975. The main purpose of the meeting was to determine how much interest there was in perpetuating nationwide access to computer-based learning materials in the health sciences

There *was* a groundswell of support, and the Health Education Network User Group (HENUG) was formed. Dr. Votaw was elected chairperson of a Steering Committee that had members from several different institutions. Task forces in the areas of networking, faculty development, and courseware evaluation were established.

In August of 1974, as a presession to the summer meeting of the Association for the Development of Computer-based Instructional Systems (ADCIS), a second meeting was held in Bellingham, Washington. It was emphasized that HENUG was intended as a nationwide organization, and users of the Experimental CAI Network from the western United States were invited to participate and become involved. This meeting reinforced the findings of the earlier session in Connecticut and the HENUG Steering Committee was confirmed. Additional persons were appointed to assure a broad geographical representation. Three days later at the ADCIS meeting which followed, HENUG was recognized as an interest group of ADCIS. This association of CAI professionals provided key financial support to foster our efforts at a critical stage in the development of the new, user-supported Network.

Subsequently, HENUG sessions were held in conjunction with the winter meeting of ADCIS (January, 1975 in Charleston, South Carolina) and the summer meeting of ADCIS (August, 1975 in Portland, Maine). HENUG also sponsored displays at the annual meetings of the Association of American Medical Colleges (November, 1974 in Chicago, and November, 1975 in Washington, D.C.). The latter involved full-scale system demonstrations, distribution of HENUG literature, availability of personnel from MGH and OSU, as well as access to persons who were regular users of the Network.

The HENUG Steering Committee met more frequently and grappled with issues relating to operating the Network in the absence of the considerable financial and moral support that had been provided by the LHNCBC. Mutually beneficial relationships with professional associations having similar concerns have been explored with the Interuniversity Communications Council (EDUCOM), the New England Regional Computer Network (NERComp), the Association of American Medical Colleges (AAMC), and the American Association of Dental Schools (AADS). Some effort was also expended to have the National Library of Medicine reconsider the LHNBC's decision to discontinue support for a nationwide network. Although there was no change in policy, some funds were made available for partial support of the position of Network Coordinator during the 11-month transitional period after cessation of federal funding. On May 31, 1975, the Experimental CAI Network terminated its activities and on June 1, 1975, the Health Education Network picked up the support role with the Network Coordinator located at the University of Connecticut Health Center under Dr. Votaw's supervision. There was no interruption of service to the users as a result of the change. During the first year of operation, there was a gradual increase both in the number of user institutions and in the number of hours of use. The peak usage of the Experimental CAI Network has not yet been surpassed, but there is every expectation that this will happen during the second year of operation.

In recognition of the need to establish a legitimate identity for the Health Education Network, Articles of Incorporation were developed and filed in the District of Columbia. The Articles specify the purpose of the organization and state that the corporation shall have members consisting of qualified institutions and organizations having a direct interest in the purposes of the corporation and which are themselves nonprofit corporations. Management of the businesss of the corporation is vested in a board of directors as defined in the statutes of the District of Columbia. Incorporation under the Nonprofit Corporation Act of that jurisdiction became effective October 24, 1975.

Bylaws for the corporation were also developed. The latter specified that all institutions which satisfied the nonprofit condition for membership prior to the adoption of the bylaws and who were users as evidenced by Letters of Agreement with one or both of the data-base hosts would be accorded membership in the corporation. At a meeting of such members in Santa Barbara, California, on January 26, 1976 the bylaws were adopted and a board of directors was elected. Members and officers of this board with their affiliations can be found in Table 2. On January 29, 1976, Thomas H. Held, Ed. S., of the University of Maryland School of Medicine was elected Chairperson of the HENUG Steering Committee. This group, with its unrestricted membership, is being retained to provide a broad interface to both the user community and professionals in the field of CAI through the affiliation with ADCIS. Unlike the board of directors of the corporation, which is charged with setting the policy to support a nationwide network, it can be expected that HENUG will provide a forum for users and potential users. Presumably HENUG will become increasingly concerned with such long-range issues as faculty development, courseware evaluation, and curricular integration.

On June 1, 1976, the Internal Revenue Service ruled that the Health Education Network, Inc., was exempt from federal income tax under section 501(c)(3) of the Internal Revenue Code. This finding sets the stage for a grant-procurement program which is considered essential if the Health Education Network, Inc., expects to achieve its mission of providing economical access to health-related CAI.

Challenges for the Future

Acceptance of the network concept on a broad scale is the fundamental challenge confronting the proponents of this technology today. In a preceding section, the advantages of networking have been presented. These advantages need to be recognized more universally throughout the medical community. Thus, until the level of computer literacy among medical faculty increases sufficiently to improve and sustain the CAI thrust, we must continue the effort initiated by the Experimental CAI Network to provide an authentic demonstration of networking benefits at costs that (a) are acceptable to current users and (b) will attract new users.

Obviously, the way in which the Network is financed is tightly coupled to this challenge; acceptance is more easily achieved when user fees are low. To bring

Table 2. Board of Directors of the Network and Data-Base Host Contact Persons

President Robert G. Votaw, Ph.D. Associate Dean for Medical Education University of Connecticut Health Center	Robert C. Hickey, Ph.D. Associate Vice Chancellor of Health Professions University of Pittsburgh School of Medicine
Secretary Barbara B. Farquhar Assistant Director of Laboratory of Computer Science Massachusetts General Hospital	Martin Kamp, M.D. Chief of Academic Computing Services School of Medicine University of California at San Francisco
Treasurer Charles S. Tidball, Ph.D., M.D. Director of Computer Assisted Education and Services George Washington University Medical Center	Harvey S. Long, Ph.D. Instructional Systems Consultant IBM Corporation Ruann E. Pengov, Ph.D. Director, Division of Computing Services College of Medicine The Ohio State University
William C. Brown, Ph.D. Head, Information Science Section National Research Council of Canada	

Karen A. Duncan, Ph.D.
Director, Office of Computer Resources
College of Dental Medicine
Medical University of South Carolina
	At Massachusetts General Hospital
	    Kathleen Famiglietti
	    Laboratory of Computer Science
	    Massachusetts General Hospital
	    Boston, MA 02114
	    (617) 726-3950

Weston D. Gardner, M.D. Professor of Anatomy Medical College of Wisconsin	

Charles M. Goldstein
Chief, Computing Technology
Lister Hill National Center for Biomedical
    Communications
National Library of Medicine
	At the Ohio State University
	    Mark H. Forman
	    Division of Computing Services
	    076 Health Science Library
	    376 W. Tenth Avenue
	    Columbus, OH 43210
	    (614) 422-6192

about low fees without substantial subvention requires distributing the services across the broadest possible base so that the fixed expenses are shared by as many institutions as possible. Acceptance is also coupled to the nature of the total data base available; this raises the issues of new data-base hosts, competition between data-base hosts, and courseware evaluation. Ultimately, a key question with regard to acceptance is whether CAI is used adjunctively or whether it is genuinely integrated into the total professional curriculum. Here we deal with such questions as faculty involvement, local authoring, and courseware maintenance. The Network has no overall solution to offer for these complex and difficult issues, but we affirm that networking is one of the tools that can help the profession cope with the increasingly awesome task of educating across such a broad information base. In the sections that follow are some specific suggestions that seem feasible and attractive to the author; they represent his personal opinions and should not be construed as Network policy.

The Data Base

Although some persons consider the current data base available to users of the Network adequate, most would agree that it can be improved. The easiest way to make substantial alterations is to add new data-base hosts. As attractive as the idea may be, there are some deterrents that are primarily economic. At the moment, neither data-base host is consistently logging more than 1000 hours of use per month. If a new data-base host reduces the hours of use at the present hosts, this would be undesirable. Under current technological considerations merely interfacing a new host to the TYMNET incurs costs of approximately $35,000 per year, which does not include the cost of installing the hardware or programming the interface between the host computer and the communications computer. By constrast, if adding a new data-base host were to increase usage at MGH and OSU, then this would be advantageous. Unfortunately, it is not always possible to predict the impact of such alterations in system configuration in advance.

Central Management

Currently, the contractual obligations reside, on the one hand, between the database hosts and the communications carrier, and on the other, by separate Letters of Agreement between the users and each data-base host. As more hosts are added to the Network, this arrangement will become increasingly burdensome. There will be some advantages in having the Network contract with the data-base hosts for access to their programs and having the Network contract for the communications. Users will then make a single agreement with the Network, and the latter will provide each user with one bill for the total service used. Multiple billing will be eliminated, but the Network will have to take on personnel, or contract to have services performed, to accomplish work now being performed by the data-base hosts. Since universities are often slow in paying their obligations, the Network will face cash flow problems without the resources of another operation to buffer the cash demands. Nevertheless, the Network will then be setting terminal connect fees that will have an advantage in terms of its mission to maintain economical access to health-related courseware. Once again, a relatively large scale of operation will be essential to provide the necessary stability of performance that will assure success for a central management effort.

Authoring versus Student Use

Local authoring is obviously advantageous from a number of points of view. Not the least of these is the favorable impact on user acceptance of having faculty who will recommend their own programs and integrate them into the curriculum more readily than those written by other authors. One of the best ways to encourage local authoring on the Network is to reduce the terminal connect fees for such activity. At current levels of use, this is not economically feasible. With central management and the Network setting the terminal fees, local authoring may become cost effective. This will require either a different way of paying for services and/or a larger scale of user acceptance.

Courseware Evaluation

The issue of courseware evaluation is unlikely to be resolved in the near further although both the LHNCBC and the AAMC are developing guidelines. Local authoring will increase the pressure to create review procedures so that there is minimal delay between the initiation of a new program and its acceptance, if of appropriate quality, for nationwide access. Whether this will be a function of the Network, the institution where the author resides, the data-base host insitution, or some as-yet-to-be identified fourth agency, remains to be seen.

Conclusions

The Health Education Network, Inc., has come into being because a dedicated group of users of the Experimental CAI Network sponsored by the LHNCBC of the National Library of Medicine refused to accept the termination of nationwide access to high-quality CAI material at reasonable costs. The Network has completed the first year of operation during which it has seen a steady growth. Further, it has developed (a) a nationwide user group (HENUG), (b) a nonprofit corporate base that has been declared exempt from federal tax by the Internal Revenue Service, and (c) a Board of Directors that is representative of several disciplines and is well-distributed geographically. There are three elements involved in achieving the goal of low-cost access to CAI materials: increasing acceptance to favor economies of operating on a larger scale; outright subvention by foundations, federal agencies, or states; and other savings brought on by centralizing Network operations. The current nationwide data base that consists of approximately 600 hours of effective interaction is adequate but can probably be improved without incurring decreased utilization by competition between data-base hosts. Remote authoring favors faculty involvement and the development of specialized courseware. Cooperation among CAI users is helpful in a variety of ways and is being nurtured by the presence of the Network. The real challenges of wider CAI acceptance remain at the level of fostering computer literacy, faculty development, courseware evaluation, and curricular integration. The Network is dedicated to helping all its members and affiliates make progress toward these elusive elements.

ACKNOWLEDGMENT

The author wishes to acknowledge the participation of all members of the original HENUG Steering Committee in the development of this chapter. More particularly, Robert G. Votaw, Barbara Farquhar, and Ruann Pengov were of especially pertinent help in the preparation of the final draft.

References

Harless, W. G., Drennon, G. G., Marxer, J. J., Root, J. A., and Miller, G. E., 1971. CASE: A computer aided simulation of the clinical encounter, *J. Med. Educ.* **46**: 443.

Health Education Network, 1975. *By-laws*, Washington, D.C., 17 pp.

Kamp, M., 1975. *Index to Computerized Teaching in the Health Sciences*, University of California, San Francisco, 183 pp.

Lefever, R. D., and Johnson, J. K., 1976. *Survey of the Use of Computers in Instruction*, Association of American Medical Colleges, Washington, D.C., 173 pp.

Tidball, C. S., 1976. *Overview of Survey of the Use of Computers in Instruction*, Association of American Medical Colleges, Washington, D.C., 8 pp.

12

Electronic Publishing and Electronic Literature

Theodor H. Nelson

No alert person, drubbed by popular magazine and TV news, can fail to have heard that we are on the threshold of some sort of new era in the use of information. Soon, we hear, we will be able to get at the Library of Congress stored on a disk, or movies in a pinky ring, and information that we want vaguely may come at us without our even having to ask.

Corporations are being formed. The hearts of investors are palpitating. Foundations and federal agencies are continuing to put out money for breakthrough showcase projects. Yet, in my estimation, we have not a state of progress but a state of confusion. Never before have so many accepted the unrefined technical fantasies of so few. Never before has so much been spent for what has been so little understood or thought out. Unfortunately, the public has no simple comprehension of the varieties of possibilities, the vast range of options. They will believe anything they are told except the whole picture, which nobody tells them.

This sort of thing happens easily in any field. Technical people create catchphrases, and people from outside, eager to be up-to-date, seize on the catchphrases as received wisdom, ideas that seem to span and comprehend all the possibilities. Those outsiders then spread the gospel to their own corners of the world, never quite sensing what an arbitrary selection has been made for them; failing to ask pointed questions, they in turn become opinion leaders for other outsiders who are even more afraid to ask. To mix parables, it is as if the blind men, after evaluating the elephant, then lead the other blind men in their several directions.

I am referring to the overblown public expectations for "video records" (which are at this writing still a fiction), for the supposed wonders of cable TV and framegrabbing, and for such brittle concepts as "computer-assisted instruction," "information retrieval," and "artificial intelligence." By brittle I mean that under pressure they shatter into many separate pieces, individual concepts lacking the collective magic of the overall name.

My objective here is not to criticize these approaches; many of them have their virtues and uses. But I want to stress the problem we face: a variety of people are

---

Theodor H. Nelson · Project Xanadu, Swarthmore, Pennsylvania.

proposing different arrangements by which *other* people, meaning we the public, should handle information in the future; and accordingly the public ought not submit with docility to just whatever may result spottily by chance.

On the other hand, wonders are indeed upon us, particularly in the area of cheap computers. The dramatic fall of equipment prices – best symbolized by the introduction in January, 1975 of the Altair, a full-fledged computer for about five hundred dollars – negates most of the previous economic assumptions about computers. Comparably cheap graphic computer displays are now available, although screens capable of fast and detailed presentations will continue to cost considerably more. The computer on every desk is within sight; the era of Computers for People has come, if only we decide what we want.

With this question in mind – what do we want? – let us consider a few basic capabilities of today's equipment and systems.

First of all, high-performance display scopes are now generally available. These are visual display terminals capable of rapidly bringing text and pictures from computer storage to the screen. By "high performance" I mean capable of holding over a thousand alphabetical characters in upper and lower case, in *more than one font*, and capable of *moving the text smoothly on the screen* – a feature many do not realize to be necessary. Such scopes also make possible animated graphical displays, with computer-generated diagrams and cartoons in motion.*

Second, instant accesses are possible. That is, the reader at such a high-power screen, making a request, may be rewarded within seconds by whatever he wants to see or read. While this level of performance is presently available only with larger computers, the problem is basically one of software – the master control programs – and rapid strides may be expected here.

Obviously, for the larger and larger amounts of material to be offered, some sort of network of storage and supply must send materials on demand, as the nearest computer cannot possibly hold everything you want to read. Here, too, developments are proceeding rapidly, with people increasingly aware that such a network can be built of small computers rather than big ones, as long as the hookup includes a lot of storage space.

Third, rapid arbitrary jumps are possible. That is, material stored in one place may offer a link, much like a footnote, to material stored in another place; a reader may choose to take such a jump between one thing and whatever has been put for him at the other end of the link. The new material arrives on the screen at once. (The NLS system of Douglas Engelbart, at Stanford, is the most well-known to offer this capability, but there are now numerous others.)

---

* This presupposes a "calligraphic" type of display equipment, not video. An exemplary unit of this type, the Model VT11 from Digital Equipment Corporation, now costs $6500 and offers all these features; it requires, in addition, a PDP-11 computer, currently costing about $5000. (It may be possible at some time in the near future to get the same effects with the "bit map" type of display, the prices of which are dropping rapidly. Such equipment has the advantage of using video signals of the normal type, rather than the more expensive electronics of the other.)

Fourth, such links may provide for automatic "windowing" between one thing and another; that is, a document on the screen may have a window into another document, or a picture on the screen may have a window into another picture. (For text, such windowing has been developed on Engelbart's and other systems. Graphical windowing usually requires special hardware but is largely the same problem.)

These are the elemental capabilities. The power and breadth of the possibilities thus opened do not seem to be widely understood, although much of CAI – the tell-and-test, multiple-choice approach – appears to be a restricted exploitation of the "jump" concept. It has long seemed to me that such linkage concepts offered much wider opportunities for education, research, and literatures of the future than have yet been put to use.

Computer storage and screen presentation can now change our relation to information fundamentally and completely. The paper world we have lived in for so long – a forest of documents (books, magazines, certificates, and whatnot, each having a certain type of paper housing) – may and perhaps should be supplanted by an electronic counterpart. But in this transformation we have a chance to improve the world – a one-time chance.

It seems to me that the way to proceed now is to look at our paper world, consider its best features, and study how to preserve, extend and improve them. Then we ought to be able to design a world of electronic documents, techniques for rapidly calling them, and techniques for working on them. This could keep everything we want of the old ways while eliminating the "paperwork." Such a general framework means basically that our reading, writing, and record-keeping may be simplified, clarified, and etherealized – the papers will be everywhere and nowhere, will need no filing, and cannot be mislaid.

According to this point of view, then, what matters is what we want on our screens, and the computer technicalities must be worked out accordingly. Such a view is not considered entirely welcome by some parts of the computer establishment, but it is obviously a legitimate approach. Some ramifications of this viewpoint for "business" programming are taken up elsewhere (Nelson, 1978).

Let us consider the possibilities of "electronic literature," some form of writing and publication that employs electronic transmissions and presentations but serves the functions literature serves now – publication, scholarship, and citation; research, education, and entertainment; and general enlightenment. My belief is that the same things can be done better on screens.

However, this will not come about accidentally. Literature as we know it has developed step-by-step, with its traditions of publication date, citation, footnote, and so forth. Yet these can only be mapped into electronic embodiment by a series of conscious decisions. Mere convention must be replaced by active design – design of the visible forms of jump, windowing, and annotation desired; and design of the hidden forms of interconnection, transmission, and look-ahead that are called for underneath.

To accompany such an electronic literature, there should somehow be built-in techniques for the general intercomparison of things in the system (comparable to looking at books side-by-side); a free anthologizing facility, allowing each user to make his own "anthologies" with windows into whatever else he wants to keep around; and the ability to quote and present modified versions, wherein one writer may show his modification of another's material.

To design in this area, we both need to know technically what is possible and to feel intuitively what different literatures have meant to people in the past. Among the questions we must ask are: What forms of organization in a nonsequential written work will be most helpful and clear? What forms of personal annotation will be most useful for making private notes on what we read? What forms of screen publication are most useful and viable? And appealing? And most important, how may we best preserve and extend the facilities – and freedoms – we have had before?

What we need is an orderly and yet truly versatile way by which a user of the screen may get around in an ever-increasing panorama of offerings – on-line documents and facilities and "thinkertoys." These will include writings, user-manipulable graphics, pathways among these things and anthologies that embrace and window them, and layer upon layer of public and private annotation and commentary by a parade of authors and users.* The problem is to find some orderly, overall meta-design that will preserve clarity while facilitating easy movement by the user (Nelson, 1965). Anybody can design a system that is complicated and confusing. The problem is how to design a system that is *general, simple,* and *clear.* Contrary to a widespread myth, generality and simplicity not only can coexist but belong together.

I have for some time promoted the term "hypertext" for nonsequential writing using such facilities. The general idea of hypertext is that, by creating pathways for readers with different interests, we can both simplify writing and make reading more appropriate to the reader's interest and level of knowledge.

However, it must be admitted that general hypertext is in itself a somewhat disorderly notion. The possibilities go in too many directions. My present concern, then, is to bring some sense of order and generality to these areas.

The approach I am presently investigating I call "structured literature," by analogy with Dijkstra's well-known concept of "structured programming". Just as programming can get you into tangles, arbitrary jumping around on screens can get you into tangles, and the same remedies used in programming may prove helpful.

The structured-literature approach is based on the idea of finding a few powerful and clear organizing techniques and employing these exclusively, with the idea of avoiding idiosyncratic and exceptional forms of connection. If properly done, this need not limit the versatility of performance of the system or its contents but may

---

* Note that blind excursions – events that the user cannot fully control, such as animated cartoons and most CAI – confuse these offerings slightly, as the user may not be able to find out precisely what he is in for.

provide an ordering, which increases the flexibility and power available to the user.

A structured literature, then, is one having defined data structures of certain generalized types – especially text and animated graphics – and allowing certain types of link structures among them. Many types of viewing and jumps may, in turn, be devised around these link types.

In my present formulation, there are several link types. These include the plain jump, the window that can open from one file to another (the quote window), and the intercomparison multilink (collateration). With the use of such a set of linkage types, documents and screen views may be nested to any degree without obscuring the fundamental simplicity of interconnection. The interesting thing is that these link structures appear to have enough generality for all desirable tasks yet confer a certain clarity upon the resulting system.

This structured-literature approach also supposes a hypothetical network of fairly definite properties. Such a network will service individual consoles that are not mere "terminals" but that will each be capable of individual, private operation. Both network and individual consoles will be set up to handle big files with arbitrary structure. The network will have techniques permitting storage of both private and public materials, including private annotations and modifications of public documents. (Thus, a "publication" method must be defined within the network. Since publishing can be instantaneous and unrestricted, merely a "publish" button on the console could do it – but the dangers of rash publication to an individual's reputation would be great. Some formalized technique would therefore be required for "committing to publish" – probably a ceremony and signature.)

One interesting scheme for copyrighting would appear to bind such a system well. Copyrighting is normally a matter of status and litigation, but such a network could establish a copyright convention *internal to the network* and agreed upon by all participants. Under one possible arrangement, each author would consent to a certain royalty – say, a few cents per screen hour – and each reader would contribute those few cents automatically as he reads along. The windowing approaches already mentioned could then automatically furnish a general solution to the "copyright problem" with regard to quotation and citation, simply by this means: authors who are windowed automatically get royalties as well.

Actually these formulations are intended simply to facilitate the extension of literature as we have previously known it into the era of cross-linked screen access. What these specific linking ideas really do is stress the singularity of each document, its external and internal borders. Thus, we focus on the integrity of the "document" as we have long known it, the "author" as we have long known him, and an extended form of "writing" as we have long done it and read it – rather than what some people, such as McLuhan and the video freaks and the CAI folk, have been telling us would be anonymous, collective, scrambled, psychometric, and/or Boolean.

And it should go without saying, but it must be said, that none of our freedoms should be sacrificed for any new advantages. Our files must be free from snooping, tampering, and censorship (the restricting of accessibility). Naturally, no absolute guarantees can be put in at the computer level; but it may be that steps can be taken to make incursions — whether by government or other source of mischief — plain and flagrant. It is our common paramount interest to do so.

References

For additional material on the topics discussed here, the reader is referred to my book *Computer Lib* (1974) available from The Distributors, 702 S. Michigan, South Bend, In. Of particular relevance in that volume are "Apparatuses of Apparition" and "Babel's in Toyland," p. 125; "The Mind's Eye," pp. 109 ff.; "No More Teachers' Dirty Looks," pp. 113 ff.; "Hypertext," pp. 84–85; "Doug Engelbart and 'The Augmentation of Intellect,'" pp. 82–83. On collateration, "Thinkertoys," p. 77 and "The Parallel Textface," pp. 75–76. On the network, see "Xanadu," pp. 72–73.

Nelson, T. H., 1965. A file structure for the complex, the changing, and the indeterminate, *in Proceedings of the Association for Computing Machinery Annual Conference*, ACM, New York.

Nelson, T. H., 1978. Data realms and magic windows, *in Proceedings of the ACPA-V Conference*, published by the Association of Computer Programmers and Analysts, in press.

13

A Self-Contained CAI Machine for Health Sciences Education

J. A. Starkweather and M. Kamp

The use of computer-based education in schools of medicine, nursing, dentistry, pharmacy, and other health sciences disciplines has traditionally been carried out with multiple computer terminals connected to a time-sharing computer system (Weinberg, 1973; Wooster and Lewis, 1973; Alpert and Bitzer, 1970). This method was developed to allow sharing of scarce computer resources and requires a complex operating system as well as some form of communication between terminals and computer. Both of these requirements can and do result in operational failures and complex access procedures, but the more efficient use of expensive computer resources has justified the potential difficulty.

Recent years have seen a dramatic increase in the computing power that can be available in small, relatively inexpensive machines based on microprocessor technology (Vacroux, 1975). It is now possible to consider avoiding the problems of telecommunications and complex operating systems by using a self-contained computer/terminal device for each student CAI station. Such a device would consist of a central processor with attached direct access memory, a bulk storage unit such as a magnetic tape cassette or disk storage unit, a keyboard for student input, and a display screen (or typewriter) for output of information from the computer.

The Self-Contained CAI Machine

The self-contained CAI machine being used at University of California in San Francisco uses the PILOT language on a Datapoint 2200 or 1100 computer/terminal, which is capable of stand-alone operation as well as communication with remote computer systems. This machine has a built-in minicomputer with direct access semiconductor memory, and the PILOT system has been written in two versions

J. A. Starkweather · Department of Psychiatry, University of California, San Francisco, California. *M. Kamp* · Scientific Computing Services, University of California School of Medicine, San Francisco, California.

for machines equipped with 8000 or 12,000 bytes of memory (Kamp and Stark-weather, 1973). The Datapoint has a standard ASCII keyboard, a cathode ray tube for character display, and two built-in magnetic tape cassette drives. This capability is housed in a single unit smaller than many cathode ray tube terminals.

In operation, the machine is first loaded with the PILOT system from a tape cassette. This goes into execution immediately and displays instructions for the student to load a program tape. The system runs as an interpreter of PILOT instructions, and occupies a section of memory as long as the machine is running PILOT programs. The remainder of memory is used for the particular instructional program in use, with a capacity of about 2000 bytes (characters) in the 8K machine and about 5000 bytes in the 12K machine.

About 130,000 characters of PILOT program code can be stored on one side of a tape cassette, and the instructional program is read into memory under control of instructions written into the PILOT program. The second cassette can be used, also under control of instructions written into the PILOT program, to collect some or all of the displayed text, some or all student responses to program questions, student comments, and program remarks as desired by the author.

With a communications adapter and suitable programs, the self-contained computer/terminal can simulate a variety of conventional terminals. The character coding, communications protocol, and different transmission speeds are all handled by a terminal simulation program. This provides access to the facilities of larger time-sharing systems when needed, such as statistical programs for the analysis of collected student data. If the self-contained machine is equipped with tape cassettes or some other bulk storage device, this can be used to transmit or receive data when connected to the time-sharing system. The ability to communicate with a time-sharing system also allows the use of its high-speed printing equipment when appropriate, as well as the use of sophisticated on-line editing systems.

The ability to operate in either a stand-alone or a communications mode allows an operational choice between relatively inexpensive and easy access to a dedicated and personal machine and more complex access to powerful computation or large data bases when this is required or would be more efficient. At the authors' institution there is a compatible version of PILOT running on our time-sharing system and providing greater capability when it is required.

Although the Datapoint self-contained machine provides a convenient packaging of central processor, character display, keyboard, and cassettes, there are also other self-contained computer/terminal devices that contain microprocessors of equal or greater capability. We can expect this type of equipment to share the progress of computer technology, in general, and the near future will probably bring new machines with much greater capability at a lower cost.

Easy Access to Instructional Computing

Health sciences students are likely to view the computer as an expected utility. They are not studying computers or computing methods, and they will consider the usual methods of computer access to be irrelevant distractions. The same applies to faculty members who are developing computerized teaching materials but are not interested in knowing the details of their implementation.

Accessing CAI programs via a time-sharing terminal requires significantly more steps than on a self-contained machine. The student must know how to use an acoustic coupler, how to carry out the dial-in procedure and establish contact with the computer, and how to sign on and begin the program he wants. The system is normally not very forgiving or helpful if even minor errors are made at any step in this process. The stand-alone machine, on the other hand, needs only to have a program tape loaded and it is ready to begin. There is no contention for access to terminal ports, which are often fully occupied at peak periods on a time-sharing system. This convenience and lack of complexity can be a very important factor to persons who are studying a subject other than the computer itself.

Reliability

The self-contained CAI machine is inherently more reliable than the time-sharing terminal because both the hardware and the software are simpler in the small machine. The small machine is dedicated to a single student and does not require a complex operating system such as the one used to allocate the resources of the larger computer. The machine itself is much simpler and smaller, and no communications equipment is needed because the input and output devices (such as keyboard and display screen) are an integral part of the computer.

Response Time

Speed is another way of comparing the two methods of delivering CAI programs. Typical response times for teleprocessing systems are in the range of ½ to 5 seconds, measured from the time the student response is terminated to the time the computer begins to display the next line of text. The response time varies, depending on the number of terminals that are being serviced, and on the load from other jobs that might be running on the same computer. With most time-sharing systems, response time is likely to be slowest at the same time the largest number of people want to use the computer, such as the frequently seen peak of activity in the middle of the afternoon.

In the self-contained CAI machine, all of the computer resources are dedicated to the single student user, and response time is almost always less than 1 second. Periodically a different portion of the CAI program must be read into the main memory from a bulk storage device such as a tape cassette. This introduces a longer delay, but the new material can often be read while the student is studying a text display that has just been presented to him. In the near future, these machines will more commonly be equipped with small disk storage units that will allow access to any part of the CAI program without appreciable delay.

Computing Power

Modern mini- and microcomputers have impressive performance, but they cannot match the storage capacity and computational power of a larger time-sharing system. The most powerful and comprehensive software is written for larger machines, and they can easily manipulate large masses of data. For most types of CAI programs, especially in the health sciences, this power is not needed since programs are primarily text-handling tasks and do not require a large amount of computing.

The amount of direct access memory is normally limited in a mini- or micro-computer. There are some CAI programs that cannot operate under that restriction if the auxiliary storage device is a low-speed unit such as a tape cassette that will not allow practical random access. An example would be a simulated clinical encounter or interview that allows the students to enter a wide variety of questions in their own words, and requires immediate access to a large matching sequence and many sets of possible responses. Still, the majority of computerized teaching programs can be run using a combination of the relatively small amount of direct access memory with the large capacity of inexpensive bulk storage devices such as a magnetic tape cassette. When small disk storage units become more common, even very complex large programs can be accomodated.

Cost Comparison

Determining the cost of using a computer is usually a complex task, and can be approached in a variety of ways. With computerized teaching systems, the most common measure is the cost per hour of computerized teaching programs delivered to a student terminal or station. For purposes of this comparison, we will assume that the computer equipment is being rented rather than purchased, and that each student station is in use 30 hours per week or 120 hours per month. We will not include the cost of personnel or facilities, since that will be similar for both approaches.

In the case of the remote time-sharing system, the cost would include about $100 per month for rental and maintenance of the computer terminal, the acoustic coupler, and the telephone. The current approximate cost of accessing CAI programs via the Health Education Network is in the range of $10.00 per hour, and this includes communications as well as computer charges. For 120 hours of student—computer interaction, the monthly cost would be $1300, or $10.83 per student hour.

With the self-contained CAI machine, the monthly cost is fixed, no matter how many student hours are provided each month. A self-contained machine currently in use at the University of California, San Francisco, can be leased for $200 per month, including the maintenance charges. At this rate, 120 hours per month of CAI usage would cost $200, or $1.67 per student hour.

The widest difference of costs between the two methods of delivering CAI programs occurs when the level of use is 100 or more hours per month. At very low levels of use, such as 10 or 20 hours per month, the hourly rates are similar. The cost of using some other time-sharing computer systems may be much less, since a large part of the cost of the CAI service provided by the Health Education Network results from the expense of allowing access to two computer systems via a nation-wide communications network. Still, time-sharing CAI services would have to be available for less than $1.00 per hour to even approach the low cost of the self-contained machine.

Expandability and Backup

The fact that each student station using a self-contained CAI machine is a dupli-cate of every other student station will affect planning for expanding the system and for providing backup for mechanical failures. In a time-sharing system, some amount of expansion can be easily accommodated by acquiring more terminals and more access ports for the central computer. Then there will be a point at which a major component of the time-sharing computer must be replaced in order to accommodate more terminals or to maintain adequate response time. This may mean new communications equipment, more disk storage or memory, or even a more powerful central processor. Thus, at some point in the growth of the system it may require an additional disk storage unit to accommodate two more student terminals, and this makes expansion difficult at times. Expanding the number of self-contained CAI machines is a simpler matter, because the cost is the same for each additional station and no large system modifications are needed.

A large student facility using self-contained CAI machines still retains the simplicity and reliability of the single small machine. If a self-contained CAI machine is used for each student station, then a mechanical failure will put only one station out of operation and a substitution can easily be made with one of the other machines. On the other hand, it is not usually possible to provide redundancy in major components of a time-sharing computer system. Then, when a major compo-nent has a breakdown, all student stations are out of operation until it can be repaired.

Program Preparation and Maintenance

For the author and programmer, both approaches provide facilities for writing and modifying the CAI programs. Most time-sharing systems offer on-line program entry and editing, and some have special-purpose programs that actively help the author with questions and prompting. The self-contained machine can be loaded with an editor system that facilitates entry and modification of programs on the local storage device, such as a magnetic tape cassette or small disk unit. The larger time-sharing systems have much more powerful editing systems and can provide program listings and other types of printouts via their high-speed printer.

The self-contained CAI machine does not have powerful editing systems for program entry and normally uses a display screen rather than having a hard copy output device. By acting as a terminal to a time-sharing system, it can take advantage of the editing and printing facilities when needed. Programs can be edited and printed by using the small machine to communicate with a larger system, and the finished program can be transmitted and stored on a tape cassette for routine use in stand-alone operation. This flexibility allows the programmer to use the facilities of the larger system when they are appropriate, and work on the inexpensive small machine the rest of the time.

Program Exchange

One of the problems of sharing computerized teaching materials between institutions is the variety of programming languages and system congfigurations that are in use. This problem occurs with all types of delivery systems and does not appear to be related to their size. Both types of systems also have the capability of making duplicate copies of their program material for distribution.

Proponents of the use of a nationwide network for delivery of health sciences CAI services argue that sharing and revision of teaching programs is greatly facilitated when only a single copy needs to be installed and maintained on the central computer. This would be a powerful argument in favor of time-shared computer use if all health sciences schools could be economically served by such a network, and if all faculties could agree to use the same teaching programs with their students.

Unless there is a single time-sharing system, the same problems of system and language differences will impede sharing CAI programs between systems. Self-contained machines are more likely to be produced in large numbers and thereby standardized. Programs can be shared via inexpensive tape cassettes and, if necessary, can be modified by local faculty members to fit the particular content and emphasis of their teaching.

Programming Languages for the CAI Machine

The easy access made possible by the self-contained CAI machine should not be compromised by the programming language that is used with it. The programming language must be easy to learn, so faculty members and students interested in writing their own programs can get started with a minimum of difficulty. At the same time, the programming language should be flexible and powerful enough to be able to run the natural-language and simulation programs that are now being used in some health sciences institutions.

In the interest of program maintenance and transportability, the programming language should have a format that is readable without constant reference to the manual. Ideally, the language would also be widespread and standardized so that only minimal alterations would enable a program to operate in many different machine environments.

The PILOT Language

The PILOT language was developed in 1968 at the University of California in San Francisco (Starkweather, 1969). PILOT stands for Programmed Inquiry, Learning Or Teaching, and was first developed as a time-sharing system for the IBM 360 computer. Since then it has been implemented on more than a dozen computers of all sizes, but one of its most successful versions to date has been on an "intelligent terminal," the Datapoint 2200 (or 1100), an example of a self-contained CAI machine.

PILOT has been particularly successful in terms of immediate ease of use by persons unfamiliar with computers, for it may be used in minimal form with only brief introductory knowledge to get started. PILOT has been used for traditional frame-oriented instructional programs as well as for providing practice with simulated clinical situations, self-evaluation testing, and simulated interviewing with natural-language input from the students (Kamp and Burnside, 1974; Brody *et al.*, 1973; Starkweather *et al.*, 1967). It has proven itself to be especially readable, allowing authors and instructors who obtain programs from other centers to make modifications without difficulty.

Summary of PILOT Language Specifications

There are four basic types of instructions in PILOT, and they perform the functions of presenting text, accepting answers, matching keywords in the answers, and transferring control (jumping) to another part of the program.

```
T: TEXT
A:
M: ITEM, ITEM, ITEM
J: *LABEL3
```

All of the core instructions have a single-letter code followed by a colon, and in the case of the T-instruction anything following the colon will be typed or displayed on the screen. The A-instruction will cause the program to stop and accept an answer from the keyboard, and the M-instruction will attempt a "match" between the item(s) following the colon and the most recent answer that has been accepted. If the match is successful a "yes" flag is set, otherwise a "no" flag is set.

The J-instruction (JUMP) will transfer control to another section of the program identified by the *LABEL. These basic instructions, in some form, are found in all CAI languages.

Any instruction in the PILOT language can be made conditional by writing a "Y" or "N" after the instruction code and before the colon. If a Y is used, such as TY: TEXT or JY: *LABEL 3, then the instruction will only be carried out if the "yes" flag is set (the last match was successful). Instructions with the N condition are only carried out if the "no" flag is set.

Any instruction can also be made conditional by using a numeric variable, in parentheses, following the instruction code and preceding the colon. Thus the instruction "J(X): *LABEL" will only be carried out if the number represented by X is greater than zero. C-instructions allow computational operations of varying complexity depending on the particular implementation of PILOT in use.

Standardization of PILOT

PILOT was developed for the IBM 360 Computer in 1969, and by 1972 several versions of the language had been written to run on other machines. Partly because of individual preferences and partly because of the requirement of different computer systems, each version of the language was somewhat different from the others. In early 1973, representatives of the major implementations of the PILOT language met and agreed on a set of core language specifications to be common among all the systems. This new standard was originally called PILOT-73, and current acceptance has shortened the name to PILOT (Starkweather and Kamp, 1976).

Complete compatibility between different implementations of the language did not seem to be a realistic goal, so a standard way of describing functions outside the core language was agreed upon. Additions or variations from the core language instructions will be written as keywords with two or more letters as an instruction code. Thus, several types of matching functions have been written for special purposes and are coded as "MW:" for "match word," "MS:" for "match squeezed string," amd "MNUM:" for "match only numeric." This method allows each installation to implement special functions in a standard manner, while the majority of the PILOT code remains common to all programs.

When a programming language is implemented on several different computers, there are always some special instructions or codes needed for the specific equipment being used. The version of PILOT written for the Datapoint 2200 or 1100 machine includes a set of commands for flexible control of the display screen and the two tape cassette drives.

Examples of Programs on the Self-Contained Machine

Many types of computerized teaching materials can be used on the self-contained CAI machine, from simple self-evaluation test questions to case-oriented tutorials in which the student enters questions in his own words and is allowed to go through the process of evaluating and treating a simulated patient. The following examples are programs that are written in the PILOT programming language and are running on a self-contained Datapoint 1100 or 2200 computer/terminal. To make the printed example clear, the student's responses are preceded by an "S" even though this does not occur in actual operation.

The first example is a self-evaluation exercise with corrective feedback for each student response. If he wishes, the student is allowed to go through each question repeatedly, so he can explore the feedback for every one of the alternatives. If his performance is being scored, only his first response to each question is collected on the data tape. The topic of this sample is psychiatry, with emphasis on the relationship between physical and mental illnesses.

WHICH OF THE FOLLOWING PSYCHOLOGICAL MECHANISMS BEST DESCRIBES THE PROCESS BY WHICH MEDICAL SYMPTOMS APPEAR IN NEUROTIC DEPRESSION:
(1) SOMATIC PREOCCUPATION   (4) IDENTIFICATION
(2) SOMATIZATION   (5) LYING
(3) CONVERSION

S: 3

CONVERSION IS THE PROCESS BY WHICH AN UNCONSCIOUS CONFLICT IS EXPRESSED AS A SYMBOLIC SOMATIC SYMPTOM, AND IT IS SEEN PRIMARILY IN HYSTERICAL NEUROSIS. CHOOSE ANOTHER.

S: 4

THIS IS AN ACCEPTABLE ANSWER SINCE PATIENTS WHO ARE DE-PRESSED IN RESPONSE TO THE ILLNESS OR DEATH OF A LOVED ONE OFTEN IDENTIFY WITH THE LOST INDIVIDUAL. THERE IS A BETTER ANSWER.

S: 1

THIS IS THE BEST ANSWER. DEPRESSION IS COMMONLY CHARACTER-IZED BY FOCUSING ATTENTION ON THE BODY AND AWAY FROM CONCERN WITH THE PSYCHOLOGICAL LOSS.

WOULD YOU LIKE TO DO THIS QUESTION AGAIN? (TYPE Y OR N)

The next example is a program with a similar format, but the subject matter is pharmacy or pharmacology. This is derived from a large data bank of test questions developed at the University of Kansas Medical Center.

ALL OF THE FOLLOWING HAVE SIGNIFICANT ANTI-INFLAMMATORY ACTION EXCEPT (WHICH ONE)?
(1) ACETAMINOPHEN   (4) INDOMETHACIN
(2) AMINOPYRINE   (5) PHENYLBUTAZONE
(3) ASPIRIN

S: 2

NO, AMINOPYRINE BELONGS TO THE PYRAZOLON GROUP OF DRUGS WHICH ALSO INCLUDES PHENYLBUTAZONE. THE PRIMARY USE OF

THIS GROUP OF AGENTS IS FOR THEIR ANTI-INFLAMMATORY ACTION.
TRY AGAIN.

S: 1

RIGHT. ACETAMINOPHEN, ACETANILIDE, AND PHENACETIN ALL
BELONG TO THE PARA AMINO PHENOL CLASS OF AGENTS THAT HAVE
ANALGESIC AND ANTIPYRETIC ACTIVITY, BUT DO NOT HAVE ANTI-
INFLAMMATORY ACTIVITY.

WOULD YOU LIKE TO DO THIS QUESTION AGAIN? (TYPE Y OR N)

Other PILOT programs use a clinical case description as the basis of the tutorial
session. This type of program allows the student to go through the steps of gathering data about a patient described by the computer, making a diagnosis of the
problem, and having a tutorial interaction about the treatment process. Unlike the
previous examples, this program does not ask the student to select an answer from a
list. The student is asked to type his query or response in his own words, so the resulting interaction has more resemblance to a real encounter with a patient.

The following example is from a program about a 6-year-old patient who has
swallowed unknown medications from the family medicine cabinet. The cabinet is
known to contain cardiac and anticonvulsant medications.

THE NURSE CALLS YOU TO THE EXAMINING ROOM, SAYING THAT THE
CHILD HAD BECOME RESTLESS AND VOMITED. LOOKING AT THE
VOMITUS CONFIRMS THE NURSE'S REPORT THAT THERE IS NO RECOG-
NIZABLE DRUG TO BE SEEN.

WHAT TEST OR PHYSICAL FINDING DO YOU WANT TO CHECK FIRST?

S: CHECK THE VITAL SIGNS

THAT IS THE RIGHT IDEA.

WHICH SINGLE OBSERVATION IS THE MOST IMPORTANT?

S: PULSE

OK, THAT OBSERVATION IS IMPORTANT AND CAN BE DONE QUICKLY,
BUT WHAT OTHER SIMPLE OBSERVATION IS EVEN MORE IMPORTANT?

S: SINCE HE HAS VOMITED YOU SHOULD CHECK HIS AIRWAY

THAT IS A GOOD CHOICE.
SINCE THE CHILD MAY BE INTOXICATED AND HAS JUST VOMITED, YOU
SHOULD CHECK HIS RESPIRATION TO MAKE SURE HE HAS NOT ASPI-
RATED ANY VOMITUS.

HERE IS THE INITIAL DATA ABOUT THE PATIENT ...

RESPIRATION IS 20 PER MINUTE, AIRWAY IS CLEAR. RADIAL PULSE
INITIALLY IRREGULAR IN STRENGTH AND RHYTHM, THEN REGULAR
AT 80 PER MINUTE.

WHAT TEST OR PHYSICAL FINDING DO YOU WANT NEXT?

S: EKG

THE CARDIOGRAM IS A GOOD CHOICE, BUT WHILE IT IS BEING SET UP
YOU SHOULD NOT FORGET TO CHECK THE BLOOD PRESSURE, WHICH IS
120/75.

This program goes on to help the student identify the probable cause of this patient's symptoms, and allows him to make decisions about important aspects of the treatment process. It is not a true simulation in the sense of being based on a computer model of the patient, but the sequence closely parallels a typical clinical experience for the student. The self-contained CAI machine, using programs stored on magnetic tape cassettes, can be successfully used for this type of flexible program with a large proportion of free-response input from the student and with the computer assuming the role of the "patient" or the "professor" at appropriate times.

Current and Future Trends

In discussing the advantages of shared versus stand-alone use of the computer for health sciences education, we have already mentioned the changing relative costs of central processor hardware (local computing logic) and of communication technology. Though some elements of data communication are becoming more efficient the costs in this area are not dropping in the dramatic fashion that is evident for central elements of the computer itself. It is apparent that future hardware costs of stand-alone computing will be determined less and less by electronic logic elements but will be dominated by whatever peripheral equipment is needed — equipment such as printers that have mechanical components.

It seems likely therefore, that one form of future self-contained computer, and one particularly attractive for CAI purposes, will be an increasingly compact keyboard/screen combination, capable of interactive instruction from programs stored in its sizeable memory. It will also be able to communicate with remote machines, however, so that it can access new program material, share that which its user has locally developed, or make use of a printer, plotter, or other special device. A central computer that can be accessed by such individual units will prove useful for storage and revision of current CAI programs and for descriptive documentation of available material.

Another changing cost relationship exists between the decreasing cost of hardware and the steadily increasing human cost of developing software. Whatever can be done to use inexpensive processors and memories as a means to avoid software costs will be an advantage. The PILOT language is of course one example of a software production aid, specialized for a particular type of interactive language-handling program. We can expect to see an increasing variety of computer-based aids for the development of programs of all types. Without such aids, the actual useful access to the cheap computer power we have predicted will be severely limited for many people.

Another trend that should be considered in our view of the future can be described as a changing public image of the computer. We are moving away from a view of the computer as an experimental instrument that a lucky student might briefly contact, to a view that expects the computer to be available as a tool. Some already view it also as a source of recreation, and this will likely expand as users are given improved access and increasing control over its actions. As students gain such control there will be more and more possibilities for self-study. Increased use will develop new problem solving capability on the part of the user, so that more complex problems become possible of solution. We can confidently expect that users of our stand-alone machine will invent ever more capable personal computers to act as their assistants.

References

Alpert, D., and Bitzer, D., 1970. Advances in computer-based education, *Science* 167: 1582.

Brody, H., Lucaccini, L., Kamp, M., and Rozen, R., 1973. Computer based simulated patient for teaching history-taking, *J. Den. Educ.* 37(8): 27.

Kamp, M., and Burnside, I., 1974. Computer-assisted learning in graduate psychiatric nursing, *J. Nurs. Educ.* 13(4): 18.

Kamp, M., and Starkweather, J., 1973. A return to a dedicated machine for computer-assisted instruction, *Comput. Biol. Med.* 3(3): 293.

Starkweather, J., 1969. A common language for a variety of programming needs, *in* R. Atkinson and H. Wilson (Eds.), *Computer Assisted Instruction – A Book of Readings*, pp. 269–304, Academic Press, New York.

Starkweather, J., and Kamp, M., 1976. PILOT for the Datapoint 2200 and 1100, available from the Computer Center, University of California, San Francisco.

Starkweather, J., Kamp, M., and Monto, A., 1967. Psychiatric Interview Simulation by Computer, *Methods of Information in Medicine* 6(1): 15.

Weinberg, A., 1973. CAI at the Ohio State University College of Medicine, *Comput. Biol. Med.* 3(3): 299.

Wooster, H., and Lewis, J., 1973. Distribution of computer-assisted instructional materials in biomedicine through the Lister Hill Experimental Network, *Comp. Biol. Med.* 3(3): 319.

Vacroux, A., 1975. Microcomputers, *Sci. Am.* 232(5): 32.

14

Using Minicomputers for Courseware Delivery

Charles S. Tidball

Introduction

Much has been written about the development of computer-based instruction in institutions where this mode of teaching is well established. The signs of a nutritive environment include administrative backing, processing on large machines, availability of special-purpose CAI languages, high-level programming support for language refinement, staff deployment to encourage faculty authoring, and evidence of extramural financial support. The present communication does not emanate from such an environment. At the Medical Center of The George Washington University, CAI is a relative newcomer and has only been developed on a small scale. Accordingly, our experience may be of particular interest to those institutions that are contemplating the addition of this capability to their educational programs and are looking for an economical approach to such implementation.

The CAI Environment

In July of 1971, the Department of Physiology acquired a Digital Equipment Corporation PDP-12 minicomputer. The original equipment order, totaling $45,000, was supported by a number of sources, since it was not then possible to justify an expenditure of that magnitude from a single academic or research budget. This point is important because, from the outset, the computer was seen as a general-purpose resource, and all parties desiring to make use of it had to compete for time on the machine. In addition to the CAI interests of the author, there was an active neurophysiology group anxious to use the PDP-12 for on-line control of experiments in real-time, several other laboratories interested in off-line processing of experimental data, and one funding source wishing to perform patient interviewing. It was also assumed that the equipment would be available to expose graduate and medical students to the rudiments of computer utilization.

By the end of the first year, the minicomputer facility was well established

---

Charles S. Tidball • Computer Assisted Education and Services, George Washington University Medical Center, Washington, D.C.

and a variety of research and academic users were sharing access to the processor. The latter was facilitated by the development of a multilanguage time-sharing system for the PDP-12 (MTS-12) which permitted not only two simultaneous users but also patient interviewing at sites remote from the computer (Tidball *et al.*, 1972). A year later, with the core memory of the processor increased from 8000 to 12,000 12-bit words, the addition of two more LINCtape drives, and two more entry ports on the communication multiplexer, it was possible to improve the power of MTS-12 and still increase the number of simultaneous users to three (Tidball and Bon, 1973). Ultimately, another 8000 words of memory were acquired as well as the necessary input ports to permit the full complement of six simultaneous users that was designed into MTS-12. It should be emphasized that this LINCtape-activated CAI environment is less than ideal: response delays of 20 to 40 seconds are occasionally experienced as a tape spins to find the next program. However, the system is functional and has the virtue of being put together from standard components at minimal cost. Thus, without in any way impairing the utility of the PDP-12 to perform real-time tasks for a single user at a time, a versatile, general-purpose time-sharing system has been created to provide an alternate mode of operation for this popular minicomputer. During regular working hours, use of the PDP-12 is scheduled for either stand-alone use or time-sharing. At night and over the weekend, MTS-12 is always available; the system runs unattended during those hours, but personnel are on call if difficulties are encountered.

The time-sharing system is multilingual in capability, but the only high-level computer language currently implemented is the general purpose computer language FOCAL (Digital Equipment Corporation, 1973). This is not a special purpose CAI language, yet it is a relatively simple computer language to learn. The coding is line-oriented, and there is an excellent editing capability built into the language. Programs are stored in a form that can be listed conveniently at the terminal without operator intervention. Thus, after a training period measured in hours, even those with no previous exposure to computer science can be writing relatively sophisticated tutorial or simulation sequences. The latter is especially facilitated if the presentation structure has already been developed by someone with more programming experience, as outlined below.

Finally, a description of the facilities available for student and author use will complete this presentation of the CAI environment. In the spring of 1973, the School of Medicine and Health Sciences occupied a new building that also housed the Paul Himmelfarb Health Sciences Library. An Audio-Visual Education Center was established in the latter including 13 student carrels and supporting library staff. Two Tektronix 4010 memory oscilliscope terminals and a Tektronix 4610 hard copy unit, which can support up to four terminals simultaneously, have been installed for student access to computer-based instruction. These terminals have been fitted with Bell Telephone System Dataphones that provide the ability to be connected to either external or internal computer equipment. The authoring area is located in proximity to the computer room which is in the portion of the building devoted to the Department of Physiology. Here, there is another Tektronix 4010 and an Execuport 300 typewriter terminal. A portable Execuport 300 has also been acquired and is convenient either for persons wishing to interact with the computer at home or for conducting demonstrations.

Major Areas of Activity

Given the general-purpose nature of the computing facility, our activity has occurred in a number of different areas. A brief description of the more important categories of computing is provided to emphasize the versatility of even a small-scale computing resource.

System Development. Development activity relates to those decisions about hardware acquisition and software development that are under constant review in any computing facility. Larger units are able to deploy one or more persons who can devote full-time effort to this activity. Of necessity, the small-scale operation will deploy whatever staff support is available. For us the total staff has varied from one to three programmers; therefore, there has never been the equivalent of one full-time person assigned to system development. Our primary projects in this area have included MTS-12 (described above); COMUSE, a program to monitor computer utilization; a LOGON program for stand-alone usage; a revision of MTS-12 to permit on-line data acquisition; the design of a second minicomputer mainframe (see below); improvements to FOCAL for use under MTS-12; experimentation with solid state memory, as well as another revision of MTS-12 to reduce dependence on LINCtape for MTS-12 utility programs, so as to improve MTS-12 reliability.

Teaching about Minicomputer Utilization. Under the auspices of the Department of Physiology, a 2-credit course entitled "Computer Utilization in Physiology and Medicine" has been offered since the fall of 1971. A graduated series of programming problems enable the student to explore the rudiments of computer processing at the assembly language level. This procedure has made it possible to remove the mysteries of how the digital computer actually accomplishes its tasks. In addition, the student learns enough FOCAL to undertake a meaningful project that is often a portion of a CAI sequence. A number of our current CAI programs have been developed and refined by successive student projects in this course.

Facilitating Access to Remote Computer Systems. During the 1972–73 academic year, The George Washington University became an active participant in the Experimental CAI Network established by the Lister Hill National Center for Biomedical Communications of the National Library of Medicine (see Chapter 8). Before encouraging students to communicate with remote computers over a nation-wide network it seemed appropriate to provide them with an introduction to terminal interaction on our internal equipment. MTS-12 was well-suited to this task and a program called TERMLEARN was developed for the purpose. At a speed of 30 characters per second the TERMLEARN sequence takes approximately 25 minutes and deals with the topics indicated in Figure 1, which is a reproduction of the initial selector frame. Note that the latter permits reentry at various places in

*** TERMLEARN *** IS WRITTEN IN SEVERAL SECTIONS TO

FACILITATE RE-ENTRY INTO THE MIDDLE OF THE PROGRAM,

IF   DESIRED.

TYPE   A   FOR INTRODUCTION

          B   FOR SEND MESSAGE KEY

          C   FOR PAGING

          D   FOR CORRECTING ERRORS

          E   FOR LEVELS OF INTERACTION

          F   FOR CHANGING LEVELS

AFTER THE COLON (:) BELOW, TYPE THE LETTER CORRESPONDING

TO YOUR CHOICE AND PRESS THE KEY MARKED RETURN, OR CR,

TO SEND THAT INFORMATION TO THE COMPUTER.

Figure 1. The initial selector frame of the TERMLEARN program which illustrates the technique used for moving about within the program.

the program without requiring a knowledge of labels, program names, or the use of FOCAL direct commands.

Patient Interviewing. In the restricted setting of an Exercise Test Facility, an automated initial patient-history sequence compatible with the MTS-12 time-sharing system was developed. The system includes such items as a self-checking patient identification number with patient name response, a "do not understand the question" response, the ability to change answers, a confirmation of patient identity at the end of the questionnaire, and the storage of patient data on magnetic tape. Information retrieval and computer-generated summaries of the history were also featured (Tidball *et al.*, 1974).

Learning a Computer Language. A tutorial program called FOCLEARN was developed to teach the computer language FOCAL. In Figure 2 can be found the Table of Contents for this learning experience. The program is highly interactive and contains numerous exercises and example programs before the final practice programs indicated in the Table of Contents. There is a carefully designed HELP sequence that has been created for each of the final practice programs. The student is instructed in how to call up the HELP subprogram that is designed to provide just enough help to get the student going again without revealing the entire solution. There are at least four different categories of help available for each of the final practice programs and, since the assistance can be interrupted at any point, the student need not see any more of the remedial sequence than is desired. The

```
** TABLE OF CONTENTS **

*** FOCLEARN *** IS WRITTEN IN SEVERAL SECTIONS TO

FACILITATE RE-ENTRY INTO THE MIDDLE OF THE PROGRAM,

AS DESIRED.

TYPE     A  FOR INTRODUCTION

         B  FOR USE OF DIRECT COMMANDS

         C  FOR RUDIMENTS OF PROGRAMMING

         D  FOR USE OF MODIFY COMMAND

         E  FOR FOCAL COMMAND & FUNCTION SUMMARY

         F  FOR FOCAL MC2K SPECIAL VARIABLES

         G  FOR PRACTICE PROGRAM A - INTEREST ON BANK LOAN

         H  FOR PRACTICE PROGRAM B - TWO QUESTION QUIZ

         I  FOR PRACTICE PROGRAM C - STATISTICAL FORMULA
```

Figure 2. Table of Contents for the FOCLEARN program. In the Introduction, the student is taught how to interrupt the program; in the section on the Use of Direct Commands, the student is taught how to call up the Table of Contents; thus this subprogram is the key to altering the sequence of presentation, if desired.

interchange depicted in Figure 3 illustrates help at the first level. Note that the assistance guides the student in what to do but does not reveal the solution. A complete sample solution is available by selecting answer choice D in the initial HELP selector frame (see Figure 3). With either answer choice B or C, a subsequent selector frame permits the assistance to be focused tightly on the area of student difficulty. In this manner, the student is spared from having to read assistance that is not related to the actual problem.

Small-Scale Statistical Processing. From the outset we developed a library of statistical programs enabling the PDP-12 under MTS-12 to be used as a data-reduction device. The implementation of new statistical routines has also been greatly assisted by the student projects referred to in an earlier section.

Data-Acquisition Procedures. Much of physiological research is based on data that are originally collected as a tracing on an oscilloscope or chart recorder. Measurement of these tracings has always been a time-consuming task. The acquisition of a spark gap digitizer (Graf/pen, manufactured by Science Accessories Corporation of Southport, Connecticut) has enabled us to make these measurements under computer control with data storage on LINCtape on the PDP 12. Modifications of MTS-12 have made it possible to support this activity under time-

INDICATE BY A SINGLE LETTER AFTER THE COLON THE KIND

OF ASSISTANCE YOU WOULD LIKE.

    A   NEED LIST OF TASKS TO BE PERFORMED

    B   NEED HELP WITH PROGRAMMING

    C   NEED HELP WITH BRANCHING TO SECOND SUBPROGRAM

    D   WOULD LIKE TO SEE SAMPLE SOLUTION

    E   TO START PRACTICE PROGRAM C

    : A

YOU MAY WISH TO USE THE FOLLOWING SEQUENCE OF STEPS

TO HELP YOU WRITE PRACTICE PROGRAM B.

    1.   CREATE A NAME FOR YOUR PROGRAM BY REPLACING THE X'S

         IN THE EXAMPLE BELOW WITH TWO OF YOUR OWN INITIALS

                  TEMPBXX1

    2.   WRITE A COMMENT IN LINE 1.01 TO INDICATE THE NAME OF

         THE PROGRAM AND THE FACT THAT IT IS TO BE STORED ON

         FILE 1.

    3.   WRITE INSTRUCTIONS TO THE STUDENT TAKING THE QUIZ

    4.   WRITE THE FIRST QUESTION

    5.   WRITE THE ANSWER CHOICES

    6.   WRITE THE 'ASK' COMMAND TO STOP THE COMPUTER FOR

         STUDENT INPUT

    7.   WRITE THE 'IF' STATEMENTS TO INTERPRET THE ANSWER

    8.   WRITE A RECOVERY ROUTINE FOR UNEXPECTED ANSWERS

    9.   WRITE THE FEEDBACK FOR THE ANSWERS

   10.   TAKE CARE OF CALLING UP THE NEXT SUBPROGRAM

   11.   SAVE YOUR PROGRAM USING THE NAME CREATED IN STEP 1

   12.   EXECUTE YOUR PROGRAM

13. DEBUG AND RESAVE AS NEEDED. YOU WILL HAVE TO

    'PROGRAM DELETE' YOUR FORMER VERSION BEFORE YOU

    CAN SAVE A REVISED VERSION UNDER THE SAME NAME.

14. REPEAT FOR SECOND SUBPROGRAM

Figure 3. Excerpts from the HELP feature associated with the final Practice Program B (see text for explanation).

sharing. The two major uses in this environment have been the determination of (a) systolic time intervals from the analysis of electrocardiograms, pulse waves, and phonocardiograms and (b) membrane permeability from the analysis of alternating current waves.

Neurophysiological Research. The group using the PDP-12 in stand-alone to process human electroencephalograph data by the signal-averaging technique are relatively independent and have undertaken several major revisions of their data-acquisition programs without our assistance. However, they still rely on us for MTS-12 usage and diagnosis of hardware difficulties they may be encountering.

Training in CAI Authoring. At our institution, CAI authoring does not come about as a result of a full-time effort on the part of a group specially organized for courseware development; on the contrary, such effort is perceived as a set of additional duties by most participants who are already heavily committed to other academic pursuits. Thus, it can be said that our development program represents one extreme of how to involve persons in CAI authoring. The benchmarks with regard to how long it takes to accomplish results should be interpreted in that light.

Two of the major units in training potential authors consist of the programs TERMLEARN and FOCLEARN, which have been previously mentioned. Although TERMLEARN is not mandatory for students wishing only to access CAI programs, it is required for prospective authors because it describes the operational levels in MTS-12. These are essential features of the courseware delivery system that every author must understand.

In teaching CAI, often the potential author has little or no experience with an interactive computer program. Thus, considerable efficiency is achieved by using the CAI technique to instruct the potential author in the computer language to be used. There are, however, two pitfalls that must be carefully circumvented. The first of these is that the potential author may be turned away from becoming involved in CAI if the computer language instruction program is perceived as either too trivial or too difficult. The second is that the instructional program may not be sufficiently sophisticated to reveal the full gamut of CAI techniques. These pitfalls can be avoided by careful attention to the CAI program used in computer language instruction, i.e., what is suitable for student use may not be ideal for prospective authors, especially if they are members of the faculty. It is also essential to provide the learner sufficient "one-on-one" contact with well-established authors during the learning period.

A third training aid developed by the author was originally intended as a computer-driven sequence but was designed for the TSS-8 time-sharing system on the Digital Equipment Corporation PDP-8 which is not currently available in our environment. Nevertheless, this aid entitled "Computer Assisted Education Using FOCAL" has been preserved in notebook form. The latter is often made available to authors seeking more information than can be found in FOCLEARN on such subjects as moving around within a CAI program; ways to code free text entry as opposed to multiple-choice responses; how to utilize quizzes to determine the entry point in lengthy tutorial programs; and means of conforming special notations, such as chemical expressions, to the limitations of the upper-case-only printing capabilities of most computer terminals.

Beyond the specific aids identified above, we now have a library of approximately 20 interactive programs in different subject areas, many of which have rather different stylistic approaches. Thus, the would-be CAI author has a number of patterns to select from in deciding how to solve any particular problem. In addition to the programs available internally, there are another one hundred or more CAI, CMI, and simulation programs available to us over the Health Education Network, Inc. (see Chapter 11), as the successor to the Lister Hill Experimental CAI Network is called, that can also be used as exemplars for developing a new learning sequence.

Launching a New CAI Program

The first step in developing a new CAI venture is to strike the spark of interest at the highest possible administrative level. Often this contact will be with the chairperson of an academic department or the director of a service unit. If a computer-based instructional experience is available in that discipline, it can be used to good advantage as a starting point. When the prospective collaborator indicates the deficiencies of the courseware being demonstrated, the stage is set for inviting the group to undertake a new program that more closely meets its needs. Further discussion establishes some major objectives, and then the entrepreneur of CAI will find it useful to offer to design a prototype program for subsequent review. If this offer is accepted, it is desirable to produce the prototype as soon as possible since this gives a favorable indication of how quickly an item of courseware can be created.

If the prototype is well-received and a decision is made to proceed with the authoring effort, the next step is an orientation session. It is possible to accomplish this for several potential authors at the same time, and this generally precedes attempts to engage either TERMLEARN or FOCLEARN. The session covers the seven major tasks involved in authoring CAI as shown in Figure 4. The point is made that the content expert need not be proficient in items #3, 4, 5, and 6. However, if that person desires to be able to perform editing (task #6), there is no better way to learn that skill than by coding and debugging one or two programs oneself.

1. Develop the objectives to be met by the course.
2. Write the program in English.
3. Understand the courseware delivery system.
4. Code the program in a suitable computer language.
5. Remove the errors in program logic so that the program performs as desired.
6. Perform the editorial tasks which keep the program current and responsive to student needs.
7. Evaluate the program by comparing it with other means to teach the same material.

Figure 4. The seven major tasks in producing a CAI program.

Thereafter, when coding becomes less challenging, it can be relegated to staff support if such is available. It is useful to bring a portable terminal to this orientation session which should preferably take place in the home territory of the potential authors' own department. The ease with which the terminal is connected to the system is demonstrated and the prototype CAI program is presented. It is essential to establish a positive tone from the outset. In dealing with busy adults who were not exposed to the benefits of CAI in their own education, the motivational thread is more fragile than even that sought for in the most recalcitrant student!

Alternatively, it may be preferable, before undertaking an orientation session for several prospective authors, to select a promising author candidate and work closely with that person for the 2 or 3 weeks required to develop an independent authoring capability. Then, when the orientation session is held, the skeptics who are concerned about being able to learn the necessary skills can be referred to one of their own members who has already succeeded.

Case History

In the spring of 1973, the author approached the chairman of the Department of Anatomy to determine how much interest was available in utilizing CAI. Although programs in Anatomy were available from Ohio State University over the Experimental CAI Network, these were primarily computer-managed instruction and did not reflect as much clinical orientation as the department desired. Accordingly, the author offered to develop a prototype for a computer-based learning experience with material supplied by the chairman that was taken from a section on clinical correlations in the latter's textbook (Snell, 1973).

After several weeks, the prototype was available for review and enthusiastically received by the chairman. At that moment the Anatomical Clinical Correlation (A-CL-COR) program was born. For his part, the chairman agreed to encourage his faculty to become involved in preparing computer programs for additional patient simulations; and the author agreed to provide the necessary training. Eventually, in that first year, in addition to the chairman and the author, three faculty members, two graduate students, and one medical student became involved in authoring.

The first member of the Department of Anatomy faculty to request training was interviewed by the author late in the summer of 1973. Some time was devoted to discussing his motivation for involvement. Clearly the chairman had made it obvious that he considered this activity part of the faculty member's total commitment to his department. Additionally, this faculty member lacked exposure to both computer technology and clinical medicine. He perceived that learning to author for the A-CL-COR program would broaden his experience and improve his effectiveness as a teacher of medical students. We agreed from the start that becoming a CAI author was a portion of his teaching activity and should not interfere with progress in his research endeavor.

Although this faculty member had ample native intelligence, computer programming did not come easily. A-CL-COR is a relatively sophisticated simulation of the patient–physician encounter. We attempted to ease the burden on new authors by isolating the code that created the shifts from history, to physical examination, to special tests and to disposition, but inability to understand these routines, or to debug improper sequencing when it occurred, created a sense of frustration for the faculty member. This was resolved when, in the spring of 1974, a first-year medical student with previous programming experience was added to the authoring team. Although it had taken the better part of 3 months for our first faculty member to complete his first patient simulation, the second went much more quickly. By this time, other faculty members in the Department of Anatomy were learning FOCAL, and a total of eight patient simulations had been completed by the fall of 1974. Toward the middle of the fall semester, the programs were made available to the first-year students as an adjunct to their other sources of information. Not all the students in the class of 150 availed themselves of this opportunity, but those who did responded favorably to the experience and were able to perceive the multiple objectives that had been designed into the computer-based learning sequences. The favorable evaluation has encouraged the department to extend this technique to other areas of its teaching, and several new patient simulations are in various stages of development.

Improving the CAI Environment

During the first two years of operating the PDP-12, two more LINCtape drives, two data-communication entry ports, and a 50% increase in core memory were undertaken. In spite of these system expansions, it was difficult to keep up with the increasing requests for access to the machine. In particular, stand-alone use was competing with time-sharing use, and since we could accommodate more users under time-sharing, scheduling became increasingly difficult. Accordingly, a decision was made to acquire a second processor – a Digital Equipment Corporation PDP-8/E. This also made it possible to take advantage of new economies in hardware design. That the new machine cost only $20,000 and yet represented significant improvements over the PDP-12 indicates how rapidly prices have fallen in the minicomputer market. The new machine is now equipped with two random-access disk cartridge drives that eliminate the slow response of the earlier system. A combination hardware—software, virtual computer, time-shared operating system called ETOS has been acquired from Educomp Corporation of Hartford, Connecticut (Cini and O'Donnell, 1974). The latter provides support for multiple computer languages without major reprogramming. We are in the process of developing a semicompiler version of the special educational computer language PILOT (Stark-weather, 1969; Rubin, 1973) for this 12-bit machine. Not only will the availability of PILOT simplify author training, but it will make it possible for us to exchange programs with other institutions since many PILOT support packages are currently running on several different computers designed by various manufacturers. The courseware developed in this environment will be capable of implementation on a variety of machines ranging from single-user minicomputers under $10,000 to full-scale, timesharing systems on multimillion-dollar mainframes.

A Frame of Reference for Making System Comparisons

The classical approaches to courseware delivery each have their own drawbacks. Maxicomputer systems involve initial equipment costs in excess of one million dollars; and though it is possible to lease these machines, it is generally necessary to justify their existence with non-CAI computing activities. In so doing, a more complicated system architecture is required, exacerbating their second disadvantage which is the need for large supporting staffs. Midicomputer systems also involve large initial equipment costs (in excess of $100,000) and are not usually able to be leased except through a third party. These systems often feature many simultaneous users at the expense of language flexibility and are therefore not easy to upgrade to a desired full capability over time. Minicomputer systems have a low entry cost, but they often are inadequate in terms of processor speed and power. Obtaining adequate bulk-storage capacity for the CAI library in the lower-priced minicomputer models is often problematic. On the other hand, the minicomputer approach is the surest way of controlling the overall cost of developing a CAI facility. Finally, system reliability is dependent on duplicating the key components of the entire system, which can be done considerably more easily at the minicomputer level.

It is legitimate to question how far one can stretch minicomputer technology to meet the requirements of a moderate-to-large educational environment. The frame of reference for such an inquiry should acknowledge other factors besides equipment costs. One disadvantage of the use of cost per instructional hour, which has been employed by some developers, is that the hidden costs to assure faculty motivation, curriculum integration, and educational program restructuring are usually ignored. Unfortunately, the real benefits of CAI can rarely be achieved until many of these hidden costs have been met or the problems they represent have been worked through. The items listed here are not exhaustive but serve to highlight practical concerns that are not easily expressed in monetary terms:

Adequacy of computational power
Computer language flexibility
Convenience for courseware authors
Ease of courseware maintenance
Flexibility for interinstitutional courseware exchange
Learner convenience and terminal versatility
Number of simultaneous users
Record keeping for student responses
System reliability
System response time

This discussion would not be complete without a brief consideration of the number of simultaneous users needed in the typical health education environment. It is instructive to recognize that at the height of the operation of the Lister Hill National Center for Biomedical Communication's Experimental CAI Network, there were over 60 institutions being served and over 3000 connect hours per month, and yet all this was being accomplished on a total of approximately one dozen entry ports. It would seem, therefore, that the average medical school could do very well with a 16-user internal system as the kingpin of the CAI operation. (This is well within the range of current minicomputer systems.) If such a system is coupled with access to a general facility like the Health Education Network or a nearby institution which is willing to encourage time-sharing on its own mainframe, both the requirements for a broad data base and improved reliability will be well-served. A recent AAMC survey on The Use of Computers in Instruction (Lefever and Johnson, 1976) confirms that many institutions are making joint use of internal and external computer facilities for CAI as recommended above.

Conclusions

On the basis of some 6 years of experience with a small-scale CAI operation we have learned the following: CAI can be performed on minicomputers. It is not necessary to have a special staff to create courseware. Faculty tend to find fault with programs written by others and wish to put their own individual stamp on teaching materials to be used by their students. Faculty can be trained in CAI authoring. It is desirable to interview prospective authors to establish grounds to support motivation and eliminate unrealistic expectations. The use of a CAI program to teach faculty authors a programming language is efficient and gives them a firsthand experience with the medium. The availability of a CAI program does not reduce the need for considerable "one-on-one" contact and training reinforcement, since faculty members can easily be distracted from learning to be CAI authors by their many other academic pursuits. Administrative support for authoring at the level of departmental chairpersons or unit chiefs is considered essential. The computer industry is moving in the direction of less expensive machinery and some universality of computer languages so that improved courseware exchange can be anticipated. The inherent economies of creating a CAI facility on minicomputer hardware yield some assurance that developmental costs can be kept to manageable proportions. For the sake of access to a broad data base and improved reliability of services, it is desirable that internal CAI capabilities be coupled with external support provided by nationwide networks or regional time-sharing arrangements.

References

Cini, A. F., and O'Donnell, J., 1974. ETOS – a multi-language timesharing system for the PDP-8, *DECUS Proceedings* Fall, **495**.

Digital Equipment Corporation, 1973. FOCAL-8, Order No. DEC-08-LFL8A-A-D, Maynard, Massachusetts.

Lefever, R. D., and Johnson, J. K., 1976. *Survey of the Use of Computers in Instruction*, American Association of Medical Colleges, Washington, D.C.

Rubin, S., 1973. A simple instructional language, *Computer Decisions* November, 17.

Snell, R. S., 1973. *Clinical Anatomy for Medical Students*, Little, Brown and Company, Boston, pp. 909.

Starkweather, J. A., 1969, A common language for a variety of conventional programming needs, *in* H. A. Wislow and R. C. Atkinson (Eds.), *Readings in Computer-Assisted Instruction*, Academic Press, New York.

Tidball, C. S., and Bon, B. B., 1973. MTS-12 revisited: Powerful interviewing capabilities for the PDP-12 through an improved time-sharing FOCAL, *DECUS Proceedings* Spring, 85.

Tidball, C. S., Crawford, J. E., III, and Bon, B. B., 1972. MTS-12: A multi-language, time-sharing system for PDP-12 computers, *DECUS Proceedings* Spring, 277.

Tidball, C. S., Smalley, D. E., Gorman, P. A., and Naughton, J. P., 1974. An automated initial medical history program for patients undergoing exercise testing, *Med. Sci. Sports*, 6: 73.

15

The Evolution and Use of Computer-Assisted Instruction (CAI) in Health Sciences Education at The Ohio State University College of Medicine

Ruann E. Pengov

Introduction

The Ohio State University College of Medicine has evolved as a leader in the field of computer applications in health sciences education. As noted in the most recent index of Kamp and Brigham (1976), the largest single collection of available computer-assisted instruction (CAI) courseware in medicine and health-related areas resides at The Ohio State University College of Medicine.

The CAI system at The Ohio State University College of Medicine did not just happen. It has grown from a one-terminal, one-course system in 1967 to the operational system of today that provides 22-hour-per-day, 7-day-per-week CAI access for students and health professionals in Columbus, in Ohio, and throughout the United States; maintains a program library of over 350 interactive hours of CAI materials; logs approximately 4000 usage hours per month; and adds CAI course materials to its library at the average rate of 5 interactive hours per month.

This chapter reviews the utilization of CAI in health sciences education at The Ohio State University College of Medicine and describes the hardware and software systems that support CAI development and utilization within the College. What is offered here is an overview; references will direct the reader to more detailed information.

At the outset, it is imperative to state the philosophy of the College in the development and use of CAI materials since this emphasis will tenor all discussions that follow. The emphasis in CAI courseware has been placed on: (a) the quality of content; (b) the applicability and usefulness of the materials in the health sciences curricula; and (c) the soundness of the educational strategy employed. The approach has been not to emphasize CAI as a technology but rather to develop CAI as

Ruann E. Pengov · Division of Computing Services for Medical Education and Research, College of Medicine, The Ohio State University, Columbus, Ohio.

an educational resource that can uniquely meet some educational needs. Throughout this chapter, emphasis is placed on the *use* of the computer rather than on the computer itself. Discussion will be organized according to arenas of application of CAI (i.e., undergraduate medical education, nursing education, allied medical education, continuing education); configurations for access to CAI; and the support environment for CAI usage and development. The above categories are not mutually exclusive nor are they intended to address all aspects of CAI; they are used here to bring some organization to the various subsystems and/or components of the operational CAI System at The Ohio State University College of Medicine.

Arenas of Application of CAI

Major arenas of application of CAI at The Ohio State University College of Medicine are (1) undergraduate medical education, (2) nursing education, (3) allied health professions education, (4) continuing health sciences education, and (5) patient and nonmedical support staff education.

Undergraduate Medical Education

Since 1964, The Ohio State University College of Medicine has been continuously reevaluating and revising its medical education curricula. Initial experience with independent study was acquired through the use of a two-track curriculum in anatomy and independent study groups in biochemistry (Graves *et al.*, 1969). CAI was first utilized in 1967, when CAI courses in anatomy and biochemistry were written to complement the independent study efforts in the classroom. These courses were used by students as self-evaluation exercises and consisted of linear sequences of multiple-choice questions with feedback to each response. In discussing his work, Graves cites evidence that "voluntary choice of learning method allows students and faculty opportunities for satisfaction, creativity and innovation as well as motivating them to achieve" (Graves *et al.*, 1969).

Later, under the direction of an oral surgeon, the first case study approach was used in a course on oral cancer recognition (Gaston, 1969). Number codes were used to interrogate the simulated patient and subsequently to enter a diagnosis. Student-controlled slide projectors were used to present color visuals.

Other faculty became interested and, in histology, a simulated laboratory experience at the CAI terminal was offered as an option to the actual laboratory in organ identification. Considerable time was saved using the CAI mode with similar student comprehension (Wismar and Christopher, 1969). Appendix A provides a sample student interaction from the histology course.

Continued individual faculty efforts resulted in the addition of more CAI courses (see Appendix B for full listing) until 1969, when a research project was undertaken to investigate the effectiveness and efficiency of utilizing independent study for the medical basic sciences portion of medical student education. The goal was to design, implement, and evaluate a preclerkship curriculum that would incorporate as its foundation certain educational principles and tenants of independent study. The Independent Study Program (ISP) was formed as a result of a grant from the U.S. Public Health Service, Bureau of Health Manpower. The grant provided for 1 year of program development and 2 years of operation and evaluation (1970–72). Basically,

> the ISP at The Ohio State University College of Medicine involves students in a self-paced individual learning experience that punctuates primary learning through books, journal articles, films, slides and tapes with periodic tutorial self-evaluation at computer terminals. The ISP provides a second pre-clinical medical school curriculum and is run parallel to the regular lecture–discussion (L/D) curriculum. (Griesen, 1973a)

Approximately 60 students per year have been admitted to the ISP. Academic performance results are encouraging in that National Board scores of ISP students were higher than National Board scores of the L/D students in anatomy, physiology, and biochemistry (Beran, 1974).

The ISP curriculum uses a body system organization and consists of three segments: "Normal Man," "Introduction to Pathophysiology and Therapeutics," and "Pathophysiology of Man." The segments are further organized into over 70 submodules or 30 modules of instructional materials, each written by an interdisciplinary team of faculty members. When the student is satisfied that he has learned the content of a given module, he can then access a computer-assisted tutorial evaluation system (TES) designed to sample his knowledge of the designated module of study. The CAI tutorial self-evaluation exercises are designed to provide the student with a gauge of his success in meeting the objectives of the modules and to delineate areas for further study and review. The TES offers an interactive learning situation in which the student must overtly respond as an active learner:

> While it would certainly be possible to conduct the ISP without the computer-based self-evaulation and instructional management systems, the faculty and students of the program are uniform in their agreement that it would be considerably more difficult and less efficient. (Griesen, 1973b)

Total utilization of the almost 2885 TES items approaches 8000 interactive hours per year with each Ohio State ISP student utilizing approximately 1.2 interactive hours per week. Since July 1972, the ISP has been financially supported by the College of Medicine as an alternative to the Lecture–Discussion curriculum. A recent publication (Beran *et al.*, 1976) discusses in-depth the philosophy and history of the curricula, offers an outline of the curriculum (including objectives), and provides a discussion of the research findings. Chapter 3 in this volume offers an update on the ISP.

The Lecture–Discussion (L/D) curriculum for medical students is also a 3-year curriculum based upon body systems. Although lecture–discussion, rather than independent study, is employed as the primary mode of instruction, CAI programs are rather extensively employed: some 52 CAI programs are used by medical students in this curriculum. The most extensive use is in physiology, in which CAI review questions have been developed to accompany the class lectures and readings. For each of 26 logical content units, two sets of questions have been developed for student demonstration of mastery of the content.

Graduate students taking a course in medical education have produced a number of the CAI programs that provide alternative learning resources for both medical and allied medical students in anatomy topics. These programs include:

ABANG, abdominal arteriographic anatomy
ELBOW, anatomy of the elbow
HANAT, anatomy of the hand
LOWEX, lower extremity anatomy
SHOJT, the anatomy of the shoulder joint
SKULL, the anatomy of the skull

The college became integrally involved in the use of clinically related CAI materials via the refinement and further development of a model for natural language simulation of the patient–physician encounter. The intial version of the CASE (Computer Assisted Simulation of the Clinical Encounter) model was developed at the University of Illinois. It was transferred to OSU for refinement and further development during the last half of 1973 and the first half of 1974, when the CAI group at the University of Illinois was disbanded. Earlier publications describe the philosophy of CASE and the accompanying GENESYS system that automatically generates COURSEWRITER (the IBM language used at OSU) CAI statements from author inputs (Harless *et al.*, 1973a). Several man-years were invested in further development and refinement of the GENESYS system (Harless *et al.*, 1973b). Currently, the authoring and creation of a "case" take less than 2 man-weeks. This is a significant improvement over the 10 to 20 man-weeks previously required. Of this time, only 10–20 hours is author time, with the remainder being support staff time.

The CASE system provides a library of simulated clinical encounters covering a wide range of disease situations in which a student or physician assumes responsibility for the simulated patient from the moment the patient seeks care until the medical problem has been resolved, either successfully or unsuccessfully. In a CASE simulation, an initial description of the patient and the setting is the only unsolicited information the student or physician receives. By typing questions at the CAI terminal using natural language, the user is able to "interview" the patient and collect *history data, laboratory data* and/or *physical examination data* as needed to diagnose and treat the patient. The user may transfer between the history, laboratory, and physical exam sections at any time to acquire needed information. A diagnosis and a treatment plan are entered when the student or physician feels he has enough information and insight into the "case." To help evaluate his performance, he receives a description of the author's diagnoses, suggested treatment plan, and listing of the critical concepts that are important in proper diagnoses and treatment of the patient. (See Appendix C for a sample CASE interaction.)

Table 1. *Summary of CAI Programs used in the Nursing Curriculum, The Ohio State University School of Nursing*

CAI program title	CAI access code	Audience	Required (R) optional (O)	Number of interactive hours
Child development between ages 2 and 5	TOTS	Sophomore	R	$1\frac{1}{4}$ hr
Reading a patient's medical record	MEDREC	Sophomore	O	$3\frac{1}{2}$ hr
Use of measurement systems and equivalents	MATH	Sophomore	R	10 hr
Care of and feeding by veins	VEINS	Junior	R	2 hr
Principles of orthopedic traction	ORTRAC	Junior	O	$1\frac{3}{4}$ hr
Principles of orthopedic surgery for the hip and knee	PROSHK	Junior	O	$\frac{3}{4}$ hr
Assessment of the patient with respiratory pathophysiology	ASSESS	Senior	R	1 hr
Closed drainage systems for the thoracic cavity	BOTTLE	Senior	R	2 hr
Basics of electrocardiography	STRIP 1	Senior	R	$1\frac{1}{2}$ hr
Cardiac arrhythmias	STRIPS	Senior	R	2 hr
Anticoagulant medication	TRUAMI	Senior	O	2 hr
Short topics for patient usage	PACARE	Senior	O[a]	$\frac{3}{4}$ hr
Review of nursing in coronary care	CCNUR	Senior	O[a]	4 hr
Anesthetic agents and adjunct drugs for nurses	AGENT	Senior	O	$1\frac{3}{4}$ hr
Psychotropic medications	PSYMED	Senior	O	$1\frac{1}{2}$ hr

[a]Required if student fails Nursing 505 (Nursing Transactions with Patients and Families in Crisis) pretest.

Nursing Education

The School of Nursing Bachelor of Science curriculum includes more than 35 interactive hours of CAI materials that are used in a variety of ways by the over 600 nursing students. Table 1 summarizes the use of the CAI programs in the School of Nursing curriculum. Eight CAI programs (20 interactive hours) are required of all nursing students and seven CAI programs (15 interactive hours) are used as optional supplemental learning materials. Faculty are considering usage of several ISP CAI program modules (Mourad and Forman, 1976).

The utilization of CAI materials in the School of Nursing has shown a dramatic increase in recent years. The overall CAI utilization for 1975 was approximately 3800 hours — 30.6% higher than that of 1974.

Allied Medical Professions Education

The School of Allied Medical Professions (SAMP) of the College of Medicine has eleven major divisions offering a Bachelor of Science in Allied Health Professions to approximately 250 undergraduates per year and a Master's degree to approximately 32 students per year. The degree of curriculum integration of CAI programs in the School of Allied Medical Professions varies by division as shown in Figure 1. Special

DIVISION	COURSE #	CAI ACCESS CODE	CAI PROGRAM TITLE	NUMBER OF INTERACTIVE HOURS
Occupational Therapy	452	'group'	Developmental Task Groups	2 hrs.
	625	'sitin'	Sensory Integrative Therapy	1 hr. 15 min.
		'percep'	Perceptual Terminology and Concepts	1 hr.
	627	'stroka'	Stroke Rehabilitation	6 hrs.
		'ccnur'	Nursing in Coronary Care	4 hrs.
		'abbrev'	Medical Record Abbreviations	15 min.
		'tots'	Child Development Between Ages 2 & 5	1 hr. 15 min.
		'sitin'	Sensory Integrative Therapy	1 hr. 15 min.
		'medrec'	Reading the Patient's Medical Record	45 min.
		'pacare'	Short Topics for Patient Use	45 min.
		'pamadi'	Patient Management of Diabetes	2 hrs.20 min.
		'peds'	Birds-eye View of Pediatrics	2 hrs.
		'quails'	Questions about Illostomy Surgery	1 hr. 30 min.
		'judi'	Juvenile Diabetes Patients	1 hr.
		'assess'	Assessment of the Patient with Respiratory Path.	45 min.
		'hibaby'	Hi Baby	30 min.
		'judiab'	Juvenile Diabetes For Health Professionals	1 hr. 30 min.
Physical Therapy	480	'bugout'	Infection Control	45 min.
		'cai'	Introduction to CAI	2 hrs.30 min.
		'signs'	Vital Signs	3 hrs.
		'rescue'	Basic Techniques of CPR	1 hr.30 min.
		'psymed'	Psychotropic Medications	1 hr.30 min.
		'shock'	Septic Shock Care	2 hrs.
		'terms'	Medical Terminology	1 hr.
		'oneaid'	First Aid	1 hr.
	495	'ganatl'	Gross Anatomy Self Evaluation	12 hrs.
		'hanat'	Hand Anatomy	1 hr. 30 min.
		'lowex'	Lower Extremity Anatomy	1 hr. 30 min.
		'elbow'	Musculature of the Elbow Joint	1 hr. 30 min.
		'shojt'	The Shoulder Joint	1 hr.
		'vesali'	Neuromuscular Morphology	2 hrs.15 min.
	542	'stroka'	Stroke Rehabilitation	6 hrs.
	585	'abbrev'	Medical Record Abbreviations	15 min.

Department	Course	Code	Program	Time
Radiation Technology	201, 420	'group' 'terms'	Developmental Task Groups Medical Terminology	2 hrs. 1 hr.
	411, 412	'radtec' 'terms'	Review of Radiologic Technology Medical Terminology	3 hrs. 1 hr.
Medical Dietetics	420, 421, 422 522, 523	'foods'	Food Item File	V
	521, 522, 523	'plan'	Clinical Simulations in Medical Dietetics (est 20/cases)	6 hrs/case
Circulation Technology	560	'pilot'	Renal and Circulation Modules	2 hrs.
	570	'pilot'	Renal and Circulation Modules	2 hrs.

V = program requires a variable amount of time depending on the food items retrieved

Figure 1. Summary of CAI programs used in the Ohio State University School of Allied Medical Professions curricula.

note must be made of the extraordinary effort expended in CAI development by faculty in the Division of Medical Dietetics. Increased student enrollment, linked with increased difficulty in finding faculty with appropriate clinical experience, and the desire to maintain a reasonable student –faculty ratio without increasing the number of faculty, led to the development of a simulation model of a patient–student encounter called PLAN. This effort was supported in part by a grant from the Department of Health, Education and Welfare in 1973 (Grant #5D12AH-00519).

The objectives of PLAN were:

1. To simulate interaction with patients who exhibit specified metabolic, nutritional, and socioeconomic needs and problems
2. To help in the assessment, planning, implementation, and evaluation in the professional development of the student in the clinical area
3. To optimize the utilization of the faculty
4. To supplement inadequate available patient resources
5. To provide additional mechanisms for strengthening patient–dietitian interaction skills

The magnitude, complexity, and success of the resulting simulation has made PLAN among the most advanced CAI programs in use at OSU today. The program itself consists of six separate sections (see Figure 2 for a sample flow):

1. Quizzes to test the student's knowledge before and after visits with the "patient"
2. A medical record that allows the student to obtain any information on the "patient" normally obtained from the hospital medical record
3. A nursing cardex that contains specific nursing instructions and notes
4. A drug formulary that allows the student to gather information on any of 106 different drugs
5. A nutrient catalog that allows the student to gather and analyze 14 nutrients for any of 320 different food items
6. A natural language simulation of the patient–student encounter

The student can ask the "patient" questions about his diet history or menu selection or the student can counsel the patient in nutrition-related areas. The answers to questions bring out the "patient's" personality to the extent that the students sometimes begin talking about the computerized "patients" as though they were real. The design of this particular section is extremely sophisticated and is one of the most advanced models presently in operation (Sentieri, 1976; Sutherland, 1976).

At present, there are ten different "patients" on-line and integrated into the Medical Dietetics curriculum in a three-course junior-year medical dietetics sequence (M.D. 521, 522, 523). When compared to a 1973 control group, students using PLAN during 1974 received seven fewer real-clinical experiences. The use of the PLAN simulations resulted in: (1) students receiving more faculty contact time in the remaining real-clinical experiences, (2) students receiving more "overall"

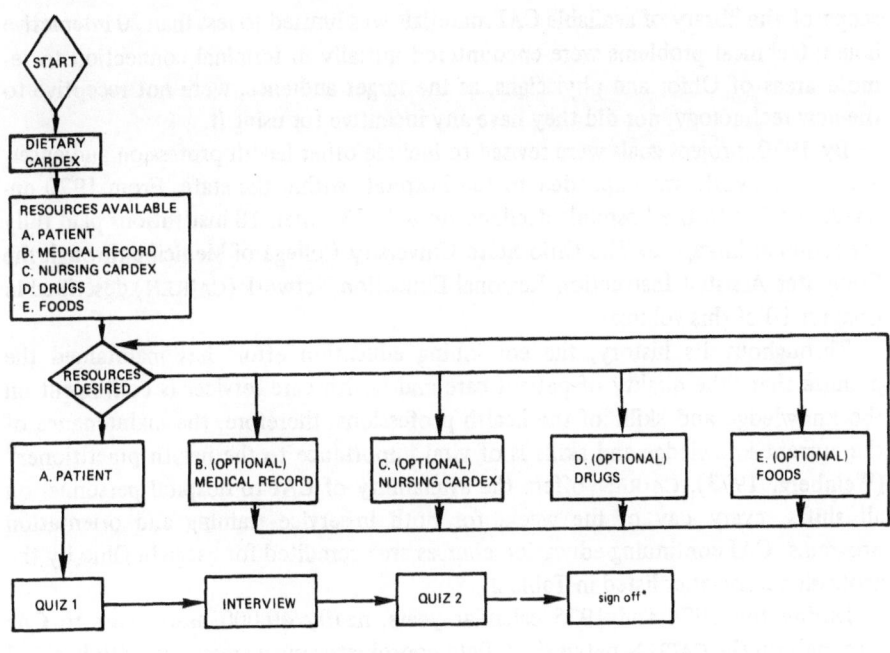

Figure 2. Flow description for clinical simulations of the patient–student encounter (PLAN). After meeting with the clinical instructor to obtain a patient assignment, the student "signs onto" the computer patient where he/she receives the dietary cardex (which is normally received from the instructor) and gathers more information as needed from one of several sources: the medical record, the nursing cardex, the drug catalogue or the foods catalogue. When the student indicates he/she is ready to interview the patient, he/she is presented with quiz 1. Following quiz 1, the student begins the simulated interview with the patient. Upon completion of the interview, the student is presented with quiz 2. This comprises the simulation of the first day's encounter. The second day's simulation is essentially the same format; i.e., quiz 3, interview, quiz 4, with all optional information updated and made available for day 2. The student then meets with the clinical instructor for an evaluation of the simulation experience and of his performance.

clinical experiences, and (3) utilization of less overall faculty time. In addition, students using PLAN simulations performed as well, and in some cases better, on comparable postacademic performance measures (Breese and Schimpfhauser, 1976).

Continuing Medical Education

Given the initial success of CAI usage in the College's primary education curriculums, the College requested and received funds (Public Health Service Grant #1 C03 RM 00070 01) to assess the feasibility of applying computer technology to the continuing education needs of Ohio's physicians. During 1968, a pilot network was established and placed in four community hospitals chosen to represent various geographical areas of the state. Success was not immediate for several reasons: the scope of the library of available CAI materials was limited to less than 20 interactive hours; technical problems were encountered initially in terminal connection to remote areas of Ohio; and physicians, as the target audience, were not receptive to the new technology, nor did they have any incentive for using it.

By 1970, project goals were revised to include other health profession audiences, and the network was expanded to ten hospitals within the state. From 1970 onward, subsidy to the hospitals declined until 1975, when 18 institutions paid fully for terminal linkage to The Ohio State University College of Medicine through the Computer Assisted Instruction Regional Education Network (CAIREN) described in Chapter 10 of this volume.

Throughout its history, the continuing education effort has maintained the premise that "the quality of patient care and health care services is contingent on the knowledge and skills of the health professions; therefore, the maintenance of the current knowledge and skills is of vital importance to the health practitioner" (Weinberg, 1973). CAIREN offers the availability of CAI to hospital personnel on all shifts, every day of the week, for both in-service training and orientation programs. CAI continuing education courses are accredited for usage in Ohio by the professional societies listed in Table 2.

During the 1974 and 1975 calendar years, nearly 40,000 users came to CAI terminals on the CAIREN network. A field coordinator meets regularly with hospital continuing education committees, administrators, and staff to assist in planning the usage and development of CAI courses for each institution. Many courses developed for the continuing education environment have proven quite useful for undergraduate training in medicine, nursing, and allied health professions; the reverse has also been true.

One of the more exciting uses of CAI in the area of continuing competency has been by the American Board of Internal Medicine (ABIM) which is exploring the use of CASE simulations in the recertification process. The project is directed by Dr. William G. Harless, of the Pacific Medical Center, San Francisco, with computer and implementation support by the Division of Computing Services for Medical Education and Research at The Ohio State University College of Medicine.

Table 2. *Accreditation of Continuing Educating Courses by Professional Societies*

	Approximate hours of CAI credit available
American Dietetic Association	108
American Medical Association	70
American Osteopathic Association	All programs eligible for Category II-A credit
Ohio Council of Medical Technology	60
Ohio Nurses Association	6
State of Ohio Board of Pharmacy	106

The project, which has assumed the acronym MERIT (Model for Evaluation and Recertification through Individualized Testing), began July 1, 1973. Specifically, the MERIT Project was designed to investigate:

1. An approach to recertification whereby the specific patient problems of each internist will be the basis for the evaluation of his skills, knowledge and clinical judgment;
2. The use of an advanced computer simulation of the physician—patient encounter (CASE) as the examination instrument for the individualized evaluation;
3. The development of a scoring system for CASE to assess various dimensions of clinical behavior;
4. The involvement of each participating internist in an evaluation process which will help him to identify deficiencies and thus allow him to plan for more meaningful individualized continuing education; and
5. Assessment of attitudes of practicing internists toward a recertification process that embraces the preceding components. (Harless, 1975)

A field test involving approximately 90 physicians was conducted in April 1976, using the CAIREN network. Physicians showed an overall positive reaction to use of the CASE in the recertification process. Chart audit of individual patient records showed that physicians interacted with the simulated patients in a manner consistent with their interactions with real patients. A national field test of the MERIT process is now being designed (Harless *et al.*, 1976).

Patient and Nonmedical Support Staff Education

As a direct result of the continuing education efforts, patient education courses were developed. For example, there are CAI courses that offer instruction to mothers in care and feeding of newborns, to the patient who wishes to assess his probability of heart attack, and to any individual wishing to explore proper menu planning.

Courses have also been developed for use by nonmedical support staff. Courses on the medical record and on medical terminology are examples of two such courses that have been useful to secretaries and medical typists in the CAIREN hospitals.

Summary of Usage

The Ohio State University College of Medicine CAI programs have proven to be useful to a variety of audiences. Table 3 summarizes the number of CAI courses relevant to each of several major audiences. An indexing of all College of Medicine CAI materials by audience is available in Appendix B. *The User's Guide to Computer Assisted Instruction at The Ohio State University College of Medicine* (Division of Computing Services, 1973a) offers a more detailed description of each CAI program.

Table 3. The Ohio State University College of Medicine CAI Programs Indexed by Audience

Audience	Number of programs
Clinical laboratory	27
Dietary	26
Dental	6
Emergency medical	14
Environmental services	8
Management	6
Medical records	8
Medical (physicians, residents, interns, and students)	113
Nursing	51
Occupational therapy	18
Optometry	5
Patients and families	10
Pharmacy	6
Physical therapy	20
Respiratory	15
Radiology	17
Secretarial	11

Configurations for Usage

Looking at The Ohio State University College of Medicine CAI System from another perspective, one can view the configurations for user access to the materials described above. Basically, two configurations for access are used: *an off-line configuration* in which the user installs a portion or portions of The Ohio State University College of Medicine System on his own computer; and *an on-line configuration* in which the user links directly to the CAI data base at The Ohio State University College of Medicine.

In efforts to facilitate sharing, the College has released materials in both configurations. Although both off-line and on-line mechanisms are used for sharing, experience has shown a higher success rate with on-line sharing. Hence, the College has channeled the major portion of its resources in the direction which encourages usage through one of the existing on-line networks.

Off-Line Configuration

Under the auspices of the College's *A Workable Policy for CAI Materials Release* (Pengov and Trzebiatowski, 1972), all CAI materials (except those restricted by the author or by copyright concerns) are available for release to other nonprofit institutions. The policy facilitates sharing while protecting the author and the College. Since January, 1974, over 110 course and program units have been distributed, using this policy, to institutions in the United States, Europe, and South America.

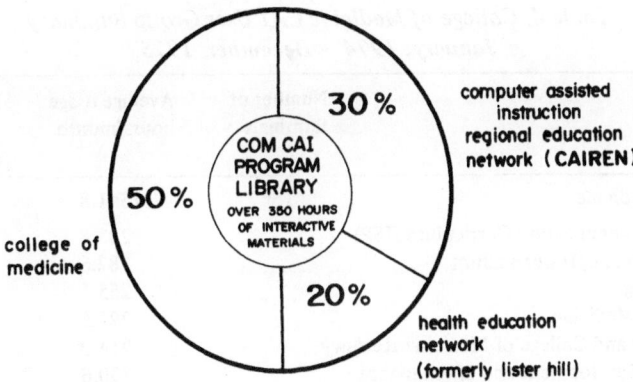

Figure 3. The Ohio State University College of Medicine CAI system data base and user group overview. Copyright 1975, Division of Computing Services for Medical Education and Research.

On-Line Configuration

The on-line configuration has three subsystems that share the central library of CAI programs or courseware (Figure 3): the College of Medicine (including M.D., Ph.D., Nursing, and Allied Medical curricula); the Computer Assisted Instruction Regional Education Network (CAIREN); and the nationwide Health Education Network (formerly the Lister Hill Experimental CAI Network).

Table 4 offers an overview of each group's average monthly usage including the number of terminals serviced. Figure 4 offers a historical view of the usage profile and the almost 140,000 cumulative usage hours from 1971 through 1975.

Local Network

In the local configuration, over 20 terminal sites exist within the city of Columbus for accessing CAI courses. The largest number of these terminals are in the CAI Learning Center in the Health Sciences Library at OSU. To use a CAI course, the student comes to the monitor's room, checks out a key and associated visuals (if needed for use in the CAI session), and proceeds to a learning carrel. Each carrel contains a silent teletypewriter-like computer terminal that furnishes the student with a complete "hard copy" record of his interactive on-line learning sessions. The carrel also contains a carousel slide projector and rear-screen projector for viewing of slides used in conjunction with several of the CAI programs.

These carrels are monitored and maintained by a staff of parttime employees who are students in the College of Medicine. These students are responsible for scheduling carrels and regulating the circulation of the associated visuals. They also are instrumental in providing technical assistance to new users in the CAI Learning Center. It is important to note that the CAI Learning Center serves students in the College of Medicine, including the School of Nursing and the School of Allied Medical Professions. Additional terminals are located in high usage areas or areas that have funds to support their own usage.

Table 4. College of Medicine CAI User Group Summary
January, 1974 – December, 1975

Category	Number of terminals	Average usage hours/month	Percentage of total system usage
College of Medicine	16[a]	1541.8	52.8%
Independent Study Curriculum (ISP)		283.8	9.7%
Medicine, L/D Curriculum		182.6	6.3%
Nursing		255.1	8.7%
Allied Medicine		221.5	7.6%
Visitor and College of Medicine Review[b]		214.9	7.4%
DCS, Development and Maintenance		330.6	11.3%
College of Optometry		52.9	1.8%
Subtotal		1541.4	52.8%
Computer Assisted Instruction Regional Education Network (CAIREN)	18	758.4	26.0%
Health Education Network	56	618.5	21.2%
Total	90	2878.3	100 %

[a]These terminals form a pool located in the Health Sciences Library.
[b]Includes College of Medicine faculty, students, and visitors who are not primary users of a course but who desire to review it.

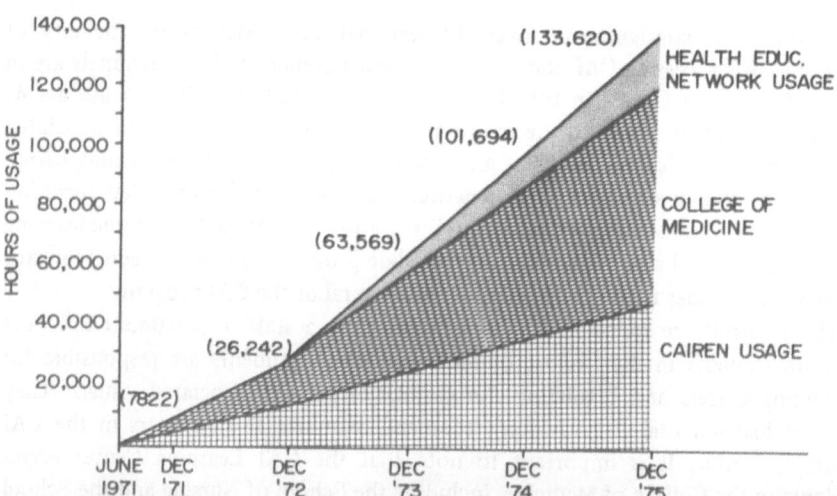

Figure 4. The Ohio State University College of Medicine CAI system hours of usage by user group. Copyright 1975, Division of Computing Services for Medical Education and Research.

State Network (CAIREN)

The State of Ohio or CAIREN configuration consists of some 20 institutions throughout Ohio linked directly via telephone to Columbus and The Ohio State University College of Medicine site. This configuration is described in more detail in Chapter 10 of this volume.

National Health Education Network (HEN)

In 1972, under a grant from the Lister Hill National Center for Biomedical Communications of the National Library of Medicine (Grant #NO1 LM 2 4717), the College linked its data base to an experimental network for CAI access. The purpose of the experimental network was to test the interinstitutional sharing of CAI materials housed at The Ohio State University College of Medicine, at Massachusetts General Hospital in Boston, and at the University of Illinois Medical Center (Lewis and Wooster, 1973). Other chapters in this volume describe the Lister Hill involvement (Chapter 8) and the national network (Chapters 7 and 11), so these aspects will not be discussed here.

The hardware network is maintained by the TYMSHARE Corporation of Cupertino, California, and is a combination of minicomputers with high-speed lines linking cities in the United States and Europe (Combs, 1973). Users on the national network vary from small hospitals to major medical centers; the type and extent of usage varies as much as does the type and size of institution. By far, the largest number of users are presently reviewing available materials with no commitment to long-range usage. But several institutions have made significant commitments for utilization. The University of Washington in Seattle has accessed The Ohio State University Independent Study Program materials and has altered them to meet local specifications. The University of Pittsburgh, in association with Pittsburgh Eye and Ear Hospital, is using ophthalmology materials and has developed its own CAI materials using the CAI support staff at The Ohio State University College of Medicine. The University of the Pacific, in cooperation with the American Board of Internal Medicine, is refining, revising, and generating new CASEs using the CAI support staff at OSU.

Support Configuration for CAI

At The Ohio State University College of Medicine there are two major sets of actors in CAI development and usage, the authors and the support staff. The authors of CAI materials are most often College faculty, although students have authored several allied medical and basic anatomy programs. Student authors may receive graduate credit for developing a viable program. Two primary support units house the second set of actors, the support staff (see Figure 5).

The Division of Research and Evaluation in Medical Education assists in research and evaluation design studies involving CAI. This division also interfaces with all College curriculum committees and helps set priorities for new CAI development.

The Division of Computing Services for Medical Education and Research:

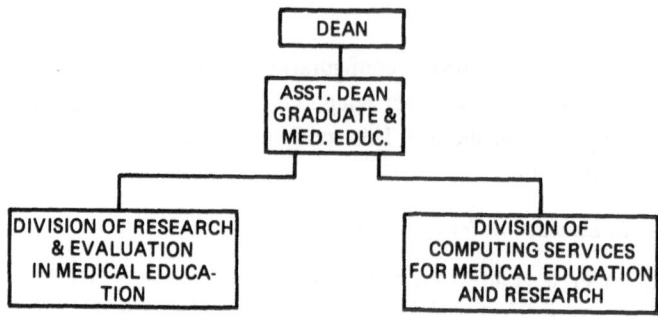

Figure 5. CAI support units.

1. Maintains and troubleshoots all hardware, including computers, terminals, telephone lines, etc.

2. Maintains and upgrades existing CAI courseware, including conversion of all courseware from 100 character-line length to 70 character-line length, and updates in course content.

3. Maintains, develops, and upgrades software for the COURSEWRITER III Language and CAI System, including addition of numerical and algebraic manipulation capabilities to the COURSEWRITER CAI System.

4. Maintains, develops, and upgrades software for the Computer Assisted Instruction Reporting System (CAIRS), which generates student and system usage reports (Pengov, 1974; Division of Computing Services, 1973b).

5. Performs all user interface functions, including: (a) on-line distribution of CAI materials via the CAI Learning Center on the OSU campus, via the Computer Assisted Instruction Regional Network (CAIREN) and via the Health Education Network (HEN); (b) provision of user interface services such as distribution of User's Guides, troubleshooting, and the coordination and distribution of monitor services, and visuals; (c) summarization and distribution of CAI usage reports, statistics, etc., to user groups; and (d) coordination of CAI demonstrations, visitors, and general requests for information.

6. Assists faculty in usage and in incorporation of CAI programs into College curriculums.

7. Develops new CAI courseware.

Further discussion of CAI support services is now offered under these subheadings: CAI Development, CAI User Services, and the CAI Hardware and Software Systems.

CAI Development

The support team for development of new CAI courses is one of the strong points of the CAI environment at The Ohio State University College of Medicine. Figure 6 schematically depicts the CAI development team. The major actors are the author and the instructional programmer (IP), who serves as the primary interface

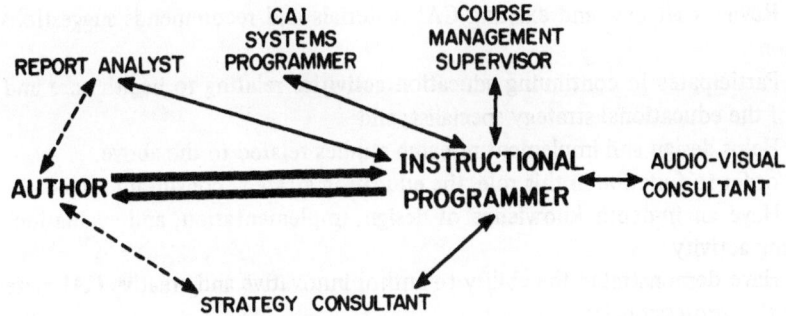

Figure 6. The Ohio State University College of Medicine CAI course development team, Copyright 1974, OSU College of Medicine.

between the author and CAI hardware and software. The author remains the content specialist, while the instructional programmer consults with the author regarding objectives, strategy, and design of the material; codes and inputs the material in the COURSEWRITER language; works with the systems programmer in design of new course facilities or systems functions to effect the course strategy; works with the systems analyst to design student reports and/or usage reports as required by the author; arranges for appropriate content reviewers; consults with the author and the audiovisual consultant on the use of audiovisuals in conjunction with the CAI courses; serves as the ongoing caretaker and troubleshooter for the course once it is released for student usage (this includes continual monitoring of student comments); and monitors and helps interpret item statistics and student usage reports for evaluation and revision of materials.

As a "jack-of-all-trades," the IP must have access to backup resources in most areas. An audiovisual consultant, educational strategy consultant, course management supervisor, systems programmer, and report analyst are all available as needed to assist the instructional programmer. The IPs, for the most part, have backgrounds in education rather than in computers or health; they are trained on the job (Burson, 1975).

The percentage of instructional programming time spent in major activities are: 50% for development of new CAI programs; 38% for revision and maintenance of existing CAI programs; and 12% for other (including administrative duties, continuing education, etc).

The educational strategy consultant is a key member of the development team and as such:

1. Participates in the planning of new materials under development;

2. Assists and helps train instructional programmers in writing objectives, selecting learning strategies, and developing appropriate evaluation mechanisms for CAI materials;

3. Helps monitor the quality of CAI programs;

4. Suggests strategies to assist the CAI staff in solving programming problems related to instructional flow or achievement of objectives;

5. Reviews all new and existing CAI materials and recommends suggestions for revision;

6. Participates in continuing education activities relating to health care and the role of the educational strategy specialist; and

7. Helps design and implement research studies related to the above.

In order to function in this role, the education strategy consultant must:

1. Have an in-depth knowledge of design, implementation, and evaluation of a learning activity;

2. Have demonstrated the ability to author innovative and creative CAI materials for health professionals;

3. Have an operational knowledge of the CAI system and language capabilities and an in-depth knowledge of all College of Medicine CAI materials;

4. Be able to apply practical judgment and sensitivity in decisions related to CAI development and utilization; and

5. Be able to analyze data, recognize flow problems, synthesize alternative strategies and/or design alternative solutions.

CAI projects often require specialized capabilities or special reports which are not currently available in the IBM COURSEWRITER III language and system. The systems programmer is responsible for alterations and extensions to the COURSE-WRITER language and system.

The report analyst, on the other hand, is primarily concerned with the collection, analysis, and reporting of data necessary to support specific projects or activities (i.e., student progress reports, CAI usage reports, line activity reports, response prints, etc.) (Pengov, 1974).

The course management supervisor is responsible for the maintenance of all CAI files and courses on the COURSEWRITER III system and does his work through the COURSEWRITER III supervisor commands.

The philosophy of providing a trained team of professionals to support the faculty/author and of alleviating the need for the faculty's and author's learning of computers, systems, or languages is a cornerstone of successful CAI program development in the College. This support has been extended to assist authors remote from OSU in the development of CAI materials on the OSU system (Harless *et al.*, 1976; Pengov *et al.*, 1976).

Of equal importance in any developmental effort is the delineation of a plan for development and utilization of each course that minimizes the possibility of fragmentation and duplication of efforts (both content and purpose). It is recognized that specific needs and availability of authors and financial resources may force development in parts. However, this does not preclude development of a master plan for the parts and a schema for prioritizing the development of CAI materials.

A number of guidelines have been used in making the decision to proceed with developmental efforts in CAI. Although programs accepted for development have been unique and each situation has been evaluated individually, answers to the following general questions have been useful in prioritizing development.

1. Is the request originating from the College of Medicine?
   a. Will students or faculty of the College of Medicine receive primary benefit?
   b. Will the program be used as part of a College course? curriculum?
2. Has the department or division reviewed and/or approved the proposed development?
3. What is the faculty/author's commitment to the proposed program?
4. What are the educational goals and objectives of the proposed usage?
5. Is CAI the proper medium to accomplish the author's educational goals?
6. Does the proposed project overlap in content with already existing CAI programs?
7. What is the time schedule (deadline, if any) for the development?
8. Is the proposed audience and usage large enough to justify the time and effort in development?
   a. How many students will take the program? During what time frame?
   b. Will the program be used for successive years?
9. Can the development be completed and ongoing usage facilitated using existing expertise, systems, and equipment?
10. Will the acceptance of the project cause slippage in other CAI projects?
11. Is the program applicable to CAIREN and HEN audiences?

CAI materials created and undergoing major revision during 1974–75 amounted to an average of 61.5 interactive hours per year or 5.1 interactive hours per month. During this time, a staff of four instructional programmers completed all development and revisions, given an average of 15.4 interactive hours of CAI produced by each instructional programmer per year (or 1.3 hours per month per instructional programmer).

A review process follows the development and/or revision of every CAI course. This review process, which is currently being studied in more depth under a grant from the National Fund for Medical Education, is an important contributor to the College's success in CAI.

Not only is it important to have direction and guidelines for continuity in development, but it is imperative that the continuing quality and correctness of the College of Medicine CAI materials be ensured. All materials (past, present and future) must be monitored by an appropriate quality control process.

A well conceived quality control process must assess the effectiveness and efficiency of the materials. An integral part of the correctness of content, and foremost to its reception, are the quality, appropriateness and efficiency of the programming flow. The process must also include the review of appropriate field test data whereby programming problems can be clearly identified before general dissemination. Aside from updating the subject matter, content errors and/or subjective interpretations must be identified and changes implemented to make the material adaptable and relevant to a variety of participants. Continuity of content must persist and creativity of programming must prevail while presenting an activity conducive to objective achievement. Therefore, a primary concern in the development, maintenance and utilization of College of Medicine

CAI materials must be that of strategies designed for effective presentation and efficient utilization of the material. (Edited from a memorandum dated January, 1975, from Jeanne Burson, Educational Strategy Consultant, to the author).

The steps of the review process are summarized below:

1. *Technical Review*. Once CAI material has been input into the system by the instructional programmer (IP), the IP checks the program to make certain that the program reflects the content and branching structure which was contained in the author-written draft materials. Careful checks are made for improper branching, closed loops, improper feedback to student responses, etc. When the IP is satisfied that no programming errors remain in the program, the educational strategy consultant and the author review the program.

2. *Educational Strategy Review*. The educational strategy consultant serves as the "first line" quality control agent reviewing aspects such as student vs. machine control, flow, cohesiveness, appropriateness of visuals, and matching of educational objectives with strategy chosen. The educational strategy consultant reviews every CAI course at several points in the development process and provides the primary quality control for educational strategy and CAI design.

3. *Content Review*. After technical and educational strategy review, the author of the program reviews the program at the terminal (usually with the assistance of the IP). This review permits the author to see the program from the standpoint of the student. Content "gaps" and logic of content flow are primary concerns in this review. After the author review, all changes are made by the IP. The author again reviews the program; if the program requires no more changes, the program passes to the next stage; otherwise, the review—reprogramming process is performed as many times as necessary. Following the author content review, several content specialists (colleagues or peers) review the program for accuracy and timeliness and react to the usefulness of the program as a teaching device. Suggested corrections and changes are reviewed by the author and IP and incorporated where appropriate.

4. *Participant Tryout*. After content review, two or three students from the target population take the program. Any remaining problems in flow and content are identified at this time. Necessary corrections are made by the author and the IP.

5. *Field Testing*. All programs produced by the CAI development staff are field tested with a small sample of the user population before being released to the general library. Revisions from field testing greatly increase the probability that the CAI course will respond correctly to a student response. Field testing permits the programs to be further individualized by anticipation of frequently occurring responses not previously considered.

Programs that are developed by authors outside of OSU are subjected to the review process delineated above. Only programs that successfully complete all the steps are released for general use.

A manual for the authoring of CAI materials, *The Author's Guide to CAI* (Burson, 1976), familiarizes the new CAI author with the potential of CAI as an individualized instructional medium. It explains the CAI program development process in an easily understood step-by-step fashion. Numerous examples of CAI materials employing a variety of strategies and branching techniques are provided as models for the new author. Special CAI authoring forms are provided to assist the author in the writing process. This guide is available to all potential authors, both local and remote.

The *Instructional Programmers Guide* (in development) is designed as a training and reference manual for IPs. It documents techniques and procedures related to the entire CAI program development process; it describes the role of the IP and the IP's relationship to other members of the CAI development staff; it delineates the resources and facilities available to the IP; it offers information on standardized coding techniques and prewritten functions; and it serves as an index to other relevant resources.

CAI User Services

The CAI User Services Unit is responsible for providing documentation of procedures and materials along with the technical assistance and adjunct visuals necessary for facilitating the access and use of the CAI data base. This area of support is critical to the provision of CAI access for College users as well as members of CAIREN and HEN. It is important to note that the coordination of these services was brought about by the obvious need to avoid duplication of effort and to make effective use of the existing resources in the Division of Computing Services for Medical Education and Research.

The services provided fall into five major areas:

1. *Documentation of the CAI Data Base. The User's Guide to Computer Assisted Instruction at The Ohio State University College of Medicine* (Division of Computing Services, 1973a) documents the CAI program library by offering detailed descriptions of each of the program entries. Several indices (alphabetical, subject, audience) have been provided to help users locate relevant CAI materials.

The dynamic nature of the CAI data base necessitates a monthly updating of the *Guide* and the automatic production of these manuals from a master data base. A computer program generates new *Guides* as well as updates (only those pages where additions, corrections, or deletions have been made). Over 300 *Guides* have been distributed to date. Copies of the *Guide* are available for student and faculty personnel in the CAI terminal area of the Health Sciences Library.

In addition to the *Guide*, a variety of handout materials have been prepared which briefly describe the programs in the CAI Library and discuss their applicability in a variety of environments.

2. *Adjunct Materials.* Many of the CAI programs require associated visuals in the form of slides or hard copy (photographs, charts, graphs, etc.) pages. The CAI User Services Unit maintains the master files for all such visuals and distributes copies as needed to all users.

3. *Troubleshooting.* Trained personnel are available throughout the working day

to facilitate the use of OSU CAI materials. The troubleshooting activity addresses user concerns with technical malfunction in the terminal, communications interface, and/or computer system.

4. *Communication Mechanisms.* A "monthly mailing packet" serves as the primary communication mechanism between the CAI User Services and all users. This packet includes:

> Monthly usage reports
> *CAI Chronicle* (newsletter)
> Updates for *CAI User's Guide*
> Program flyers for new CAI offerings
> Updates in associated visual materials
> Monitor notes

5. *User Education.* Slide–tape presentations, handouts, and demonstrations are all made available to new users who are interested in learning about CAI and to faculty who wish to orient entire classes or groups of students to CAI. These presentations and promotional materials are developed and distributed by the CAI User Services Unit.

The CAI Hardware and Software System

The usage described previously is supported by central hardware, software, and systems support personnel. Appendix D gives a concise summary of the software and hardware which keeps CAI "running." More detailed documentation of this on-line IBM COURSEWRITER system is available (Division of Computing Services, 1973c). The Ohio State University College of Medicine CAI system operates 22 hours per day with a stability rate of 93% to 100%. With up to 25–30 persons utilizing the system simultaneously, user response time is less than one second. During these peak usage periods, as many as 70,000 students and system-recording records may be logged per week. These records and the system of background programs which process them are called the Computer Assisted Instruction Reporting System (CAIRS) (Pengov, 1974). This system provides feedback regarding CAI utilization and effectiveness to (1) students, (2) educators, (3) faculty advisers and tutors, (4) programmers and analysts, (5) authors of CAI materials, (6) managers of CAI operations, and (7) administrators.

In addition to daily maintenance, backup, and operation of the CAI on-line system and CAIRS, the CAI system support staff has effected or helped effect major software and hardware developments such as:

1. Conversion of all CAI courseware from 100 to 70 characterlines
2. Installation and maintenance of the TYMNET national network interface
3. Implementation of authoring improvements such as: "See student record, br*+, and multiple word modifier"
4. Development of a program to automatically compress COURSEWRITER course files

5. Development of a cross reference for labels, counters, switches, buffers, and registers in the print program

6. Installation of a secure course file backup procedure

Summary

Several factors that have been significant in the history of CAI growth and development at The Ohio State University College of Medicine are still significant today:

1. Educational strategy and content application of the CAI materials is given first priority in CAI materials development. The current strength of the College of Medicine CAI System is the breadth and depth of its courseware, not the elegance of its hardware.

2. Definition of what is to be developed comes from outside of the CAI support unit, thus alleviating any tendency for the support unit to breed a life of its own. Decisions on the priorities for new CAI development come from directors of the curricular areas, from the field coordinator for the CAIREN and HEN networks and from the faculty. The support unit functions according to the needs and priorities of the content areas.

3. Introduction and gradual incorporation of CAI materials into existing college curricula is effected by credible faculty in each area. Although the integration often moves slowly and is facilitated by support units, it will not move at all without involvement of faculty within the content area.

4. Each CAI project, curricular effort, or program utilizes staff and expertise in existing College support units. Each new effort builds upon the knowledge and expertise of past efforts of the central support staff. Lessons learned by support staff or authors on one project are applied immediately to other projects. Personnel and system resources are shared by all projects in a cost effective and coordinated fashion. This alleviates formation of small support "fiefdoms," each "recreating the wheel" of CAI.

5. The structure and process of the CAI course development team has maximized the quality and quantity of CAI development while minimizing faculty time expended.

6. The College has maintained a commitment to an operational system with continuous uptime and usage. This environment facilitates growth and integration of CAI into the College curriculums without prohibiting research and development. It has also paved the way for transition of CAI support from "soft" to "hard" dollars. This essay would be remiss if it did not stress the importance of outside funding for large-scale CAI development (ISP, CASE, PLAN). The costs in staff time alone for such developmental efforts are so high that few institutions could afford the initial capital investment. As equally important, however, is the need to approach CAI usage and development with the eventual goal of transferring on-going usage and maintenance costs (even if only on paper) to the various audience groups. Close attention has been given at OSU to accurate CAI costing and to

development of a system of user payment for CAI usage and services. This point is particularly important in helping users realistically access the costs and benefits of CAI usage in their learning environment. Such a cost approach avoids the all too common syndrome of using CAI because it is available rather than because it allows the use of learning strategies (i.e., simulations) and facilitates learning approaches (i.e., independent self-paced study) which other learning systems cannot provide. Currently, a rather extensive system exists within the College's Division of Computing Services for Medical Education and Research to accurately determine costs of CAI development, maintenance, and usage by a given user group (Pengov, 1975). Monthly and hourly access rates are available with varying levels of user support services provided according to category of access chosen.

7. *Administrative support for the CAI effort has been present within the College* (this is especially important in the early development stages). Administrative support is a necessary (but not sufficient) condition for consideration of issues such as faculty incentives for involvement in CAI.

In summary, The Ohio State University College of Medicine has found CAI to be a valuable alternative learning resource that can be used for cost effective enhancement of the medical education process.

ACKNOWLEDGMENTS

Many of the data used in this chapter are drawn from the 1974–1975 *Progress Report of the Division of Computing Services for Medical Education and Research*, College of Medicine, The Ohio State University, January 1976. The contributions of Division Managers Verl Dennis and Mark Forman in compiling data for this chapter, and of EDUCOM for allowing reproduction of portions of an earlier publication, are acknowledged.

Appendix A. Sample of Student Dialogue: Histology Course

EXAMPLE 1: STUDENT FLOW
HISTL

COMPUTER: 1. STUDY SLIDES 1 AND 2. THEN TYPE THE NAME OF THE ORGAN.
STUDENT: STOMACH
COMPUTER: NO. THE LAMIN PROPRIA OF THE STOMACH IS PACKED WITH TUBULAR GLANDS AND THE EPITHELIUM IS OF A SINGLE CELL TYPE. TRY AGAIN.
STUDENT: SMALL BOWEL
COMPUTER: NO. LOOK CLOSELY AT SLIDE 2. WHAT YOU PROBABLY ASSUMED WERE VILLI ARE STRAIGHT TUBULAR GLANDS. NOTICE THE NUMEROUS LIGHT STAINING CELLS IN THE EPITHELIUM. TRY AGAIN TO NAME THE ORGAN.

STUDENT: ANAL CANAL

COMPUTER: NO. OBSERVE THE FOUR LAYERS IN THE WALL OF THIS ORGAN –
             MUCOSA, SUBMUCOSA, MUSCULARIS, AND SEROSA. THIS IS HIGHLY
             INDICATIVE OF THE ALIMENTARY CANAL. NAME THE ORGAN.

STUDENT: ESOPHAGUS

COMPUTER: NO. NOTICE THE LARGE NUMBER OF GOBLET CELLS IN THE
             MUCOSA AND THE ABSENCE OF VILLI. TRY AGAIN.

STUDENT: LARGE INTESTINE

COMPUTER: CORRECT. THE CHARACTERISTICS YOU SHOULD HAVE OBSERVED
             WERE CRYPTS OF LIEBERKUHN WITH A LARGE NUMBER OF GOBLET
             CELLS PRESENT AS WELL AS THE ABSENCE OF VILLI.

EXAMPLE 2: STUDENT FLOW
HISTL

COMPUTER: 12. THE FOLLOWING IS A LIST OF TISSUES AND STRUCTURES THAT
             ARE PRESENT IN THIS TUBULAR ORGAN. STUDY THE LIST AND
             NAME THE ORGAN DESCRIBED.
             (1) NONCORNIFIED STRATIFIED SQUAMOUS EPITHELIUM
             (2) A LAYER OF LONGITUDINAL MUSCLE BUNDLES
             (3) GLANDS SOMETIMES PRESENT IN THE LAMINA PROPRIA AND/
                 OR SUBMUCOSA
             (4) CIRCULAR AND LONGITUDINAL MUSCLE LAYERS IN THE
                 OUTER COAT

STUDENT: VAGINA

COMPUTER: WRONG. THE VAGINA CONTAINS STRATIFIED SQUAMOUS EPITHE-
             LIUM BUT THE MUSCULAR COAT IN THE VAGINA IS COMPOSED OF
             INTERLACING LONGITUDINAL, CIRCULAR, AND OBLIQUE MUSCLE
             FIBERS RATHER THAN TWO DISTINCT LAYERS AS IN THIS ORGAN.
             ALSO, THERE IS NO MUSCULARIS MUCOSA IN THE VAGINA. TRY
             AGAIN.

STUDENT: ESOPHAGUS

COMPUTER: YOU ARE CORRECT. LOOK AT SLIDES 16 AND 17. REMEMBER THAT
             MOST OF THE SECTIONS OF ESOPHAGUS YOU WILL SEE HAVE ONLY
             ONE TYPE OF GLAND AND OFTEN THERE ARE NO GLANDS PRESENT.

Appendix B. CAI Courses: Audience Listing

THIS INDEX LISTS ALL OHIO STATE UNIVERSITY COLLEGE OF MEDICINE CAI
COURSES (RELEASABLE AND RESTRICTED) WHICH ARE CURRENTLY OPERATIONAL.
NON-OSU COLLEGE OF MEDICINE USERS CAN NOTE VIA THE ALPHABETICAL LIST
THE COURSES RELEASABLE TO THEM.

CLINICAL LABORATORY

ABBREV	MEDICAL ABBREVIATIONS
ABEL	ACID BASE AND ELECTROLYTES
ACIBA	ACID BASE BALANCE
BUGOUT	HOSPITAL INFECTION CONTROL
CVTERM	CARDIOVASCULAR TERMINOLOGY
ENDO	THE ENDOCRINE METABOLIC SYSTEM
ENZICS	ENZYME IDENTIFICATION, CLASSIFICATION AND SIGNIFICANCE
JUDI	JUVENILE DIABETES
MATH	MATHEMATICS FOR HEALTH PERSONNEL
OBTERM	OBSTETRIC TERMINOLOGY
ONEAID	FIRST AID
PAMADI	PATIENT MANAGEMENT OF DIABETES
PACARE	SHORT TOPICS FOR PATIENT USE
PCHEM1	PHYSIOLOGIC CHEMISTRY
PHASE4	DISEASES OF THE APPENDIX
PILOT	INDEPENDENT STUDY PROGRAM
PUZZLE	HEALTHWORD PUZZLES
QUCOST	STATISTICS FOR QUALITY CONTROL
RESCUE	BASIC TECHNIQUES OF CARDIOPULMONARY RESUSCITATION
REVIEW	REVIEW TOPICS (SECTIONS C AND D)
TERMS	MEDICAL TERMINOLOGY
TOADS	TECHNIQUE, OBSERVATION AND DISCUSSION OF STAINS
TRUAMI	ANTICOAGULANT MEDICATION
UANDME	COMMUNICATIONS
URAL	URINALYSIS
VEINS	CARE OF AND FEEDING BY VEINS

DIETITIANS

ABBREV	MEDICAL ABBREVIATIONS
ACIBA	ACID BASE BALANCE
AFEPI	ASSESSMENT OF FLUID,ENERGY AND PROTEIN INTAKE IN INFANTS
ALTRAC	ALIMENTARY OBSTRUCTIONS OF THE NEWBORN
BUGOUT	HOSPITAL INFECTION CONTROL
DIETAN	ANATOMY FOR DIETITIANS
FOODS	FOOD ITEM NUTRIENT FILE
JUDI	DIABETES FOR TEENAGERS
MATH	MATHEMATICS FOR HEALTH PERSONNEL
NUTRO	PHYSIOLOGIC CHEMISTRY OF NUTRITION
PCHEM1	PHYSIOLOGIC CHEMISTRY
QUAILS	QUESTIONS ABOUT ILEOSTOMY SURGERY
QUCOST	STATISTICS FOR QUALITY CONTROL
RECIPE	COST AND QUANTITY CALCULATIONS
REVIEW	REVIEW TOPICS (SECTION: A)
TERMS	MEDICAL TERMINOLOGY
UANDME	COMMUNICATIONS

DENTAL PERSONNEL

ORALCA	ORAL CANCER RECOGNITION
ORPAIN	APPROACH TO DIAGNOSIS OF OROFACIAL PAIN
PHARMA	DENTAL PHARMACOLOGY REVIEW
TOOTHA	DIFFERENTIAL DIAGNOSIS OF TOOTHACHE
TRETPA	TREATMENT PLANNING FOR THE RELIEF OF REGIONAL PAIN

EMERGENCY MEDICAL TECHNICIANS

ABBREV	MEDICAL ABBREVIATIONS
CVTERM	CARDIOVASCULAR TERMINOLOGY
INTUBE	ENDOTRACHEAL INTUBATION
MATH	MATHEMATICS FOR HEALTH PERSONNEL
OBTERM	OBSTETRIC TERMINOLOGY
ONEAID	FIRST AID
RESCUE	BASIC TECHNIQUES OF CARDIOPULMONARY RESUSCITATION
REVIEW	REVIEW TOPICS (SECTION H SUCTIONING)
SHOCK	SEPTIC SHOCK
SIGNS	VITAL SIGNS
STRIP1	BASICS OF ELECTROCARDIOLOGY
STRIPS	ARRHYTHMIA STRIPS
VEINS	CARE OF AND FEEDING BY VEINS
VENTAR	VENTRICULAR ARRHYTHMIAS

ENVIRONMENTAL SERVICES

BUGOUT	HOSPITAL INFECTION CONTROL
PACARE	SHORT TOPICS FOR PATIENT USE
PAMADI	PATIENT MANAGEMENT OF DIABETES
RESTUP	YOU'VE GOT TO HAVE HEART
SIGNS	VITAL SIGNS
TERMS	MEDICAL TERMINOLOGY
TOTS	CHILD DEVELOPMENT AGES 2-5
UANDME	COMMUNICATIONS

MANAGEMENT

ABBREV	MEDICAL ABBREVIATIONS
BUGOUT	HOSPITAL INFECTION CONTROL
CALC	MATHEMATICAL CALCULATIONS SERVICE
QUCOST	STATISTICS FOR QUALITY CONTROL
TERMS	MEDICAL TERMINOLOGY
UANDME	COMMUNICATIONS

MEDICAL RECORDS

AGENT	ANESTHETIC AGENTS AND ADJUNCT DRUGS (SECTION: ANESTHETIC RECORD)
ABBREV	MEDICAL ABBREVIATIONS
BUGOUT	HOSPITAL INFECTION CONTROL
CVTERM	CARDIOVASCULAR TERMINOLOGY
OBTERM	OBSTETRICAL TERMINOLOGY
PUZZLE	HEALTHWORD PUZZLES
TERMS	MEDICAL TERMINOLOGY
UANDME	COMMUNICATIONS

MEDICAL STUDENTS, RESIDENTS AND INTERNS

ABANG	ABDOMINAL ARTERIOGRAPHIC ANATOMY
ABBREV	MEDICAL ABBREVIATIONS
ABEL	ACID BASE AND ELECTROLYTES
ACIBA	ACID BASE BALANCE
ALTRAC	ALIMENTARY OBSTRUCTIONS OF THE NEWBORN
BREECH	CAI IN BREECH DELIVERY
BUGOUT	HOSPITAL INFECTION CONTROL
CASE	COMPUTER AIDED SIMULATION OF THE CLINICAL ENCOUNTER
CVTERM	CARDIOVASCULAR TERMINOLOGY
ELBOW	MUSCULATURE OF THE ELBOW JOINT
ENDO	THE ENDOCRINE-METABOLIC SYSTEM
FUNDUS	OPHTHALMOSCOPIC INTERPRETATION
GANAT1	GROSS ANATOMY
GANAT2	GROSS ANATOMY
GASEM	OXYGEN THERAPY EQUIPMENT
HANAT	HAND ANATOMY
HIST1	HISTOLOGY
INTUBE	ENDOTRACHEAL INTUBATION
IONIZE	INTRODUCTION TO RADIATION THERAPY
JUDI	JUVENILE DIABETES
JUDIAB	JUVENILE DIABETES
LOWEX	LOWER EXTREMITY ANATOMY
LUMBUM	ORTHOPEDIC LESIONS
MATH	MATHEMATICS FOR HEALTH PERSONNEL
MEDREC	READING THE PATIENT'S MEDICAL RECORD
MORPHO	MUSCULOSKELETAL SYSTEM
NEURO	NEURO ANATOMY
NUTRO	PHYSIOLOGICAL CHEMISTRY OF NUTRITION
OPHTHA	EXAMINATION OF THE FUNDUS
PCHEM1	PHYSIOLOGICAL CHEMISTRY
PEDS	A BIRD'S EYE VIEW OF PEDIATRICS
PERCEP	BASIC PERCEPTUAL TERMINOLOGY AND CONCEPTS
PHASE4	DISEASES OF THE APPENDIX
PILOT	INDEPENDENT STUDY PROGRAM
PROSHK	PRINCIPLES OF ORTHOPEDIC SURGERY FOR THE HIP AND KNEE
PSYMED	PSYCHOTROPIC MEDICATION
RADIO	CLINICAL ORGAN SCANNING
REDEYE	DIAGNOSIS OF REDEYE
RESCUE	BASIC TECHNIQUES OF CARDIOPULMONARY RESUSCITATION
RESTUP	YOU'VE GOT TO HAVE HEART
REVIEW	REVIEW TOPICS FOR MEDICAL PERSONNEL
SEXED	HUMAN SEXUALITY EDUCATION
SHOCK	SEPTIC SHOCK
SIGNS	VITAL SIGNS
SITIN	SENSORY INTEGRATIVE THERAPY
SKULL	ANATOMY OF THE SKULL
STRIP1	BASICS OF ELECTROCARDIOLOGY
STRIPS	ARRHYTHMIA STRIPS
STROKA	STROKE REHABILITATION
TERMS	MEDICAL TERMINOLOGY
THERM	PHYSIOLOGY AND DISORDERS OF BODY TEMPERATURE REGULATION
TRUAMI	ANTICOAGULANT THERAPY
UANOME	COMMUNICATIONS

NURSING

ABEL	ACID BASE AND ELECTROLYTES
ABBREV	MEDICAL ABBREVIATIONS
AFEPI	FLUID, ENERGY, AND PROTEIN INTAKE IN INFANTS
AGENT	ANESTHETIC AGENTS AND ADJUNCT DRUGS
ALTRAC	ALIMENTARY OBSTRUCTIONS OF THE NEWBORN
ASSESS	NURSING ASSESSMENT OF THE PATIENT WITH RESPIRATORY PATHOPHYSIOLOGY
BOTTLE	CLOSED DRAINAGE SYSTEMS OF THE THORACIC CAVITY
BREECH	CAI IN BREECH DELIVERY
BUGOUT	HOSPITAL INFECTION CONTROL
CCNUR	NURSING CARE OF THE PATIENT WITH CORONARY HEART DISEASE
ELBOW	MUSCULATURE OF THE ELBOW JOINT
ENDO	THE ENDOCRINE-METABOLIC SYSTEM
ENZICS	ENZYME: IDENTIFICATION, CLASSIFICATION AND SIGNIFICANCE
GROUP	DEVELOPMENTAL TASK GROUPS
HANAT	HAND ANATOMY
HIBABY	HI BABY
INTUBE	ENDOTRACHEAL INTUBATION
JUDI	JUVENILE DIABETES
MATH	MATHEMATICS FOR HEALTH PERSONNEL
MEDREC	READING THE PATIENT'S MEDICAL RECORD
NUCTEC	NUCLEAR MEDICINE TECHNOLOGY
OBTERM	OBSTETRIC TERMINOLOGY
OBTOX	TOXEMIA OF PREGNANCY
ORTRAC	PRINCIPLES OF ORTHOPEDIC CARE
PAMADI	PATIENT MANAGEMENT OF DIABETES
PEDS	A BIRD'S EYE VIEW OF PEDIATRICS
PERCEP	BASIC PERCEPTUAL TERMINOLOGY AND CONCEPTS
PILOT	INDEPENDENT STUDY PROGRAM
PROSHK	PRINCIPLES OF ORTHOPEDIC SURGERY FOR THE HIP AND KNEE
PSYMED	PSYCHOTROPIC MEDICATION
QUAILS	QUESTIONS ABOUT ILEOSTOMY SURGERY
QUCOST	STATISTICS FOR QUALITY CONTROL
RESTUP	YOU'VE GOT TO HAVE HEART
REVIEW	REVIEW TOPICS
SEXED	HUMAN SEXUALITY EDUCATION
SHOCK	SEPTIC SHOCK
SHOJT	THE SHOULDER JOINT
SIGNS	VITAL SIGNS
SITIN	SENSORY INTEGRATIVE THERAPY
SKULL	ANATOMY OF THE SKULL
STRIP1	BASICS OF ELECTROCARDIOLOGY
STRIPS	ARRHYTHMIA STRIPS
STROKA	STROKE REHABILITATION
TERMS	MEDICAL TERMINOLOGY
THERM	PHYSIOLOGY AND DISORDERS OF BODY TEMPERATURE REGULATION
TOTS	CHILD DEVELOPMENT AGES 2-5
UANDME	COMMUNICATIONS
UREME	MEASURING AND RECORDING OF URINARY OUTPUT
URAL	REVIEW IN URINALYSIS
VEINS	CARE OF AND FEEDING BY VEINS
VENTAR	VENTRICULAR ARRHYTHMIAS
VESAL1	NEUROMUSCULAR MORPHOLOGY

OCCUPATIONAL THERAPY

ABBREV	MEDICAL ABBREVIATIONS
BUGOUT	HOSPITAL INFECTION CONTROL
ELBOW	MUSCULATURE OF THE ELBOW JOINT

```
GANAT1    GROSS ANATOMY
GROUP     DEVELOPMENTAL TASK GROUPS
HANAT     HAND ANATOMY
LOWEX     ANATOMY OF THE LOWER EXTREMITIES
VESALI    NEUROMUSCULAR MORPHOLOGY
ONEAID    FIRST AID
PAMADI    PATIENT MANAGEMENT OF DIABETES
PERCEP    BASIC CONCEPTS AND TERMINOLOGY OF PERCEPTION
RESCUE    BASIC TECHNIQUES OF CARDIOPULMONARY RESUSCITATION
QUAILS    QUESTIONS ABOUT ILEOSTOMY SURGERY
STROKA    STROKE REHABILITATION
SHOJT     SHOULDER JOINT ANATOMY
SITIN     SENSORY INTEGRATIVE THERAPY
UANDME    COMMUNICATIONS
VESALI    NEUROMUSCULAR MORPHOLOGY
```

OPTOMETRY

```
FUNDUS    OPHTHALMOSCOPIC INTERPRETATION
OPCLIN    OPTOMETRY CLINIC
OPHTHA    EXAMINATION OF THE FUNDUS
OPTOM     OPTOMETRY
REDEYE    DIAGNOSIS OF REDEYE
```

PATIENTS & FAMILIES

```
FOODS     FOOD ITEM NUTRIENT FILE
HIBABY    HI BABY
JUDI      JUVENILE DIABETES
ONEAID    FIRST AID
PACARE    SHORT TOPICS FOR PATIENT USE
PAMADI    PATIENT MANAGEMENT OF DIABETES
QUAILS    QUESTIONS ABOUT ILEOSTOMY SURGERY
RESCUE    BASIC TECHNIQUES OF CARDIOPULMONARY RESUSCITATION
RESTUP    YOU'VE GOT TO HAVE HEART
TOTS      CHILD DEVELOPMENT AGES 2-5
```

PHARMACY

```
AGENT     ANESTHETIC AGENTS AND ADJUNCT DRUGS
CALC      MATHEMATICS CALCULATIONS SERVICE
MATH      MATHEMATICS FOR HEALTH PERSONNEL
QUCOST    STATISTICS FOR QUALITY CONTROL
TRUAMI    ANTICOAGULANT THERAPY
VEINS     CARE OF AND FEEDING BY VEINS
```

PHYSICAL THERAPY

```
ABBREV    MEDICAL ABBREVIATIONS
BUGOUT    HOSPITAL INFECTION CONTROL
CVTERM    CARDIOVASCULAR TERMINOLOGY
ELBOW     MUSCULATURE OF THE ELBOW JOINT
GANAT1    GROSS ANATOMY
GROUP     DEVELOPMENTAL TASK GROUPS
HANAT     HAND ANATOMY
LOWEX     ANATOMY OF THE LOWER EXTREMITIES
ONEAID    FIRST AID
PERCEP    BASIC CONCEPTS AND TERMINOLOGY OF PERCEPTION
PUZZLE    HEALTHWORD PUZZLES
QUAILS    QUESTIONS ABOUT ILEOSTOMY SURGERY
RESCUE    BASIC TECHNIQUES OF CARDIOPULMONARY RESUSCITATION
```

```
SHOJT     THE SHOULDER JOINT
SIGNS     VITAL SIGNS
SITIN     SENSORY INTEGRATIVE THERAPY
STROKA    STROKE REHABILITATION
TERMS     MEDICAL TERMINOLOGY
UANDME    COMMUNICATIONS
VESALI    NEUROMUSCULAR MORPHOLOGY
```

RESPIRATORY

```
ABEL      ACID BASE BALANCE AND ELECTROLYTES
ACIBA     ACID BASE BALANCE
ASSESS    NURSING ASSESSMENT OF THE PATIENT WITH RESPIRATORY
             PATHOPHYSIOLOGY
BOTTLE    CLOSED DRAINAGE SYSTEMS OF THE THORACIC CAVITY
CALC      MATHEMATICS CALCULATIONS SERVICE
CVTERM    CARDIOVASCULAR TERMINOLOGY
GASEM     OXYGEN THERAPY EQUIPMENT
INTUBE    ENDOTRACHEAL INTUBATION
MATH      MATHEMATICS FOR HEALTH PERSONNEL
PCHEM1    PHYSIOLOGIC CHEMISTRY
QUCOST    STATISTICS FOR QUALITY CONTROL
RESCUE    BASIC TECHNIQUES OF CARDIOPULMONARY RESUSCITATION
SIGNS     VITAL SIGNS
TERMS     MEDICAL TERMINOLOGY
UANDME    COMMUNICATIONS
VEINS     CARE OF AND FEEDING BY VEINS
```

RADIOLOGY

```
ABANG     ABDOMINAL ARTERIOGRAPHIC ANATOMY
ABBREV    MEDICAL ABBREVIATIONS
BUGOUT    HOSPITAL INFECTION CONTROL
CALC      MATHEMATICS CALCULATIONS SERVICE
ELBOW     MUSCULATURE OF THE ELBOW JOINT
HANAT     HAND ANATOMY
LOWEX     ANATOMY OF THE LOWER EXTREMITIES
MATH      MATHEMATICS FOR HEALTH PERSONNEL
NUCTEC    NUCLEAR MEDICINE TECHNOLOGY
QUCOST    STATISTICS FOR QUALITY CONTROL
RADIO     CLINICAL ORGAN SCANNING
RADTEC    REVIEW IN RADIOLOGIC TECHNOLOGY
SHOJT     THE SHOULDER JOINT
SIGNS     VITAL SIGNS
SKULL     ANATOMY OF THE SKULL
TERMS     MEDICAL TERMINOLOGY
UANDME    COMMUNICATIONS
```

SECRETARIAL

```
ABBREV    MEDICAL ABBREVIATIONS
BUGOUT    HOSPITAL INFECTION CONTROL
CAI       CAI TECHNIQUES AND CONCEPTS
CVTERM    CARDIOVASCULAR TERMINOLOGY
OBTERM    OBSTETRIC TERMINOLOGY
ONEAID    FIRST AID
PACARE    SHORT TOPICS FOR PATIENT CARE
PUZZLE    HEALTHWORD PUZZLES
TERMS     MEDICAL TERMINOLOGY
TOTS      CHILD DEVELOPMENT AGES 2-5
UANDME    COMMUNICATIONS
```

Appendix C. A *CASE* Sample Interaction

The statements preceded by a question mark are questions and comments made by the learner. Users are given the following codes for accessing various sections of Computer Assisted Simulation of the Clinical Encounter (CASE) and are told that they can freely move between the first three sections as they desire; any time a question appears the learner may ask a question or change sections.

TO ACCESS SEPARATE SECTIONS

H, HISTORY SECTION
P, PHYSICAL EXAMINATION SECTION
L, LABORATORY SECTION
T, USER'S TREATMENT AND DIAGNOSIS

The first paragraph below is the learner's introduction to the "patient."

YOU HAVE JUST ENTERED YOUR OFFICE AND HAVE BEEN APPRISED THAT A PATIENT IS WAITING FOR YOU. HIS NAME IS JOHN JONES. YOU ENTER THE INNER OFFICE AND FIND HIM WAITING FOR YOU TO BEGIN THE INTERVIEW.

? WHAT SEEMS TO BE YOUR PROBLEM
I'M NOT FEELING SO GREAT. FOR ABOUT A MONTH NOW I'VE BEEN FEELING SO TIRED AND RUN DOWN. I FIGURED IT WAS TIME I SAW ANOTHER DOC ABOUT IT.

? HAVE YOU SEEN A DOCTOR ALREADY
I HAVEN'T SEEN ANY OTHER DOCTOR. I'M A CHIROPRACTOR MYSELF, BUT YOU'RE THE FIRST DOCTOR I'VE GONE TO ABOUT MY PROBLEM. I HOPE YOU CAN HELP ME.

? HOW OLD ARE YOU
I HAD A BIRTHDAY LAST MONTH AND THAT MADE ME 44 YEARS OLD.

? DO YOU SMOKE
I'VE BEEN SMOKING CIGARS FOR A LONG TIME. I KNOW YOU GUYS SAY THAT SMOKING IS BAD AND THAT CIGARS ARE TOO STRONG IF YOU INHALE BUT I JUST ENJOY IT TOO DAMN MUCH TO QUIT.

? P
** PHYSICAL EXAM**
? VITAL SIGNS
VITAL SIGNS –
TEMPERATURE: 100.5 DEGREES, ORAL; PULSE: 92 AND REGULAR; RESPIRATION: 18 PER MINUTE; BP: 120/80 BILATERALLY SUPINE AND ERECT.

? EYE
EYE INSPECTION –
PUPILS ARE EQUAL AND REACT WELL TO LIGHT AND ACCOMMODATION. CON-

JUNCTIVA APPEAR WHITE IN COLOR. A PETECHIAL HEMORRHAGE IS NOTED IN THE LEFT INFERIOR CONJUCTIVAL SURFACE. FUNDUSCOPIC EXAMINATION REVEALS NORMAL DISC SIZE AND APPEARANCE. THERE ARE NO HEMORRHAGES OR EXUDATES. VEIN TO ARTERY RATIO IS NORMAL.

?L
LABORATORY

? CBC
COMPLETE BLOOD COUNT
RBC: 3.8 MIL.; WBC: 12.5 THOUSAND HGB: 12.8 GM.; HCT: 34%
RBC MORPHOLOGY
MCV: 87 U3; MCH: 29 UUG; MCHC: 34%
DIFFERENTIAL:
POLY. 78%; STAB. 7%; LYMPH. 5% MONO. 9%; EOS. 1%; BASO. 0%
NRBC/100 WBC: NONE. NO EVIDENCE OF ANISOCYTOSIS. NO EVIDENCE OF POIKILOCYTOSIS.
NORMAL CHROMICITY.

? BLOOD SUGAR
FASTING BLOOD SUGAR: 85 B/100 ML.

? BUN
BLOOD UREA NITROGEN: 13 MG/100 ML.

? T
TREATMENT AND DIAGNOSIS
PLEASE TYPE YOUR DIAGNOSIS AT THIS TIME.

? ENDOCARDITIS
AT THIS POINT YOU MAY DESCRIBE YOUR TREATMENT PLAN
                                    OR
YOU MAY RETURN TO ASK MORE QUESTIONS OR GATHER MORE LABORATORY OR PHYSICAL DATA.

? REST
THE AUTHOR OF THIS CASE, DR. S. MEDICINE, NOTED THE FOLLOWING DIAGNOSIS FOR MR. JOHN JONES . . .

1.   SUBACUTE BACTERIAL EDOCARDITIS
2.   CONGESTIVE HEART FAILURE
3.   RHEUMATIC HEART DISEASE WITH MITRAL INSUFFICIENCY

DR. MEDICINE PRESCRIBED THE FOLLOWING TREATMENT:
1.   BED REST, METHICILLIN OR CEPHALOTHIN AND PROBENECID
2.   BED REST, DIGOXIN 0.25 MGM TID FOR TWO DAYS, QUAM THEREAFTER, MERCURHYDRIN 1 CC OR 2 CC STAT OR HYDRODIURIL 50 MGM. QAM.
3.   BENZATHINE PENICILLIN 1,200,000 UNITS MONTHLY.

AUTHOR'S CRITICAL CONCEPTS – HISTORY

SMOKING	PAST ILLNESSES	CHEST
DRINKING	TIREDNESS	HEART
BREATHING	COUGHING	JOINTS
RHEUMATIC FEVER	FEVER AND CHILLS	

AUTHOR'S CRITICAL CONCEPTS – LABORATORY
RED CELL MORPHOLOGY
RETIC COUNT
MICROSCOPIC URINALYSIS
BLOOD CULT. AND SENS.
URINE CULT. AND SENS.
ELECTROCARDIOGRAM
CHEST X-RAY

AUTHOR'S CRITICAL CONCEPTS – PHYSICAL EXAMINATION
VITAL SIGNS
CHEST
HEART
LUNGS
CONJUNCTIVAE
HANDS

Appendix D. The Ohio State University College of Medicine CAI System Facilities Description

1. Software: IBM Package Program: COURSEWRITER III, V 2.1 under VS/MVT
2. Core Storage: Ranges from approximately 65K upward depending on:
   a. Number of line data areas (LDA) (2K each)
   b. Subroutine areas (2K each)
   c. Lines (require approx. 550 bytes for each new line)
   d. Teleprocessing buffers (128 bytes each)

   As of 12/30/75 OSU COM CORE requirement is approximately 84K (5 Sub areas and 8 line data areas; 25 teleprocessing buffers).

   Above estimates do not include BTAM, BSAM, and BDAM access methods which require about 15K.
3. Hardware: IBM 370/158
   - 1   3705 Teleprocessing control unit
   - 1   3330 Disk Pack, approx. 1 pack with 8 course files
   - 9091 Tracks for course files, with 180 courses
   - 209 Tracks for libraries
   - 883 Tracks for student recording and line activity data
   - 570 Tracks for work areas

NO Tape drives required

30 TTY terminals on a dial-up rotary, with 26 ports

5 Ports on a dial-up rotary for Health Education Network

2 Portable Texas Instruments teletypewriter terminals with built-in accoustic coupler

1 Portable digilog terminal (CRT)

4. System performance:

    a. Scheduled "up" from 3:30 a.m. to 3:00 a.m. daily

    b. CPU time used per hour of "up" time averages less than 2 minutes

    c. Average system response time (from time student hits the Return key until his feedback from the terminal begins): .5—1.0 seconds

    d. Average number of terminal usage hours per day:
       89.5 hours (this figure was computed from Jan.—Sept., 1976)

    e. Average number of lines active:
       10—12 during prime time (8:00 a.m. to 9:00 p.m. EST) with a peak of 31 in use at any one time

    f. Average number of student recording records per day:
       11,252

    g. Average number of log-ons per day:
       175

    h. Average number of system—student interactions per hour:
       674

5. OSU COM Additions to the IBM Package Program:

    a. Control program changes

       (1) Utility files converted from tape to disk

       (2) Student recording and line activity files converted from tape to disk

       (3) Addition of the operator message routine

       (4) Expansion of translate tables to allow for printing of special characters

       (5) Expansion of available monitor commands

       (6) Addition of an abbreviated "lines" command for supervisors and monitors

       (7) Addition of support for IBM 2741 terminals and ASCII-coded terminals

       (8) Addition of interface between OSU and a national communications network

    b. Subroutines and functions:

       FN STDATA: gives the course author access to special student information (student name, date, etc.)

       FN FSTNAM: allows the author to say "Type your name" from which this function will select the first name only

       FN RMP: permits the system to keep trace of multiple users within a single sign-on number

       FN PMS: handles student management for the Independent Study Program

FN SET: gives the author extensive mathematical and algebraic manipulation

FN STRING: permits concatenation and manipulation of data strings

FN RECORD: allows the author to record a message to himself on the Student Recording File

CALC   is made up of subroutines but operates like HELP; it is transparent to the program and gives the student access to the computational ability of the computer

DEFINE   is constructed like CALC and HELP; it gives the student access to an on-line medical dictionary.

Many additional, useful functions have been added to our system. Also, a full series of remote processing programs have been written to generate various student performance and system monitoring reports.

References

Beran, R. L., 1974. Students in independent study program score higher than similar group going via traditional lecture–discussion route, *AAMC Education News* 2(2), 1, 6.

Beran, R. L., Folk, R. L., Griesen, J. V., and Camiscioni, J. S., (Eds.), 1976. *Individualizing the Study of Medicine, The Ohio State University College of Medicine Indpendent Study Program*, Westinghouse Learning Corporation, New York, 10017.

Breese, M. S., and Schimpfhauser, F., 1977. Computer-simulated clinical encounters – Part I: Development, utilization and evaluation, *Journal of The American Dietetic Association*, 70(4): 382–388.

Burson, J. L., 1975. Learning outcomes: Criteria for accountability in the training and functions of instructional programmers, *Journal of Computer-Based Instruction* 2(2): 40–47 (November).

Burson, J. L., (Ed.), 1976. *The Author's Guide to CAI*, The Ohio State University College of Medicine, Division of Computing Services, 4th ed.

Combs, B., 1973. TYMNET: A distributed network, *Datamation* 19(7): 40–44.

Division of Computing Services for Medical Education and Research, 1973a. *The User's Guide to Computer Assisted Instruction at The Ohio State University College of Medicine*, 376 West Tenth Avenue, Columbus, Ohio 43210.

Division of Computing Services for Medical Education and Research, 1973b. *Technical Documentation for the Computer Assisted Instruction Reporting System (CAIRS)*, The Ohio State University College of Medicine, 376 West Tenth Avenue, Columbus, Ohio 43210.

Division of Computing Services for Medical Education and Research, 1973c. *Additions and Modifications to IBM COURSE WRITER III*, Version 2. 1, The Ohio State University College of Medicine, 376 West Tenth Avenue, Columbus, Ohio 43210.

Gaston, G. W., 1969. Oral cancer recognition (ORALCA): A CAI program documented *in The User's Guide to Computer Assisted Instruction at The Ohio State University College of Medicine*, 376 West Tenth Avenue, Columbus, Ohio 43210.

Gaston, G. W., 1975. Critical review of the use of computer-assisted instruction in clinical encounter simulations, *Biosciences Communications* 1(3): 146–158.

Graves, G. O., Evans, L. E., Ingersoll, R. W., and Camiscioni, J. S., 1969. Need for a multiple-track system in medical education, *J. Med. Educ.* 44(5): 344–348.

Griesen, J. V., 1973a. Computer assisted independent study, *J. Clin. Comput.* 2(4): 68–76.

Griesen, J. V., 1973b. Independent Study Program at Ohio State based on "computer managed instruction," *Communications News* (November).

Harless, W. G., Drennon, G. G., Marxer, J. J., Root, J. A., Wilson, L. L., and Miller, G. E., 1973a. CASE – A natural language computer model, *Comput. Biol. Med.* 3(3): 227–246 (October).

Harless, W. G., Drennon, G. G., Marxer, J. J., Root, J. A., Wilson, L. L., and Miller, G. E., 1973b. GENESYS – A generating system for the CASE natural language model, *Comput. Biol. Med.* 3(3): 247–268 (October).

Harless, W. G., 1975. MERIT – A model for evaluation and recertification through individualized testing, *Proceedings of the Fourteenth Annual Conference on Research in Medical Education* November, 1975, Association of American Medical Colleges, Washington, D.C.

Harless, W. G., Dean, B., Farr, N., Zier, and Gamble, J., 1976. MERIT Progress Report – Ohio Field Study (October), MERIT Project Staff, Pacific Medical Center, San Francisco, California 94120.

Kamp, M., and Brigham, C., 1974. Current status of computer assisted instruction in the health sciences, *J. Med. Educ.* 49(3): 279.

Lewis, J. F., and Wooster, H., 1973. Description and utilization of the Lister Hill Center CAI Experimental Network, presented at the Association for the Development of Computer Based Instructional Systems, August, 1973, unpublished.

Mourad, L. and Forman, M., 1976. The role of CAI in nursing education at The Ohio State University, *American Journal of Nursing*, submitted.

National Library of Medicine, "Data Communication Service Contract Proposal," NO1 LM 2 47.7, National Institutes of Health, June, 1972.

Pengov, R. E., and Trzebiatowski, G. L., 1972. A Workable Policy for CAI Materials Release, Association for Development of Instructional Systems (ADCIS), August 9, 1972, Quebec, Canada.

Pengov, R. E., A modularly-designed computer assisted instruction reporting system (CAIRS), 1974. *MEDINFO 74 (Proceedings of the First World Conference on Medical Informatics, Stockholm, August 5–10, 1974)*, North-Holland Publishing Company, Amsterdam, The Netherlands.

Pengov, R. E., 1975. Philosophy for Determination of a Rate Structure for Access to Computer Assisted Instruction (CAI), Internal Document at The Ohio State University College of Medicine's Division of Computing Services for Medical Education of Medicine's Division of Computing Services for Medical Education and Research, 376 West Tenth Avenue, Columbus, Ohio 43210.

Pengov, R. E., *et al*, 1976. OSU participation in the LHNCBC Experimental Network, June 1, 1972–November 30, 1976, *Final Report to the Lister Hill National Center for Biomedical Communications*, National Library of Medicine, National Institute of Health, Public Health Service, and Department of Health, Education and Welfare, Washington, D.C.

Public Health Service, Development and Evaluation of: Computer Simulated Case Studies in Clinical Dietetics, National Institutes of Health, NIH 1D12-8H-0051901, Public Health Service, Department of Health, Education and Welfare, Washington, D.C.

Public Health Service, Proposed Planning for the Use of CAI in Meeting Information Needs of Local Community Health Practitioners, Division of Regional Medical Program 1 CO3 RM 00070 01, Public Health Service, Department of Health, Education and Welfare, Washington, D.C.

Sentieri, J. C., 1976. Simulation – Dialogue and teaching style, *Proceedings of The 1976 Winter Meeting of The Association for the Development of Computer-based Instructional Systems*, Santa Barbara, California, January 26–29, 1976.

Sutherland, J. C., 1976. NATLAN – A model for a natural language interpreter, *Proceedings of The 1976 Winter Meeting of the Association for the Development of Computer-based Instructional Systems*, Santa Barbara, California, January 26–29, 1976.

Weinberg, A. D., 1973. CAI at The Ohio State University College of Medicine (1973), *Comput. Biol. Med.* 3(3): 299–305 (October).

Wismar, B. L., and Christopher, G. R., 1969. Computerized histology, *Proceedings of the 8th Annual Conference on Research in Medical Education*, pp. 87–89, Association of American Medical Colleges, Washington, D.C.

16

Computer Applications in Self-Paced Medical Education in the Basic Sciences: The University of Washington Experience

Ralph E. Cutler and Arden W. Forrey

The Medical Student Teaching Program

The Changing Medical Curriculum

The starting point for the present medical curriculum at the University of Washington School of Medicine is generally regarded as beginning with the 1965 report of an *ad hoc* committee which contained the following paragraphs:

> A basic curriculum for medical students should provide:
> 1. Sufficient flexibility to meet the diverse demands for varied training of medical specialists (including practitioners and academicians), [and] medical scientists...
> 2. Sufficient breadth and depth of subject material to prepare the end-product to meet the many demands of our changing society.

This report was followed by the establishment of the Committee for Major Curricular Change. Three groups of faculty were enlisted to study basic science, clinical, and behavioral aspects of the medical curriculum. Their reports were combined in 1967 and included a Basic Curriculum which was approved by the faculty in 1968.

Basic Curriculum and Clerkship Pathways

Originally, the Basic Curriculum consisted of 20 courses all bearing the name Human Biology and numbered sequentially through the first six quarters. Student instruction during the first five quarters was confined to afternoons and Saturday mornings; in the sixth quarter, the Basic Hospital Clerkship was full-time. A total of 1139 contact hours were assigned during these 2 years. This represented a reduction of 44% from the former total of 2030 contact hours. The half-time Basic Curriculum schedule allowed students to elect one or more additional courses each quarter during the Basic Curriculum years.

Ralph E. Cutler and Arden W. Forrey · Department of Medicine, Harborview Medical Center, University of Washington School of Medicine, Seattle, Washington.

During the second year of the Basic Curriculum, students were requested to select one of four clinical pathways which they would pursue in the subsequent 2 years. New clinical advisers were also assigned at this time to aid students in their clinical career development elective choices. Four pathways were defined in the elective curriculum: behavioral specialists, family-medicine practitioners, medical scientists, and clinical specialists. Each pathway provided general guidelines only and each student had the ability to develop a unique program.

The Basic Curriculum has undergone continuous modification since 1968. Until 1972, the only style of presentation was that described as lecture–discussion. This referred to a format in which medical subjects were presented by lecture or small group discussions or both. This approach could be considered as typical of that used in most medical schools in this country and will not be further discussed. The curricular sequence for this program is outlined in Table I.

The Initiation of Independent Study

However, members of the entering class of 1972 were offered another way to complete their preclinical clerkship requirements via independent study. The Washington Independent Study Program (WISP) was instituted to allow greater flexibility in curricular scheduling for a diverse student body who entered with a wide variety of undergraduate education.

From an administrative viewpoint, WISP, fortuitously, offered another unexpected benefit to the medical school. At a time when classroom space was becoming scarce and scheduling was evermore restricted due to a rapidly expanding class size, the removal of 50–60 students from a classroom setting provided an unplanned boon.

WISP Educational Philosophy

The general concept of independent study and its advantages to students was well expressed by Ben Green (1971), while at MIT's Education Research Center:

> From the student's point of view, he (1) works at his own rate; (2) works when he wants to; (3) knows what he is responsible for; (4) can get personal help; (5) is not rushed past the hard parts; (6) is not held back on material he already knows; (7) gets over being afraid of tests; (8) knows where he stands; and (9) enjoys being actively involved in learning instead of just listening to lectures.

In the medical school setting, "independent" study does not apply. Rather, the term "self-paced supervised study" is a better description. Since the self-paced course combines both teacher and student control, the disjunction between teacher-centered v. student-centered instruction does not apply. The educational philosophy that is important, however, is the value given to the individual student rather than to "the class" as the unit of instruction.

Whatever the specific variations might be, we feel that the following concepts are basic to self-paced supervised study:

Table 1. The Basic Curriculum

		Hours
First Quarter (Autumn)		
Introduction to Medicine and the Curriculum		
Orientation		
Hu Bio 511	Anatomy	127
Hu Bio 512	Mechanisms in Physiology and Pharmacology	55
Hu Bio 513	Introduction to Clinical Medicine	15
Hu Bio 514	Molecular and Cellular Biology I	41
Hu Bio 515	The Ages of Man	40
		278
Second Quarter (Winter)		
Hu Bio 520	Cell and Tissue Response to Injury	62
Hu Bio 521	Natural History of Infectious Diseases and Chemotherapy.	72
Hu Bio 522	Introduction to Clinical Medicine	36
Hu Bio 523	Systems of Human Behavior I	30
Hu Bio 524	Molecular and Cellular Biology II	26
		226
Third Quarter (Spring)		
Hu Bio 530	Epidemiology	20
Hu Bio 531	Head, Neck, Ear, Nose, and Throat	40
Hu Bio 532	Nervous System	80
Hu Bio 533	Medicine, Health, and Society	20
Hu Bio 534	Endocrine System	30
Hu Bio 535	Introduction to Clinical Medicine	30
		220
Fourth Quarter (Autumn)		
Hu Bio 540	Cardiovascular Respiratory System	110
Hu Bio 541	Gastrointestinal System	62
Hu Bio 542	Introduction to Clinical Medicine	36
Hu Bio 543	Medicine, Health, and Society	22
Hu Bio 549	Genetics	10
		240
Fifth Quarter (Winter)		
Hu Bio 550	Introduction to Clinical Medicine	80
Hu Bio 551	Skin System	20
Hu Bio 552	Reproductive Biology	64
Hu Bio 553	Musculoskeletal System	56
		220
Sixth Quarter (Spring)		
Hu Bio 560	Introduction to Clinical Medicine	100
Hu Bio 561	Hematology	46
Hu Bio 562	Urinary System	62
Hu Bio 563	Systems of Human Behavior II	30
		238

1. Teachers, along with books, slides and audiovisual aids, function through the active participation of the learner. Instruction is successful when it systematically directs the student through participation activities.
2. Self-direction and responsibility are learned. They are acquired from experience – from being given opportunities to be self-directing and responsible.
3. Learning is promoted when the required outcomes of instruction are carefully explained and understood.
4. Student motivation is increased when the importance and relevance of subject content are made clear.
5. Ability to profit from instruction is impaired by inadequate preparation for the learning task. Specifying prerequisites increases chances for success.
6. Motivation increases to the degree that the learner perceives himself in control of the learning situation. Independent choice of instructional activities along with self-pacing contribute to a sense of control.
7. Learning styles vary. Basic styles are acquired at an early age and are not subject to fundamental change. A choice of instructional modes varying in their sensory and interactive dimensions allows for individual preference.
8. Learning is enhanced by small logical step presentation of instructional paths.
9. Practice of newly acquired skills and opportunities to use new knowledge are important to learning success.
10. Frequent self-testing with immediate feedback increases the effectiveness of instruction.

The Establishment of WISP

The Pilot Medical School as a Model

WISP is an outgrowth of the Pilot Medical School (Folk *et al.*, 1975; Beran and Folk, 1975; Griesen and Camiscioni, 1975) program begun in 1969 at the Ohio State University Medical School. The Pilot Medical School (PMS) was a research project investigating the effectiveness and efficiency of utilizing selected concepts of independent study in medical education. The PMS was formed as a result of a 3-year grant from the U.S. Public Health Service, Division of Physician Manpower. The first class of 32 students began their medical studies under this "independent study" curriculum in July of 1970. The PMS curriculum was divided into five parts. Part I was an Introduction to Medicine and placed emphasis on the processes common to all body systems. Part II was entitled Normal Man and was organized into seven body systems. Part III was entitled Introduction to Pathophysiology and Therapeutics. This included the topics of general pathology, immunology, biostatistics, preventive medicine concepts, drug mechanisms, and microbiology. Part IV was entitled Pathophysiology of Man and covered diseases of organ systems. Part V was entitled Physical Diagnosis and began in the second week of medical school. This was one part of the curriculum that maintained a definite schedule and was conducted on an individual or small group basis throughout the program.

An integral part of the program was use of a computer-based tutorial evaluation system (TES). The PMS did not employ computer-assisted instruction in a primary instructional role. The students' use of the computer was for self-evaluation. Exercises were designed to provide the student an opportunity to gauge his progress and determine his success in satisfying the objectives of the study unit.

A TES program was available for each instructional unit. These exercises were designed by the faculty to test comprehension of the instructional objectives for each module. Items in the exercise included constructed response, true-false, multiple choice, matching, or ranking questions. The computer presents the student with a question and then immediately evaluates his response. Correct answers receive a reinforcing type of feedback, while wrong ones trigger corrective feedback and another chance to respond to the question. The computer will also respond to unanticipated answers and attempt to coach the student through a series of statements to the correct answer. The computer programs have also been designed to indicate to a student when he is not doing well. In this instance, the computer will alert him to his deficiencies with study prescriptions. Study prescriptions may appear as an additional study assignment, a review of previously suggested material, or a simple statement suggesting a faculty conference. At the completion of his TES exercise, the student keeps the computer printout for study, reference, or review.

Curricular logistics are as follows. When a student begins an instructional unit, he examines the educational objectives for that module and begins study of the learning resources provided or any other resources he desires to pursue to meet the stated objectives. He may wish to consult with a faculty member during his study to clarify certain points he does not understand. When a student feels he has mastered the educational objectives, he signs on the computer terminal for the self-evaluation exercise. His own judgment of his performance determines whether he reviews any deficiencies, seeks out faculty for assistance, or proceeds to the module posttest.

By 1972, the PMS faculty, based on evaluation of their students, was convinced that student academic achievement was similar to that in the regular curriculum and was interested in disseminating this educational approach to other institutions. At this point, ten faculty members from the University of Washington (UW) School of Medicine visited and evaluated PMS and recommended that UW compete for the opportunity of being selected as the second school. This suggestion was accepted by both UW and OSU. Faculty were rapidly recruited, largely on the basis of expressed interest. By using, in the initial year, much of the OSU material, the WISP curriculum was instituted in a period of 4 months for the entering class of 1972. This rapid start-up could not have been accomplished without the encouragement of the PMS faculty and the free use of the materials which they had generated.

The Role of the NLM Network

Another fortuitous circumstance aided in the transplantation of independent study to the University of Washington, namely, the availability of the telecommunication network subsidized by the National Library of Medicine. At that time, the Lister Hill National Center for Biomedical Communication (LHNCBC) had established, through a commercial timesharing vendor, a program whereby selected medical schools could access via local telephone lines the computer-based programs which were available at the University of Illinois, Ohio State University, and Massachusetts General Hospital. The convenience of a communication node in Seattle made access to the computer-based materials (TES) at OSU readily available as WISP was begun.

Faculty Acceptance of External Courseware

Although the educational material from OSU was initially accepted by the faculty and students as a necessity to initiate WISP, dissatisfactions were quickly noted because PMS goals, objectives, and learning resources often differed from those of the UW faculty. This quickly resulted in a metamorphosis of most of the OSU module guidelines and a desire to modify the computer-based material to bring it in line with the new module objectives. The present WISP curriculum (Table I) is similar to the Basic Curriculum except that modules may be taken in any sequence the student desires. Few prerequisites are present except that first year modules dealing with normal biology should precede those dealing with pathophysiology.

OSU agreed with our modification of computer-based material and allowed us to reprogram on their system a computer-assisted evaluation (CAE) which more appropriately met student needs for self-assessment. Currently, less than 50% of the original TES material from OSU is used in WISP and, even then, in a modified format. It is well to point out at this time, based on our experience, that during the next few years, until the strategies and techniques of using computers in instructional settings become established, access by "have-not" institutions to resources at "have" institutions will be an important way of providing the "have-nots" with the resources by which they are able to demonstrate the technical ability and instructional importance of this kind of instruction by allowing the creation of instructional materials at off-campus sites. Moreover, access by all schools belonging to such a network to different kinds of software resources at other institutions is an important way of testing the effect of different approaches to instruction before heavy investment is attempted. The programmed instructional material used by WISP was largely created during the initial 2 years of the program, starting from the work of the PMS program and remodeling it to meet the structure and needs of WISP. It is important to recognize that this restructuring will take place at any acquiring institution because there will be, rightly so, different curricular objectives upon which any programmed instruction is based.

The rewriting of CAE material began almost at once and in many instances, almost total revision of the TES material was necessary. The revision consumed a considerable amount of faculty time and this effort is a source of a large part of the resistance of basic science faculty to expand the use of this mode of instruction. It is possible that more extensive commitment by the school to the use of this instructional medium and the availability of a greater variety of computer support facilities and services available to the faculty may displace a major portion of this resistance but it must be accepted that a certain level of objection due to unfamiliarity with the best goals, uses, and evaluations of this medium will remain for some time. This is true of any new technologic advance.

Transfer of WISP Computer Courseware to Local Facilities

In late 1974, it was clear that if a reliable computing service were available on our campus, the quality of interactive instructional computing could be raised and costs could be reduced. This awareness was given additional emphasis by the termination of the network support of the National Library of Medicine in May, 1975. Fortunately, a local computing service became available through the Cardiovascular Research and Training Center which purchased, with the help of the School of Medicine, a Digital Equipment Corporation (DEC) system-1060 computer. This equipment possessed adequate machine resources including a number of high-level programming languages which included FORTRAN, BASIC, ALGOL, SAIL, SIMULA-67, SNOBOL, and LISP, as well as a large number of utility packages. The machine was configured initially with 196K words of core and 120M characters of disk storage with 10 dial-up ports. These resources were more than adequate to initiate the level of services needed to support WISP.

The next choice we needed to make was the programming language which we would use for development of WISP courseware. COURSEWRITER III (CWIII) was the language in which the WISP courseware was written on the OSU computer. Neither this language nor MUMPS, the language used for the MGH based programs, were available on the DEC-10 system. Thus, the direct transport of computer courseware to the local equipment could not easily and directly be accomplished.

After consideration of the problem, we decided not to implement CWIII on the DEC-10 system. Although CWIII was the first major language developed for computer-assisted instruction and a large amount of courseware had been written in that language, it appeared to have a number of shortcomings which were not presented in other CAI languages available today. In CWIII, only very simple branching instructions are possible, and these can make use of only the limited number of switches and counters provided by the system. A minor degree of logical complexity results in a great deal of program complexity, and consequently leads to problems in debugging, updating and documentation, which in turn requires the investment of increased amounts of expensive human time. Perhaps the greatest weakness of CWIII results from the philosophy of its design, namely that *implicit* actions are good. As a consequence, most of the commands available contain implicit assumptions and perform automatic and sometimes invisible actions; for example, to assist in specifying that a question is to be asked until correctly answered, and then the next question in line is to be asked. This is ideal for simple programmed-learning type materials, but obstructs the programming of more complex questions, as the programmer must continually determine what happens behind the scenes and turn off automatic features which are supposedly there for convenience. Indeed, the design of CWIII obstructs even the conception of certain more sophisticated question structures.

Our decision was to acquire and use the PILOT (Programmed Inquiry, Learning, Or Teaching) language. PILOT has a number of features to recommend it. It is in the mainstream of CAI work, making previous PILOT work available and transfer of subsequent work possible. It is *explicit*, so that it does exactly as told and nothing more, and is consequently largely self-documenting. Also, it is orthogonal, which is to say that there are no *ad hoc* cases — if a construct is valid, it is valid everywhere. PILOT is simple to learn and to read, concise, arbitrarily flexible, and ideally suited to programming anything involving large amounts of interactive dialogue with the user.

Based on our observation of the experience at Western Washington State College (WWSC), we decided to convert CWIII material which we had programmed on the OSU computer to PILOT via a machine translator. This allowed us to automatically translate about 90% of any CWIII program. The remainder was easily and rapidly completed by hand. This technique has allowed us to shift our computer-based material from the OSU system with minimum expense and maximum speed. In general, a CAE program can be converted, debugged, and run within a single working week.

Although the machine translator approach worked well for CWIII material, it did not solve the problem of transporting the MUMPS programs which we were using in WISP. Few MGH programs were used directly in WISP, but we did see the potential for such programs in clinical clerkship and continuing medical education. Therefore, we also decided to develop the capability of using MUMPS on the DEC-10 system. This decision to utilize MUMPS was also heavily influenced by the success of the language-standardization effort jointly sponsored by the Health Resources Administration/HEW and the National Bureau of Standards. Had a standard dialect of MUMPS not been available, the potential availability to share useful instructional materials and application programs would not have been present. The University of Washington has paid greater costs in this software development than subsequent DEC-10 systems users because of its role as an initiator of this approach. In the near future, however, the availability of many application programs from the MUMPS Users Group library and the sharing of instructional programs through the National Library of Medicine should make the development of programs of instruction which are tailored to the needs of the user institutions a relatively more straight-forward process and much less costly.

The Computer in WISP

General Areas of Application

In WISP, the computer has been found useful in six areas: (1) physiological model simulation, (2) CAE for student self-assessment, (3) learning resource management, (4) student progress monitoring, (5) computer-assisted test construction (CATC), and (6) module posttesting. The first four areas are currently functional while the latter two are in developmental stages.

Physiological Model Simulations

The current curriculum of most medical schools contains few laboratory experiences. This has occurred for a variety of reasons related to cost as well as teaching relevance and effectiveness. The computer does offer, for certain disciplines such as physiology, a cost-effective way of demonstrating and reinforcing concepts via model simulations. This has been effectively applied by Harold Modell in WISP through a computer model which he and his colleagues have developed to exercise concepts in the field of respiratory mechanics and ventilation. The computer model is used in a highly structured teaching format but does allow ample student opportunity to manipulate different parameters and note the resultant effect on patient gas exchange and acid—base parameters. In addition, the ready availability and endless way in which the model can be manipulated allows adequate opportunity for "discovery" learning in totally unexpected ways and areas.

Student reaction to this computer application has been extremely enthusiastic. The faculty, in turn, are convinced of its usefulness in fulfilling their teaching objectives. Other models in the area of fluid—electrolyte balance and pharmacokinetics are currently being developed for curricular trial.

Computer-Assisted Evaluations

In self-paced study, students lack the frequent interaction with peers and faculty that is forced upon them by the nature of a time-oriented lecture—discussion curriculum. They feel the need, therefore, to test their knowledge and problem-solving skills prior to modular posttesting. The CAE offers a way for students to achieve self-assessement to evaluate if they are learning what they are supposed to learn as they proceed through each module. Some faculty have disdain for computer-based material and have elected to use paper and pencil media. In our experience, this is satisfactory for many needs but does not have the rich feedback, branching, and diagnostic capability of a good CAE.

What are the characteristics of a "good" CAE in the student's opinion (see Appendix)? First, it must test all the concepts and skills the faculty tutor feels are important. Second, the feedback from all questions should expand knowledge and be reinforcing rather than be just a simple negative or affirmative answer. Thus, such a CAE is a long and arduous exercise covering all significant modular objectives. However, in all student questionnaires, a shortening of CAE material has been disdained. Third, the objectives stressed by the CAE must exactly replicate that found in both the module guidelines and module posttest. Total congruity should exist and the module posttest should offer no conceptual surprises. Some instructors, in fact, have chosen to use some of the CAE material on their module posttest.

Learning Resource Management

The principal source for conveying factual material in WISP is the printed page (textbooks, syllabi, reprints, etc.). In addition, because student learning styles are diverse and not easily changed, multiple other media are used such as audiotapes, slides or microfiche with text, videotapes, CAI programs, etc. Keeping track of this material, which is constantly changing as modules are modified, was a major problem until a computer-based management system was developed. This system allows the WISP administrative secretary to interactively retrieve, add, modify, or delete any item desired in a computer file via a terminal. Because most material is stored in the reserve section of the Health Sciences Library, the necessary library identification is included in the file with each item. The system is set up in such a way that items can be retrieved by any of its identifiers (title, call number, module, authors, etc.). This technique has enabled the easy production of a current list of learning resources for any or all modules for a variety of purposes and has enabled us to keep orderly material which was previously in a chaotic state.

Student Progress Monitoring

In WISP, students finish modules in varying sequences and at different times. This makes evaluation of student progress difficult. A pragmatic solution has been to record satisfactory completion of the module posttest as the time of module completion. Currently, a record of all WISP students is kept in a large computer-based table. Each student is alphabetically ranked by last name in a group with other WISP students who entered medical school in the same year. This forms the left-hand column of the table. Along the top of the table is listed each WISP module. When a module is satisfactorily completed, a number is registered indicating the school quarter in which the completion occurred. Unsatisfactory performance is indicated by other symbols, and so forth. Being computer-based, the table is easily updated and multiple copies are generated as required on a monthly basis for advisers and other faculty members.

Currently, the system is kept updated by secretarial interaction via computer terminal. It is hoped, as computer-based module posttests are developed, that these will be graded and automatically update the student progress file, thus obviating the need for secretarial input.

Module Posttesting and CATC

Although some independent study programs have chosen to deemphasize student testing, the WISP approach has been to apply the concepts of mastery teaching (Block and Anderson, 1975) and allow frequent testing of modular contents. In this system, modules are divided into sub-units which contain about one week's worth of student work. Master exams are then given at the completion of one or more sub-units. In most cases, a comprehensive module posttest also is given, covering the entire module contents.

Two problems are inherent in a self-paced program which uses frequent testing: (1) availability of adequate testing items, and (2) security of tests. The first problem is not difficult to solve if the instructional objectives for each module have been delineated and two or more test items are developed for each objective. However, as the number of test items increases, accessibility and review of all items at the time of test construction becomes more arduous and time-consuming. In order to solve this dilemma, we are evaluating several types of software for CATC. Although current experience in WISP is small, CATC has already demonstrated its efficiency in preparing hard-copy parallel-forms of a test, thus allowing rapid preparation of tests using random or highly selected items from the test-item data bank.

CATC should also help us solve the problem of security. Although there has been little evidence of abuse of the student honor system in WISP, the faculty continues to be concerned. If the test-item data bank is large enough, CATC could allow an individualized test for each student. At the worst, two or more parallel-forms of a test could be generated, which should enhance security.

As a further enhancement of CATC, we are considering on-line testing. This has already been carried out successfully in some CAI courses. It does allow security if (1) several parallel-forms of the test are available, or (2) each test is individualized by random selections from the test-item data bank. Additionally, it allows automated scoring of a tutor—student conference to discuss the test, and (2) storing of all student responses for test-item analysis at some future date.

Projections Based on the WISP Experience

Acceptance of Computers in Medical Instruction

Objective measurement of the effectiveness of computer tools in instruction, particularly higher education, is sadly lacking. The existing measures of their acceptance in instructional settings are gross ones, such as enrollment figures or brief attitude surveys. At the University of Washington Medical School, students in WISP are enthusiastic about self-assessment examinations and consider them a necessary component of independent study. However, they are not totally committed to the concept that these exercises need to be computer-based. However, as programs have become more sophisticated, this media has been increasingly accepted and praised by our students. The early criticism of computer-based material was mainly based upon frequent failure of the telecommunication or computer systems. As these problems have resolved, student attitudes have improved. On the other hand, faculty attitudes have not shown any unusual swing toward the use of computer-based instruction. In large part, this stems from their lack of experience with this instructional medium and unwillingness to allocate sufficient priority in their teaching to develop material for this educational tool. It is hoped that faculty attitudes will change as computer tools become more reliable, easier to use, and are more widely available. However, it is interesting to note that Hoffer (1975) does not expect this change to occur rapidly. The situation at our medical school may be different, however, in that there has been and will continue to be a major administrative commitment to an educational program which will eventually pervade all aspects of medical training, including continuing medical education. It is expected that, at some point, a threshold reaction of both student and faculty acceptance of computer methods will occur which will make its presence as an appropriate work tool in both basic science and clinical medicine an accepted fact. At that point, a self-sustaining steady growth in its use can be expected to occur undramatically.

Measurement of the factors relating to faculty acceptance and their views regarding the mode and direction of computer use will, hopefully, be forthcoming, but are not yet present. Additionally, it has been difficult, perhaps impossible, to obtain agreed-upon criteria for judging the various factors which modify the medical education process. Certainly, agreement upon the criteria to be used in evaluating the effect of various educational media will be required before reliable statistics can be obtained which will enhance either the acceptance or the effectiveness of computers in medical education.

Transportability

In recent years, it has become clear that in order to control the cost of computer-based instruction in higher education, the ability to transport quality instructional materials among a variety of users will be very important. Program movement can only be considered if standard nomenclature and classification schemes for medical information and standard programming, and author/student languages for instructional computing are developed and are commonly understood. Thus, achievement of our goals will be directly dependent upon the use of commonly adopted conventions. The process of adoption of common conventions in all fields, not only in instructional computing, can potentially involve larger costs than can be borne by any one user for the development of the needed systems and instructional and testing tools required to provide services to a major fraction of a medical class. Partial control of these costs may, therefore, be possible by sharing the instructional resources themselves, but we also recognize that this step will only be possible if standard languages and their generalized software support systems are available to many users.

To demonstrate the practicality of transportability of instructional segments, we are, as noted above, not only importing instructional programs, but are also planning that all of our new instructional modules will be written in transportable standard languages. Moreover, we will be building our catalogs of instructional materials, both print and non print (Spedick *et al.*, 1975), along general and extensible lines, using transportable software. Specifically, we are importing MUMPS programs, either in the standard dialect or by translating the acquired programs into that dialect for use in all phases of teaching. We have, in addition, translated our existing CWIII instructional modules into the PILOT instructional language, as noted above, so that they are now, or will shortly be, compatible with *ad hoc* standard conventions now being encouraged by the National Library of Medicine for that language. These PILOT programs will also be runnable on Standard MUMPS machines using PILOT/MUMPS software that we have created. We feel that these steps will enhance the effectiveness and will decrease the costs of sharing modules with others or developing our own instructional modules.

Appendix. WISP CAE Evaluation

Introduction. During the winter quarter of 1976, a questionnaire survey about CAE was conducted among the current WISP students. About 60% of those polled responded. Many comments were made, but only a small representative sample are included.

1. Should a self-assessment exam, whether oral, pencil and paper, or computer-assisted, be available for all modules?

Definitely Yes	1	2	3	4	5	Definitely Not
Frequency	29	2	—	1	1	
Percent	88	6	—	3	3	

$$X = 1.27 \quad SD = .88$$

Comments:

I find practice tests very helpful in focusing on my areas of weakness. A good way to know what to study when you feel you're almost ready for the final exam.

Without a testing situation, self-evaluation cannot be meaningful.

Self-assessment, along with definite learning objectives, makes learning more fun and more efficient, especially in a professional school.

Allow me to evaluate his [instructor's] organization and sense of importance of material in a way that is an alternative to lectures.

2. If a self-test is available, should it be computerized?

Definitely Yes	1	2	3	4	5	Definitely Not
Frequency	—	3	17	10	3	
Percent	—	9	52	30	9	

$$X = 3.39 \quad SD = .79$$

Comments:

CAE has the advantage of multiple feedback for answers that you just can't get otherwise.

Sometimes beneficial to have computer feedback loops and sometimes not.

3. When CAEs are available for modules, how often do you use them?

Never	1	2	3	4	5	Always
Frequency	1	2	5	14	11	
Percent	3	6	15	42	33	

$$X = 3.97 \quad SD = 1.02$$

4. When you do use a CAE, what percent of the time do you use it as a:

a. Pretest

	0–20	21–40	41–60	61–80	81–100	42% of respon-
Frequency	2	1	2	2	7	dents utilized
Percent	14	7	14	14	51	the CAE in this

$$X = 69.64 \quad SD = 34.92 \qquad \text{manner}$$

b. Intermediate progress check

	0–20	21–40	41–60	61–80	81–100	24% of respon-
Frequency	3	2	2	1	—	dents utilized
Percent	38	25	25	12	—	the CAE in this

$$X = 35.62 \quad SD = 21.62 \qquad \text{manner}$$

c. Late progress check

	0–20	21–40	41–60	61–80	81–100	70% of the res-
Frequency	4	3	6	5	5	pondents utilized
Percent	17	13	26	22	22	the CAE in this

$$X = 56.6 \quad SD = 29.88 \qquad \text{manner}$$

d. Study guide

	0–20	21–40	41–60	61–80	81–100	45% of the res-
Frequency	4	4	2	3	2	pondents utilized
Percent	27	27	13	20	13	the CAE in this

$$X = 47.13 \quad SD = 30.70 \qquad \text{manner}$$

Please explain your distribution:

I do the CAE when I feel I have a fair idea of what's going on in the module. The CAE helps me know if I do or if I don't, and what areas I need to study more.

Depends on the subject; often I want to have an idea of the kinds of things I'll have to learn. Sometimes as outright pretest, but usually after I've looked over the syllabus and have started to take in some of the material. A good CAE at this level may turn into a study guide.

The module author should specify his purpose for the CAE – whether to test mastery of the specified objectives – or to present new information. I mostly use it to get some idea of what is expected for the posttest regarding depth.

5. Should there be any "rule" (or strong suggestion) on the use of CAEs? If yes,

please elaborate.

	Yes	No
Frequency	3	26
Percent	10	90

It's silly to waste computer time on CAEs that give little or no feedback. The advantage of the computer is in the feedback.

Everyone's study and learning needs vary. No rules, please.

6. What could be done to make CAEs a better evaluation instrument?

Supply useful feedback with all CAEs.

The more closely it fits the module material and format, the better. No CAE can make up for a poorly organized module, though.

More feedback loops.

(1) Always print out percentages at the end of the exam. (2) Require CAEs of all modules. (3) Have CAEs reflect course objectives – some don't.

References

Beran, R. L., and Folk, R. L., 1975. Part II. The curriculum, *in Individualizing the Study of Medicine: The Ohio State University College of Medicine 1975, Independent Study Program*, Westinghouse Learning Corp., New York.

Block, J. H., and Anderson, L. W., 1975. *Mastery Learning in Classroom Instruction*, MacMillan, New York.

Folk, R. L., Griesen, J. V., and Beran, R. L., 1975. Part I. Learning system, *in Individualizing the Study of Medicine: The Ohio State University College of Medicine 1975, Independent Study Program*, Westinghouse Learning Corp., New York.

Green, B. A., 1971. *Mastery Learning: Theory and Practice*, Holt, Rinehart and Winston, New York.

Griesen, J. V., and Camiscioni, J., 1975. Part III. The outcome, *in Individualizing the Study of Medicine: The Ohio State University College of Medicine 1975, Independent Study Program*, Westinghouse Learning Corp., New York.

Hoffer, E. P., 1975. CAI: While it has many advantages, let's not forget that it has problems, *AAMC News* 13(2): 6.

Spedick, M., Ingalls, E., and Walters, R., 1975. A Curriculum-Oriented Catalog of Multimedia Learning Resources, *Proceedings of the MUMPS Users' Group Meeting 1975*, p. 163, MUMPS Users' Group, St. Louis.

17

A Tutorial System

Jane B. Hirsch, Wilbur D. Hagamen, Suzanne S. Murphy, and John C. Weber

Introduction

A Tutorial System (ATS) was developed by members of the Anatomy Department of Cornell University Medical College (CUMC). The system was designed to enable teachers to converse with students through a natural language computer-mediated dialogue (tutorial). ATS consists of two major parts, an author-interrogation program (used in preparing tutorials) and a tutorial supervisory program (used during the student—teacher dialogue). ATS, in turn, is based on the computer language APL.

Over the 7 years of its development, ATS has progressed to an integrated program that includes 65 tutorials used at CUMC in Gross Anatomy, Microscopic Anatomy, Neuroscience, Biochemistry, and Pharmacology. The tutorials are used by first- and second-year medical students.

The ATS author-interrogation program allows a teacher to write tutorials without any computer programming knowledge. Conversational in approach, it asks the author what he wants to do, states some of his options for him, prevents him from making certain errors, and leads him through a logical authoring sequence. The authoring program includes interactive editing, computer-drawn flowcharts of branching logic, automatic, detailed, easily understandable documentation, and many other aids.

The ATS tutorial supervisory program has the syntactic abilities to understand when a student is asking rather than answering a question, to determine the referents of pronouns used by students, and to correct student misspellings or typographical errors. It also handles partially correct answers and answers that combine the distinctive features of right and wrong answers. This artificial intelligence is part of the tutorial supervisory program and therefore operates independently of the author, who needs only to be concerned with course content.

In addition to the two major parts of ATS, the system also includes programs for analysis of student performance and attitudinal data. These analyses include summaries of the data from on-line student evaluations of the tutorials and summaries of all student responses.

Jane B. Hirsch, Wilbur D. Hagemen, Suzanne S. Murphy, and John C. Weber · Department of Anatomy, Laboratory of Computer Science, Cornell University Medical College, Ithaca, New York.

Development

Changing Attitudes

ATS has followed a classic pattern of CAI (computer-assisted instruction) development. It was first accepted by the students, then by the administration, and last by the faculty.

The development of ATS started in 1967, funded by a grant from the National Fund for Medical Education. In the middle years of its development, it was supported by being paired with other, cost-justified computer applications, such as accounting and budget programs for CUMC. Terminals were available for ATS development when not in use for other applications. In 1975, the College administration decided to support terminals specifically for use by students taking ATS tutorials.

Student use of ATS varies widely but has increased over the years to 1585 sessions during the 1974–75 school year, when 40 tutorials were offered in three subjects: Gross Anatomy, Microscopic Anatomy, and Neuroscience. During that year, 90% of the first-year class of 102 students tried at least one tutorial. Two-thirds of the class were frequent users of computer tutorials.

Faculty acceptance of ATS, or, indeed, of any form of computer-assisted instruction, has developed more slowly. Teachers as well as students need to be motivated. Students can look to CAI as an aid to learning. For teachers, on the other hand, it may be seen as merely a demand on their time, with few apparent benefits. Faculty acceptance is increasing, however, as CAI begins to prove its value as a means of increasing teaching productivity and as administrators offer greater encouragement and support.

Course Development

In order to use a teacher's time in the most efficient way, CUMC has developed a team approach to authoring (writing) computer tutorials. Medical students, supported by fellowships, write tutorials during the summer. The student-author works with a faculty member as content advisor and with a member of the ATS staff as technical adviser. This system has proven an effective method for CUMC. Some of the tutorials written by student-authors have been among the tutorials best received by the class, probably because of the well-known principle that someone who has just learned a topic is very sensitive to the difficulties encountered. For the student-authors, this method provides the opportunity to learn a topic in depth from an expert on that topic. For the faculty member, there is the opportunity to implement additional educational materials in their courses.

Simulating Human Discourse

ATS is designed to create both the illusion and the pedagogical utility of conversing, via a terminal, with one's own individual tutor. For this desired result to occur, not only must the teacher's factual knowledge be put into the computer but his reasoning and conversational abilities as well.

ATS facilitates the inputting of factual material. However, this is the easiest part of the task. If one accepts the premise that the output should be conditioned by the student's input, other problems arise.

This premise presupposes that the computer understands what the student is saying. This is one reason that so many computer-mediated "tutorials" have a multiple choice format. If a student is restricted to choosing among A, B, or C, analyzing his answer is quite easy. On the other hand, if one wants to permit a truly free-format discussion, many fairly complex decisions must be made. Fortunately, most of these decisions are common to every tutorial. For this reason, ATS has a general-purpose program to supervise every tutorial. Built into this program is a knowledge of the basic rules of human discourse so the author does not have to worry about them. Present and future work on ATS is directed toward the expansion of these artificial verbal intelligence features of the tutorial supervisory program.

In discussing ATS we shall look at it in its normal environment – the teaching of medical students. To illustrate it with trivial examples would fail to show many of the powerful and intelligent features that are the substance of ATS.

For this reason we shall now examine ATS in student mode and use excerpts from actual medical tutorials. (Although you will not actually be interacting with these tutorials, perhaps you will be in a better position to evaluate whether or not they could teach, and the importance of the techniques employed, by struggling through examples that may be new to some of you.)

In the following excerpts from terminal sessions, everything the computer prints is indented two spaces except for the "□:." This symbol signals the student that it is his turn to type. What the student types is not indented.

Pronouns in Student Questions

If what we produce deserves the name of a tutorial discussion, then the students should be able to interrupt the conversation at any point to ask questions of their own.

    A CHILD HAS A CONGENITAL WEAKNESS OF HIS RIGHT SUPERIOR RECTUS.
    HOW WOULD YOU TEST THIS MUSCLE?

□:

WHAT IS CONGENITAL
    I DON'T UNDERSTAND WHAT YOU WANT TO KNOW ABOUT CONGENITAL.

□:

WHAT DOES IT MEAN?
    CONGENITAL MEANS PRESENT FROM BIRTH.

    NOW WE'LL RETURN TO WHERE YOU WERE BEFORE ASKING YOUR
    QUESTION.

How did the program know the student was asking a question, rather than answering one, since the input did not contain a question mark? It simply looks for the presence of certain interrogative pronouns or verbs beginning the response. This is the way we recognize questions in ordinary conversation. We also have the ability to turn even declarative sentences into questions in oral conversation by the inflection of our voice. Similarly in ATS any response is converted to a question if it ends in a "?."

When the student asked, "What is congenital?," it was fairly clear that he meant, "What is the meaning of congenital?" However, the word "is" can imply other relations. Thus, the program interpreted the question as being ambiguous and gave the student an opportunity to make it more explicit. Sometimes students are too verbose or are really asking more than one question, in which case the program will again try to keep the student in normal conversation until he can make his question specific enough to be answered.

Perhaps of more interest is the use of the word "it" in the second question the student asked. How did the program know that the pronoun referred to "congenital"? It did so by a means similar to that employed by you or me, simply keeping track of the subject under discussion. This meaning of the indefinite pronoun resulted from the fact that the student had just used the word in his previous question. The supervisory program inferred this reference with no effort, or even awareness, on the part of the author of the tutorial.

Reasoning Through the Answer to a Question

       A CHILD HAS A CONGENITAL WEAKNESS OF HIS RIGHT SUPERIOR RECTUS.
       HOW WOULD YOU TEST THIS MUSCLE?
□:

HOW WOULD YOU TEST IT
       WHAT IS THE ACTION OF THE SUPERIOR RECTUS?
□:

There are two main points to notice here. The student again used the word "it," but here it clearly was not interpreted as meaning "congenital." Rather, the program assumed that it meant "superior rectus," since that is the subject currently under discussion, and it is quite likely that you, the reader, would have interpreted it the same way.

This time the student was not given a direct answer to his question. Rather, he was asked another question in return. We consider his question to be a conceptual one and shall try to show him how to reason through the answer to his own problem. This is an attempt to give the student a new way of looking at problems so that, if he is ever faced with a similar question, he should be able to think it through.

A fact that should be stressed is that the program, not the author, decided which question or series of questions the student should be asked to show him the most logical approach to his problem. To avoid misunderstanding, we will elaborate upon this important point.

The program does not generate questions. It can do no more than utilize the information the author has provided, since it has no other source of knowledge about the muscles of the eye. How then does it make this selection? Again the answer, or at least the way we implemented it in ATS, is probably the way you would make the selection. We assume that when a student asks us a question, this is comparable in many cases to our having asked him that question and his replying with the equivalent of "I don't know." For every question the author enters into the program, he is required to provide an "I don't know" type branch, or what we call the UN branch, where UN stands for unanticipated answer.

Thus, all the program does is search through the list of questions that the author provided until it finds the closest match, and then it selects the UN branch to present to the student. In this case, it did not have to look very far, since he was essentially repeating, (if you consider the evaluation of "it") the question he had just been asked. However, when necessary it will search every question in the tutorial. If the tutorial supervisor finds no match, it will tell the student it does not understand his question. Whether or not the program performed its job well can be evaluated in the following sequence. When the program thinks it has either extracted from the student, or given to the student, enough information for him to answer his question, it will return him to the question he avoided answering.

> A CHILD HAS A CONGENITAL WEAKNESS OF HIS RIGHT SUPERIOR RECTUS. HOW WOULD YOU TEST THIS MUSCLE?

□:

IT MOVES THE EYE SUPERIORLY, MEDIALLY, AND ROTATES IT INTERNALLY
> IF THE PATIENT IS LOOKING STRAIGHT AHEAD (FIG. 1A), CONTRACTION OF THE SUPERIOR RECTUS WILL ADDUCT THE EYE (FIG. 2A), MAKE IT LOOK SUPERIORLY (FIG. 3A), AND ROTATE IT INTERNALLY (FIG. 4A).

For those readers who may not be familiar with the muscles of the eye, the student here gives a typical textbook answer. Medical students are very adept at memorizing the printed word. Just how much good it may have done him in this case, you may judge for yourself, but his answer is correct. The program merely paraphrases his correct answer and suggests by implication that "adduct" is synonymous with "look medially."

> ASSUME THAT HE STARTS WITH HIS EYE ADDUCTED, WHAT IS THE ACTION OF THE SUPERIOR RECTUS (FIG. 5A)?

□:

INTERNAL ROTATION
> IT CAUSES PURE ROTATION, SINCE THE LONG AXIS OF THE EYEBALL AND THE LONG AXIS OF THE MUSCLE ARE AT RIGHT ANGLES.

> ASSUME THAT HE STARTS WITH HIS EYE ABDUCTED, WHAT IS THE ACTION OF THE SUPERIOR RECTUS (FIG. 6A)?

□:

MOVES THE EYE SUPERIORLY
> IT CAUSES THE EYE TO LOOK SUPERIORLY, SINCE THE LONG AXIS OF THE MUSCLE AND THE LONG AXIS OF THE EYEBALL ARE PARALLEL.

Here the student is asked two more questions which the author considered important for a student who had missed the initial question. In this example he answered them both correctly. If he had missed either one of them, the reasoning behind each of his answers would have been explored.

> HOW WOULD YOU TEST THE SUPERIOR RECTUS, I.E., WHAT WOULD YOU ASK THE PATIENT TO DO?

□:

ASK HIM TO LOOK MEDIALLY, INFERIORLY AND ROTATE HIS EYE INTERNALLY.

Here is the crux of the student's misunderstanding. He is parroting back the well-learned textbook description. Rotation of the eye means torsion around the long axis of the eyeball. It is not under a person's voluntary control.

> TO TEST ANY OF THE EXTRINSIC MUSCLES OF THE EYE YOU FIRST ASK THE PATIENT TO LOOK IN A DIRECTION THAT WILL MAKE THE LONG AXIS OF THE EYEBALL PARALLEL TO THE LONG AXIS OF THE MUSCLE. WHAT DIREC- TION WOULD THIS BE FOR THE SUPERIOR RECTUS (FIG. 1A)?

□:

LATERALLY
> YOU WOULD GET HIM TO ABDUCT THAT EYE OR MOVE IT IN A LATERAL DIRECTION (FIG. 6A)?

□:

SUPERIORLY
> YOU WOULD ASK HIM TO LOOK SUPERIORLY TO TEST THE MUSCLE.

Here the program is asking the student two very important questions that almost tell him, if he answers them correctly, how to test not only this muscle but any eye muscle. The principle is first to get the eye in a position where the action of a single muscle is isolated and to reduce the request of the patient to movements he can easily perform. The student answers correctly in both cases.

> HOW WOULD YOU TEST THE SUPERIOR RECTUS, I.E., WHAT WOULD YOU ASK THE PATIENT TO DO?

□:

LOOK LATERALLY, THEN SUPERIORLY
> YOU WOULD ASK HIM FIRST TO ABDUCT HIS EYE, TO MAKE THE LONG AXIS OF THE EYEBALL AND LONG AXIS OF THE MUSCLE PARALLEL, AND THEN ASK HIM TO LOOK SUPERIORLY TO TEST THE MUSCLE. NOW WE'LL RETURN TO WHERE YOU WERE BEFORE ASKING YOUR QUESTION.

Now the program (as predetermined by the author) feels that the student should know how to test this muscle. Apparently, with this student the judgment was borne out, as shown by the fact that he gave the correct answer. Whether it is equally true of you, the reader, is by no means certain. However, if you had been actively involved in the tutorial process, with as many additional questions and responses as you happened to need, and had reached this point, we feel from experience that you would. If your level of understanding were less than that of the student, you would not have reached this point by so direct a route. This is the nature of the tutorial process.

Key-Word Analysis

Whether one is conversing with a computer or another person, each participant must have some means of understanding what the other is saying. The method ATS currently uses is key-word analysis. Thus, when a teacher is asked by the author-interrogation program to supply the answers he anticipates students may give to a question, he does not usually type in the anticipated answer verbatim. Rather he selects certain (key) words which, if they occur in the proper relationship to each other and in the proper context, will extract the essential meaning of what was said.

Misspelled Words

We have to consider not only the author but the student as well. Even though a misspelled word requires only that a student retype his answer, this can become tiresome for a student who happens to be a poor typist, especially if the question requires long answers. Thus ATS makes an attempt to correct the student's spelling whenever a person reading his answer would have the same ability. This mechanism, built into all ATS tutorials, accounts for the following sequence:

> HOW WOULD YOU TEST THE SUPERIOR RECTUS, I.E., WHAT WOULD YOU ASK THE PATIENT TO DO?

□:

LOOK LATERALLY, THEN SUPERRIORLY
> I ASSUME YOU MEAN SUPERIORLY INSTEAD OF SUPERRIORLY.

> YOU WOULD ASK HIM FIRST TO ABDUCT HIS EYE, TO MAKE THE LONG AXIS OF THE EYEBALL AND LONG AXIS OF THE MUSCLE PARALLEL, AND THEN ASK HIM TO LOOK SUPERIORLY TO TEST THE MUSCLE.

The ATS algorithm for correcting misspellings takes care of over 95% of the typographical errors students make and is greatly appreciated for this reason. When the student is so far off that it does not match, he must reenter his answer.

Negating and Contradictory Words

> HOW WOULD YOU TEST THE SUPERIOR RECTUS, I.E., WHAT WOULD YOU ASK THE PATIENT TO DO?

□:

LOOK LATERALLY, BUT NOT SUPERIORLY

If the program were looking only for the two key words "laterally" and "superiorly," then this incorrect answer would have been treated as if it were correct. Thus, there must be some provision for words such as "not" that would negate the meaning of an otherwise correct answer.

Therefore, there is a list of standard negating words built into every ATS tutorial. This list may be modified (additions and/or deletions made) by the author for any part of the tutorial.

HOW WOULD YOU TEST THE SUPERIOR RECTUS, I.E., WHAT WOULD YOU ASK THE PATIENT TO DO?

□:

LOOK LATERALLY, THEN SUPERIORLY OR INFERIORLY
SUPERIORLY AND INFERIORLY ARE CONTRADICTORY TERMS.

□:

"Superiorly" and "inferiorly" of course have opposite meanings.

Such hedging by students, or use of two contradictory words as the answer, may also be handled by the author's adding to the standard list of negating words antonyms to the correct answer.

Synonymous Words

HOW WOULD YOU TEST THE SUPERIOR RECTUS, I.E., WHAT WOULD YOU ASK THE PATIENT TO DO?

□:

ABDUCT HIS EYE, THEN LOOK SUPERIORLY
YOU WOULD ASK HIM FIRST TO ABDUCT HIS EYE, TO MAKE THE LONG AXIS OF THE EYEBALL AND LONG AXIS OF THE MUSCLE PARALLEL, AND THEN ASK HIM TO LOOK SUPERIORLY TO TEST THE MUSCLE.

"Abduct his eye" is synonymous with "look laterally." Every time an author indicates an anticipated answer, he is asked by the author-interrogation program whether there are any equivalent ways of saying the same thing. In this case, the words "lateral," "laterally," and "abduct" have all been made equivalent.

Phrases Treated as Single Words

THE EXTRINSIC OCULAR MUSCLES TEND TO WORK CONJUGATELY OR IN PAIRS. WHAT MUSCLE WOULD YOU BE TESTING IN THE LEFT EYE WHILE YOU WERE TESTING THE RIGHT INFERIOR OBLIQUE?

□:

LEFT SUPERIOR OBLIQUE RECTUS
NOW LET'S DISCUSS SOME OF THE ANATOMICAL POINTS RELATED TO THIS QUESTION.

The correct answer to this question is "left superior rectus." The program was sufficiently informed not to let "left superior oblique rectus" slip by. The reason is that the author was asked whether any of the words in his answer should be treated as single terms. He indicated that "superior rectus" should be considered as a single term or "word." Not only do we not want the word "oblique" slipped in the middle, we do not want anything separating these two words "superior rectus."

Word Sequence

HOW WOULD YOU TEST THE SUPERIOR RECTUS, I.E., WHAT WOULD YOU ASK THE PATIENT TO DO?

□:

LOOK SUPERIORLY, THEN LATERALLY
    YOUR ANSWER IS OUT OF SEQUENCE.
□:

Although this answer contains the correct words, the fact that they are not in the proper sequence makes the answer very incorrect. Thus, this answer is not the same in meaning as the paraphrase of the answer the author wanted:

YOU WOULD ASK HIM FIRST TO ABDUCT HIS EYE, TO MAKE THE LONG AXIS OF THE EYEBALL AND LONG AXIS OF THE MUSCLE PARALLEL, AND THEN ASK HIM TO LOOK SUPERIORLY TO TEST THE MUSCLE.

For this reason, whenever an anticipated answer contains more than a single key word, or more than a single term, as defined above, the program asks the author whether or not the order between words or terms matters. If he indicates that it does, then the student will automatically get this response to an improperly sequenced answer and then have the opportunity to answer again.

This is such a serious error that in this case the author might well want to make special provision for it, i.e., if the student confused sequence of tests, discuss with him the significance of this mistake. As with all these examples that illustrate what ATS will do automatically for an author, the author may overrule the program. However, the fact that these automatic features exist can save the experienced author a lot of time and cover for the inexperience of others.

Partially Correct Answers

HOW WOULD YOU TEST THE SUPERIOR RECTUS, I.E., WHAT WOULD YOU ASK THE PATIENT TO DO?
□:

LOOK LATERALLY
    LATERALLY IS CORRECT, BUT INCOMPLETE. PLEASE REPHRASE YOUR ANSWER.

The complete answer should have been, "Have the patient abduct his eye and then look laterally." The author may want to make special provision for a number of partially correct answers that frequently occur in his experience. However, if he does not, ATS will automatically handle them in this way. Since this could result in an endless loop if the student did not know what was missing from his answer, he is only given such a message twice for any one question before the program proceeds with the conversation.

Summary of Syntactic Analysis in ATS

ATS is unique in the degree to which it can carry on a free-format discussion with students. Extensive knowledge of the rules of human discourse is built into the supervisor program that interfaces with the students and becomes part of every tutorial without any effort on the part of the author. Such features of artificial intelligence include the ability to distinguish a question from an answer based on the syntax of the response, the ability to answer questions not specifically anticipated by the author, a spelling algorithm that will correctly interpret typographical errors with about the same degree of accuracy as a person, and the ability to assign meaning to personal pronouns according to the context of the discussion at any given moment. Figure 1 summarizes these features of artificial intelligence.

Authoring in ATS

Interactive Authoring and Editing

ATS is designed for experienced teachers who want to write sophisticated computer-mediated tutorials, but who neither know nor want to learn anything about computer programming. This is almost a prerequisite if we expect to recruit the best qualified teachers to author tutorials. To this end ATS contains an author-interrogation program that reviews the teacher's grammar. Figure 2 illustrates an author interacting with the program to edit his tutorial.

```
    A CHILD HAS A CONGENITAL WEAKNESS OF HIS RIGHT INFERIOR

    RECTUS.  HOW WOULD YOU TEST HIS MUSCLE?

▯:

WHAT IS CONGENITAL?(*1)

    I DON'T UNDERSTAND WHAT YOU WANT TO KNOW ABOUT CONGENITAL

▯:

WHAT IT MEANS (*2)

    CONGENITAL MEANS SOMETHING THAT EXISTS FROM BIRTH.

    NOW WE'LL RETURN TO WHERE YOU WERE BEFORE ASKING YOUR

    QUESTION (*3)

    A CHILD HAS A CONGENITAL WEAKNESS OF HIS RIGHT INFERIOR

    RECTUS.  HOW WOULD YOU TEST THIS MUSCLE?

▯:

I WOULD HAVE THE PATIENT ADUCT HIS EYE AND LOOK INFERIORLY

    BY ADUCT, DO YOU MEAN ADDUCT OR ABDUCT (*4)

▯:

ABDUCT
```

YOU WOULD ASK HIM FIRST TO ABDUCT HIS EYE, TO MAKE THE LONG

AXIS OF THE EYEBALL AND LONG AXIS OF THE MUSCLE PARALLEL,

AND THEN ASK HIM TO LOOK INFERIORLY TO TEST THE MUSCLE.

THE EXTRINSIC OCULAR MUSCLES TEND TO WORK CONJUGATELY OR IN

PAIRS. WHAT MUSCLE WOULD YOU BE TESTING IN THE LEFT EYE

WHILE YOU WERE TESTING THE RIGHT INFERIOR OBLIQUE?

⊓:

I WOULD BE TESTING THE LEFT RECTUS

    I WAS EXPECTING RECTUS WITH SOME OTHER WORDS (*5)

    PLEASE REPHRASE YOUR WHOLE ANSWER

◻:

I WOULD BE TESTING THE LEFT SUPERIOR RECTUS.

Figure 1. Sample student interaction illustrating artificial intelligence. (*1) ATS understands that student is asking, not answering a question, and keeps him in conversation until a common ground or discussion can be reached. (*2) ATS understands student's question even though he has abbreviated his discourse by (a) not using a question mark, and (b) using a pronoun. The program remembers the referent of the pronoun. (*3) ATS keeps track of where the student was, so that student can direct his own session by asking questions, but when the student's questioning ends, it returns to control of the program for determination of the most appropriate sequence of questions. (*4) Spelling or typographical errors are automatically handled by the program, without the author's having to plan for them. (*5) When an answer is partially correct, the program intervenes as it does in all cases of default by the author. In this instance, the program prompts the student to give a more complete answer. These features of artificial intelligence are intrinsic to the program. The author needs only be concerned with content.

Some Additional Authoring Aids

Some of the features designed to aid the author were mentioned in the preceding section. Here we will illustrate a few others. Our purpose is to present an overall feeling for the authoring process, not the details.

Correcting Spelling Errors

A time-saving feature for the author is the ability to correct every occurrence of a misspelled word with a single entry by using the ATS CHANGE command:

◻:
CHANGE
    ENTER WORD
◻:

EDIT

    WHICH AQ? 0=OUT (*1)

☐:

3

     (AQ 3) OUT, QUESTION, SUBJECT, ANSWER, ABRANCH, ACORRECT?

        (*2)

☐:

QUESTION

     AQ:

     OUT, DISPLAY, INSERT, ERASE, CUT, REPLACE? (*3)

☐:

DISPLAY

      WHAT ARE THE 2 SUBSTITUENTS?

      OUT, DISPLAY, INSERT, ERASE, CUT, REPLACE? (*4)

☐:

REPLACE

      WHICH WORDS?

☐:

2

      ENTER WORDS:

☐:

3

      OUT, DISPLAY, INSERT, ERASE CUT, REPLACE?

☐:

DISPLAY (* 5)

      WHAT ARE THE 3 SUBSTITUENTS?

      OUT, DISPLAY, INSERT, ERASE, CUT,REPLACE?

Figure 2. Interactive editing. (*1) Program asks author which Author's Question he wants to edit. (*2) Program presents author with his options. At this point, he can work on any of these parts of the question. He chooses to work on the question itself, rather than the student's answer, his response to that student, etc. (*3) Program prompts author with his options. Author displays the question. (*4) Program again informs author of his options. He chooses to replace a number with another number. (*5) Author displays the question. His replacement of "3" for "2" has been made.

SUPERIORRLY
    ENTER REPLACEMENT:
□:
SUPERIORLY

Here we replaced (corrected the spelling of) the word "superiorrly."

The FIND Command

A time-consuming part of authoring is obtaining up-to-date listings (displays) of the tutorial. For a long tutorial, this could require up to 2 hours, but the need for such a listing is eliminated in ATS. If one wants to know the location of any block of text, e.g., a question, anticipated answer, comment, etc., and remembers only the general content of the text, he may locate it by typing in those words that he remembers. The FIND command will then locate every block of text containing those words.

In the following examples of terminal interactions with the authoring program, the formatting is changed somewhat. Everything that the computer prints is indented four spaces. What the author types is indented two spaces or less.

FIND
    ENTER TEXT:
ACTION SUPERIOR RECTUS
    (ORDER)? (Y/N)
Y
    QUESTION, ANSWER, RESPONSE, UN? O = OUT
Q
    THE TEXT IS FOUND IN QUESTION 2
    DISPLAY? (Y/N)
Y
    QUESTION 2:
    WHAT IS THE ACTION OF THE SUPERIOR RECTUS?
    CONTINUE WITH THIS TEXT? (Y/N)
N

The author has asked the program to locate the words, "action superior rectus," in that order. The program responded that it was found in question 2 and displayed the entire question.

Learning from Experience with Students

In order to improve the quality of tutorials, one must have a means of evaluating their effectiveness. This is equally true of other teaching media. It is difficult to assess the efficiency of lectures and other conventional methods of instruction except by performance on exams and by soliciting student evaluation via questionnaires. The uniqueness of computer-based instruction is the ability to monitor every step of the learning process.

Student Performance

Any teacher learns from his experience with students. At present ATS tutorials do not improve automatically from experience with students. However, every student who takes a tutorial leaves a trace or record of his interaction. This can be retrieved and given to the author at any time he desires.

The "trace" consists of the sequence of questions the student was asked and those that he asked of the computer. In addition, it also records the following three types of information verbatim and the context in which they occurred: (a) any questions the student asked that the program could not answer, (b) every answer a student gave that was not anticipated by the author, and (c) any comments the student made during the course of his interaction with the computer.

As the number of sessions has risen into the hundreds and thousands, the need has become obvious for looking at grouped, rather than individual, data. Figure 3 is an excerpt from a report summarizing such grouped data.

EXCERPT FROM PERFORMANCE DISPLAYALL OF 'CNERVE'(*1)

AQ. 1.2:

A PATIENT HAS LIMITED   FACIAL PARALYSIS ALONG   WITH SOME MOTOR   IMPAIRMENT OF THE   UPPER LEFT   EXTREMITY.   HE CANNOT MOVE MUSCLES IN THE LEFT LOWER PART   OF HIS   FACE THOUGH HE CAN FROWN AND WILL SOMETIMES SMILE AND LAUGH AT A JOKE.   HE CAN CLOSE HIS EYES   AND   FURROW   HIS BROW.   HIS   SPEECH   IS SOMEWHAT IMPAIRED.   EYE MOVEMENTS ARE INTACT.   WHERE MIGHT A SMALL LOCALIZED LESION MOST LIKELY PRODUCE THESE SYMPTOMS?

TOTAL FREQUENCY: 52

PERCENT GIVEN: 96

1:   50

2:   1

AA1:   RIGHT CAPSULE

FREQUENCY: 8

PERCENT: 15

AA2: *LEFT CAPSULE*

FREQUENCY: 1

PERCENT: 1

AA3: *CAPSULE*

FREQUENCY: 8

PERCENT: 15

AA4: *V11 NUCLEUS*

FREQUENCY: 6

PERCENT: 11

AA5: *CORTEX*

FREQUENCY: 5

PERCENT: 9

AA6: *LEFT CORTICOBULABAR*

FREQUENCY: 6

PERCENT: 11

AA8: *CORTICOSPINAL*

FREQUENCY: 0

AA9: *PEDUNCLE*

FREQUENCY: 4

PERCENT: 7

UN RESP: *THIS LESION INVOLVES CRANIAL NERVE V11.*

FREQUENCY: 14

PERCENT: 26

UN RESPONSES:

RIGHT PRECENTRAL CYRUS MEDIALLY (887)

LEFT SIDE AT C2 TO C7 (887)

I DON'T KNOW (892)

X (908)

UPPER MOTOR NEURON (918)

DONT KNOW (924) LESION IN NUCLEUS AMBIGUS(935)

I DONOT KNOW (935)

PRECENTRAL GURUS IN FACE REGION , LATERAL

(993)

UPPER CERVICAL CORD (1021)

IN THE PONS NEAR THE FACIAL AND VAGUS

NERVES (1140)

Figure 3. Summary of student response data. (*1) A display of a tutorial (of CNERVE), including item analyses of all student answers and the text of all unanticipated student answers. Author's Question 1.2 was given 52 times, to 96% of the students who took the tutorial. One student was asked this question twice; the other 50 students, once. Of the 9 answers which the author anticipated, there was a rather even distribution of students' matching on 8 of them. AA1 (the first answer anticipated by the author), "right capsule," was given by 8 students, or 15% of those who answered this question. The UN Response, "This lesion involves cranial nerve V11," was given by the author to the 14 students whose answers he had not anticipated. The text of the students' unanticipated answers may be used by the author to build additional teaching sequences into his tutorial, or they may be used as a source of information for teachers of the course.

These reports of student feedback become the basis for editing the tutorials. Often, the students' answers that were originally unanticipated prove to have been correct but phrased in a novel way. In that case, these answers are added as synonyms for the correct answer. If many students give the same, unanticipated answer which is wrong, then we make this a new anticipated answer, with a special response or remedial routine for those students who give that answer, in order to be more specifically responsive to more students in the future.

Student Attitudes

We presently obtain several types of student appraisals of teaching quality. Students using the computer are assigned anonymous identification numbers so that the performance of a single student can be followed throughout the course. However, the student need not be reluctant to answer freely or give his honest opinion of the teaching ability of that tutorial.

At the end of the trimester, students are given a detailed attitudinal questionnaire in each course in which computer tutorials are used. It asks for a rating (1–10) of the comparative value of the different teaching methods that were used in the course, e.g., lectures, laboratories, self-study slides, computer tutorials, clinical case presentations, etc. This is really our only means of comparing the effectiveness of one instructional medium with another, since we do not selectively present certain material only in one form so it could be correlated with exam performance – although we may move to that. On the computer side, they are also asked to answer on a scale of 1–10 questions about technical problems, tutorial format and quality, system use, the role of computer-assisted instruction, and their attitude toward computer tutorials, in general. Students enter their identification numbers on these questionnaires so that we can correlate attitudinal variables with performance variables (such as how many and which tutorials they have taken) and what their scores and experiences were on those tutorials. Figure 4 is an excerpt from a report summarizing students' on-line evaluations of a tutorial.

At the end of every computer tutorial, the student is required to answer a series of questions before he can sign off. These include a rating of the tutorial, a checklist of specific problems encountered, and open-ended questions on the best and worst features of the tutorials. The results here are more consistent and statistically significant, probably because the experience is still fresh in the students' minds. Their responses are stored on disks and automatically collated. The two quantified parts of this evaluation (the rating and the checklist) can be statistically analyzed and correlated with factors we think influence tutorial success, which are obtained by methods described under the headings to follow.

Students are permitted to make comments at any point in the computer tutorials. The comments are stored and can be retrieved by tutorial and by student. However, they are also immediately brought to the attention of the author or program supervisor. When a teacher signs on his user number, all new comments from all the tutorials for which he has responsibility are automatically displayed. He may then reply to those comments via the system so that the next time the student signs on, he has the author's response displayed for him. This relatively rapid feedback system encourages the students to utilize comments to resolve their personal difficulties and to contribute toward improving the tutorials.

Students may also ask questions at any point in the discussion. The ability to answer the majority of student questions is built into the system. However, all questions that the program could not handle are recorded and printed out for the author. If the questions are deemed relevant and important, the author then adds to the tutorial the information necessary to answer the question.

Evaluating Teaching Strategy

Using Students' Time Efficiently

The student is not given a numerical grade at the end of a tutorial, although this facility exists in ATS and is often used when students are given self-evaluation

COMA

TOTAL NUMBER OF SESSIONS: 49

RATING:

10: (31) 1079 1097 1107 1108 1109 1119 1132 1146 1164 1166 1191
    1213 1214 1215 1216 1229 1250 1260 1375 1418 1447 1519 1520 1536 1554
    1576 1583 1587 1608 1612 1650
9: (4) 1077 1198 1354 1661
8: (7) 1161 1228 1300 1301 1432 1457 1548
7: (1) 1416
6: (3) 1124 1391 1441
5: (3) 1181 1526 1567
4: (0)
3: (0)
2: (0)
1: (0)
0: (0)

MEAN RATING: 9

MEDIAN RATING: 10

BEST FEATURES:

COMPLETE, INTERESTING, GOOD EXPLANATIONS   1077

SO FAR, IT'S GREAT. I JUST HAD TO LEAVE EARLY.   1097

*EXCELLENT REVIEW OF NUEROLOGY NEUROANATOMU, PHYSIOLOGY, AND GROSS
ANATOMY*   1119
EXCELLENT EXPLANATION OF EACH SIGN   1132

INTERESTING INFORMATIVE   1146

*IT WAS AN EXCELLENT IDEA TO ASK THE STUDENT WHICH POINTS HE/SHE
WOULD LIKE TO DISCUSS FURTHER. MY ONLY CRITICISM OF THE TUTORIAL*
1161
ANS PROMPTLY   1164

ITS COMPLETENESS   1166

VERY WELL DONE   1191

GOOD MATERIAL   1198

GAVE YOU A WORKOUT   1213

* * *

Figure 4. Report of the summarized student evaluation data on the tutorial on coma. Between March 1 and July 1, 1975, a total of 51 sessions were conducted. A total of 32 students rated the tutorial 10 and the numbers of their sessions appear to the right. (These numbers can be used to retrieve the individual student records of those sessions.) The mean rating was 9, and the median rating was 10. The best features problems encountered (as listed on the terminal), technical problems and suggested improvements follow, in the full report, each with the session number after the entry.

exams. Rather, in a true tutorial, the program tells the student when he or she has demonstrated sufficient understanding of the material. Students who already know the material can demonstrate their competence in 2–3 minutes, while slower students can stay on the same tutorial for 2 hours without completely retracing their steps. With the increasing demands on a medical student's time, it is appropriate that he spend it only where it is needed.

One of the advantages of the tutorial format is that it is possible to evaluate a student's level of competence quickly and skim over areas where he is already knowledgeable. This is achieved in ATS by having a large number of application-type questions. If a teacher were talking to a student, he would probably ask him some questions which, if the student answered them satisfactorily, would demonstrate not only that he knew the factual material the teacher wanted to cover, but also that he understood how to apply this knowledge in practical situations. Also, it is unlikely that the teacher would begin with the same question with each student but would probably intuitively select from a whole repertoire of questions. Thus, the ATS manual suggests that the author start with comprehensive questions and only go down to simpler levels as students show an individual need.

Figure 5 shows a computer-drawn flowchart that enables the author to analyze his teaching logic at a glance to see whether or not he has: (1) individualized his tutorial and (2) provided specific, efficient teaching.

Future Directions

Interactive Graphics

During the school year 1975–76, CUMC began integrating ATS with interactive graphics so that, in the near future, it should become possible for authors to present to students such pictures as molecular models, diagrams of neural pathways or brain slices, and graphs of drug response. These would be modified according to the degree of understanding shown in response to questions about them. Another dimension will thus be added to the capabilities of ATS.

Modeling

Two working versions of brain models have been developed by W. D. Hagamen, Director of the CUMC Laboratory of Computer Science, a neuroanatomist, and one of the chief developers of ATS. One of these is a neuronal model that enables the person using the program to designate neural tracts and lesions and model the results of stimulating or blocking the tracts. The other brain model takes as Input a series of signs and symptoms and gives as output a computer-drawn diagram of a brain slice identifying the site of the lesion. Both of these models can be used either for diagnosis or for teaching purposes. When their development is complete, they will become part of ATS. The models will provide students with needed practice in diagnosis. The tutorials will reason with them about points they have difficulty learning.

FLOWCHART OF 'NEURO'
SEGMENT 1

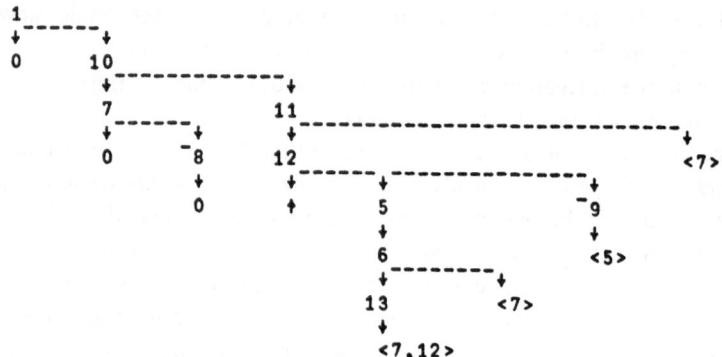

FLOWCHART OF 'NEURO'
SEGMENT 2

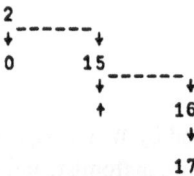

Figure 5. Flowchart of teaching strategy. (A) Rapid exit after demonstration of mastery on a comprehensive test question makes tutorial flexible, able to individualize, and uses student's time efficiently. (B) Multiple question pre- and posttest: provides variety if retest is needed. These questions within one segment should all test the same topic and same skill level. (C) Segmentation. Each segment covers one topic. Segments can be added or deleted. (D) Width of branching. Different responses for three types of anticipated answers. Provides for variety of student knowledge. Legend: 0, out of segment; <>, numbers found elsewhere on this page; ↑, question is re-asked, after clarification.

Interface with Hospital Data Bases

Concurrently with the development of ATS, a system for allowing hospital administrators to store patient records in the computer has been developed at CUMC. Each computer tutorial now pretests the student, drawing upon a small bank of test questions, usually clinical cases, written by the author. However, it is difficult, artificial, and time-consuming for teachers to make up these cases. It is therefore desirable to draw upon real clinical cases stored in the computer's hospital record files and selected for the combinations of attributes relevant to the point being taught in a given tutorial. This capability will be added to ATS in the near future.

Further Development of Artificial Intelligence

Linguists are making great strides in analyzing both the surface and the deep structures of English sentences. Although ATS already contains considerable ability to understand what the student says, further development will enable it to become even more sensitive to the nuances of student responses.

Further Development of Evaluation Standards

As part of a study of the authoring process, one of the authors of this chapter (Murphy, 1975) has developed a system for analyzing the pedagogical moves in a computer tutorial. Differences in authoring style were studied, using such parameters as style, type of reinforcement, branching logic, question type, and degree of individualization. These factors in the authoring process will be correlated with measures of student performance and attitudes, in order to determine what structural or pedagogical features are associated with teaching effectiveness. When these factors have been isolated, we will automate their incorporation in future tutorials at the time of authoring.

Networking

Considering the relatively large initial investment of time necessary to develop tutorials and the fact that the cost of development per student contact hour decreases as the number of students increases, it is desirable for medical schools to share both the cost of development and the curricula produced. At some times in the past, CUMC has not been able to share its computer tutorials because we have had unique software. However, CUMC has joined a national network, TELENET, with nodes throughout the country, which will make possible both joint curriculum development efforts and sharing of tutorials developed at CUMC.

Summary

Since there is perhaps no single area in which a written description can mislead a reader more than in the realm of computer-assisted instruction, there is no real substitute for actually using the system. In lieu of this, we have tried to illustrate some of the features of the author-interviewing program and the supervisor program by means of sample terminal interactions. The two features that make ATS unique among instructional systems are the ease of authoring and the aspects of machine intelligence (actual knowledge of the rules of human discourse) built into the program.

The results of the analyses made to date on student evaluation and performance and on author style and strategy have shown ATS to be a powerful, computer-teaching tool. Lines of development now underway or in the planning stages promise to enhance the system considerably and to make it readily accessible to other institutions.

References

Murphy, S. S., 1975. Author Styles in Programming for a Computer Assisted Instruction Language (ATS: A Tutorial System), Columbia University, Teachers' College. Unpublished doctoral dissertation.

18

The Use of Computer-Assisted Teaching Systems (CATS) in Pharmacology

John Doull and Edward J. Walaszek

The general rule of study is that time is a constant and achievement a variable. Since the study of drugs by physicians must be a lifetime endeavor we will begin by instituting achievement as the constant and time as a variable.

Introduction

Computers are now used extensively in education at the primary, secondary, and collegiate level but relatively infrequently in medical education, and it has been suggested that this is because computers are not applicable to medical education. However, several such programs have been developed in the past five years in internal medicine and a few in biochemistry, pharmacology, and anatomy (Abelson, 1972; Alpert and Bitzer, 1970; Hyatt *et al.*, 1972; Murray *et al.*, 1976; Norton *et al.*, 1972; Smith and Sherwood, 1976; Stolurow *et al.*, 1970). Associated with the growing interest in this area, several professional groups, such as ADCIS (The Association for the Development of Computer-Based Instructional Systems), and governmental agencies, such as the Lister Hill Center for Biomedical Communications of the National Library of Medicine, have arranged meetings, workshops, and various other programs designed to encourage, support, and coordinate some of these activities. It is now evident that computers can support medical education directly through computer-assisted instruction (CAI) and through computer-managed instruction (CMI) and indirectly through the establishment and maintenance of exam question data banks, machine scoring of examinations, and the availability of sophisticated programs for analyzing student and faculty performance and the effectiveness of different educational methodologies, as well as other educational problems. It is equally clear that the use of computers in medical education will increase dramatically during the next decade and that this growth will be accompanied by technological advances that will have an even greater impact on all aspects of the education of health professionals (microprocessors, intelligent terminals, inexpensive communication networks, massive storage devices, combined video—CAI techniques, etc.).

John Doull and Edward J. Walaszek · Department of Pharmacology, University of Kansas Medical Center, Kansas City, Kansas.

The purpose of this chapter is to describe a computer-assisted teaching system (CATS) that was developed in the Department of Pharmacology at the University of Kansas Medical Center in 1970 and that has been subsequently used and further developed by a group of cooperating United States and European medical schools.

Prior to 1970, the pharmacology courses at the University of Kansas Medical Center for both the medical and the nursing students utilized a conventional approach (a series of lectures, laboratories, and one or more examinations). The stimulus to change our teaching approach resulted from several factors: an increase in the medical student class size from 115 to 200 students, a switch from a 4-year to a 3-year medical school curriculum, and a growing demand for additional courses in pharmacology from nursing and allied health and from outside the institution. These requests for additional instruction in pharmacology, and particularly the demands for more continuing education and in-service training programs, are typical of the current trend among health professionals at all levels to seek new and more effective ways to improve their skills and to anticipate new relicensing requirements. In designing a system, therefore, to handle both our current and projected teaching needs in pharmacology, we were seeking not only a more effective way to teach pharmacology to medical and nursing students, but also an effective and innovative method for meeting the needs of medical technicians, hearing and speech therapists, graduate students, pharmacists, house staff, and other health professional groups, both within and outside of the Medical Center.

Five major objectives were identified as being essential for our teaching program.

1. The pharmacology courses must be easily available at any time throughout the year to students within and outside of our institution.
2. The programs must be able to handle students with different levels of preparation.
3. Students must be able to progress through the courses at varying speeds (self-paced).
4. The system must provide for frequent and rapid feedback on progress through each course.
5. The teaching program should utilize newer educational technology and techniques to provide optimal flexibility in the student approach to learning pharmacology.

It was anticipated that a teaching program which fulfilled these objectives would provide a satisfactory answer to one of the major criticisms of basic science teaching in the medical schools, namely, lack of flexibility or lock-step curricula. We were also concerned, however, about a second common criticism of basic science teaching, which is the so-called gap in knowledge problem. In a conventional pharmacology program with one or two examinations, it is possible, for example, for a student who is well versed in the pharmacology of morphine to pass the examinations even though he has a deficiency or a gap in his knowledge about penicillin. Many medical school programs have attempted to solve this problem by defining a series of educational objectives for each course and requiring students to meet each of these objectives. We have adopted a similar approach, which is to subdivide the course material into a number of modules or units and to then require the students to demonstrate competence in each of these modules or units. An important advantage of this approach (a modularized course with a pass—fail system for each module) is that it provides the department with a mechanism to offer minicourses in each of the different areas of pharmacology for students with specialized interests. We now provide, for example, a course in antibiotic pharmacology or chemotherapy for medical technologists in the bacteriology lab, a course in cardiovascular pharmacology for respiratory technicians, and a course in adverse reactions for nursing floor supervisors in addition to the regular series of course offerings in pharmacology.

The name selected for our new pharmacology teaching program was CATS, which stands for Computer-Assisted Teaching Systems, and the two computer-supported parts of the system are commonly referred to as the CAI or computer-assisted instruction part and CMI or computer-managed instruction part of the CATS system. CATS was used on a pilot basis in 1971 and 1972 to teach pharmacology to medical students and was fully implemented and extended to other teaching areas in pharmacology in 1973. Subsequently, we have shared the philosophy and the teaching material of the CATS system with other interested medical schools, and in 1974 a Consortium of CATS system users was created with 29 active members (listed in Table 1). At the present time there are over fifty medical school members with CATS Consortium. There are, in addition, over a dozen medical schools in Europe that are considering the use of the CATS system either in English or translated into the appropriate language. The purpose of the CATS Consortium is to provide a mechanism whereby participating schools can: (1) cooperate in the development of new educational approaches to medical education, (2) share and exchange educational material, and (3) generally encourage the development of innovative

Table 1. CATS Consortium Members

1. University of Kansas	16. Texas Tech University
2. Thomas Jefferson University	17. University of Washington
3. University of Arkansas	18. University of Illinois (PLATO)
4. University of Arizona	19. Texas A & M University
5. University of Hawaii	20. Rush Medical School
6. Michigan State University	21. University of California
7. Mayo Clinic Medical School	(San Francisco)
8. University of Wisconsin	22. University of Kentucky
9. Southern Illinois University	23. Duke University
10. Meharry Medical College	24. Wayne University
11. University of Cincinnati	25. Chicago Medical School
12. University of North Carolina	26. McGill University
13. University of Maryland	27. Eastern Virginia Medical School
14. University of Minnesota (Duluth)	28. University of California (Davis)
15. University of Texas (Dallas)	29. Ohio State University

teaching in pharmacology. During the last 2 years the Consortium has also functioned in an advisory role to government agencies that are interested in and responsible for policy decisions regarding the use of computers in medical education.

CATS Computer-Managed Instruction

The CMI portion of the CATS system consists of three major parts, the test-question file and the associated software to create and maintain this file, the test-generating system, and the test-grading and -evaluation system. The programs associated with each of these three parts of the CMI system (Table 2) are all written in standard COBOL and are designed so that in addition to supporting the educational objectives of the Pharmacology Department they are also suitable for maintaining test question files and for the generating, grading, and evaluating of examinations in other departments. At the present time, there are about 26,000 items in the total test-question file, which is stored as a variable length VSAM file on approximately 28 cylinders of an IBM 3330 disk. At the University of Kansas Medical Center the CMI system is available on an IBM 370/158 (DOS/VS), but the system is also in use with other IBM computers and with Sigma 7, DEC 10, Cyber 70, and Univac and Burroughs 6700 equipment. With some adaptation it has also been possible to support the CMI system on several types of minicomputers. Most of the CATS Consortium users run the CMI programs exclusively in the batch mode, although the system contains an on-line question-editing program and some schools also use an on-line examination administration and grading program.

Table 2. CATS-CMI VS Programs

Program	Description
VS-01:	An on-line update program under CICS/VS to update, delete, and add questions
VS-06:	A utility program for tape-to-disk or disk-to-tape transfers of the question file
VS-09:	Key program of the present system. Generates exam evaluation from input selection cards, COURSEWRITER III tapes, exam decks for further use, proof copy, etc. Scrambles the order of exam questions within question type (Subroutine RANDOM) and links these scrambled versions to VS-10 for final output.
VS-10:	Prints exams for student use
VS-15:	Card input update, deletion, or addition program. Will handle new questions or individual lines of old questions
VS-21:	File printing program. Prints all or selected portions of the question file on individual cards
VS-25:	OpScan answer-sheet printing program. Uses OpScan answer sheet DC 33-687 and prints student name, number, box number, exam number, date, and comments
VS-27:	Modification of VS-21 to prepare tape of the question file by category or sequentially for preparation of microfiche
VS-11:	Transfer program for preparing COURSEWRITER III course-off tapes from selected segments of the question file
VS-12:	Student response processor. Record-keeping program for CATS-CAI system
VS-40:	Abbreviated on-line grading program

In describing each of the sections of the CMI system, we will discuss primarily the way in which the CMI system is used at the University of Kansas in the medical school and nursing pharmacology courses.

Test-Question File

Before soliciting questions to be included in the test-question file, it was necessary to consider two questions. First, what limitations should be imposed in terms of question format, and second, what information in addition to the text of the question should be included in the test-question file? It was decided that we would use only objective type questions in order to simplify the programming requirements for the CMI system, and that we would use the five question formats commonly employed in State and National Board examinations. Examples of each of these types and the associated instructions to the students are shown in Table 3. Subsequently, we have added three additional question formats; two of these are modifications of the above formats that enable us to use textual, graphic, or photo-

Table 3. Question Type Formats Used in Pharmacology CATS-CMI File

Type A: Multiple choice
For each of the following multiple choice questions, choose the most appropriate answer.

Type B: Select best answer(s)
Select (A) if 1, 2, and 3 are correct
Select (B) if 1 and 3 are correct
Select (C) if 2 and 4 are correct
Select (D) if only 4 is correct
Select (E) if all four are correct

Type C: Cause and effect
Answer the following using the key outlined below:
A. If both statement and reason are true and related as to cause and effect.
B. If both statement and reason are true but not related as to cause and effect.
C. If statement is true but reason is false.
D. If statement is false but reason is true.
E. If both statement and reason are false.

Type D: Greater-than—less-than
Select choice (A) if (A) is greater than (B).
Select choice (B) if (B) is greater than (A).
Select choice (C) if (A) and (B) are equal or nearly equal.

Type E: Association
Answer the following questions by using the key outlined below:
A. If the item is associated with (A) only.
B. If the item is associated with (B) only.
C. If the item is associated with both (A) and (B).
D. If the item is associated with neither (A) nor (B).

Type F: Chained questions
These types of questions are questions that can relate back to a single diagram, case history, etc.

graphic information as a part of individual questions or with a series of related questions. The third type is a simple true–false question format that was added at the request of several allied health users of our system. In setting up the CMI system, it was also decided that each question should be identified by a unique item number and that appropriate coding would be included with each question to identify the source of the question, the question format, the correct answer, and a category classification that would enable questions to be selected on the basis of individual drugs, classes of drugs, or on pharmacologic principles. File space was also provided to store with each question statistical performance data related to the type of student, year of use, and participating school from which the data were obtained.

The source of the pharmacology question in the CMI test-question file has been mainly from recent examinations given by the various Consortium members and other pharmacologic colleagues. Since several of the Consortium member schools teach pharmacology to veterinary, nursing, dental, and allied health students in addition to medical and osteopathic students, this selection process has provided diversity both in the type and orientation of the questions and also in the difficulty level of the items in the file. It has been necessary, however, particularly in the allied health and nursing areas, to utilize additional collections and lists of questions to insure adequate coverage in all of the different category areas. When new questions are added to the file, they are subjected to a preliminary screen to insure that they fit into one of the acceptable question-type formats, that they are appropriate for inclusion in the pharmacology file, and that they represent a level of difficulty which will be usable with at least one of the student populations for which examinations need to be constructed. Since questions in pharmacology tend to become outdated rather rapidly as new drugs are developed and new therapeutic approaches occur, it is necessary to maintain an input of new questions and to periodically review the existing file items to insure that they are consistent with current therapeutics and to correct erroneous and duplicate entries. In our system, this review process takes place at the time the questions are selected from the file for inclusion in examinations rather than at the time the questions are initially added to the pharmacology test-question file.

Updating of the CMI test question file can be accomplished in any of three ways: (1) by using VS-15, which is a batch program with card input, (2) through VS-01, which is an on-line update program operating under the IBM terminal handling program, CICS/VS, and (3) by using TEXTED II which is a locally produced on-line text-editing system operating under COURSEWRITER III. The principal advantage of the batch process card input system (VS-15) is that it does not require a time-sharing capability and that additions, deletions, or changes to questions can be carried out remotely and at times when the computer is not available. The advantage of the on-line system (VS-01) is that it enables last-minute changes to be made in the question film before printing examinations or answer changes to be made immediately prior to the grading of an examination. In general, the on-line update system is less efficient for entering batches of new questions than either the card input or text-editing methods and some care must be exercised in its use in order to avoid destroying segments of the test-question file. For this reason, we use a password system which limits access to the on-line update system (VS-01) to the test chairman, system programmer, and to the supporting personnel who have direct responsibility for file maintenance. As an additional precautionary measure, the on-line disk file containing the test questions is periodically transferred to tape and one copy of this tape is stored in the pharmacology department. The use of the TEXTED II system for adding groups of new questions and for other purposes will be described elsewhere in this report.

The classification system used for the pharmacology test-question file is shown in Table 4 where it can be seen that it consists of a major category designation, which correlates with the unit or module of the pharmacology course, and a minor category designation, which indicates the various classes of drugs within each unit. It may be noted that there are eight major categories in the test-question file whereas there are only five units in our pharmacology course. The reason for this is to enable the test-question file to be used to prepare exams in other courses which are more sharply defined than the units in the medical student pharmacology course. For example, toxicology and endocrinology are combined as one unit in the pharmacology course whereas these two subjects are separated in the test-question file. Similarly, the drugs affecting the autonomic nervous system are considered as a single unit in the pharmacology course but are subdivided in the test question file into major categories 1 and 2. This classification system was established initially by combining the lecture schedule of the pharmacology courses at several medical schools and the index terms used in the major pharmacology textbooks. Although this system has proven to be generally satisfactory for our purposes and those of the other CATS Consortium users, it should be pointed out that in many cases the assignment of questions to one or another of these categories is somewhat arbitrary and that in these situations the decision is usually made on the basis of the drug class of the correct answer. Currently, we are in the process of adding additional levels of coding to this classification system which will permit us to search the test-question file for individual drugs by trade or generic name and for the pharmacologic characteristics of individual drugs (general information, pharmacokinetics, efficacy, adverse effects, and therapeutics). The purpose of this additional coding is to enable us to link the pharmacology test-question file with either an on-line pharmacology syllabus or the drug-information system which we are developing.

Whenever questions from the pharmacology test-question file are used in an examination, it is desirable to capture any available statistical information resulting from their use and to store this information with each question. At the present time, we are recording the last date on which the question was used, the number of students who were exposed to the question, and the difficulty and discrimination factors. Separate statistics are being maintained for the medical students and the nursing students and provision has been made to include statistics from various other groups. It is anticipated that similar sets of statistics will be accumulated for

Table 4. Classification of Pharmacology Question File

1A	ANS GEN PRIN	5A	BLOOD DRUGS
1B	CHOLINESTERASE	5B	ANTICOAGULANTS
1C	MUSCARINIC	5C	ANTACIDS
1D	NICOTINICS	5D	CATHARTICS
1E	NMJ AGENTS	5E	VITAMINS
1F	CATECHOLAMINES	5F	ANTILIPID DRUGS
1G	ADRENERGIC		
1H	ALPHA ADRENERGICS	6A	TOX GEN PRIN
1I	BETA ADRENERGICS	6B	CLINICAL TOX
		6C	ASPIRIN
2A	POLYPEPTIDES	6D	CORROSIVES
2B	SEROTONIN	6E	PHOSPHORUS
2C	HISTAMINE	6F	SOLVENTS
2D	OTHER DIURETICS	6G	ALCOHOL
2E	MERCURIAL DIURETICS	6H	PLANT TOXINS
2F	THIAZIDE DIURETICS	6I	ANIMAL TOXINS
2G	GLYCOSIDES	6J	PESTICIDES
3H	VASODILATORS	6K	RADIATION
2I	ANTIHYPERTENSIVES	6L	GASES
2J	ANTIARRHYTHMICS	6M	DUSTS
		6N	METALS
3A	CNS GEN PRIN		
3B	STIMULANTS	7A	ENDO GEN PRIN
3C	HALLUCINOGENS	7B	PITUITARY
3D	HYPNOTICS	7C	INSULIN
3E	SEDATIVES	7D	OXYTOXICS
3F	ANTICONVULSANTS	7E	ADRENAL STEROIDS
3G	GENERAL ANESTHESIA	7F	ANTIINFLAMMATORY AGENTS
3H	LOCAL ANESTHESIA	7G	THYROID
3I	ANTIDEPRESSANTS	7H	SEX HORMONES
3J	ANTIPARKINSON		
3K	ANALGESICS	8A	MISCELLANEOUS
3L	MAJOR TRANQUILLIZERS	8B	ABSORPTION
3M	MINOR TRANQUILLIZERS	8C	DISTRIBUTION
		8D	BIOTRANSFORMATION
4A	CHEMO GEN PRIN	8E	EXCRETION
4B	SULFAS	8F	DOSE RESPONSE
4C	ANTISEPTICS	8G	RECEPTORS
4D	PENICILLINS	8H	INTERACTIONS
4E	GRAM POS ANTIBIOTICS		
4F	ANTITUBERCULOSIS		
4G	ANTILEPROSY		
4H	GRAM NEG ANTIBIOTICS		
4I	BROAD SPECTRUM AGENTS		
4J	ANTIFUNGALS		
4K	ANTICANCER		
4L	ANTIVIRAL		
4M	ANTIMALARIALS		
4N	AMEBICIDES		
4P	HELMINTICS		

student groups at other CATS Consortium schools, but the implementation of this task has been delayed until all of the members of the Consortium can agree on a standard format for collecting and storing the student performance statistics.

Test Preparation

In our system each of the instructors who is involved in teaching any of the pharmacology courses in our department is provided with all of the questions in each of the areas with which he is involved. The instructor goes through this set of questions and indicates those which he wishes to use on examinations or which need to be modified or replaced and those which he would like to have deleted from the file or designated for use with a special group. To facilitate this selection process, a computer program (VS-21) is used to print each of the questions in the pharmacology file on individual cards and examples of these are shown in Figure 1. The faculty responsible for the teaching in each unit then decide how many exams they wish to prepare and how many questions from each minor category they wish to include in each exam. The approved questions are then assigned to each exam and reassigned until they meet the area coverage and difficulty objectives of the unit faculty. In some cases, the unit faculty may rely heavily on the statistical information to select questions for exams whereas other groups may rely more on topic coverage or other learning objectives. VS-21 will also prepare a computer tape which can be transferred to microfiche so that all of the questions in a unit or category are available for selection by this method. Regardless of the method used to select the test questions, it is the unit faculty in our system that is responsible for both the teaching in that unit and for selecting the exam questions to be used with their unit. In contrast to this system, some CATS Consortium users allow the computer to select questions for an exam using either the statistical information or a random-number generator to select the desired number of questions in each category. It is evident that when this procedure is used, the question file must be prescreened to remove duplicate questions and those which cover essentially the same material.

After the questions are selected and updated (if necessary), the item or question numbers are submitted to the computer using the program VS-09, which will generate either a proof copy of the exam or a final version with appropriate instructions to the student for answering each of the different types of question formats. In the proof copy of the exam, all of the questions from a single category are arranged together so that the instructor can evaluate the coverage within the exam, and information is provided concerning the number of questions in each category, the predicted average score and discrimination factors for the exam and each section, the number of questions utilizing each of the different question formats, and various other types of information. If the proof copy is satisfactory, the final versions of the exam are produced by another program, VS-10, which scrambles the questions within each question type to provide several versions of the same test which are used to minimize cheating. If only a few copies of the exam are needed,

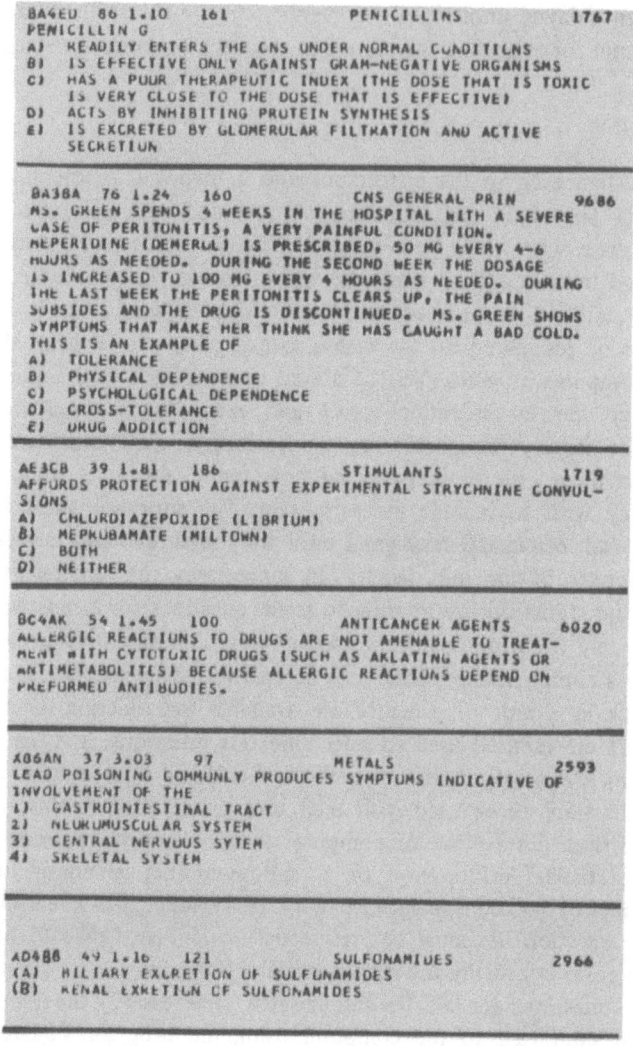

```
BASED   86 1.10    161              PENICILLINS              1767
PENICILLIN G
A)   READILY ENTERS THE CNS UNDER NORMAL CONDITIONS
B)   IS EFFECTIVE ONLY AGAINST GRAM-NEGATIVE ORGANISMS
C)   HAS A POOR THERAPEUTIC INDEX (THE DOSE THAT IS TOXIC
     IS VERY CLOSE TO THE DOSE THAT IS EFFECTIVE)
D)   ACTS BY INHIBITING PROTEIN SYNTHESIS
E)   IS EXCRETED BY GLOMERULAR FILTRATION AND ACTIVE
     SECRETION


BA38A   76 1.24    160              CNS GENERAL PRIN        9686
MS. GREEN SPENDS 4 WEEKS IN THE HOSPITAL WITH A SEVERE
CASE OF PERITONITIS, A VERY PAINFUL CONDITION.
MEPERIDINE (DEMEROL) IS PRESCRIBED, 50 MG EVERY 4-6
HOURS AS NEEDED.  DURING THE SECOND WEEK THE DOSAGE
IS INCREASED TO 100 MG EVERY 4 HOURS AS NEEDED.  DURING
THE LAST WEEK THE PERITONITIS CLEARS UP, THE PAIN
SUBSIDES AND THE DRUG IS DISCONTINUED.  MS. GREEN SHOWS
SYMPTOMS THAT MAKE HER THINK SHE HAS CAUGHT A BAD COLD.
THIS IS AN EXAMPLE OF
A)   TOLERANCE
B)   PHYSICAL DEPENDENCE
C)   PSYCHOLOGICAL DEPENDENCE
D)   CROSS-TOLERANCE
E)   DRUG ADDICTION


AE3CB   39 1.81    186              STIMULANTS              1719
AFFORDS PROTECTION AGAINST EXPERIMENTAL STRYCHNINE CONVUL-
SIONS
A)   CHLORDIAZEPOXIDE (LIBRIUM)
B)   MEPROBAMATE (MILTOWN)
C)   BOTH
D)   NEITHER


BC4AK   54 1.45    100              ANTICANCER AGENTS       6020
ALLERGIC REACTIONS TO DRUGS ARE NOT AMENABLE TO TREAT-
MENT WITH CYTOTOXIC DRUGS (SUCH AS AKLATING AGENTS OR
ANTIMETABOLITES) BECAUSE ALLERGIC REACTIONS DEPEND ON
PREFORMED ANTIBODIES.


X06AN   37 3.03    97               METALS                  2593
LEAD POISONING COMMONLY PRODUCES SYMPTOMS INDICATIVE OF
INVOLVEMENT OF THE
1)   GASTROINTESTINAL TRACT
2)   NEUROMUSCULAR SYSTEM
3)   CENTRAL NERVOUS SYTEM
4)   SKELETAL SYSTEM


AD488   49 1.16    121              SULFONAMIDES            2966
(A)  BILIARY EXCRETION OF SULFONAMIDES
(B)  RENAL EXRETION OF SULFONAMIDES
```

Figure 1. Examples of questions from pharmacology test-item file. Information contained in the first line of each question includes: source of the question, question type, major category, answer and minor category, per cent of students choosing correct answer, discrimination factor and number of students encountering this question, the name of the minor category and the unique question number.

the computer can be used to print all of these; however, in most cases the final versions of the exam are run on multilith paper or in a form that is suitable for reproduction or subsequent printing. In those cases in which graphs or figures are required in the exam, these are added before the exam is duplicated or printed. A sample of a page from one of these exams is shown in Figure 2.

In the medical school pharmacology course at the University of Kansas, we

```
                              6  EXAM 51053

*   FOR EACH OF THE FOLLOWING MULTIPLE CHOICE QUESTIONS, CHOOSE    *
*   THE MOST APPROPRIATE ANSWER.                                   *
********************************************************************

   26  WHICH OF THE FOLLOWING STATEMENTS CONCERNING PENICILLIN AND
       ITS SEMISYNTHETIC DERIVATIVES IS FALSE?
       A)  ACID RESISTANT PENICILLINS ARE COMMONLY GIVEN BY
           THE ORAL ROUTE
       B)  PENICILLINASE RESISTANT PENICILLINS ARE USEFUL IN THE
           TREATMENT OF PENICILLIN RESISTANT STAPHYLOCOCCAL INFEC-
           TIONS
       C)  LONG-ACTING PENICILLINS ARE LESS ALLERGENIC THAN
           PENICILLIN-G
       D)  PENICILLINS ARE USUALLY ELIMINATED FROM THE BODY BY
           TUBULAR SECRETION
       E)  NONE OF THE ABOVE

   27  A MAJOR DISADVANTAGE TO THE DETERGENT TYPE OF ANTISEPTICS IS
       THAT
       A)  THEY REDUCE SURFACE TENSION
       B)  THEY ARE HIGHLY TOXIC TO WOUND SURFACES
       C)  THEY CAUSE SURGICAL INSTRUMENT TO RUST
       D)  THEY ARE INACTIVATED IN ACID SOLUTIONS
       E)  THEY CAUSE HYPER-SENSITIVITY

   28  USED SYSTEMICALLY FOR DERMATOMYCOSIS TREATMENT
       A)  GRISEOFULVIN
       B)  AMPHOTERICIN
       C)  NYSTATIN
       D)  TOLNAFTATE (TINACTIN)
       E)  DEMECLOCYCLINE

   29  EFFECTIVE ANTIFUNGAL AGENT IN THE TREATMENT OF RINGWORM OF
       SKIN AND NAILS
       A)  AMPHOTERICIN B
       B)  NYSTATIN
       C)  NEOMYCIN
       D)  GRISEOFULVIN
       E)  BACITRACIN

   30  SULFISOXAZOLE
       A)  INHIBITS PROTEIN SYNTHESIS
       B)  INHIBITS NUCLEIC ACID SYNTHESIS
       C)  INHIBITS CELL WALL SYNTHESIS
       D)  IS A NEUROMUSCULAR BLOCKER
       E)  INHIBITS FOLIC ACID SYNTHESIS
```

Figure 2. Sample page from a computer-generated student exam.

offer examinations containing 100 questions in each of the 5 units of the pharmacology course at weekly intervals throughout the 20-week teaching period, and the advantages of the large pharmacology question file and the computer-generated exam system in meeting this task are obvious.

Exam Grading and Evaluation

This portion of the CMI system includes a number of programs that print the student answer sheet, machine score the examinations, write a diagnostic letter to the student, print an exam evaluation for the faculty, and carry out the associated statistical evaluation and appropriate record keeping. Each student who registers in one of the pharmacology courses is given a packet of Phelix cards (Figure 3) that are prepunched with the student name, number, mail box number, course number, and section. Whenever the student wishes to take an examination, he submits one of these Phelix cards, on which is indicated the unit in which he wishes to take the exam and the date for the exam. Program VS-25 then uses these cards to preprint the optical scanning answer sheets with the information from the Phelix card plus any comments or information which the unit staff wishes to give to the individual

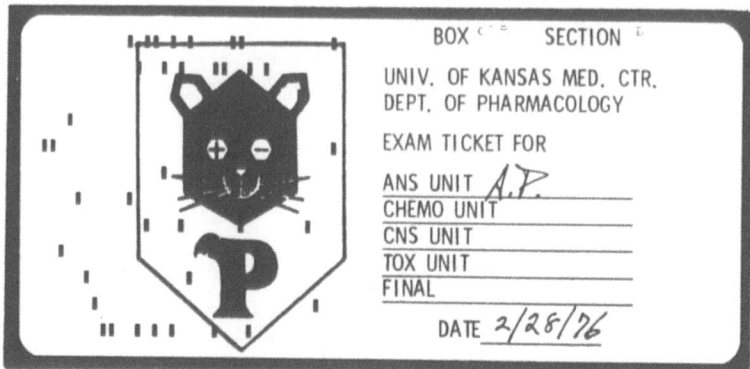

Figure 3. "Phelix card" used by students to register for exams in each unit and used by computer to print answer sheet for each student.

student. An example of an examination sheet is shown in Figure 4, where it can be seen that space is also provided for a student's signature which is used, together with student photographs, to ensure that the correct student has actually taken the exam.

Machine scoring of the answer sheets is accomplished in our institution by means of an OpScan 17 that can be linked to a keypunch to provide card output or operated directly on-line to the computer. If there are only a few exams to be graded, we use an abbreviated grading program (VS-40) in which the OpScan data are evaluated and the results transmitted to an IBM 2741 typewriter, which is located in the student testing area. In most cases, however, the information from the OpScan 17, together with the exam decks generated by VS-10 and the student master record tapes, are used as input for a series of programs that generate the student letters, prepare the evaluation for the unit chairmen, and the grading reports for the test system chairman. A list of the LR (learning resource) programs that are used to support the exam-grading and -analysis system is shown in Table 5 and a flow chart for the interaction of these programs is shown in Figure 5. Samples of the student letter output generated by the LR system is shown in Figure 6, and it can be seen that in addition to indicating the exam grade and the questions that were missed on the exam, this letter also provides diagnostic information for each student on his areas of weakness in the material covered by that exam. The letter also tells the student how much of the course he has completed. Similar letters are sent weekly to those students who do not take an examination in order to remind them of their progress in the course. The LR program evaluation for the unit chairmen faculty includes an item analysis of the questions used on the test (difficulty, discrimination factors, etc.), a listing of the number of students who performed poorly in each of the various segments of the unit (Figure 7), and a listing of all of the students who have obtained grades of superior, satisfactory, or unsatisfactory in the unit plus those who have not yet taken any examinations in that unit (Figure 8). The statistical information from this report (number of students, difficulty index and discrimination factor, etc.) is tabulated after each exam in

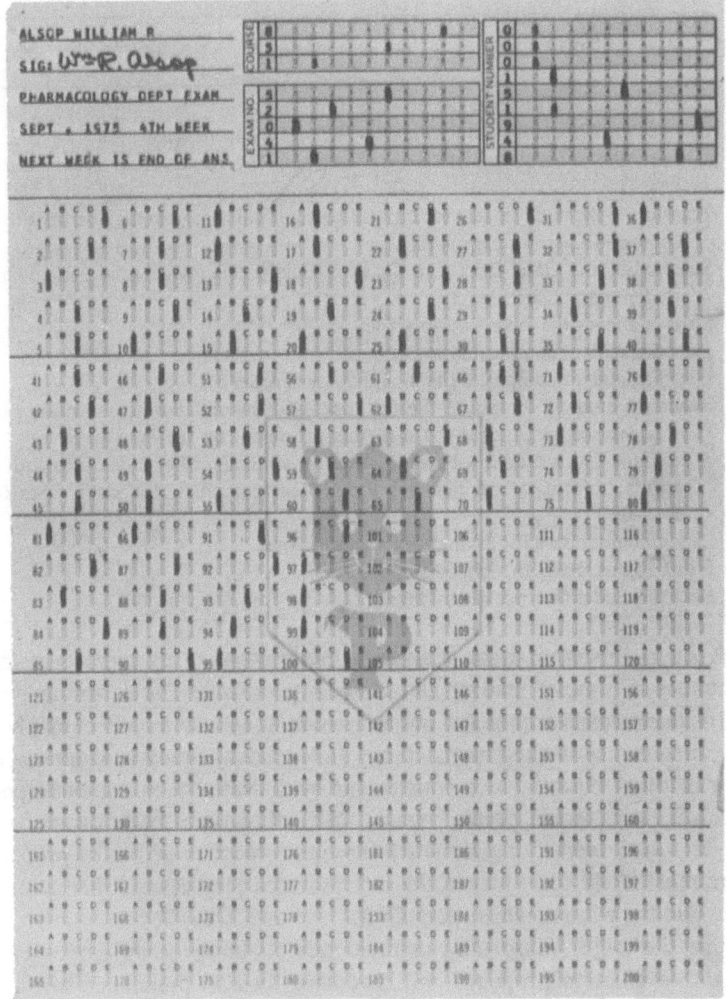

Figure 4. OpScan student answer sheet (ready for machine scoring).

either card or tape format in a form that is suitable for input to the exam-question file. Finally, the LR programs generate a test chairman's report which is a current summary of the weekly performance of each student in the course, and an example of this is shown in Figure 9. At the end of the course, or sooner if required, the LR programs will also prepare various types of summaries of student performance, test question usage, and other types of information obtained from the student master tape and the appropriate card decks.

In addition to the LR grading system described above, various other types of grading and evaluation programs are available and used in some of the pharmacology courses and in the grading programs of other departments. These include the

Table 5. CATS-CMI LR Programs

Program	Description
LR-60	Creates the student master file on tape from cards
LR-61	Updates or corrects the student master file on tape from cards
LR-62	Updates the student master file on tape with the results from processing student tests (LR-70)
LR-69	Transfers OpScan-CICS records on disk to tape. This program may be used to backup OpScan-CICS transmission failures
LR-70	Fuses/edits the data from the OpScan/backup tape/cards into a single file, the student composite file
LR-71	Edits and loads the exam category file
LR-72	Lists the student composite file
LR-73	Lists the student composite file in alphabetical order
LR-74	Reads the student composite file (on disk) and the updated student master tape and creates a sorted file on disk for further processing by LR-75
LR-75	A program that writes unit-based analysis for a number of examinations with student results; reformats and punches the student composite file onto cards for later analysis
LR-76	Lists student letters for a variety of examinations
LR-77	Prints absent letters in alphabetical order
LR-78	Lists the student master file on tape

revised Kocher—Oosterhof item analysis, a modified point by serial type analysis, and a number of simpler grading and analysis programs. The Learning Resource Division of this medical school also has a program underway to collect and compare data on performance in the Pharmacology Independent Study programs with performance in other basic science courses and with National Board exam performance, MCAT scores, grade point averages, and other types of information which may be useful in identifying some of the characteristics in health professionals which are most likely to influence the rate at which they achieve their educational objectives and the ways in which they do so.

Many of the CATS Consortium member schools have locally developed exam-grading and -evaluation programs and have used these in preference to the LR or other systems. In other cases, CATS Consortium members have modified the LR programs to fit their local requirements. At the University of Hawaii, for example, the LR programs have been rewritten so that they can be used on a minicomputer that is under departmental control. However, even in those schools in which the use of the LR system has been patterned after the use at Kansas, the actual system in use is usually substantially different than that employed here.

To summarize the CATS-CMI section on this chapter, several observations can be made.

1. The CMI is the most attractive, or at least useful, part of the CATS system since all of the CATS Consortium members, with the exception of PLATO at the University of Illinois, use the CMI portion of CATS.

2. The CMI is the least expensive part of CATS to implement since the entire system can be operated in batch mode and the storage costs can be minimized by using tapes or removable disk packages.

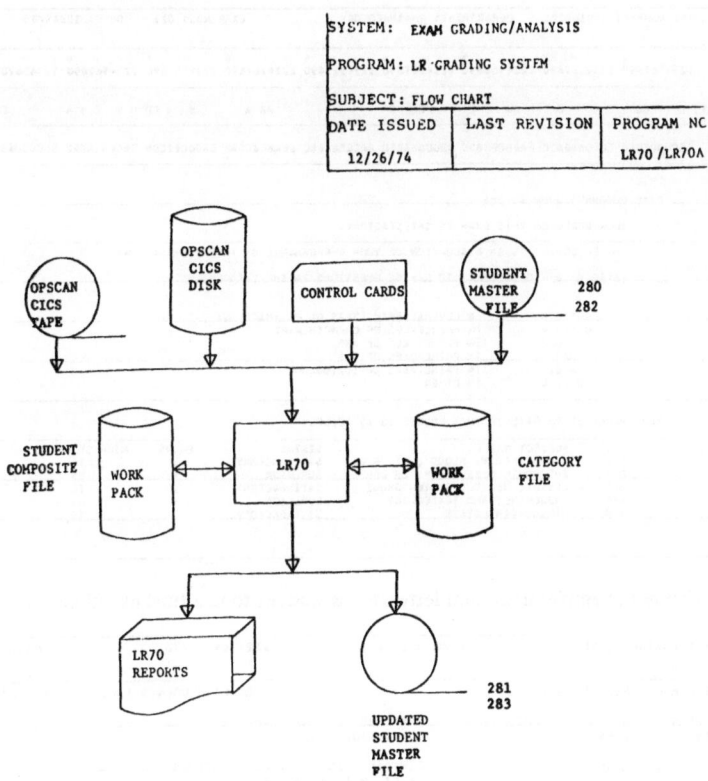

Figure 5. Flow chart for LR programs (exam grading and evaluation system).

3. Since the CMI system is written in standard COBOL, it is transportable to virtually any computer system.

4. The CATS-CMI programs can be used to create, support, and maintain question banks and to grade and evaluate examinations in disciplines other than pharmacology.

5. Although the pharmacology test-question bank was created to support medical student pharmacology teaching, it has proven to be equally useful with other groups of health professionals.

6. Since the pharmacology question file represents a rather widespread concensus of the material that pharmacologists feel should be included in a pharmacology course, this question file provides a useful yardstick for individual schools to evaluate both the content of their courses and the quality of their teaching.

CATS Computer-Assisted Instruction

The CATS-CAI system was developed initially by Professor Stata Norton of the Department of Pharmacology at the University of Kansas to serve as an enrichment or adjunct to the medical student pharmacology course. Since there were only a

```
STUDENT NUMBER: 000168225    DEPARTMENT: PHARMACOLOGY          EXAM NO.: 021    DATE: 12/19/75    GRADE: 078
```

```
              1          2          3          4          5          6          7          8          9         10
        1234567890 1234567890 1234567890 1234567890 1234567890 1234567890 1234567890 1234567890 1234567890 1234567890
```

```
CORRECT   D   BC        D    DA    E     E    B              AB  A        B  A BD D B  C B A            C
ANSWERS
```

```
YOUR       AEDDDDEFRB EDEDAABACC EABBCEDBBD ADDDDDBAEED BACCBBABEC EEABCBDDBB BADDCEECDB CBCCBEAEAE BBDDDDABAB DDDAABACAB
ANSWERS
```

```
        DEAR WOODHAMS JOHN T  366

            YOUR GRADE ON THIS EXAM IS SATISFACTORY.

            THE FOLLOWING IS AN EVALUATION OF YOUR PERFORMANCE ON THIS EXAMINATION:

            RATIO OF NBR OF CORRECT TO NBR OF QUESTIONS IN THE CATAGORY.

                005/010      IN GENERAL PRINCIPLES OF PHARMACOLOGY
                021/024      IN PRINCIPLES OF CHEMOTHERAPY
                020/022      IN PRINCIPLES OF ANS
                016/022      IN PRINCIPLES OF CNS
                016/022      IN PRINCIPLES OF TOXICOLOGY
                000/000      IN OTHER

        YOUR PROGRESS TO DATE IN THIS COURSE IS AS FOLLOWS:

            UNIT   SUBJECT MATTER                       STATUS         EXAMS   HIGHEST GRADE
            1-6    CHEMOTHERAPY, BLOOD & GI DRUGS        SATISFACTORY     2         71
            2-7    AUTONOMIC NERVOUS SYSTEM DRUGS        SUPERIOR         4         85
            3-8    CENTRAL NERVOUS SYSTEM DRUGS          SATISFACTORY     2         78
            4-9    ENDOCRINES AND TOXICOLOGY             SUPERIOR         4         80
            5-0    FINAL EXAMINATION                     SATISFACTORY     1         78
```

Figure 6. Sample of student letter. (This student took a final examination.)

```
UNIT CHAIRMANS REPORT              EXAM NO.: 151          DATE: 04/08/76               PAGE   6
```

```
STUDENT PERFORMANCE BY CATEGORY                          NO. OF STUDENTS TAKING EXAM:  23
```

NO. OF WEAK STUDENTS	NO. OF QUES.	CAT.-SYM.	CATEGORY-CONTENTS/NAME & CAT.-GROUPING.
8	10	A	GENERAL PRINCIPLES OF CHEMOTHERAPY 4A 8A 8B 8C 8D 8E 8F 8G 8H
17	10	B	SULFONAMIDES AND ANTISEPTICS 4B 4C
17	16	C	PENICILLIN AND GRAM & ANTIBIOTICS 4D 4E
15	9	D	TB, LEPROSY AND GRAM – ANTIBIOTICS 4F 4G 4H
11	10	E	BROAD SPECTRUM AND ANTIFUNGAL AGENTS 4I 4J
12	15	F	ANTICANCER AND ANTIVIRAL AGENTS 4K 4L
18	10	G	ANTIPROTOZOAN AND ANTIHELMINTIC DRUGS 4M 4N 4P
8	10	H	BLOOD DRUGS AND ANTICOAGULANTS 5A 5B
13	9	I	GI DRUGS, VITAMINS AND ANTILIPID AGENTS 5C 5D 5E 5F
16	1	J	OTHER Ħ

```
                151                          MEAN: 62.56     SD: 13.26    RANGE: 41 TO 84
```

Figure 7. Sample of student performance data from unit faculty report. The number of weak students is the number of students failing to achieve a grade of 71 on this exam in the chemotherapy unit. Eighty-six students took this exam.

```
UNIT CHAIRMANS REPORT    EXAM NO.: 152    DATE: 04/08/76    MEAN: 58.62    SD: 10.10    RANGE: 40 TO 75         PAGE 7

  PERFORMANCE ANALYSIS BY HIGHEST-SCORE IN THIS UNIT:
  NO.-OF-EXAMS / HIGHEST-GRADE / NAME.

SUPERIOR IN THIS UNIT      SATISFACTORY IN THIS UNIT      UNSATISFACTORY IN THIS UNIT    INCOMPLETE IN THIS UNIT

01 087 DILLON  STEVEN C 054  01 074 ALLEN   MARK J   001   02 070 ALVERIO NELSON MO03    ALLRED  CHARLES  T002
01 084 DREILING ROGER JO58   01 072 COCK   BRUCE A   060   01 062 ARNOLD  PAUL N   005    ANDES   ELIZABETH 004
01 094 GILLAN DALE F JR069   01 075 GAY   RICHARD G JR067  01 064 HERRY   SUSAN A   015    APPIGHI DAVID A  006
02 083 WILSON JOHN A   208   01 073 GRENCH LAWRENCE  073   01 057 BILLINGTON CHARLO16    ATWOOD  STEVEN D 007
                             01 073 HALLERAN WILLIAM078     01 043 BLANK   ELLEN L   017    BAKER   DARRELL L 008
                             01 071 LAFFERTY WILLIAM103     01 064 BCREL   TERRY C   022    BALFS   DENNY L  009
                             01 072 MAYER  FRANK E   123     01 052 BRAMBLE JOHN W   028    BARCLAY PAULA J  010
                             01 074 SHFADER CHARLES  176     01 053 CONAN   JOHN H    043    BARNARD WILLIAM  011
                             02 079 SMITH  MICHAEL G 180     01 061 DAVIS   SCOTT H   049    BELL    RANDALL C 012
                             01 073 WEAGER JONELL    209     01 063 DEMOTT  JOHN D JR052     BENNETT RICHARD  013
                                                            01 065 GARNER WARREN L  066    BERNASEK ROBERT  014
                                                            01 053 GRAHAM RAPNEY S  071    BLUM    CAROL A  018
                                                            01 041 GRENE  ROBERT R  074    BODEMANN MICHAEL019
                                                            01 040 HALL   ERNEST B JR077    BOEHM   MINDY    020
                                                            01 047 HARTUNG TORY J   080    BOHO    GREGORY L 021
                                                            01 047 HENRY  CLARKE L  084    BOSSEMEYER CHARLO23
                                                            01 045 HUSTEAD RUSSELL  089    BOWLER  LARRY D  024
                                                            01 049 JACKSON WARREN K093     BOWLER  ULYSSES S025
                                                            01 062 JAKOWATZ JAMES G094     BOWLUS  THOMAS L 026
                                                            01 061 MCLAUGHLIN PEGGY130     BUXBERGER GREGORO27
                                                            01 054 MORITZ CARL A   138     BRUWN   JAMES O  029
                                                            01 046 NOHINEK BARBARA 145     BROWN   SCOTT S  030
                                                            01 063 O'BRIEN JOHN L   147     BROWNING JIMMIE  031
                                                            01 050 PIERSALL GEORGE  152     BURGE   G WAYNE  032
```

Figure 8. Sample of student distribution section of unit faculty report: lists number of exams taken by each student in this unit, highest grade, and status in the unit.

few programs available during the first 2 years, these programs were first used in a pilot fashion to evaluate student acceptance of this mode of teaching and the effectiveness of the CAI programs as teaching tools in pharmacology. Although the use of the CAI programs was optional during this period, 98% of the students ran all of the programs and virtually all of the students were enthusiastically in favor of expanding this teaching approach. Further, by comparing student performance on exam questions covering material that had been included in CAI programs with performance on exam questions covering material that was not included in the CAI programs, Dr. Norton was able to demonstrate a significant increase in student performance in both of the units of the pharmacology course for which CAI material was available (Norton *et al.*, 1972). Some of the data which Dr. Norton has presented elsewhere in support of this conclusion is reproduced in Table 6, where it can be seen that the use of CAI increased student performance by 4% in the autonomic nervous system unit examinations and by 13% in the central nervous system unit examinations. Using a similar approach, she also evaluated the ability of the different CAI programs to teach, and the results of these studies are shown in Table 7. It can be seen that the programs differed appreciably in their apparent ability to teach pharmacology and that, whereas seven of the nine programs increased student performance, two of these programs actually decreased student performance on the pharmacology unit exams. Encouraged by these studies and the positive

```
LXTAJUG4              TEST CHAIRMAN'S REPORT                          12/22/75   PAGE   2

STUDENT NAME        STUDENT ID  1/15  2/16  3/17  4/18  5/19  6/20  7/21  8/22  9/23  10/24 11/25 12/26 13/27 14/28
                                /29   /30   /31   /32   /33   /34   /35   /36   /37   /38   /39   /40

ARTHUR DOUGLAS R  240  000142989  ABSENT ABSENT ABSENT ABSENT ABSENT 223051 232071 ABSENT 252069 ABSENT ABSENT 342053 362078 121065
                                   102072 472061 481073 081077 ABSENT ABSENT ABSENT ABSENT ABSENT        LAB085

AUSTER PAUL F     241  000225271  ABSENT ABSENT ABSENT ABSENT ABSENT 222040 231064 243063 252075 ABSENT 311053 342080 ABSENT 122043
                                   102064 112074 ABSENT 491072 092064 ABSENT 001072 ABSENT ABSENT        LAB087

HANNAN PATRICK S  242  000126707  642050 ABSENT ABSENT 662062 ABSENT ABSENT 231069 243076 321074 121076 421071 ABSENT 031376 211070
                                   ABSENT ABSENT ABSENT ABSENT ABSENT ABSENT ABSENT ABSENT ABSENT        LAB091
                                   ACV085 SATIS

BRANDENBERGER WM  594  000225272  ABSENT ABSENT ABSENT ABSENT ABSENT ABSENT 232044 242056 251063 261079 ABSENT 342050 362058 371068
                                   381072 111046 162055 191075 402044 441053 451072 012071 ABSENT        LAB082

BRIAR DAVID K     243  000144835  ABSENT ABSENT ABSENT ABSENT ABSENT 223067 231071 ABSENT 321050 352065 313060 342071 ABSENT 122057
                                   101071 ABSENT ABSENT 492071 092064 ABSENT 002072 ABSENT ABSENT        LAB090

BRICKMAN M DOUGLAS 244 000225675  642066 ABSENT ABSENT ABSENT 211054 222072 331056 ABSENT 321069 353068 312070 141076 441075 041065
                                   051072 ABSENT ABSENT ABSENT ABSENT ABSENT ABSENT ABSENT ABSENT        LAB073

BROWN SHARON           000225473  631081 441084 431071 421066 411064 CHEMUA TOX-A- ABSENT ABSENT ABSENT ABSENT ABSENT ABSENT ABSENT
                                   ABSENT ABSENT ABSENT ABSENT ABSENT ABSENT ABSENT ABSENT ABSENT

BRUNFELDT JOAN K  245  000142130  641072 211058 ABSENT ABSENT 211056 223074 ABSENT ABSENT 322073 ABSENT 421075 ABSENT ABSENT 452063
                                   101076 061077 ABSENT ABSENT ABSENT ABSENT ABSENT ABSENT ABSENT        LAB090
                                   ADV092 SUPER

BUCHNER DAVID M   246  000225275  ABSENT 651051 ABSENT 662077 211047 221080 331072 ABSENT 951080 ABSENT 312064 141080 031074 ABSENT
                                   ABSENT 061079 ABSENT ABSENT ABSENT ABSENT ABSENT ABSENT        ORAL86 LAB096              SUPER
                                   ADV089 SUPER

BUDD GEORGE T     247  000141641  641052 ABSENT ABSENT ABSENT ABSENT 222076 331065 ABSENT 322074 ABSENT 131064 141071 441076 ABSENT
                                   051069 061076 ABSENT ABSENT ABSENT ABSENT ABSENT ABSENT ABSENT        LAB080
                                   ADV088 SUPER

BUESING RUSSELL   248  000143170  ABSENT 652074 ABSENT 222079 ABSENT ABSENT ABSENT ABSENT ABSENT ABSENT ABSENT ABSENT 362083 ABSENT
                                   ABSENT ABSENT ABSENT 491066 401076 ABSENT 001079 ABSENT ABSENT        LAB080

BUKATS TERRY      249  000225125  ABSENT ABSENT ABSENT ABSENT 211044 ABSENT 232062 241053 251062 261073 ABSENT 341057 361075 121030
                                   ABSENT 111074 ABSENT 491074 091060 ABSENT 002064 011073 ABSENT        LAB080

BUTTERFIELD MARI  250  000225126  ABSENT 652072 671083 ABSENT 212061 223070 231083 ABSENT ABSENT ABSENT 351077 ABSENT ABSENT 441083 371087
                                   ABSENT 061081 ABSENT ABSENT ABSENT ABSENT ABSENT ABSENT        ORAL89 LAB085              SUPER
```

Figure 9. Sample of a section of the weekly grading report for the medical student pharmacology course. Includes number and grade of each exam taken and the laboratory grade. Also includes oral exam grade for students seeking a superior grade in the course.

student response to our CAI programs, a major effort was undertaken to expand the number of programs available for these units and to develop additional CAI programs for the rest of the pharmacology course. At the present time, the CATS-CAI pharmacology system contains over 120 programs, and it is anticipated that the system will grow even more rapidly as the faculty of the other pharmacology departments in the CATS Consortium begin to participate in the development of new course material.

Type of Programs

There are three types of CAI programs available in the CATS system. These are designated as self-instruction, case history, and review-question programs. The self-instruction programs are intended to be used by the students in much the same way that textbooks and lectures are used to acquire knowledge, and each CAI course is roughly equivalent to a lecture on one topic, such as cholinergic mechanisms or antihypertensives. The format of the self-instruction CAI course is similar to that of a programmed text in that the computer presents text or didactic information and then asks the student a series of questions. Depending on the

Table 6. Effect of CAI on Student Performance in Unit Examinations

Questions	Right	Wrong	Total
ANS Pharmacology (Unit I)			
In CAI	5,173	2,110	7,283
Not in CAI	13,811	6,706	20,517
Total	18,984	8,816	27,800

Percent of exam questions in CAI: 26%
Percent of correct answers on exam questions in CAI: 71%
Percent of correct answers on exam questions not in CAI: 67%
Chi square for Unit I data: 34.065; P = <.01

CNS Pharmacology (Unit II)			
In CAI	7,528	1,747	9,275
Not in CAI	9,012	4,213	13,225
Total	16,540	5,960	22,500

Percent of exam questions in CAI: 41%
Percent of correct answers on exam questions in CAI: 81%
Percent of correct answers on exam questions not in CAI: 68%
Chi square for Unit II data: 447.205; P = <.001

student response, the computer may branch to a simpler or remedial section of the program or continue with the regular program, or jump ahead to a more difficult section of the CAI lesson. Some of the programs of this type contain both a pre- and a posttest that can be used to evaluate the effectiveness of the program in imparting information. The complexity of the branching decisions used in this type of program is, in part, dependent on the educational objectives of the instructor

Table 7. Evaluation of Individual CAI Programs

	Performance on exam questions with information in a CAI program			Performance on all other exam questions		
	Right answers	Total questions	Percent right	Right answers	Total questions	Percent right
ANS Unit Programs						
PH-02 Review questions	426	760	56	18558	27040	69
PH-03 Self-instruction	430	597	72	18554	27203	68
PH-04 Case history	1203	1678	72	17781	26122	68
PH-07 Review questions	3114	4248	73	15870	23552	67
CNS Unit Programs						
PH-01 Self-instruction	1743	2057	85	14797	20443	72
PH-06 Review questions	2576	3245	79	13964	19255	72
PH-07 Review questions	2374	2870	83	14166	19630	72
PH-10 Review questions	675	792	85	15865	21708	73
PH-11 Case history	160	311	52	16380	22189	74

writing the program, but is also heavily dependent on the skill of the instructor in devising ways to utilize the more sophisticated branching logic in constructing such programs.

The second type of CAI program is the case history or simulated patient encounter. In general, these case history programs are based on actual therapeutic or toxicologic problems that have been encountered in our emergency room or in one of the clinical services. These programs are primarily problem-solving exercises and are intended for use by students who already have some mastery of a topic. Although the general format is the same as with the self-instruction programs, the case history programs utilize more sophisticated logic and permit greater flexibility in response. In some of these programs, the computer starts a clock at a critical point in the program to stimulate a greater sense of urgency in the student response. In one of our toxicology cases, for example, the student can "kill" a patient in six ways but can only "save" him in one. One difference in this case between the computer simulation and the emergency room situation is that students who "kill" the patient are given a second chance to "save" him by the computer. The third type of program in the CATS-CAI system is the review-questions program. The logic for these is relatively simple (question → response → text → question → response → text, etc.). There is little or no branching, but the computer does keep track of the student's performance and gives him a score and evaluation at the end of each section.

Initially, all of the CAI programs in the CATS system were written by staff members in their areas of expertise. For example, a staff member responsible for lecturing on analgesia might write a program on the pharmacology and therapeutic uses of morphine or write a case history that involved the use of analgesics. The programs are written in English with questions and appropriate responses for both correct and incorrect answers interspersed with the text. The English version of the program is then coded into the COURSEWRITER III format by support personnel in the Learning Resources facility and placed in a test area of the computer for subsequent revision and updating by the author. Some authors prefer to learn the COURSEWRITER commands and do their own programming but most do not and would, in fact, regard a requirement to learn any time-sharing language as an unreasonable restriction and inefficient use of faculty time. During the early development of this CAI system, we used a locally produced CAI driver that was written specifically for the pharmacology CAI programs by C. Allen and is, therefore, smaller, simpler, and less expensive than COURSEWRITER III. Our decision to switch to a vendor-supported time-sharing language was made primarily to facilitate the maintenance of the system by computer services personnel. However, the original KUCAI driver is still used by one of the CATS Consortium members with apparently satisfactory results. During the past 2 years, we have also treated the possibility of having students write CAI programs, and we now have four programs that were written by medical students with varying amounts of faculty consultation. The rewards to the student for this effort include: (1) credit toward a medical school requirement to demonstrate writing skills prior to graduation, (2) the knowledge that their program will aid future classes to learn pharmacology, and (3) a token cash award.

As mentioned previously, we are currently in the process of developing a new CAI package that can be used as an on-line pharmacology syllabus or a drug information file. This file would contain concise statements about the history, chemistry, pharmacokinetics, efficacy, adverse effects, and therapeutic usage of a large number of drugs, and this information would be categorized in a way that would enable the user to search the file to obtain pharmacological information about a specific drug or to compare a specific pharmacologic characteristic, such as biliary excretion, within a class of drugs. With appropriate coding it will be possible to use this file to obtain therapeutic recommendations for specific diseases as well as recommended dosage regimes and adverse-reaction possibilities for each type of therapy. The major use of this new CAI option as a teaching tool will result from linking it with the pharmacology test-question file. In this combined system, a student who wishes to review his knowledge in a specific area of pharmacology would ask the computer to select questions from that portion of the exam bank. If the student is unable to provide the right answer for a question, the computer will then display the appropriate text from the syllabus or drug information file containing the answer to the question. In most CAI review-question programs the computer simply tells the student whether his answer is correct or incorrect and in some cases adds an appropriate comment. Our purpose in developing this new system (CAI-PASS) is to force the student to search out the correct answer from appropriate reference material in the hope that this effort will result in better retention.

Use of CAI

Student usage of each of the three types of programs depends somewhat on the level of training. Medical students in the pharmacology course use the self-instructional programs most heavily during the early part of each unit, whereas they use the review-question program most extensively just before taking exams in each unit. Medical students tend to use the case history programs less frequently and often will run these program as a kind of relaxation. House staff and practicing physicians, on the other hand, take the case history programs very seriously and will, in fact, become physically agitated when a case they are treating on the computer begins to "go sour." Since all of our CAI programs were designed initially to be used by sophomore medical students, it was anticipated that these programs would not be suitable for teaching pharmacology to nursing students, graduate students, or other groups. Our experience has demonstrated, however, that this is not the case and that almost all of the programs can be effectively used to teach pharmacology to any group of health professionals and that the programs are even useful for individuals who have what we would consider to be an inadequate background in biology and chemistry.

The CATS-CAI system is operated at the University of Kansas Medical School under the control of COURSEWRITER III, an IBM time-sharing program that occupies one of the five partitions in our IBM 370/158. A second partition is occupied by the IBM CICS/VS on-line system, which supports an extensive hospital information system that includes on-line programs for patient interviewing, pharmacy control, medical records, patient histories, tumor registry, etc. There are twelve IBM 3270 CRT terminals available for student use of the CAI programs daily from 8:00 A.M. to 12:00 P.M. We are considering combining COURSEWRITER III and CICS to enable our students to utilize some of the 60 additional terminals that are now dedicated to the hospital information system. Student usage of CATS-CAI averages about 60,000 cpu seconds per month, and although this usage varies greatly throughout the year, the response time only rarely exceeds 3 seconds and is generally less than 1 second.

There are currently over 800 students registered in the KUCAI system, and these include, in addition to the 200 medical students and 100 nursing students from the current classes, an equal number of students from previous classes who are continuing to utilize the system. The remaining 200 students include medical technicians, physical therapy technicians, respiratory therapy technicians, emergency medical training technicians, hearing and speech students, X-ray technicians, hospital pharmacists, interns and residents in several clinical areas, and graduate students in the Master's nursing program and in the basic science disciplines. Our system also has three "dial-up" TTY ports that are used by physicians, nurses, and other health professionals to access the CAI programs from outside of the institution. It is anticipated that the CAI usage by outside users will markedly increase in the future as a result of the recent adoption of a statewide Centrex telephone system which will significantly reduce communication costs for many of these users. The CAI system can also be accessed remotely with an IBM 2741 typewriter or comparable equipment, and we have a few outside users who employ this option. The main advantage of the typewriter terminal is that it provides the user with hard copy. Although some of our students would prefer to use the typewriter terminal to obtain hard copy for subsequent study, we actively discourage this practice since we feel that it obviates the interactive characteristic of CAI learning.

To illustrate how the student encounters the CAI programs in the Kansas system, hard copy printouts representative of 3270 screen images are presented in Figures 10 through 13. Figure 10a shows the KUCAI menu which is a list of the CAI courses available to all of the different health professional groups in our institution. If the student wishes to study pharmacology and types PHARM, the computer then shows him the pharmacology menu (Figure 10b) that lists the five units available in the pharmacology course. If he then selects the ANS unit, he is provided with a listing of the courses available in that unit (Figure 11a). It can be seen here that the KUCAI package also contains courses in Spanish, French, and German. These translations have been carried out primarily to demonstrate the CATS-CAI system to pharmacologists in other countries. The course listing for the General Pharmacology unit (Figure 10c), the CNS unit (Figure 11b), the Chemotherapy unit (Figure 12a), the Toxicology–Endocrinology unit (Figure 12b) and

```
DUULL    04/20/76   15.27.37

                   THE FOLLOWING COURSES ARE AVAILABLE ON KUCAI:
         ANATOMY (ANAT)            EMERG. MED. TECH (EMT)
         BIOCHEMISTRY (BIOCHM)     HEARING AND SPEECH (HS)
         MICROBIOLOGY (MICRO)      MEDICAL TECHNOLOGY (MTECH)
         NEUROLOGY (NEURO)         RESPIRATORY THERAPY (RTHRPY)
         NURSING (NURSE)           RHEUMATOLOGY (RHEUM)
         PATHOLOGY (PATH)          X-RAY TECHNOLOGY (XRAY)
         PHARMACOLOGY (PHARM)      CHEMISTRY REVIEW (CHEM)
         PHYSIOLOGY (PHYS)         CAI FOR AUTHORS (CAICWR)
         PHYSICAL DIAGNOSIS (CASE) STATISTICS (STAT)
         FUN AND GAMES (GAME)      COBOL (COBOL)


         (HIGH INTENSITY MEANS THE COURSE IS AVAILABLE)

         PLEASE ENTER THE CODE-WORD FCR THE COURSE YOU WISH TO RUN

         (TO REVIEW HOW TC USE THE SYSTEM, TYPE REVIEW)



         THE UNITS AVAILABLE IN PHARM ARE:
         GEN--GENERAL PRINCIPLES
         ANS--AUTONOMICS AND CARDIOVASCULAR
         CNS--CENTRAL NERVOUS SYSTEM
         CHEMO--CHEMOTHERAPY
         TOX--TOXICOLOGY AND ENDOCRINOLOGY
         EXAM--THE CHEMO EXAM GIVEN 4/3/76 IS NOW UP (NO HARDCOPY)

         PLEASE ENTER THE UNIT YOU WOULD LIKE TO TAKE.



                   THE COURSES IN THE GEN UNIT INCLUDE:
         01   INTRODUCTION TO GENERAL PHARMACOLOGY
         02   PHARMACOKINETICS I
         03   PHARMACOKINETICS II
         04   FETAL PHARMACOLOGY
         05   REVIEW QUESTIONS
         90   GENERAL PRINCIPLES EXAM (NO HARDCOPY)
     PLEASE ENTER THE TWO-DIGIT NUMBER OF THE COURSE YOU WOULD LIKE TO TAKE
```

Figure 10. Hard copy printout of the IBM 3270 presentation of the KUCAI library of programs, the units in pharmacology, and the programs in the General Unit.

representative examples of course material from some of the 96 programs that are currently available in the pharmacology CAI programs (Figure 13) are shown as hard copy printouts of the IBM 3270 terminal presentation. It should be pointed out that all of the programs in our CAI system are designed to be usable on any TTY terminal as well as the IBM 3270 and that wherever special terminal characteristics such as light pen options, high–low intensity, etc. are included in the program, the instructions for these features are coded so that they do not interfere in any way with the use of the program on other terminals. For this reason, our programs make minimal use of graphics or matching-type responses since these are difficult to use effectively with regular TTY terminals. It should also be pointed out that we make every attempt in writing the CAI programs to avoid situations that require the use of supplemental material (photographs, workbooks, figures, etc.). In our experience the advantage of having all of the necessary material and information included within the actual CAI program outweighs significantly the educational enhancement that may result from the use of such supplemental forms of instruc tional material.

Several observations can be made to summarize the CATS-CAI section of this chapter.

```
        THE COURSES IN THE ANS UNIT INCLUDE:
01  AUTONOMICS I:  GENERAL                  30  TREATMENT OF CARDIAC ARRHYTHMIAS
02  AUTONOMICS II:  NEUROTRANSMITTERS        31  MANAGEMENT OF HYPERTENSION
03  AUTONOMICS III:  CHOLINERGICS            32  POISIONING FROM "HEART PREPARATIONS"
04  AUTONOMICS IV:  ADRENERGICS                  IN THE HOME MEDICINE CHEST
05  AUTONOMICS V:  REVIEW QUESTIONS          33  CARDIOLOGY REVIEW QUESTIONS
06  CASE:  UNEXPECTED DRUG REACTION          34  DIGITALIS GLYCOSIDES
07  AUTONOMIC DRUG MATCHING QUIZ             35  TREATMENT OF ANGINA
08  ANS REVIEW QUESTIONS                     90  ANS EXAM (NO HARDCOPY)
09  ARTERIAL BLOOD PRESSURE IN
    THE ANESTHETIZED DOG
20  DIURETICS INTRO:  RENAL REVIEW
21  DIURETICS:  MECHANISMS OF ACTION
22  DIURETICS:  QUIZ


91  PHARMACOLOGIE DU SYSTEME NERVEAUX AUTONOME I
92  FARMACOLOGIA DEL SISTEMA NERVIOIO AUTONOMO I
93  CHOLINERGE MECHANISMEN UND ANWENDUNGEN
PLEASE ENTER THE TWO-DIGIT NUMBER OF THE COURSE YOU WISH TO RUN


        THE COURSES IN THE CNS UNIT INCLUDE:
01  NEUROPHYSIOLOGY REVIEW                   40  CASE:  CONVULSION WITH COMA
02  REVIEW QUESTIONS                         41  ANTICONVULSANT QUIZ
03  CNS REVIEW QUESTIONS                     50  ANTIDEPRESSANT QUIZ
10  GENERAL ANESTHESIA                       90  CNS EXAM (NO HARDCOPY)
11  CASE:  GENERAL ANESTHESIA
12  LOCAL ANESTHETIC DRUGS
13  LOCAL ANESTHETIC REVIEW               PLEASE ENTER THE TWO-DIGIT NUMBER OF
14  ANESTHESIA QUIZ                         THE COURSE YOU WOULD LIKE TO TAKE
20  HYPNOTICS AND SEDATIVES
21  STIMULANTS AND HALLUCINOGENS
22  TRANQUILIZERS
30  REVIEW OF ANALGESICS
31  ANALGESIC QUIZ
```

Figure 11. Hard copy printout of the IBM 3270 presentation of the program listing for the ANS and CNS units.

1. The major educational advantage of CAI when compared to passive learning techniques such as slides, movies, videotapes, etc. is that CAI accelerates learning by forcing the student to interact with the teaching system.

2. Most of the other advantages of CAI are related to its flexibility. Our experience and that of other CATS Consortium users demonstrates that the CAI programs can be used effectively to support independent study programs in pharmacology or as enrichment for a conventionally taught course. The availability of the CAI programs at times when the staff is not available, the nonjudgmental nature of the computer response in contrast to the usual faculty response, and the patience of the computer in repeating material for student review are general attributes of CAI rather than specific attributes of the CATS-CAI system.

3. The major disadvantage of the CATS-CAI system is the difficulty of transporting the system to another medical school which does not have compatible equipment (IBM hardware with COURSEWRITER III). Although the CATS-CAI programs have been translated into TUTOR for use on the PLATO system and into CATYLIST-PHIL and GNOSIS for use on a DEC-10, it is evident that what is most needed at the present time is a "universal compiler" which would accept programs in any standard time-sharing language and provide appropriate output.

4. CAI is relatively expensive. The rental of terminals, controllers, and the dedication of computer resources amounts to over $3,000 per month in our institution. During a 4-month period in 1975, the medical student class (160

```
                 THE COURSES IN THE CHEMO UNIT INCLUDE:
   01  GENERAL CHEMOTHERAPY                 30  CHEMOTHERAPY AND MALIGNANT NEOPLASMS
   02  HEMATINICS (THERAPY IN ANEMIAS)          SOME BASIC CONCEPTS
   03  CHEMOTHERAPY REVIEW QUESTIONS        31  CHEMOTHERAPY AND MALIGNANT NEOPLASMS
   10  CASE SERIES                              DRUG MECHANISMS
   11  CONSULT 1                            32  CHEMOTHERAPY AND MALIGNANT NEOPLASMS
   12  CONSULT 1A                               TREATMENT OF SOME DISEASE STATES
   13  CONSULT 2                            40  TETRACYCLINE AND ERYTHROMYCIN QUIZ
   14  CONSULT 3                            50  SUBACUTE BACTERIAL ENDOCARDITIS
   15  CONSULT 4                            90  CHEMO EXAM (NO HARDCOPY)
   16  CONSULT 5
   20  VITAMINS I
   21  VITAMINS II




   91  CONFERER 2
   PLEASE ENTER THE TWO-DIGIT NUMBER OF THE COURSE YOU WOULD LIKE TO TAKE




                 THE COURSES IN THE TOX UNIT INCLUDE:
   01  REVIEW QUESTIONS, GENERAL TOXICOLOGY
   02  REVIEW QUESTIONS
   03  ASBESTOS
   10  TOXICOLOGY CASE I
   11  TOXICOLOGY CASE II
   20  ASPIRIN-TYPE ANALGESICS AND ANTI-INFLAMMATORY AGENTS
   21  ANTI-INFLAMMATORY QUIZ
   30  ORAL CONTRACEPTIVES
   31  THYROID AGENTS
   32  ADRENAL STEROIDS
   33  CORTICOSTEROID QUIZ
   40  INSULIN
   41  DIABETES CASE HISTORY
   99  TOX EXAM (NO HARDCOPY)
   PLEASE ENTER THE TWO-DIGIT NUMBER OF THE COURSE YOU WOULD LIKE TO TAKE
```

Figure 12. Hard copy printout of the IBM 3270 presentation of the program listing for the CHEMO and TOX-ENDO units.

students) spent 3466 hours at the CAI terminals. Excluding other student usage, this would amount to over $3 per student hour and if the other student usage during this period is included, the cost is still over $2 per student hour. While it is evident that the cost effectiveness of CAI teaching is directly related to the size of the student population involved, our experience has clearly demonstrated that it is possible for students to learn pharmacology in an independent study program at an average cost of less than $100 per student in CAI expenses.

The Use of CATS in Pharmacology Teaching

The pharmacology teaching program at the University of Kansas is based on the concept that no two students learn at the same rate or will derive the same benefit from any single educational technique. Our teaching programs are designed, therefore, to provide each student with a number of ways to learn pharmacology and they are self-paced insofar as this is possible within the scheduling limitations of the curricula. Students in the regularly scheduled courses may learn the material by attending lectures, laboratories, discussion groups, or ward rounds, or they may learn the material on their own using textbooks, the unit syllabus, and the CAI

a NOW LET'S CONSIDER THE GENERAL SYSTEMIC EFFECTS OF MORPHINE. MORPHINE
IS VERY GOOD IN CONTROLLING MANY KINDS OF PAIN BUT IT HAS SOME SERIOUS
SIDE EFFECTS. HOW DO THERAPEUTIC DOSES OF MORPHINE AFFECT RESPIRATION?
   A. INCREASE RATE AND DEPTH
   B. DECREASE RATE PRIMARILY
   C. DECREASE DEPTH PRIMARILY
   D. DECREASE BOTH RATE AND DEPTH
   D
SLOWING OF RATE IS THE PRIMARY EFFECT OF MORPHINE AND SIMILAR ANAL-
GESICS. DEPTH MAY EVEN INCREASE IF RATE SLOWS MARKEDLY. IN FATAL
DOSES BOTH RATE AND DEPTH ARE DECREASED.

IS MORPHINE USEFUL IN CONTROLLING DIARRHEA?(YES OR NO)
   YES
RIGHT YOU ARE.
MORPHINE IS THE ACTIVE INGREDIENT OF PAREGORIC, AN OLD STANDBY FOR
DIARRHEA IN INFANTS.' (IT WORKS IN ADULTS, TOO).

b ARTERIAL BLOOD PRESSURE (DIASTOLIC) IN AN ANESTHESIZED DUG

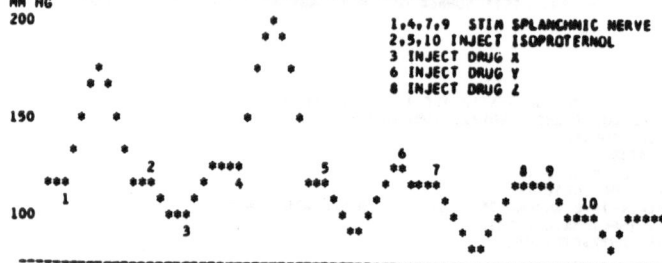

```
MN HG
200                           *
                             * *        1,4,7,9  STIM SPLANCHNIC NERVE
                                        2,5,10 INJECT ISOPROTERNOL
                   *                    3 INJECT DRUG X
                  * *                   6 INJECT DRUG Y
                 * *                    8 INJECT DRUG Z
150    *   *              *    *
          *         2   ****      5     ** 7        8 9
      ***      ***       4      ***   * ****     *****
100    1          ***                    *     10
                  ***       * *     *     *****  *****
                   3         **     * *        *
                             **           *
```

FROM THE EVIDENCE OF THE ABOVE TRACING, IS DRUG X:
A) ATROPINE; B) PROPRANOLOL; C)HEXANETHONIUM; D) PHYSIOSTIGMINE?
CORRECT. PHYSIOSTIGMINE POTENTIATES NERVE STIMULATION BY REDUCING ACH AT THE
SYNAPSE. MORE ACH CAUSES THE RELEASE OF MORE CATECHOLAMINES.
PRESS ENTER TO CONTINUE

c   CASE HISTORY: MANAGEMENT OF HYPERTENSION

   DOCTOR, WOULD YOU PLEASE HELP ME IN TREATING ONE OF
MY PATIENTS WHO COMES TO ME FOR A PHYSICAL EXAMINATION THAT HE
NEEDS FOR HIS LIFE INSURANCE. HE IS A 25-YEAR OLD BLACK MALE WHO
APPEARS TO BE IN GOOD HEALTH. I MEASURED HIS BLOOD PRESSURE WHILE
HE WAS SITTING CALMLY AND IT WAS 160/100.
WHAT SHOULD I DO NOW?
(A) BEGIN TREATMENT OF HIS HYPERTENSION.
(B) GET SOME MORE HISTORY FROM THE PATIENT.
(C) ORDER LAB TESTS.
(D) GET SOME MORE PHYSICAL FINDINGS.
(E) DO NOTHING SINCE HIS BLOOD PRESSURE ISN'T THAT
      HIGH.   E
I THINK THAT WOULD BE A SERIOUS MISTAKE, DOCTOR. IT IS CURRENTLY
ACCEPTED THAT ALL CASES OF HYPERTENSION WITH A BLOOD
PRESSURE GREATER THAN 160/95 ARE IN A GRAY AREA
IT IS NOT CLEAR WHETHER THE ADVANTAGES OF REDUCING THE
BLOOD PRESSURE OUTWEIGH THE DISADVANTAGES OF HAVING
TO TAKE POTENT DRUGS FOR A LIFETIME. AS SAFER AND BETTER
DRUGS COME OUT, THOSE PATIENTS IN THE GRAY AREA WILL
PROBABLY BE MORE OFTEN TREATED.

d THESE ARE THE DRUGS YOU HAVE   WHICH OF THESE DRUGS MOST NEARLY
       JUST STUDIED.   MATCHES THE ONE STARRED AT LEFT?
   *   1. ACETYLCHOLINE   C   A. METHOXAMINE
       2. PILOCARPINE   B. COCAINE
       3. ATROPINE   C. METHACHOLINE
       4. ISOPROTERENOL   D. NEOSTIGMINE
       5. PHENYLEPHRINE   E. PHENTOLAMINE
       6. PHYSOSTIGMINE   F. SCOPOLAMINE
       7. PROPRANOLOL   G. MECAMYLAMINE
       8. PHENOXYBENZAMINE   H. EPINEPHRINE
       9. HEXAMETHONIUM   I. DICHLORISUPROTERENOL
      10. IMIPRAMINE   J. BETHANECHOL

RIGHT, DOULL. METHACHOLINE (MECHOLYL) STIMULATES MUSCARINIC RECEPTORS AND
MIMICS THE ACTIONS OF ACETYCHOLINE. ALTHOUGH IT IS RESISTANT TO PSEUDOCHOLIN-
ESTERASE, METHACHOLINE IS SLOWLY HYDROLYZED BY TRUE ACETYLCHOLINESTERASE.

WHICH OF THE ABOVE DRUGS WOULD POTENTIATE OR PROLONG THE ACTION
OF METHACHOLINE? D
OF COURSE. NEOSTIGMINE INHIBITS THE BREAKDOWN OF METHACHOLINE.

              PRESS ENTER TO CONTINUE

```
● WHILE WE HAVE BEEN TALKING TO YOU, OUR PATIENT HAS GOTTEN
  WORSE. SHE IS NOW ATAXIC AND SAYS SHE IS "TOO TIRED TO
  STAND UP ANY MORE." SHE IS STILL CONSIOUS BUT APPEARS
  TO BE LOSING TOUCH WITH HER SURROUNDINGS. AT THIS POINT
  HER BP IS 110/70, PULSE IS 110/MIN, RESP IS 15/MIN, AND
  WE HAVE 38 DEGREES AS A RECTAL TEMPERATURE.
       DOCTOR DOULL,
  FROM HERE ON IN WE REGARD THIS GIRL AS YOUR PATIENT AND
  WILL FOLLOW YOUR INSTRUCTIONS. WHAT IS YOUR ADVICE AT THIS
  POINT?
           SEND HER HOME? (TYPE DISCHARGE)
           GET MORE HISTORY? (TYPE HISTORY)
           TREAT THE PATIENT? (TYPE TREAT)
           CONTINUE PHYSICAL EXAMINATION? (TYPE EXAM)
  WE THINK THIS GIRL IS SEVERELY POISONED AND WILL DIE IF
  NOT PROPERLY TREATED. IS YOUR MALPRACTICE INSURANCE
  PAID UP?
  PLEASE TRY ANOTHER OPTION.


f WHAT ARE YOU GOING TO DO ABOUT THE FEVER?
  SOME METHODS FOR LOWERING BODY TEMPERATURE ARE:
  A.  COOLING BLANKET.
  B.  ICE WATER BATH.
  C.  ORAL SALICYLATE
  D.  INTRAVENOUS SALICYLATE
  E.  ADMINISTER A BARBITURATE OR PHENOTHIAZINE.

  WHICH METHOD WILL YOU USE? (TYPE ONE LETTER).
  E
  THE ONSET OF ACTION IS TOO SLOW AND UNCERTAIN. WHAT IS THE MOST
  RAPID WAY?
  B
  GOOD. I HAVE PLACED HIM IN AN ICE WATER BATH FOR YOU.

  WHAT ABOUT ORAL SALICYLATE? TOO SLOW?
  YES
  RIGHT.

  IT TAKES ABOUT 30 MINUTES TO ACHIEVE AN EFFECTIVE BLOOD LEVEL.
  COULD YOU GIVE A SLOW INTRAVENOUS INJECTION OF SALICYLATE FOR
  ANTIPYRETIC ACTION.
```

Figure 13. Hard copy printout of the IBM 3270 presentation of representative CAI program material: (a) didactic (text → question → answer → response) format; (b) use of graphic information; (c) case history format; (d) matching question format with light-pen option; (e) and (f), toxicology case history.

programs and audiovisual materials, or they may request tutorial sessions with the staff. With the exception of the lectures and laboratories, all of these options are also available or can be scheduled for students enrolled in the pharmacology independent study programs (PISP). Each student can use as much or as little of the material in each of these options as he needs to achieve his objective, which is to demonstrate competence in an area of pharmacology by passing an examination over the material covered in one unit of the course.

The schedule for the medical student pharmacology course is shown in Table 8. It can be seen that there are 9 weeks of scheduled formal teaching and 10 weeks of nonscheduled teaching. In order to derive the greatest benefit from the course, students are required to progress through the units in sequence. Since the material in Unit 0 (General Principles of Pharmacology) is basic to all of the subsequent units, thereis no Unit 0 exam, but the material from this unit is included in all of the other unit examinations. The mechanics of this system are diagramed in Figure 14. Students use the various teaching options to learn the material covered in Unit 0 and Unit 1, and when they feel they are ready, they take a Unit 1 examination. If they pass this examination, they then progress to Unit 2, and this process is repeated until they have obtained satisfactory grades in all four units

Table 8. Medical Student Pharmacology Course Schedule (1976)

Unit 0	General Principles of Pharmacology	1 week (8 lectures)
Unit 1	ANS and Cardiovascular Pharmacology	2 weeks (12 lectures, 2 labs)
Unit 2	CNS Pharmacology	2 weeks (12 lectures, 1 lab)
Unit 3	Chemotherapy and Blood Drugs	2 weeks (12 lectures, no lab)
Unit 4	Toxicology and Endocrine Pharmacology	2 weeks (12 lectures, 1 lab)
	Review, Remedial, Final Eaxmination	10 weeks
	Advanced Pharmacology	8 weeks (16 lectures, 8 weeks of ward rounds)

and in a final examination. Since the exams are given at weekly intervals, it is evident that a bright student or one who has had previous training in pharmacology could complete the medical student pharmacology course in 5 weeks, there are routinely several students in each medical student class who achieve this goal. Students who do not pass the examination one week may take another exam (100 new questions) the following week or at any time thereafter. The only requirement in this course is that the student pass an examination in each of the four units and a final during the 19-week period. In previous years, when the scheduled teaching period was 14 weeks, over half of the students finished the course by the end of the 14th week. Students who complete the pharmacology course early have the

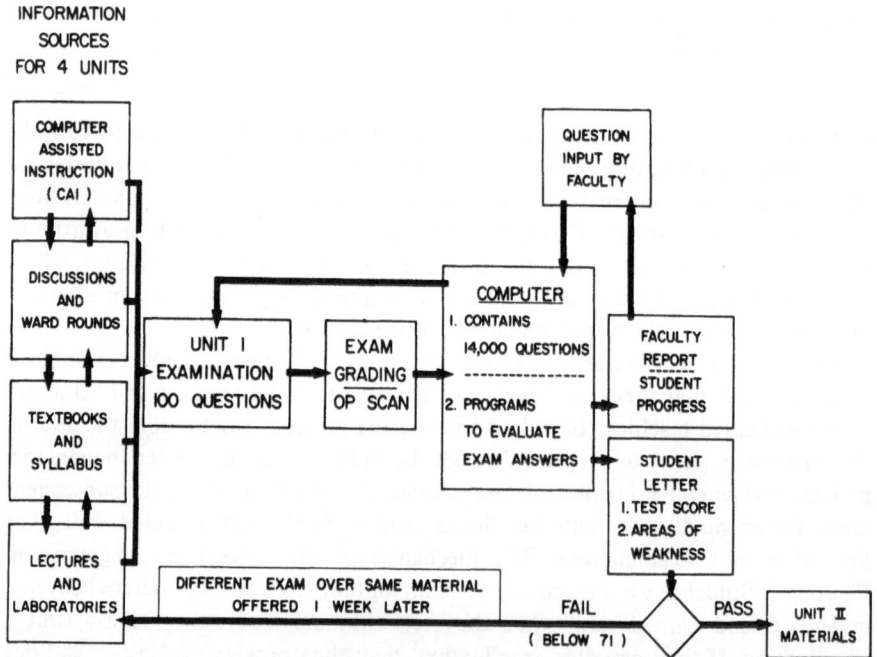

Figure 14. Flow chart of student–instructor–computer interactions in the CATS system.

option of enrolling in the advanced pharmacology course, which is offered during the last 8 weeks of the scheduled pharmacology time, or using the time available from pharmacology to study for another course. Since the advanced pharmacology course is a regularly scheduled elective, medical students can use this course to partially fulfill their elective course requirements for graduation. This advanced course in pharmacology has also proven to be useful and attractive to graduate students, residents in various clinical specialties, practicing physicians and other health professionals seeking a high-level clinically oriented short course in pharmacology.

A grade of 71 or better is required to pass each of the unit and final examinations. This passing level was established on the basis of the medical student class mean for the previous 6 years and is approximately 14% higher than the average score needed to pass the National Board examinations in pharmacology. As shown in Figure 15, since only grades above the median are passing in this system, it can be argued that the entire class is in the upper half of the distribution curve. However, less than 10% reach this level in 10 weeks and less than 5% fail to reach this level within 19 weeks. In addition to the pass—fail grade, students may also qualify for a Superior grade in pharmacology. To achieve this grade, the student must attain a grade of 80 or more on each of the unit and final examinations and must demonstrate by means of an oral examination that he has a superior knowledge in all areas of pharmacology. Since the computer records only the highest grade attained in each exam, the student is encouraged to work for a Superior grade by retaking examinations in those units where he had his lowest grades. The main advantage of this system from the students' point of view is that it retains the value of the examination as a learning tool but dissociates the trauma normally associated with "taking an exam." Students will frequently retake unit examinations as a mechanism to review for the final exam. We also have many students in clinical rotations and house staff who return to take unit or final examinations as a review mechanism to prepare for State or National Board examinations. An advantage of this system for the faculty is that it eliminates the need for makeup examinations, since the decision of whether or not to take an exam in any specific week is clearly the student's responsibility.

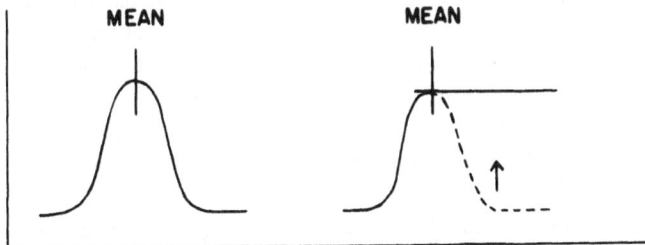

Figure 15. Effect of pass—fail grading. Normal distribution curve on left, alteration of curve by CATS system on right.

In a system such as this one, in which the student is not penalized for failing to pass an exam or for failing to take an exam, it is evident that there will be some students who neglect pharmacology because they are poorly motivated or unable to organize their time appropriately, or are overly responsive to pressure from other courses. In an effort to help this type of individual, each student in the pharmacology course is assigned to an adviser or "management consultant" who monitors the student's progress and arranges for special tutoring and guidance, if necessary. This adviser system is also important as a mechanism for maintaining person-to-person relationships which become increasingly important in any system which relies heavily on machine teaching. Many of the students who have had difficulty in other basic science courses do well in pharmacolofy, and they attribute this mainly to the extra time provided by the system and the individualized attention and concern of their adviser. Some of our minority students, for example, have commented that these factors and the fact that "Phelix is color blind" are the most important characteristics of the pharmacology teaching program.

As would be anticipated, a few of the medical students in the pharmacology course do not use the CAI programs. In our last class of 160 students, there were five students who did not use the CAI programs and four who used less than 2 hours of terminal time. In contrast to this, there were ten students who used more than 40 hours of terminal time and three of these used over 60 hours. The average for the entire class was 20 hours of CAI terminal usage. Each year at the end of the scheduled course an evaluation questionnaire is sent to each student and the information from this questionnaire is used in planning the course for the subsequent year. The data from this questionnaire indicate that our students are overwhelmingly in favor of CAI teaching (88%), the unit syllabus (91%), and our examination philosophy (96%). Although our students felt that the pharmacology faculty were excellent lecturers, they were not enthusiastic about lectures as a teaching tool. In fact, over half of the students (63%) felt that the course could be taught just as well without any formal lectures. Almost all of the students (96%) felt that the pharmacology teaching philosophy could and should be applied to other basic science disciplines. About half of the students reacted favorably to the laboratory exercises but over 80% of the students felt that the poisoning laboratories were particularly beneficial. These laboratories are emergency room simulations (in dogs) in which the students diagnose and manage several types of commonly encountered poisoning. Over 90% of the students who were enrolled in the Advanced Pharmacology course responded favorably when asked to evaluate the ward rounds and clinical lectures which make up most of this course. Not only does the Department of Pharmacology routinely win the sophomore medical student award for excellence in teaching, but in 1974 the class gave a special award to Phelix, which is the name we use for the computer, and is the basis for the CATS system logo shown in Figure 16.

Faculty response to the pharmacology teaching program has also been quite positive although none of our faculty feel that CAI teaching or the CATS system provides the ultimate answer to pharmacology or basic science teaching in the

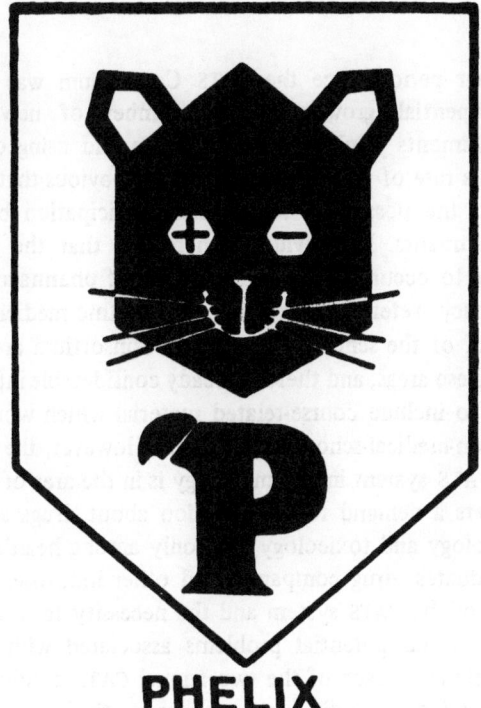

PHELIX

Figure 16. CATS system logo.

medical environment. In contrast to the students, the faculty is more evenly divided on the question of the value of the lecture as a teaching tool. When a faculty member has spent hours in preparing a lecture, it is disappointing to have only a handful of students attend, even though these are frequently the best students in the class. Some faculty members are also uncomfortable with the fact that this system involves much more small-group discussion and one-to-one interaction than conventional lecture-based courses. One unique characteristic of the system, however, which is in contrast to the usual adversary role of teacher and student, is that the instructor and the student share the same goal, which is to ensure that each student has sufficient pharmacologic information from all of his sources to pass the unit. Our examination philosophy not only puts the teacher and the student on the same "side of the fence," but it also reduces competitiveness among the medical students. In addition, since the terminal room facility is shared by medical students, nurses, pharmacists, house staff and a variety of other health professionals, this environment encourages the idea that a team effort is not only an effective way to learn pharmacology but also to deliver good health care. Much of the success of this program has come about because the participants, both faculty and students, have felt that they were involved in an experiment to improve the quality of medical education.

The Future of CATS

During the 4-year period since the CATS Consortium was organized, it has exhibited an exponential growth in the number of new medical school pharmacology departments joining the Consortium and using one or both parts of the system. If this rate of growth continues, it is obvious that in a few years we will have exhausted the possibility for further participation by medical school pharmacology departments. It is evident, therefore, that the future growth of CATS is most likely to occur through the addition of pharmacology departments in schools of pharmacy, veterinary medicine, osteopathic medicine, dentistry, and allied health. Several of the schools in the CATS Consortium are already teaching in one or more of these areas, and there is already considerable interest in expanding the CATS program to include course-related material which would be specifically tailored for these non-medical-school applications. However, the greatest potential for growth of the CATS system in pharmacology is in the area of continuing education. One encounters a demand for information about drugs and environmental problems (pharmacology and toxicology) not only among health professionals but also from undergraduates, drug companies and other industries, and even the lay public. The growth of the CATS system and the necessity to direct it according to the anticipated needs and potential problems associated with this growth have been major agenda items at each of the two annual CATS conferences. Since these conferences are attended by individuals who are actively involved in both the educational and the computer activities at each of the participating schools, they have provided an excellent opportunity for a cross-sectional analysis of the current status of CAI generally and of where it seems to be going nationally. Some of the problems, questions, and controversial areas which have been considered as agenda items at the CATS Consortium meetings are discussed below.

Distribution of Programs

CAI programs in medical education are generally provided to other institutions in one of two ways. First, the host institution sends the tapes, documentation, and other materials to the new school, which then installs the material and runs it on its own computer system, or, second, the host institution permits the new school to access the material on the host computer, either directly or through some type of network arrangement. The main advantage of the first method is that it allows each school to have full control of both the use and the content of the programs. Individual instructors can "tailor" the material to fit their courses or can eliminate or change material they do not find suitable for their students. The advantages of the second or network approach are that it can be used in schools which do not have appropriate computer facilities and it is easier to update or add new material since this involves only the host computer. The first approach has been adopted for the CATS system because we have found that pharmacologists will not readily accept and use a system over which they have limited control.

In the network approach, for example, one user cannot demand that a program be changed if several other users of the program find it acceptable, and the end result is likely to be discouraged and disgruntled users. Another major problem with the network approach is the communication costs of this system, which are prohibitive unless the user is close to the host computer. Feedback from the schools using the CATS system indicate clearly that the instructor must be more than the middleman in the system. If the staff member does not participate in selecting CAI programs for his course and accept responsibility for their content, CAI is likely to end up as an "enrichment gadget' rather than as a real part of his teaching program. One of the major differences between the schools using the CATS system and those participating in the "network" programs (MUMPS, Ohio, and PLATO) is that student usage is required in most of the CATS system schools, whereas the material is usually voluntary and is therefore peripheral to the teaching effort in other institutions and is, in fact, often available through some type of learning resource facility rather than through the teaching department.

Peer Review

Although peer review is of less concern to users of the CATS system than to network users where there is a need for majority approval, we are concerned about both student and faculty reaction to the material included in the CMI and CAI portions of the CATS system. Our experience demonstrates that student usage of different programs is a fairly accurate indicator of the teaching value of individual CAI programs. Similarly, faculty usage of questions from the CMI test file rapidly sorts out "good" questions, which are selected repeatedly, from "poor" questions, which receive little use and are discarded after 2 or 3 years. Since the students using the CATS system at the University of Kansas have several alternate ways to study pharmacology, we feel that it is significant that terminal use is exceptionally heavy on the nights before exams are given. We also feel that it is significant that after thoroughly investigating all the parts of the CATS system most of the CATS Consortium members have been willing to spend their own departmental funds to purchase the system. It is probably inevitable that there will eventually be some type of pharmacology board which will approve the content of CAI programs in much the same manner as is now done for the National Board examinations in pharmacology, but it is probably also inevitable that this system will lead to the same type of complaints and objections which are leveled at the National Board examinations. Users of the CATS-CMI system have pointed out, for example, that the CATS-CMI file is more current, larger, and more representative of what pharmacologists across the country feel is important in their discipline. Conversely, several CATS Consortium schools claim that their use of the CATS-CMI test-question file significantly improved the performance of their students on the National Board pharmacology examinations.

There appear to be three general objections to the use of the CATS system and specifically to the use of the CAI programs by pharmacology faculty. First is the complaint that the library of programs is too small to be of great value in an independent study program in pharmacology. Although this was a valid criticism when the system was new, it is much less valid and less frequently encountered with the current system. The second argument is that machine teaching will take away jobs from pharmacologists. Although some administrators perpetuate this concern by linking the use of CAI to reduced budgets and staff, the experience of the CATS Consortium users is that the use of CAI does not reduce the need for faculty but rather that it permits better teaching with the existing faculty level. The third argument is that the CATS system encourages students to learn the answers to questions rather than learning pharmacology. This is a more difficult criticism to answer since the argument that students exposed to the CATS system do better on National Board examinations in pharmacology is compromised by the fact that these exams use the same objective-type format as do most of the CAI programs. There are, however, many problem-solving questions in our exam file and in the CAI case histories, and the appropriate response to this criticism would appear to be to encourage the users of the system to contribute more of the type of material which meets their teaching objectives. In the final analysis, the teaching value of a textbook, syllabus, lecture, laboratory, or a CAI program depends mainly on the skill and ability of the teacher and is not an inherent property of the teaching tool.

Hardware and Software Problems

As mentioned previously, a major current problem for the exchange of CAI material between institutions with different computer hardware is the lack of appropriate compilers to carry out this conversion. Commercial time-sharing languages such as COURSEWRITER III and GNOSIS are rigidly machine-dependent, and this is true of other compilers (TUTOR, MUMPS, CATALYST, etc.). Although there are limitations associated with the use of time-sharing FORTRAN and BASIC, some of the CATS Consortium users have translated CATS-CAI programs into these languages. CATS-CAI programs have also been translated into PILOT by Dr. John Starkweather for use at the University of California at San Francisco. In addition, several CATS Consortium users with DEC-10 equipment are considering the use of PILOT to support the CATS-CAI programs since a compiler is available which will convert COURSEWRITER III material into this language.

Another question which has been of concern to CATS Consortium users is the feasibility of supporting the CAI portion of CATS on minicomputers or "stand-alone" intelligent terminals. Since the CATS programs which have been translated into PILOT run nicely on this type of terminal, it is evident that this is a viable alternative to the conventional big-machine support of CAI. Other areas in which members of the CATS Consortium have expressed particular interest include the use of computer-generated graphics and the ability to combine CAI programming with audiovisual material such as videotape. Although there are currently available systems in which CAI material can be combined with microfiche presentations

(PLATO) or presented sequentially with videotape (TICCIT), these systems require complex technology and special hardware and are not generally applicable to the CATS system. From the instructor's point of view, it would be helpful in presenting case history material on CAI if it were possible to show the student a section of videotape of the patient and to intersperse additional segments of videotape with appropriate sections of the CAI program. It is evident that this type of system would not only be useful in some areas of pharmacology teaching, but would also be particularly advantageous for teaching other basic science disciplines such as anatomy, histology, pathology, etc. Further, with the availability of this type of system which could be used on a commercial TV receiver and a low-cost keyboard or response device, there would be virtually unlimited possibilities for a new era in continuing education.

Summary

The CATS system in pharmacology provides an exciting and innovative teaching approach which is applicable to the needs of health professionals at all levels of preparation and training. It serves as the basis for an educational approach which is applicable not only to pharmacology but to other basic science disciplines. The CATS system provides the student with an interactive approach for learning basic information and improving his problem-solving skills and frees the instructor from many of the routine and record-keeping aspects of his position. Finally, the CATS system provides the pharmacologist with a way to maintain quality in education in the face of increasing class size, shrinking budgets, and administrative demands for innovative teaching methodology and additional teaching responsibility in allied health and continuing education.

Appendix: Additional Information about CATS-CMI Programs

VSAM File Description

```
01  VSAM-FILE LABEL RECORDS ARE STANDARD

      05  L PIC S9(4) COMP.
      05  REC-KEY
          10  DEPT PIC XXXX.
          10  DEPT-NUM REDEFINES DEPT PIC S9(7) COMP-3.
          10  QNUM PIC XXX.
          10  QNUM-NUM REDEFINES QNUM PIC S9(5) COMP-3.
          10  QSEQ PIC XX.
          10  QSEQ-NUM REDEFINES QSEQ PIC S999 COMP-3.
      05  Q-DATA
          10  Q-DA OCCURS 1 TO 439 TIMES DEPENDING ON L PIC X.

Record Types:
      1)  DEPT numeric greater than 0, QNUM numeric greater than 0, QSEQ
          numeric greater than 0: line of text in a question
      2)  DEPT numeric gt 0, QNUM numeric gt 0, QSEQ numeric = 0: calling
          card record
```

3) DEPT numeric gt 0, QNUM numeric lt 0, QSEQ numeric gt 0: line of text in an f-type question header
4) DEPT numeric gt 0, QNUM numeric lt 0, QSEQ numeric = 0: f-type control info
5) DEPT numeric lt 0, QNUM binary (193 = A, 194 = B, etc.), QSEQ numeric gt 0: line of text in a type-header
6) DEPT numeric gt 0, QNUM binary high-values, QSEQ alphameric (1st pos = major category; 2nd pos = minor category): category name designator

To Initialize System:
1) separate file from programs
2) compile VSØ6, define cluster for VSAM file, use VSØ6 to load file (no input data cards)
3) compile program VS1Ø, obtaining a deck (//OPTION deck)
4) compile program VSØ9, INCLUDE the deck from VS1Ø
5) punch the following cards and use them as input to VSØ9:

```
          OPTION E1
          00001
          00002
             .
             .
             .
          00100
          END OF TEST EXAM
          LAST
```

This should generate a sample exam.

VSØ9 Instructions

VSØ9 accepts numeric input cards, OPTION cards, END OF cards, and LAST cards.

Numeric input cards: 2 formats: format 1, one to five digit number, right justified in card cols 1 to 5; format 2, in card cols 8 to 12.

END OF name: follows all exams, signifies the last input card for a particular exam and the name of the exam (30 char max).

LAST: follows the last exam, just before the end-of-data card.

OPTION n, OPTION nxxxxxxx, or OPTION nx: various options (default are OPTION 1, EVAL, category order proof, no deck, no link).

```
OPTION n
n = 1: use format 1 question selection cards
n = 2: use format 2 question selection cards
n = 3: no evaluation (EVAL)
n = 4: punch numeric order (by type) deck
n = 5: no proof
n = 6: print numeric order proof
n = 7: no ordering of input deck of any kind
n = 8: order input deck by types only
n = 9: reset options 3 to 8 to default
n = Axxxxxxx: use xxxxxxx as the department number (0226000 assumed
         by default)
n = B: create COURSEWRITER auto-insert tape for all following exams
```

n = C: end the COURSEWRITER tape and lock the tape drive (also done
        by LAST card)

n = Dx: generate x random-order decks (x = 1,2,...9)

n = Ex: generate x random-order exams (x = 1,2,...9); i.e. link to VS1∅

VS15 Instructions

VS15 allows adding, deleting, updating of question texts, calling card
records, type headers, F headers, F texts. It accepts input cards, orders
them, and updates the file.

1--78	--12	13	14-17	18----------------------77	78--80	comment
dept #	ques #	ß	ßßßß	text line of question	ßßß	text lines must be in order
		C	ßßßß	STMAM		calling card record, 18-22 contain Source, Type, Major category, Answer, Minor category
		D	ßßßß			deletes question
		U	nnnß	revised question text		updates line nnn of the question
		U	nnnH	revised header text		updates line nnn of type header
		U	ßßßC	revised calling card record		updates calling card
		T	Xßßß	type header text		establishes type header for question type X
		G	ßßßß	nnnnnAB		f reference data: f reference # nnnnn; replace A with T for text, G for graph; replace B with the real type of the question
		F	ßßßß	text line of F question header		establishes F header for question

Prepare a deck of cards with this format, the program will order these
cards and make the appropriate changes in the file.

VS21. Prints White Cards on Double-Card Stock

Sorts file on four fields according to the following order: 1) usage
(only if designated, see below), 2) major category, 3) minor category,
4) question number.

Category selection card (one per printing):

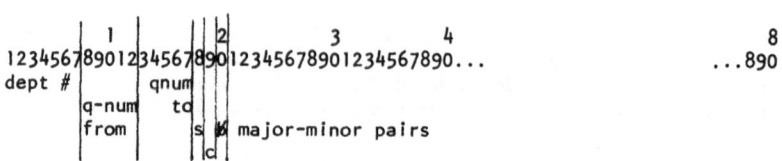

dept # = 7-digit department number
q-num from = the question number to begin from (00001 if at the beginning)
qnum to = the question number to end with (99999 if to the file end)
s = Ø if double printing on both left and right card; 1 if push-pull (q1 on
    left, q2 on right)
c = Ø if want all categories; major category n (n from 1 to 8) to get only
    that major category; * to select by major-minor pairs
major-minor pairs = pairs in cols 21-22, 23-24, etc. (up to 30 pairs); can
    select either a major-minor category combination (e.g. 1H) or an entire
    major category (i.e. 8*) by using an * in the second part of the pair
examples: to select categories 1, 2, and 8A punch: 02260000000199999Ø*Ø*2*8A
    to select only major category 7 punch: 02260000000199999Ø7

usage designation: AAAn in cols 1-4 means the quest ons indicated in the
    following deck should all be of usage n (i.e., sort on usage n to get
    a division of the file). The following cards should have a question #
    (1 per card) in cols 1-5 or 8-12. A card with BBB in cols 1-3 terminates
    this selection. The next category selection card will use the usage
    table just prepared.

VS25. OpScan Sheet Preparer

This program pre-prints OpScan continuous forms with the student name,
    number, exam number, course number, and any three lines of text.

Valid input cards:
    comment cards (the three lines of text): line 1--col 1 to 25;
                                              line 2--col 26 to 50;
                                              line 3--col 51 to 75;
                                              *** required in col 78-80.

    exam cards: exam number in col 1-5; /// required in col 78-80.

    student cards: course number in col 1-3;
                    student number in col 4 to 9;
                    student name in col 11 to 30.

The first exam must have both a comment card and an exam card before any
    student cards. Whenever another exam card is in the input stream, the
    following students are assumed to be taking the new exam; whenever
    another comment card is found in the input stream, all the following
    students will have the new set of comments.

The output is in alphabetical order within exams.

TEXTED II. Don Walter and Fred DeFeo

INSTRUCTION CODES

    i   means INSERT AFTER
    t   means TYPE (with line numbers)

p	means	PRINT (without numbers)
d	means	DELETE
r	means	REPLACE with new line(s)
m	means	MOVE
c	means	CORRECT
s	means	SEARCH for all lines with desired text
f	means	FIND only FIRST line with desired text
margin	means	set new line length
password	means	change password
help	means	show valid instruction formats
calc	means	go to calculate mode

SPECIAL CODES

Procedure codes (used during the TEXTED Procedures)

end	end of Insert Procedure; end of Calculate Mode
///	end of Insert; terminate Correction; resume Insert
+++	move next line up (during Correction)
$pbn	page backward n pages on the display screen
$lbn	line backward n lines (during Insert or Correction)
*	replaces a single character for match during Search
&	replaces any characters for match during Search

Execution codes (stores with text and executed during Print)

¢¢¢	continue line (overrides carriage return)
#¢¢	pause at end of line (during Print)
¢¢	same as ¢¢¢
#¢	same as #¢¢
)(	skip this line during Print
_ _	automatic underline

References

Abelson, P. H, 1972. The fourth revolution, *Science 177*:121.

Alpert, D., and Bitzer, D. L., 1970. Advances in computer-based education, *Science 167*:1582–1590 (March).

Hyatt, G. W., Eades, D. C., and Tenczar, P., 1972. Computer-based education in biology, *BioScience 22*:401–409.

Murray, T. W., Barber, J. H., Cupples, R. W., Hannay, D. R., and Scott, D. B., 1976. Computer-assisted learning in undergraduate medical teaching, *Lancet 1*:474–476.

Norton, S., Doull, J., and Walaszek, E. J., 1972. A computer assisted teaching system for medical pharmacology. Presented at the Fifth International Congress of Pharmacology, San Francisco, 1972.

Smith, S. G., and Sherwood, B. A., 1976. Educational uses of the PLATO computer system, *Science 192*:344–352.

Stolurow, L. M., Peterson, T. L., and Cunningham, A. C. (Eds.), 1970. *Computer-Assisted Instruction in the Health Professions*, Entelec, Newburyport, Mass.

19

Some PLATO Applications in Health Sciences Education

D. K. Bloomfield, G. L. Hody, and A. H. Levy

Introduction

The University of Illinois PLATO system has a unique flavor because it is a large network — over 950 terminals spread throughout the United States connect to the same processing facility and can access the same collection of instructional materials and communication facilities. Teaching programs in health sciences have been a feature of the system library from its early inception (see for example Bitzer and Boudreaux, 1969) and there is now an extensive catalog of lessons in health-related subjects including biology, pharmacy, veterinary medicine, nursing, and allied health. In addition, there exists a large body of instructional materials at the college level in mathematics, physical sciences, and behavioral sciences, much of which is useful as remedial or supplementary resources for health science students.

The PLATO network is not just a collection of equipment and lessons but rather, due to its rich communication facilities, can be viewed as a model of an "on-line intellectual community" beginning to come into existence, much as envisioned by project MAC at MIT and project INTREX over 11 years ago. Because the group of PLATO health science users is composed for the most part of new arrivals, it is difficult to describe it comprehensively. This chapter, then, will emphasize one particular established PLATO project in medical education, although it is our belief that it is the development of a *national community* of health science educators which is the immense promise of the current PLATO work.

In July, 1973, extensive efforts began at the University of Illinois College of Medicine, School of Basic Medical Sciences, Urbana–Champaign (SBMS/UC) to develop for delivery by the PLATO system a computer-based core curriculum in

D. K. Bloomfield, G. L. Hody, and A. H. Levy · School of Basic Medical Sciences, University of Illinois College of Medicine, Urbana, Illinois. The PLATO system has been supported by the State of Illinois, the National Science Foundation, the Control Data Corporation, and the Advanced Research Projects Agency (ARPA) of the Department of Defense. This work was supported, in part, by Contract number NO1-PE-34068 between the University of Illinois College of Medicine and the Health Resources Administration, Department of Health, Education, and Welfare.

the basic medical sciences. Substantial financial support for this work was received from the Department of Health, Education and Welfare and from the state of Illinois. Much of the subsequent discussion will deal with the accomplishments and findings of this project after which some general status information about other PLATO health science activities will be briefly presented.

Background

The School of Basic Medical Sciences at Urbana–Champaign has taken an innovative approach to first-year medical education. Its objectives are to produce, at a lower-than-average cost, clinically oriented students skilled in problem solving. The students pace and test themselves within reasonable time guidelines and with the aid of the PLATO system as they progress through a set of unit "learning packages" based on ten clinical problems. Twelve basic science disciplines have been organized so that learning objectives for each are arranged in units related closely to the relevant clinical problems. Students proceed through the 1-year basic science curriculum at their own rate; faculty serve as individual advisers and provide conventional instruction through lectures and small discussion groups. Physicians, serving as clinical associates, work with students to integrate the basic science material into a clinical experience.

This setting has seemed natural for the integration of computer-based education with its potential for a tutorial approach. Ideally, with such a system, students at differing levels of achievement would have the opportunity to learn at optimum speed with special attention to their specific needs and deficiencies. Integral and sophisticated self-assessment features would allow both the student and his or her faculty adviser to gain timely knowledge of that student's strengths and weaknesses. While these are not original observations, the juxtaposition of the defined curriculum of SBMS-UC with advanced technology of the PLATO system may well be unique at this time.

The PLATO system has been described in Chapter 9. It is especially suited for the health sciences because it is designed to simplify the human-to-machine interface — an essential consideration for many health professionals who have little time and no computer or typing skills. The PLATO system also recognizes that a collection of user aids for both student and authors is even more important than convenient equipment. Students are normally able to use the system after only a few minutes of special instruction. While author training is still measured in weeks or months, an increasing repertoire of on-line assistance for them is steadily decreasing the learning period.

Objectives of the SBMS/UC Project

The concerns of the group at SBMS/UC have been essentially the same as those of other individuals engaged in the creation of computer-assisted instruction for health professions education – except for cases where the technical characteristics of PLATO have placed somewhat different dimensions on specific factors. The issues which have been faced and those which are yet unresolved are mainly in the sphere of the medical educational process itself, secondly, in the application of computer-based systems to health science education, and, last of all, the actual problems of computer implementation of the curriculum.

Medical education, a complex undertaking, has elements of the cognitive, the overwhelming, the charismatic, and the elementary. Students are often exposed to lectures in which huge quantities of facts are dispensed in endless succession while at the same time they are emphatically told that the important thing is for them to develop their problem-solving abilities. How, they ask, can they do this when they are seldom presented with examples of such behavior and when they so often find themselves in highly charged emotional situations for which their previous training has scarcely equippped them? The amazing thing is that during the course of their medical education, they learn enough information, develop adequate work habits, and in general achieve well enough so that the American system, nonsystematized and far from optimum though it is, manages to produce physicians who are substantially competent.

Precise evaluation of competencies, the assessment of strengths and weaknesses, and the molding of curriculum to them are challenges which have not been well met by American medical education. There is little disagreement that the physician as now trained is competent, but it may well be that the degree of motivation of medical students is so high and their abilities are in general so strong that their competence is developed irrespective of the mode of education offered. Few would defend many of the individual elements in our present medical educational system or would suggest that the lecture system is an effective tool for the dissemination of information. Few would suggest that the disorganized sequence of clinical experience is an optimum way to develop problem-solving skills in students. Curricular organization into narrow specialities is, even in the clinical years, an awkward system. Yet, a central fact which must be considered in any evaluation of ancillary or innovative resources is that the educational system for the most part works. Thus, any new innovative technique must be measured as only one additional modality in an extremely complicated total system. The system itself is far from integrated; evaluation of any one component is extremely difficult.

With respect to the application of computer-based systems to medical education, it was possible to recognize from the experience of others important pitfalls to be avoided in the development of the curriculum. The potential difficulties which the project identified and desired to address included:

1. Poor coverage of curriculum due to both redundancy of programs in "popular" areas and to insufficient amounts of materials in other fields – attributable to a combination of the absence of a development plan and the tendencies of lesson authors to give preference to subjects with which they are most comfortable.

2. Inconsistent programming methods and programming errors resulting from inadequate author training, insufficient technical support from programming experts, and lack of systematic testing of finished lessons.

3. Errors in content or strategy pursuant to the absence of a formal process of appraisal, review, and general quality control.

4. Student frustration occasioned by confusing catalog and access protocols, equipment and program malfunctions, long service intervals for broken terminals.

5. A failure to take advantage of the economy and enhancement of programs which widespread interinstitutional sharing of programs could bring because programs developed on one system could not readily be made to run on a dissimilar machine at another institution.

Amazingly enough, even after the above list was compiled (with the aid of the work of Casbergue, 1974; Hickey, 1974; and Rubin *et al.*, 1975), it was extremely difficult to circumvent the known hazards in computer-based curriculum development. Nevertheless, significant progress was made on a number of major tasks.

Planning, Implementation, and Quality Control Methods

During the first 3 project years, a moderately large amount of lesson material was constructed in several disciplines of basic medical sciences. Several young doctoral level scientists were employed full-time in the design of these lessons and were supported by programmers, instructional designers, an illustrator, and a rhetoric specialist. Early in the project's history, flexible but detailed guidelines were derived to guide the lesson development process. Activities were concentrated in microbiology, pharmacology, biochemistry, and anatomy. Within these areas, advance planning limited duplication of efforts.

Quality control was performed during many stages of the lesson development. Formative evaluation/appraisal was always initiated before lessons were placed on the student catalog and was mainly conducted by project members. Ideally, each new lesson was reviewed in entirety by two content specialists and by a programming specialist before any students were allowed to use it. As with other similar projects, obtaining true "peer" review proved difficult. As an interim measure, graduate students, faculty volunteers, and others with special skills were pressed into service so that by the start of 1976, 46% of the lesson modules had undergone a journal-style "expert" review of this type. Direct feedback from students, by means of on-line notefiles, comment-writing facilities, or more conventional means also supplied a great deal of useful corrective information.

After sufficient experience had been accumulated, a set of programming style standards was assembled. The emphasis of these suggestions was on the appearance of the instructional materials as seen by students rather than on specific directives for writing TUTOR computer programs. The essential elements included a call for aesthetic use of the graphic features of PLATO (see examples in Figure 1), fast

Figure 1 (a–d) demonstrates the application of PLATO graphics to illustrate lessons in the basic medical sciences. Just as visual aids such as blackboards and color slides are essential to classroom instruction, the authors believe a full graphics capability is necessary for effective computer-based instruction in the health sciences. Illustrations from PLATO reproductive physiology lesson (a) by B. Katzenellenbogen and D. Chirolas; microbiology lessons (b, c) by M. Gabridge, K. Wagner, and K. Pechman; and genetics sequence (d) by W. Daniels and D. Chirolas.

ENDOMETRIUM of the UTERUS

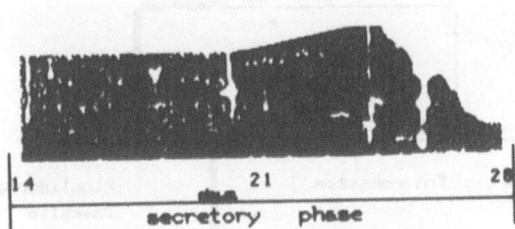

secretory phase

Uterine secretions are important in
nourishment of the early embryo if
fertilization should occur.

During the luteal phase of the cycle (day 15-28) the
corpus luteum produces estrogen, as well as another steriod
hormone that is primarily responsible for the conversion
of the endometrium from a proliferative to a secretory
state.
2.   What is the name of the hormone?

> progesterone ok

   Press -NEXT-.

b

o = white/colorless
   colony

● = pink/red colony

▌ = mixed

a ___
d ___
e ___
f ___
g
c
b
h

      This is a diagrammatic representation of a mixed
culture, similar to that seen in slide #924 and #1813.
Which area would you use to get an inoculation for
further tests on our suspected pathogen ?
   > b

      Never pick an inoculum from colonies which are
likely to be contaminated. You want a pure culture,
so you should choose an isolated, non-fermenting
colony.

c

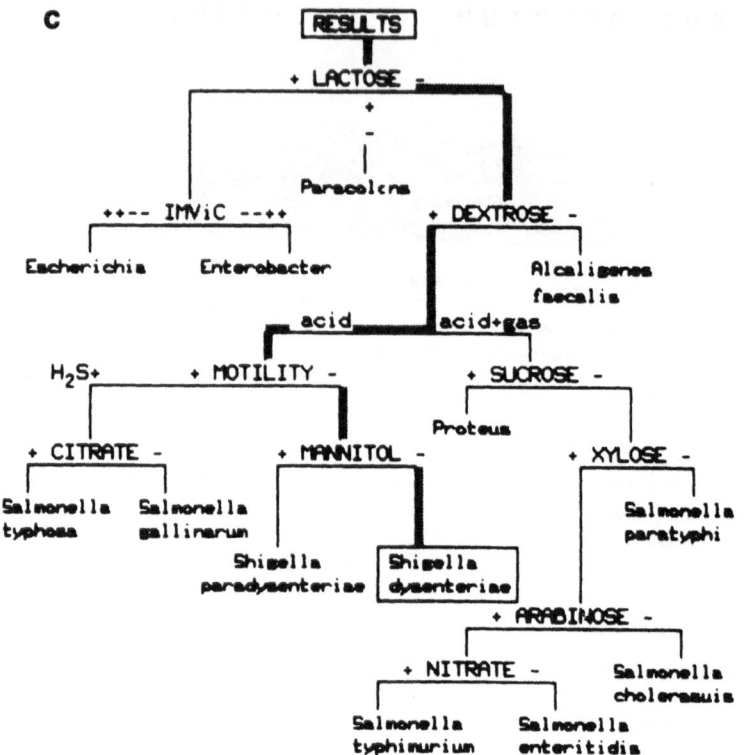

This is the path we followed......

d   This is Mr. Jones' family tree, if you need help with
this pedigree press -HELP-.

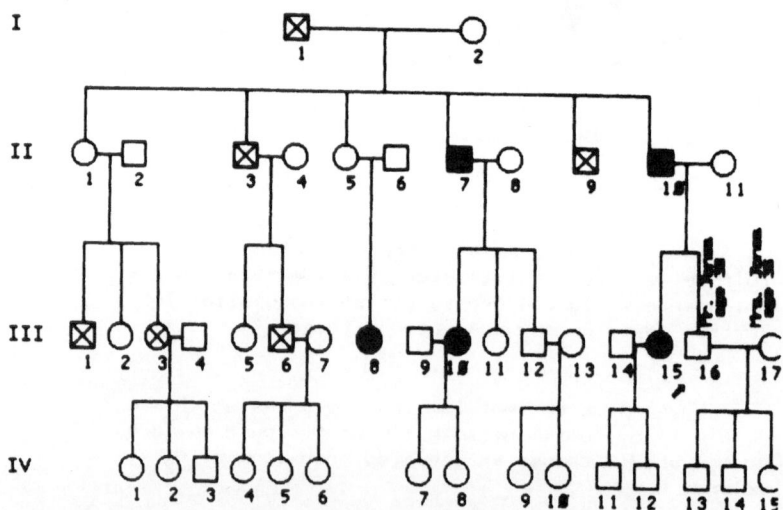

Average age of onset was 31 yr. No cases have appeared
after age 37 if normal retinal morphology.

To see Mrs. Jones' family tree press -NEXT-.

plotting of displays, an absolute absence of "dead ends" or interminable loops, consistent use of the PLATO keyset (particularly the "function" keys), and subdivision and indexing of long lessons into easily located segments. Authors were strongly urged to include specific objectives and prerequisites in their lesson and to cite off-line references wherever relevant (Hody *et al.*, 1974).

Lesson Materials

The lessons have generally followed the outline of the SBMS curriculum, but it has been found that computer-based lesson design could not be approached or organized in the same mold as the traditional text-based curriculum. Lessons have been fashioned in the several general modes that follow.

1. *Interactive, Primary Instructional Material.* These lessons have been designed to teach a student who has not been exposed to the subject via any other medium. These lessons are "information-rich," contain a substantial amount of text, capitalize heavily on graphic displays for reinforcing basic concepts, and provide for special HELP sequences for students who manifest difficulty during progression through a lesson. A large number of lessons in basic parasitology have been constructed in this manner.

2. *Basic Supplementary Instructional Material.* Many of the lessons, while suitable for primary instruction, are used by students who have had some previous contact with a topic, either through reading or through lecture. These lessons will generally be less didactic, more interactive, and will present less text and graphical material. They will have HELP sequences for students who are having difficulty, and will often provide the student with a comparative score of how s/he did in relation to others taking the lesson. These lessons, simpler in design than the first category, are produced with less professional effort. A large series of such lessons is available in pharmacology.

3. *Drills and Vocabulary Builders.* A problem faced by many students in the first year of medical school is that of needing to rapidly build a large, new, and strange vocabulary. Especially for those with some verbal-ability limitations, this may prove to be an impediment to their understanding of the relationships which the new vocabulary is designed to express. Thus, these students with initial difficulty in vocabulary have their troubles compounded as they are unable to learn the principles embodied in the words.

To assist these students, we have prepared a series of lessons, primarily drill in nature, but differing from conventional word-learning exercises in that the paradigms on which the drills are based are only possible to carry forth with computer monitoring of performance. We have engaged the collaboration of educational specialists in this area. The resulting lessons, mainly concerned with anatomical terminology, are moderately popular with students. Although we are as yet unable to appraise the effectiveness of this technique, there is reasonable expectation that it may be of substantial value, and may achieve a greater degree of usefulness in the supplementary education and the remediation of educationally disadvantaged health sciences students.

4. *Simulations*. A number of lessons in pharmacology and in the clinical sciences are designed as models of the problem under study. For example, students can, via a PLATO terminal, simulate the infusion of a dog with various doses of drugs active on the autonomic system and note graphically the effects on the affected physiological functions.

In the clinical area, both through our own efforts and through the efforts of Dr. George Miller, and now Dr. Philip Forman, at the Center for Educational Development of the University of Illinois College of Medicine in Chicago, we are continuing the development of what is now a moderately extensive series of computer-based case studies for self-assessment. Several new models have supplemented the older CASE model, originally developed by Miller and Harless (Harless *et al.*, 1973). Exercises are now available which involve social counseling, differential diagnosis, physician attitudes toward the dying patient, as well as traditional case studies regarding specific types of disease entities.

5. *Computer-Based Self-Assessment*. In addition to the primary instructional material, the School of Basic Medical Sciences at Urbana—Champaign has devised a PLATO-based diagnostic examination system. These "Level-3" exams, originally written in COURSEWRITER and later converted and expanded on PLATO, provide the students a means for individualized self-assessment. Although the examinations are primarily diagnostic instruments, they serve, to some extent, as learning instruments as well. They are of major value in providing faculty with information useful for counseling and remediation.

Students are encouraged to take an examination via the PLATO terminal after they complete each of the ten clinical problems. Each exam lasts about 2½ hours. The system allows the student an opportunity to retry questions missed on the first round, and also gives the student the correct answer after multiple incorrect responses.

An important feature of the system is a computer-generated hard copy report, given to both the student and his adviser immediately following the completion of the test. This highlights the questions that the student was unable to answer correctly and provides a literature reference pertaining to the incorrect response. A comprehensive software package for summary statistical reports, test-item analysis, on-line examination construction, and system monitoring round out this computer-based instruction-management system.

The PLATO-based examination system appears to be substantially acceptable to students, and many have expressed their preference for it over a standard paper system. Their reasons include the ability to retry questions and the individualized summary report. From an administrative standpoint, the ability to update and edit examinations, to dynamically monitor overall class performance and to examine individual performance in a timely fashion is a distinct advantage (Jones and Sorlie, 1976; Sorlie and Jones, 1975).

6. *Supplementary and Remedial Lessons*. Through the cooperation of a number of institutions and author groups, over 400 PLATO instructional modules are available for the use of health science students. These include content areas of chemistry,

physics, mathematics, statistics, psychology, nursing, veterinary medicine, and pharmacy.

Following the initial lag due to the training period of the new authors, the number of basic science lessons grew from 14 in December 1974 to 59 in December 1975 to approximately 90 in December 1976. Added to these are about 60 other lessons converted from other computer systems making a total in 1976 of about 150 modules in the basic medical sciences. The rate of addition of new materials varies, currently running about 8 per month.

Sharing Resources: The PLATO Health Sciences Network

When we began our activities on PLATO, it was already clear that the needs for a large body of lesson material could not be completely handled at a single institution, even with the assistance of the special faculty group and support staff that was funded under contract. It also seemed evident that interinstitutional participation would lead to a broader perspective of needs and more approaches to fulfilling them and a more diverse cadre of students could react to the educational material created. These were all seen as distinct advantages. On the other hand, it was recognized that wider participation might well lead to more diffuseness of educational objectives, through resulting attempts to tailor the lessons to the differently perceived needs of varying institutions. Also, there would be additional costs in terms of training authors at remote sites, communication costs between outlying institutions and Urbana, and, not the least important, the considerable overhead in faculty time in planning and administering such an informal consortium. However, it was felt that the advantages clearly outweighed the problems, and beginning in 1974, PLATO terminals were loaned by the University of Illinois to a number of other medical schools that agreed to undertake the authoring of lessons and to give their students access to the developing library of health sciences lessons (Hody, 1974).

Outside participants paid a share of the PLATO service costs as well as the actual communication costs. Since 1974, seven institutions have participated in this effort in an organized fashion. These schools have included Northeast Ohio Universities School of Medicine (campuses at Kent, Youngstown, and Akron), University of Maryland, University of Southern California, University of Oklahoma, University of Tennessee, Southern Illinois University (Carbondale and Springfield medical campuses), and The John Hopkins University. A terminal has also been located at the Lister Hill Center for Biomedical Communications of the National Library of Medicine for their use in observing the network.

The results of sharing have largely borne out our prior expectations: sharing of terminals and efforts has been a limited success. Reaction from students at most institutions has been favorable; many have become enthusiastic users; some have started authoring lessons under faculty supervision. Faculty involvement at the participating schools has resulted in the creation of a number of new lessons. We do not yet have adequate information to judge faculty reaction at schools outside of the University of Illinois, but from our limited information, the lack of recognition of computer-based lesson construction as a legitimate teaching activity has resulted in somewhat equivocal involvement. This problem is far from unique in health sciences – see for example Hudson's letter to *Science*, the antecedent article, and subsequent dicussion (Hudson, 1976).

The generally tight economic situation has discouraged the undertaking and continuation of projects with significant capital costs (as is the case with computer-based education). Also, communication costs at remote sites have been quite high in relation to the number of terminals. It is primarily for these reasons, we believe, that the Northeast Ohio Universities School of Medicine and USC have had to discontinue their participation.

The potential advantages of networking appear substantially to outweigh the problems. The burdens of administration needed for effective coordination are not trivial, but they appear small in comparison to the incremental gain in faculty involvement. The developmental expense of a lesson decreases inversely with the number of students using the lesson. In addition, there appears to be an unequivocal synergistic effect in widespread national participation.

Rate of Use

The academic year 1975–1976 can be considered the first one in which the number of health sciences lessons on PLATO was at more than a minor level; hence our usage rates for this year are the first that have any real meaning. We believe that levels of use are far below what will be achieved in the next few years: lessons are appearing at a rate greater than linear and student use is correspondingly accelerating. However, even considering these limitations, over 17,000 student instructional hours were logged by the Health Sciences Network. This is a rather substantial degree of instruction. Of course, volume alone is but one parameter of educational utility: we fully recognize the need for multidimensional evaluation. In this context, we are conducting a full-scale evaluation of the effectiveness of our activities. We are comparing the performance of "high-frequency" PLATO users to "low-frequency" users on the College's standard comprehensive examinations. In addition, faculty and student behavior patterns with respect to computer-based education are being studied to determine the principal impediments to more effective use of technology in education.

With respect to the University of Illinois PLATO system as a whole, the Health Science Network occupies a subset of 80 out of 950 terminals and typically exhibits a total of 10,000 "gross" contact hours per month (of the 120,000 hours per month characteristically amassed by the whole network). Thus, by these two rather crude measures, about 10% of the current PLATO system is more or less devoted to health science activity. (Authoring, student testing, self-assessment, communications, browsing, and recreational activity are all included in the "gross" figures, in contrast to the 17,000 contact hours per year instructional time cited above which includes only carefully measured studying activities.)

Transportation of Programs between Dissimilar Systems

It has often been said that the major impediment to realization of the potential advantages of interinstitutional sharing of computer-based lessons is the inability of programs written for one system to be readily run on another machine. While the optimal conversion method would be entirely computer-mediated, practically, the problems of accommodating differences in data formats, display technology, and most important, the implicit assumptions and features of the systems involving their basic logical structure, make this approach impossible at this time. However, in the particular case of health science materials most of the cost of lesson production resides in the development of strategy and content rather than in the computer coding itself. On this basis, the SBMS-UC project group initiated a cooperative exploratory effort with other institutions to acquire and convert programs from several other systems so that they would run on PLATO. Lesson materials for conversion were supplied by the Kansas University Medical Center (KUMC) Department of Pharmacology, The Cornell Medical College Department of Anatomy, the University of California College of Medicine at San Francisco, and the Center for Educational Development of the University of Illinois College of Medicine. Programs and languages were, respectively, about 60 pharmacology lessons written in COURSEWRITER, an antomy lesson in "A Tutorial System" (ATS), a pharmacology lesson in PILOT, and a "CASE" in COURSEWRITER.

At the conclusion of the conversion effort, it was found that this type of sharing is highly cost effective and extremely practical if the recipient system has the capability to accept the donor programs without extensive modifications – as was the case with PLATO and the languages and lessons listed above. The cost of reprogramming the materials was estimated to be less than 20% of the cost of writing them afresh – a task in many cases beyond the capability of the available staff at SBMS-UC even had funds been available. The PLATO versions of the lessons were of high quality and even though they might not appear to the user precisely the same as they had on the original host system, they proved completely satisfactory. In no case was reprogramming of the lessons particularly difficult or time-consuming except for the CASE series. For the COURSEWRITER-to-PLATO conversion, semi-automated routines were developed which made the conversion of tutorial-type lessons primarily one of retyping.

It appeared to us that such efforts had not been commonplace before because most systems are not as good recipients as PLATO and because suitable guidelines for insuring proper credits, updates, and feedback of student comments and data to the authors had not been supplied (Hody *et al.*, 1975).

Other PLATO Health Science Activities

A growing number of institutions have recently expressed interest in extending or initiating use of the PLATO system for health science instruction – either by connection to the University of Illinois system, by arrangements with the Control Data Corporation or by the use of "multiTUTOR," a language which can be used to run certain PLATO-like programs on other computer systems (Schuyler, 1974). Because their activities compose a rapidly changing and complex scenario, it is only possible to indicate in general where these groups are so that the interested reader can pursue the matter on his or her own. Some of the institutions interested in PLATO at this time include:

The University of Delaware (possibly in nursing education); The University of Florida (in dentistry and possibly medicine); The School of Health Care Science at Sheppard Air Force Base, Texas (for physician assistants); The School of Pharmacy at Purdue University (in pharmacy); The Medical College of Georgia (in nursing); and the University of Nebraska (in dentistry). This is, of course, in addition to the University of Illinois and Health Sciences Network participants.

Future Plans

Several areas appear to be of the first priority in the next 3 years:

1. Continued Development of Additional Instructional Material. It is clear that we have just started providing students with an adequate amount of health science instructional material through PLATO. Translating educational objectives into computer-based form is and will remain a costly process. However, we believe that it is *cost effective* in comparison with other capital expenditures in medical education. There is little doubt that such an effort must provide a national resource, and that federal support will be an important component in reaching this goal. Individual schools are already beginning to participate in the funding, but further support is needed to produce what is essentially a national product.

2. Developing the Mechanisms for More Effective Sharing. We have been convinced both of the value of a network of participating institutions, and of the counter part interest of many of our colleagues in participating in such efforts. To date, we have worked in this area with no formal funding, and although we have accomplished a good deal, we know that much better performance could be achieved with staff at middle-management levels to handle many details of interinstitutional cooperation that are frequently the critical determinants of success or failure. Specifically, we need to have resources for "startup" costs for new participants, to enable them to begin with a limited local institutional commitment. Additional personnel for training of faculty at new participating institutions is needed. We have already developed extensive computer programs for reporting use by individual schools, but we need the clerical staff to produce and distribute such reports.

3. Communications Costs. This is a vexing problem in that leased-line telephone line costs are increasing. New multiplexers now under development will soon increase the number of PLATO terminals which can be connected through a single line from 4 to 8. Another factor is increased utilization — since PLATO costs are all billed independently of the rate of use of the system, it is possible to bring the hourly costs down sharply by using the system as efficiently as possible.

Long-term possible solutions include the use of communication satellites, but these may introduce objectionable transmission delays due to the limited speed of light combined with the long transmission paths. Another approach is the use of microwave communications — extremely inexpensive but very limited in distance. Yet another possibility is a distributed network of minicomputers as is discussed below. However, to exploit the present technology, any expansion effort will have to bear the admittedly non-cost-effective conventional long-distance ground communications costs for the immediate future.

4. A Distributed Minicomputer Network for Medical Education. Recent technical advances in computer hardware have reduced central processor and logical units costs manyfold and have substantially reduced the costs of disk storage and other similar devices. The old principle of economy of scale may soon be invalid where the functional units of activities are geographically widely distributed. Although the word revolutionary is applied to many developing technologies, it usually overstates the case: the altered impact of new microprocessor technology on information processing, the term revolutionary is probably conservative.

The principal obstacle to the wider use of mini- and microcomputers in computer-based education has been the limited availability of software and the relatively low level of man—machine grace that minicomputer systems have manifested. We have worked with this problem for the last 3 years in an effort to make the *economical* minicomputer an *effective* instrument for health sciences education. Our efforts have now reached the point where significant results are seen. Using a minicomputer (MODCOMP IV, Modular Computer Corporation), a small developmental group in our school has created an emulation of many typical PLATO functions which runs on the small machine. With such a system, the costs of communication are drastically lowered, as a local computer must only be in contact with a central base for updating of curriculum and exchanging of records. In addition, the advantages of local administration and autonomy are obtainable. This development effort is partially completed, to the point where its success appears to be highly probable.

Conclusions

1. Computer-based medical education is a teaching tool worthy of renewed and expanded interest. Enhanced techniques of student—computer interaction, with graphics, touch input, and microfiche image projection have substantially increased its usefulness. Experience with defined curriculum design has provided a sound educational base for its use.

2. National pooling of efforts and sharing of resources has been, and will continue to be, an important instrument in making any substantial progress.

3. Efforts should be directed toward: increasing the available lesson material,

decreasing costs – particularly communications, facilitating interschool cooperation, and exploiting newer minicomputer potentials.

Additional information about the PLATO system may be obtained from the Director, Computer-based Education Laboratory, University of Illinois, Urbana, Illinois 61801. Inquiries about health science applications should be addressed to the Director, Medical Information Science Department, School of Basic Medical Sciences, University of Illinois, Urbana, Illinois 61801. The commercial version of PLATO is available from the Control Data Corporation, P.O. Box 0, Minneapolis, Minnesota 55440.

References

Bitzer M. D., and Boudreaux, M. D., 1969. Using a computer to teach nursing. *Nurs. Forum* 8:234–254.

Casbergue, J. P., 1974. Computer-Assisted Instruction in Health Professions Education: Guidelines for Utilization, Doctoral thesis, Michigan State University.

Harless, W., Drennon, G. G., Marxer, J. J., Root, J. A., Wilson, L. L., amd Miller, G. E., 1973. CASE – A natural language computer model, *Comput. Biol. Med.* 3:227–246.

Hickey, A. E., 1974. Research Guidelines for CAI, presented at the meeting of the Association for the Development of Computer-based Instructional Systems (ADCIS), Washington, D.C., January, 1974.

Hody, G. L., 1974. Introduction to PLATO IV for Health Science New Authors and Programming Style Suggestions, University of Illinois College of Medicine, SBMS/UC Report, 1974, written with members of the Basic Sciences Author Group.

Hody, G. L., A Basic Science PLATO Network for Medicine and Allied Health Instruction, 1974 Summer Conference of the Association for the Advancement of Computer-based Instruction (ADCIS), Bellingham, Washington, August 13–15, 1974.

Hody, G. L., Stull, R. E., Cohen, B., and Cohen, P., 1975. Transporation of Health Science Computer-Based Lessons Between Dissimilar Systems at the Program Listing Level, Summer meetings of the Association for the Development of Computer-based Instructional Systems (ADCIS), Portland, Maine.

Hudson, H. T., 1976. Paper mills and campus ethics, *Science* 193:274.

Jones, L. A., and Sorlie, W. E., 1976. Increasing medical student performance with an interactive computer-assisted appraisal system, *Journal of Computer-based Instruction*, 2:57–72 (also presented at the 13th Annual Conference on Research in Medical Education, November, 1974).

Rubin, M. L., Hunter, B., and Knetsch, M., Evaulation of the Experimental CAI Network (1973–1975) of the Lister Hill National Center for Biomedical Communications, National Library of Medicine, HumRRO report LHNCBC 75–03, The Human Resources Research Organization, Alexandria, Va.

Schuyler, J., 1974. The Complete Guide to HYPERTUTOR, June, 1974 (available from Computers and Teachings, Northwestern University, 2003 Sheridan Road, Evanston, Illinois 60201).

Sorlie, W. E., and Jones, L. A., 1975. Descriptions of a computer-assisted testing system in an independent study program, *J. Med. Educ.* 50(1):81–83.

20

CAI at the Michigan State University Medical Schools

Eric D. Zemper

Introduction

This chapter will discuss some fundamental aspects of computer-assisted instruction (CAI) from the perspective of the Office of Medical Education Research and Development (OMERAD) at Michigan State University, as well as research being conducted by OMERAD related to computer applications in medical education. OMERAD is in the unique position of serving two recently established medical schools, the College of Human Medicine (CHM) and the College of Osteopathic Medicine (COM), as well as a College of Veterinary Medicine and a School of Nursing. Both CHM and COM offer a curriculum which is oriented toward flexible, individualized instruction. CHM uses a combination of discipline-based courses and interdisciplinary teams to teach the basic sciences through analysis and discussion of a series of common medical problems, while COM uses an interdisciplinary approach based on systems biology. Both schools emphasize the training of primary care or family physicians. Clinical training is provided in community hospitals throughout the state, rather than in a university medical center. In such a diverse environment, OMERAD is in a position to explore many aspects of medical education, among them the potential for the use of computers in training medical personnel.

Computer-assisted instruction is a blanket term used to cover a number of teaching techniques designed to enhance learning through utilization of a computer which interacts directly with a student. As with any such innovation, the reader is cautioned to take an objective and sensible approach to it. It is most important that anyone acquainting themselves with CAI, or considering its use, maintain an objective approach and avoid overly optimistic claims of success or unwarranted bitter pessimism. CAI should be viewed as a potentially successful adjunct to other forms of teaching in certain areas. "Potentially successful" means that, based on its utilization during the last several years, it is reasonable to expect that CAI can teach effectively when *properly designed* and *applied.* "Adjunct to other forms of

Eric D. Zemper • Office of Medical Education Research and Development, Michigan State University, East Lansing, Michigan.

teaching" means that CAI is *not* designed to *replace* instructors and their standard teaching tools, but only to *supplement* them and permit instructors to be used more effectively. Although some CAI systems are designed with the ambitious purpose of completely replacing human instructors (and indeed some people seem to define CAI in this manner), such projects, with certain exceptions, have generally not proven to be cost effective in comparison with alternative modes of instruction. Therefore, we do not consider CAI as a replacement of the human instructor, but instead use the term in a broader sense which includes *any* application of computers in the instructional process. "In certain areas" means there is nothing in the past or immediate future of CAI to suggest that it is universally and equally applicable to all content areas, types of learning, and school conditions.

In terms of the types of learning to which CAI can be applied, it is finding its greatest use in the content domain; learning definitions, facts, procedures, concepts, etc. As will be seen later, CAI can be especially useful in applying content knowledge to learning problem-solving techniques in medicine. Psychomotor learning, involving any type of physical manipulation is not a prime area for potential CAI applications, since present capabilities do not allow the computer to "see" just what a student is doing in three-dimensional space. A notable exception to this generalization is SIM-1, a computer-controlled mannequin used for teaching anesthesiology procedures (Abrahamson *et al.*, 1969). Affective learning, or the acquisition of particular attitudes, is not generally considered to be a fruitful area of application of CAI. Any affective changes in students usually are a secondary result of learning through CAI.

Types of CAI Programs in Medical Education

Over the past few years there has been a proliferation of terminology in the literature related to CAI. Authors from different developmental centers seem to have their own pet terminology for essentially the same thing (i.e., "computer-assisted instruction," "computer-based instruction," or "computer-based education"), while others may use the same term to mean something entirely different. This lack of generally agreed upon definitions is probably one reason for the apparent confusion and controversy in much of the literature in this field. We use the general term "computer-assisted instruction", or CAI, because it is the most frequently used in the literature, and because it best expresses the idea of *assisting* rather than replacing an instructor. The types of CAI programs fall into several categories across a spectrum of sophistication of application, where sophistication refers to how much of the potential capability of the computer is used. Thus, certain types of drill-and-practice programs, which are little more than automated page-turners, would be on the low end of the spectrum, while at the opposite end would be programs which present simulated patients whose conditions change with time and in response to treatments prescribed by the student. Since each type, or mode, of CAI is best utilized in certain types of educational situations, it is important to understand each of them.

Drill-and-Practice Mode

The drill-and-practice mode is probably one of the more common CAI forms in use today in general education. The term drill-and-practice has come into common use, which is unfortunate since it tends to evoke visions of rigid, heavy-handed teaching methods. This is not necessarily an accurate picture of this mode of CAI, but it is the term which is predominantly used in the literature, so it is the term which will be used here. Drill-and-practice is ideally suited to the learning of information and skills which require practice. The most publicized use of this mode has been the teaching of arithmetic (Suppes and Morningstar, 1970) and reading skills (Atkinson and Hanson, 1966; Atkinson and Fletcher, 1972) in elementary school. In this mode the computer presents a series of practice problems which the student must solve in order to develop the desired skill. Individual progress is closely monitored by the program. Some students require less practice and advance quickly, while slower learners may remain at one level longer or be routed to remedial sections of the program when they have trouble. As the name drill-and-practice implies, this mode demands a great deal of activity from the student.

Diagnostic Mode

In the diagnostic mode the computer is used to assess a student's aptitude or performance level. When the computer is used primarily as a testing device it is often referred to as Computer-assisted testing (CAT) (Harman *et al.*, 1968; Woods, 1970). In this mode the student is tested on information acquired through reading or other conventional means, and feedback is immediately available to both the student and the instructor from the large body of data which can be accumulated on each student. It is possible to program specific remedial material to be presented during the testing, if the student's performance indicates it is necessary. If properly designed, this mode can result in considerable savings in an instructor's time spent on clerical chores and test administration. It is also possible to program adaptive testing, in which the difficulty of each new test item depends on the student's previous responses. Adaptive testing is especially useful in discriminating at the upper and lower ends of the ability scale (Hanson, 1969; see also Lord, 1970; Green, 1970). In most cases, though, the diagnostic mode is incorporated into teaching programs, to assess entry levels and help guide the student to remedial work in his weak areas as he moves through the program.

Tutorial Mode

Further along toward the more sophisticated end of the CAI spectrum is the tutorial mode, characterized by a greater emphasis on presenting new information to the student. It is well suited to teaching concepts, principles, and bodies of knowledge. It is one of the most common modes of CAI used in postsecondary education, and examples of it can be found in other chapters in this book. A well-designed tutorial program will also incorporate drill-and-practice and some diagnostic components, and will be able to constantly probe, test, adjust, and correct as the student progresses through the learning sequence. Based on all of his responses, the student can receive specific review material in his weak areas; and again, a large amount of student data can be made available to the instructor. Another unique aspect of CAI which should be mentioned here is the ease of updating course material. When new information or procedures become available, updating is a relatively simple matter of changing the relevant portion of the computer program, and the new material is immediately available to all students.

Simulation Mode

At the more sophisticated end of the spectrum of types of CAI is the simulation mode. This mode is used primarily to develop and practice reasoning, problem-solving, and decision-making skills. The other modes we have discussed were mainly concerned with learning and testing new information and concepts, and student responses were directed by the CAI program. In simulation, however, a problem is presented, and the student directs his own path toward the solution by asking questions and collecting data. With a little imagination, a computer simulation can duplicate the most relevant aspects of a dynamic problem situation.

The most common type of computer simulation seen in medical education is the patient simulation, where the student assumes the role of the physician and the computer is programmed to simulate the patient. The student is presented with a chief complaint and possibly a brief history, and then must collect history, lab, and physical findings to arrive at a diagnosis and treatment plan. Patient simulations can be categorized by the way in which the computer models the patient (Hoffer *et al.*, 1975). In the *static* patient model the patient's condition does not change. Every time the student asks for a CBC or a pulse rate, the computer returns the same values no matter when these values are requested. The static patient model is the most common type currently in use, and is exemplified by the early simulated patients developed by Feurzeig *et al.* (1964) and the more recent CASE simulations developed by Harless *et al.* (1971). The simulations developed by Feurzeig limit input to certain terms contained in a list which is provided to the student. The simulations developed by Harless utilize a sophisticated text analyzer which allows the student to ask questions in his own manner without limiting him. This is a more realistic approach, since a list of acceptable terms can possibly provide clues which would not be present in the real environment. A more complex approach is seen in the *dynamic* patient model, where the values for any piece of requested data may change with the passage of time and in response to the student's treatment regimen. An example of the dynamic model is the patient simulations developed by Friedman (1973). Friedman's simulation programs are also described in Chapter 23 of this book, and other examples of this CAI mode in other chapters.

For reasons which will be discussed later, simulation is one of the more important modes of CAI in medical education. Computer patient simulations are now also being developed for use in certification and recertification exams by such groups as the Royal College of Physicians and Surgeons of Canada (Taylor *et al.*, 1976; Grace *et al.*, 1975), and the American Board of Internal Medicine (Harless *et al.*, 1975).

Management and Support Modes

All of the CAI modes we have discussed up to this point have involved direct interaction with the student in a learning situation. There are also several other types of educational applications which do not necessarily involve direct contact with the student, such as computer-managed or computer-supported instruction (CMI or CSI).

CMI or CSI may be viewed as the administrative complement of CAI (Bell and Sargent, 1971). In this type of application the computer is used as a resource center for educational materials and to store and analyze student records. The instructor can request class materials on a specific topic, specify any limitations he wishes to set, and receive lists of resources, suggested readings, class and individual projects, or whatever else the system designers and instructors have felt was appropriate to be included. When student records are kept by computer, in more advanced systems, analyses of class progress and individual progress are easily and quickly obtainable; and individualized study guides and quizzes can be generated by the computer based on past student performances. Such a comprehensive and complex application of computers in medical education is being developed at OMERAD in the Student Information System Project, which will be discussed later in this chapter.

The applications mentioned in this section represent some of the more prominent types of CAI. It is not meant to be a complete coverage of the field, but merely an introduction. For a more comprehensive review of CAI educational applications, see Chapters 7–9 of Vinsonhaler (1976).

Background of CAI

Now that we have discussed the different types of CAI and some of the ways they can be applied, it is appropriate to take a quick look at the background of CAI. It did not just suddenly appear on the educational scene 10 or 15 years ago. CAI can be considered as probably having descended from three major lines of educational and technological development.

Programmed Instruction

First, CAI can be considered an outgrowth of programmed instruction (PI). The main impetus for much of the developmental work in PI in the 50s came from the work of B. F. Skinner (1963, 1968). This work, plus that of Pressey in teaching machines beginning in the 20s, and Crowder's development of the principles of "branching," has resulted in the modern PI text (Smith and Smith, 1966).

A good PI text utilizes four important learning principles: organization, motivation, activity, and individualization. CAI also utilizes these four principles, and is capable of extending them even further, particularly individualization. The computer's ability to store and act upon the basis of all a learner's previous responses makes CAI capable of individualization at a level far beyond anything previously available. Much of the early development of CAI was directly related to the field of programmed instruction. While contributing a great deal to the evolution of CAI, this close association with PI technology has been somewhat disadvantageous in that it tends to stereotype thinking about CAI in terms of the old concepts of programmed instruction and teaching machines; i.e., as a glorified teaching machine which merely presents stimuli, records responses, and sequences instruction. While computers can do this very well, they are capable of much more. Recently the fuller potential of the computer in education has begun to be utilized, as exemplified in the simulation mode.

Systems Analysis

A second important ancestor of CAI is what might be called a "systems approach" to curriculum or course design. A simple example of a systems approach in this case is to set up a course of instruction by following a comprehensive, orderly set of steps. Naturally, anyone who took part in designing curricula thought of himself as being logical and orderly in his work. Some even used the topical outline to lay out the essential areas to be covered in a course before beginning. But with the development of PI, curriculum designers became aware of the critical importance of defining and stating objectives as an initial step in designing teaching programs. The idea that teaching programs should have specific, formal self-corrective procedures built into them, so their weak points could be identified and improved, also finally gained prominence. These developments made it clear to the educational world that there was really very little in the way of basic scientific knowledge which could be easily and usefully applied to the actual process of writing a course. As a result, much has been written during the last 15 years or so concerning the analysis and classification of learning tasks, the nature of various kinds of learning, and many other areas of concern to course development.

All of this has led to the development of an orderly set of procedures to help educators design and analyze instructional sequences, or "educational systems." A typical set of such procedures is shown in simplified form in the flowchart in Figure 1. In this diagram one starts at the top and works down through the steps in sequence. Notice the arrows leading back to previous steps; these are the "feedback loops" which are built in to help assure that the instructional design does what was originally intended. It is entirely possible, for instance, to design a course

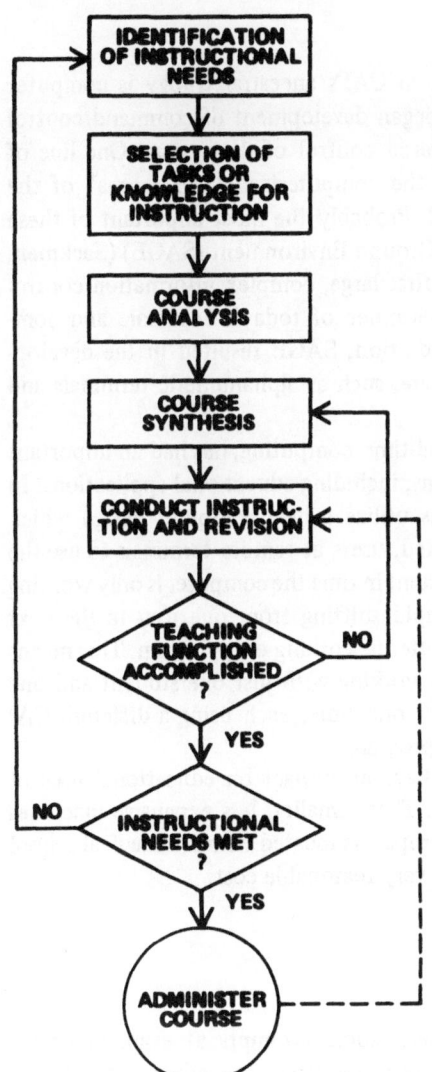

Figure 1. Suggested steps in the "systems approach" to course design (from Zemper, 1973).

that does a very effective job of teaching but teaches the wrong objectives. Notice also that once the course is being administered there is a dotted line leading back to the course-revision step. This indicates there should be a continuous process of checking and revising for improvement of the course as it is being used. One never gets all the "bugs" out the first couple of times through the course. It was quickly realized that CAI, with its step-by-step sequencing of learning, must be designed in accordance with systematic procedures such as this. The systems analysis approach was therefore incorporated into the process of CAI course construction, and has been a major factor in the successful development of CAI.

Computer Technology

The third, and most obvious, element in CAI's ancestral trilogy is computer technology. In the early 50s the military began development of command/control systems, in which computers and men shared control of the system. One line of such research led to the development of the computerized "war rooms" of the Pentagon and the Strategic Air Command. Probably the most important of these early projects was SAC's Semi-Automatic Ground Environment (SAGE) (Sackman, 1967). The SAGE project developed the first large, complex information control system, and was probably the direct forerunner of today's academic and commercial on-line time-sharing systems. In addition, SAGE resulted in the development of much of today's standard hardware, such as alphanumeric terminals and graphic terminals.

The development of time-sharing, or real-time computing, has had an important impact on all types of computer applications, including educational applications. In simple terms, time-sharing on-line systems utilize a new computer design which allows several dozen, or even several hundred, users at remote terminals to use the computer at the same time. At any one instant in time the computer is only working on one user's input, but the extremely rapid shifting from one user to the next makes it appear to each user that the computer is working only for him. This means that the computer no longer is limited to working with just one student and one program, but can handle many students at one time, each using a different CAI program, or different portions of the same program.

Another new development which will have an impact on educational uses of computers is the advent of minicomputers. These smaller, less expensive machines will make it possible to have one or two computers located within a medical school for administrative and educational uses at a very reasonable cost.

Evaluation of CAI

Over the past few years there have been some attempts at evaluating CAI, although these attempts have been relatively infrequent when compared with the number of CAI systems and programs which have been put into operation. One of the most frequent findings of these evaluations has been "no significant difference" between CAI and more traditional instruction. It is quite possible that such findings are most often the result of trying to make comparisons using different types of CAI and different student groups under many different conditions. Such results would seem inevitable when studies lump together drill-and-practice with tutorial, first graders with senior high school students, and such diverse topics as reading and chemistry, and then attempt to compare them with traditional instruction. Lack of proper evaluation standards does not seem to be unique to CAI. In his review of PI evaluation, Hartley (1966, quoted in Hickey, 1968) found that only 6 out of 112 studies comparing PI with traditional instruction met four minimum criteria involving size of test groups, length of test period, completion times, and reporting pre- and posttest results.

The message in all this should be evident: Any CAI evaluation results which are reported, especially those which are extremely negative (or extremely positive), should be examined closely as to the various parameters involved. A study which is of any value would not involve the variety of applications such as indicated above; rather, it should be limited and specific. Vinsonhaler and Bass (1972) have reviewed several major studies which used standardized tests for evaluation and followed minimally acceptable experimental procedures involving drill-and-practice for grade school children in mathematics and in language arts. The language arts studies involved about 2000 students and the mathematics studies involved 8000 students in California, Michigan, Mississippi, and New York. In both subject areas the results showed significant and substantial gains for students using the CAI drill-and-practice. One study tested for a Hawthorne effect and found it to be playing no significant part in the results (Wilson and Fitzgibbons, 1970).

While these results are not necessarily generalizable to college students, and medical students in particular, they should serve to illustrate the kind of evaluation which is necessary, but which unfortunately has been almost nonexistent in the literature purporting to "evaluate" CAI v. traditional instruction. At the moment it appears that most of the good evaluations involve the drill-and-practice mode, with very few good studies of the other modes.

One good example of a well-designed evaluation of the tutorial mode is the work of Cartwright and Mitzel at Pennsylvania State University on the CARE Project (Cartwright and Cartwright, 1972; Cartwright and Mitzel, 1971). The CARE Project (Computer Assisted Remedial Education) was designed to fill a specific need in training teachers to recognize children with educational handicaps. The package is a self-contained three-credit college-level CAI course which uses several modes of instruction, but it is primarily a tutorial program. An unusual feature of the CARE Project is that it is designed to be taken to the teacher in the field, where it is most needed. The computer and 15 terminals are located in an expandable van which is hauled by a truck to remote parts of Appalachia to be set up at various locations for 6 to 8 weeks at a time. The teachers take the course at their own convenience, close to their own school, rather than having to take a semester back at the University. In the evaluation of this course, students taking the CAI course were compared with students who take the same course, but using the traditional 10 weeks of lecture. The CAI and non-CAI groups were compared on the basis of time to complete the course and scores on identical 75-item final exams. It was found that the CAI group scored 24% higher on the final exam than the non-CAI group ($p < .001$); and the CAI group finished the course in a mean time of 25.2 hours compared with 37.5 hours for the non-CAI group. The operational costs of the system, discounting developmental costs, were comparable to costs of traditional instruction. Therefore, this application appears to be very cost effective, especially for the in-service teacher. This example should serve to illustrate that a well-designed CAI program, developed toward specific objectives and specific educational needs, can prove to be a valuable educational tool. The concept of a portable CAI lab suggests possibilities for use in continuing medical education. In fact, the Pennsylvania State University CAI Laboratory already has developed a van-mounted system to provide in-service registered nurses with college-credit courses toward earning a baccalaureate degree in nursing (Estes, 1976; Tamowski, 1976; Hall, 1976).

The CARE Project results bring out another frequent finding when comparing CAI and traditional instruction. While many studies indicate that there may be no significant differences in achievement levels, they usually do show a very significant reduction in the amount of time a student must spend learning the material using CAI. See, for instance, the review by Jamison *et al.* (1974) covering evaluation of CAI and other new modes of instruction. In some cases this reduction in time necessary for learning can be an important consideration.

Again, it should be emphasized that most evaluation of CAI has not been consistently uniform and well-designed, and results should not be taken at face value unless the experimental design has been thoroughly checked and found to meet minimal criteria. (See Markle, 1967, and DAVI, 1966, for recommendations on evaluation design.)

Economics of CAI

Cost is probably one of the more prominent questions when considering the use of CAI; and, as with evaluation, there seems to be a singular lack of usable papers in the literature on this subject. Another problem is the proper application of the tools of cost evaluation. A good introduction to this subject for educational administrators can be found in Wilkinson (1973). One fully researched paper on cost evaluation of CAI is that of Kopstein and Seidel (1968), in which they consider many factors in comparing CAI costs with those of traditional instruction. Realizing they are taking cost data from an older field (traditional instruction), where overall costs are well established but not broken down into specific categories, and trying to compare them with costs in a brand new field (CAI), where insufficient cost experience is available and costs in specific categories have been changing with new developments, Kopstein and Seidel have utilized quite conservative assumptions favoring traditional instruction in developing their comparisons. Their results indicate that CAI is considerably more expensive than traditional instruction at the elementary and secondary school levels and would have to be several times as efficient as traditional instruction in order to be cost effective. However, the situation in college and professional education is entirely different. The cost per student hour for traditional undergraduate education was estimated at $2.76 (from USOE and NEA figures), while the estimate for CAI was $2.61 per student hour.

It should be pointed out that these estimates were made in 1968, for nonprofessional undergraduate education. Costs for professional education are higher, and have risen since then. In 1973, the Association of American Medical Colleges estimated the average "full resource cost" of undergraduate medical education at $16,000 to $26,000 per year (AAMC, 1974). The actual educational costs, after subtracting contributed services and income from research and clinical activities, ranged from $9,000 to $19,000 or an average of $12,500 per student per year. At 30 to 35 hours per week of class time, for 43 weeks per year, training a medical student costs in the range of $8.50 to $10 per hour (in 1972 dollars). No doubt CAI costs have changed also, rising in some categories and dropping in others, but these figures indicate CAI can be economically competitive in medical education. It should also be mentioned that Kopstein and Seidel's estimates were based on the assumption of starting from nothing and developing an entire large-scale computer facility solely for CAI, rather than using previously existing facilities. Another cost-saving possibility which was not considered was the use of minicomputer systems, which is rapidly becoming more feasible. See, for instance, Kamp and Starkweather (1973) for such an application in medical education.

One final observation might be appropriate here. In many ways CAI seems to be presently caught in a sort of circular problem, which runs somewhat as follows: (1) There is a need to provide complete evidence of the effectiveness of CAI, but to do so requires complete and convincing demonstrations. (2) To provide complete and convincing demonstrations requires good programs. (3) To provide good programs requires well-trained personnel and a good computer system. (4) To provide well-trained personnel and a good computer system requires adequate funding. (5) To get adequate funding for CAI requires evidence of its effectiveness. And so back to (1). It appears that, in order for CAI to break out of this bind, educational (or commercial) groups around the country are going to have to be willing to invest some money in order to open up the potential of CAI.

CAI's Future in Medical Education

In deciding whether or not CAI should be used in a particular setting, Seltzer (1971) has proposed the following guidelines: (1) If CAI offers a unique solution to a major educational problem, it should be used no matter how much it costs. (2) If CAI is a more efficient or effective alternative at a reasonable cost, it should be used. (3) If the cost of development and use of CAI is relatively high, and its efficiency or effectiveness is marginal, then it should not be used.

The drill-and-practice, diagnostic, and tutorial modes of CAI are capable of providing many applications in medical education which meet the second criterion listed above, if not the first, considering the findings that students using CAI generally require much less time to reach a particular achievement level and that CAI's costs can be competitive with traditional methods of instruction at the professional education level. The use of these modes of CAI should, if properly designed, have no problem proving their worth in teaching, review, and self-evaluation, as indicated by the use of the CAI facilities at The Ohio State University and Massachusetts General Hospital (see Chapters 15 and 21). But, as with any application of a new technology, it is very critical that they be properly designed and properly applied. It cannot be overemphasized that any implementation of CAI must be carefully and systematically handled. Too many computer applications have failed because the people involved in the development did not realize all the complexities involved, and this is the fault of people, not the computer. Any application must involve a careful look at the needs and objectives of the curriculum. There can be many pitfalls for the unwary, one of which was pointed out by Jason (1971):

> Of greatest concern is the propensity of many teachers to regard new *devices* as equivalent to new *ideas*. The act of accommodating old instructional notions to new packages, such as putting an old lecture on television or on a computer, can prove to be worse than no change at all. The glossy new packaging tends to deceive both the student and the teacher into believing that something new, and assumedly, better is happening. . .
>
> There have already been repeated examples in medicine of live lectures, poorly delivered and stultifying in person, which became even more evidently so on the TV monitor. One can now find a small but growing number of computer-based instructional units which are, in actuality, electronic reincarnations of the pompous, arrogant professor whose instructional strategy is the demand of compliance from the student rather than the promotion of independent skills. Simply put: bad instruction isn't made good by inclusion in a new medium.

Applications of the simulation mode are being developed in many places around the country, and may prove to be one of the most important uses of CAI in medical education, since such applications can frequently meet Seltzer's first criterion listed above. As mentioned earlier, the most common use of the simulation mode is the patient simulation. These simulations can be used to teach and evaluate a key aspect of the training of a physician, the problem-solving and decision-making skills of clinical care and diagnosis, in a manner which has not before been possible. The preclinical years are spent in a well-structured learning environment, while clinical learning experiences are much more haphazard in comparison, because of the pragmatics of working in a clinic with real patients with real problems. Although there is no substitute for such experiences, an element of educational structure can be introduced by the use of computerized patient simulations as an intermediate or transitional stage between classroom learning and handling real patients. This gives the student the opportunity to try his problem-solving techniques in a nonpunitive atmosphere and without the fear of causing harm to a live patient. He has the complete responsibility for a "patient" which he could never be given in the clinic or emergency room, and any mistakes he does make can be very vivid learning experiences. Anyone who has worked with patient simulators probably has anecdotes such as overhearing students discussing their "patient" who "died" and saying, "I'll never make that mistake again!"

Another advantage in using computer patient simulations is, given an adequate library of problem types, it is easy to insure that each student has experience with a wide variety of medical problems. This is hard to do in a clinical setting, where there is little control over what patients come in at any particular time. With the aid of such simulations it will be much easier for the student to make the traumatic transition from classroom to clinic with the increased confidence in his own abilities and knowledge which is so important in good patient care.

Guidelines for Utilization of CAI

Granted that CAI can make an important contribution to medical education, what factors inhibit or facilitate its utilization, and how should such a change be approached by medical school administrators? Precise answers to questions such as these have not been available in the literature, so in 1972–1974 Dr. John Casbergue, of OMERAD, undertook a study to provide this much needed information (Casbergue, 1974, 1975, 1978). The specific purposes of the study were to: (1) identify the critical factors which facilitate or inhibit the development and utilization of CAI, as perceived by experienced users and developers in health professions education; and (2) develop a set of guidelines to be used by health professions administrators and faculty in planning for the adoption of CAI as an instructional medium. A complete description of this important study and its results is presented by Casbergue in Chapter 5 of this book; therefore, it will be only briefly covered here.

Casbergue surveyed experienced and nonexperienced users of CAI in health professions education to rate the critical factors facilitating or inhibiting the use of CAI. These factors were defined by the experienced users. From this work a set of seven guidelines were developed by Casbergue. In condensed form, they are: (I) The high initial investment costs of CAI must be weighed against the potential gains in learning effectiveness, rate of learning, and overall cost effectiveness of the total curriculum. (II) Reliable computer facilities and services must be made available. (III) The institution must make a commitment to the development and utilization of CAI. (IV) The faculty must make a commitment to use of CAI. (V) The utilization of CAI is facilitated by development of collaborative efforts between faculty and CAI technical staff. (VI) CAI must be made an integral part of the health professions curriculum. (VII) Educational workshops, programs, and processes must be provided to prepare faculty, students, and staff for change due to the utilization of CAI. The complete set of guidelines is presented in Chapter 5, and contains specific factors that should be considered in connection with each guideline.

The results of the survey also lead to some interesting conclusions concerning general perceptions of CAI by medical educators, which were not previously evident. Most noticeable, from the results of inhibiting-factors' ranking, was the tendency of the inexperienced group to place more emphasis on some inhibiting factors which were not perceived as important to those who had been through the process of adopting CAI (see the tables in Chapter 5). Hopefully, this study will help deans and other administrators to focus their attention on the aspects of implementing CAI which have been found to be more important.

The most important considerations in successful implementation of CAI were found to be access to a reliable computer system; and institutional (administrative) commitment to the use and development of CAI; and educational programs for faculty, administrators, and technical personnel, since they must understand how CAI can be integrated with other instructional modalities. The high initial investment costs were found to be a major inhibiting factor; but Casbergue points out that proper planning, the availability of networks such as the Health Education Network, and the experienced users' feeling that reduced learning time and probable increased learning effectiveness need to be considered, all tend to reduce the magnitude of this problem. Also, as mentioned previously, the recent advances in minicomputers and "intelligent terminals" has the potential of reducing these initial costs even further.

The results of Casbergue's work provide a very useful tool to aid a dean or other medical school administrator in deciding whether or not to commit resources to the development or utilization of CAI. Such guidelines, developed specifically for health professions education, have not previously been available in the literature.

Current CAI Activities at the MSU Medical Schools

The medical schools at MSU have not been involved in utilization of CAI to the extent seen at other institutions, such as The Ohio State University and Massachusetts General Hospital. For various reasons, not the least of which is the recent severe budget cuts from the state legislature, the introduction of computers in medical education here has taken a slower approach, out of the limelight. An example of this gradual process is seen in the Student Information System, the first of several computer-related activities being carried out by OMERAD which will be discussed in the remainder of this chapter.

The Student Information System

A comprehensive management and support application of computers is being developed at OMERAD in the Student Information System (SIS) Project, under the direction of Dr. Sui-Wah Chan. This system is evolving into a curriculum-management tool for use with curricula based on specific instructional objectives and which can allow more flexible individualized instruction. Briefly, the basic unit of SIS is the OCTL, an acronym for Objectives, performance Criteria, Testing, and Learning activities and resources (Chan, 1973a; Chan *et al.*, 1975). The interrelationships among the components of the OCTL can be visualized as shown in Figure 2. Most CSI or CMI programs only involve the relationship between objectives and testing, and a few may also involve learning resources. As can be seen in Figure 2, SIS also contains a Student Records System, a Program

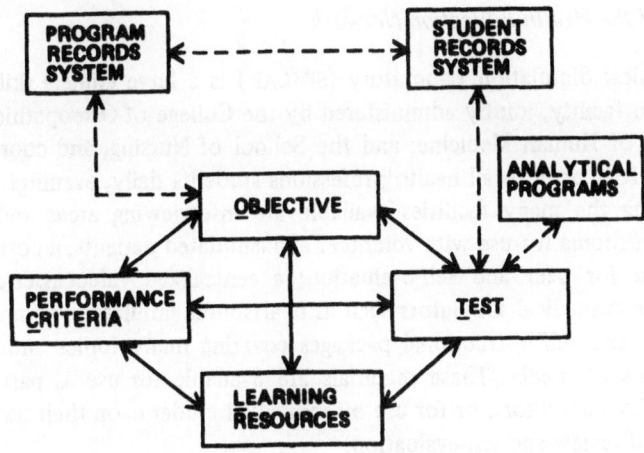

Figure 2. Components of the OCTL and the Student Information System.

Records System, and a set of Analytical Programs which oversees the operation of the information system.

There are three major functions of SIS: (1) provide a test-instrument library, with an automated test construction aid which will generate criterion-referenced tests, based on specific curriculum objectives, and produce a master copy with the test items sorted according to question type (i.e., true—false, single-answer multiple choice, multiple-answer multiple choice, matching, etc.) and grouped under appropriate headings and instructions for the students; (2) provide learning guidelines and resources for students, based on curriculum objectives and the students' individual needs; (3) provide a mechanism for comprehensive review of curriculum content and structure. This is possible because each OCTL requires well-defined relationships among its objectives, criteria, and learning resources, and among other OCTLs. This results in an extensive "road map" of the total curriculum, which can be a powerful tool for administrators and curriculum committees.

This system also provides some useful spinoffs, such as a complete inventory of learning resources from across the whole school, which can help in avoiding unnecessary duplication of resources; and it provides a unique means of making the evaluation program sensitive to curricular needs. The major components of SIS are now operating, and it is being utilized with a portion of the College of Human Medicine (CHM) curriculum at MSU. The remainder of the curriculum is being implemented as OCTLs. on the system; and, when completed, SIS will form a major component of the College-Wide Evaluation Program, a summative evaluation program being developed within CHM. It is anticipated that the curriculum of the College of Osteopathic Medicine at MSU will also be implemented on SIS, and this single system will then provide evaluation and instructional development services for students, instructors and administrators of both medical schools (Chan, personal communication).

SIMLAB and the Health Education Network

The Clinical Simulation Laboratory (SIMLAB) is a large clinical skills teaching and research facility, jointly administered by the College of Osteopathic Medicine, the College of Human Medicine, and the School of Nursing, and coordinated by OMERAD. It is open to all health professions students daily, evenings, and weekends. Among the many facilities available are interviewing areas and complete examination rooms for use with volunteer and simulated patients; a portable videotape system for peer and self-evaluation; a centralized videocassette and film library; various medical simulators such as heartsound simulators, Gynny, Resusci-Annie, etc.; and self-instructional packages covering many topics and employing various types of media. These materials are available for use as part of a class assignment by instructors, or for use by individual students on their own initiative as a means of review and self-evaluation.

Also available in the SIMLAB are two portable computer terminals and phone lines for access to the many CAI programs available at Ohio State through the Health Education Network. Before the SIMLAB was opened, in the summer of 1975, a small CAI Laboratory, under the direction of Dr. J. Thomas Parmeter, was maintained for student use during the 1974—1975 school year by the College of Human Medicine, with access to all the programs available through the Lister Hill Center CAI Experimental Network (the forerunner of the Health Education Network). A select group of students, involved in an independent study track, were notified as to what CAI programs were available, and were surveyed to find what lab hours would be most convenient for them. The CAI lab was open during these periods, with a monitor always present to help students whenever necessary. A log was kept of student usage and comments. Student reaction to the CAI programs was uniformly positive among those who used them; but, despite periodic reminders of its availability, after a moderate amount of initial interest, usage soon dwindled to a few individuals who continued to utilize the facility. Interviews with students indicated an interest in CAI; but an unwillingness to use a learning resource not assigned by an instructor, while under a heavy workload, was the reason most often cited for not utilizing the CAI lab (Zemper, unpublished data). This result is not surprising, and tends to verify Casbergue's finding that, in order for CAI to be perceived as important, it must be an integral part of the instructional system, not just an additional resource. (see Guideline IV, F; Chapter 5).

During the 1975—76 school year, CAI was available only on a limited basis in the SIMLAB, while we undertook a process of matching the CAI programs available at Ohio State with elements of our medical and nursing curricula, and then demonstrated specific usages to individual instructors in an attempt to integrate CAI into the curricula as more than an optional resource. In summary, our experience indicates the use of a national CAI resource such as the Health Education Network is a quick and relatively inexpensive way to make CAI available to medical students, but it will not be used without the same careful planning that is necessary when developing an in-house system.

Adoption of Programs Developed at Other Institutions

In addition to using a network to reduce costs of implementing CAI, there is also the expedient of obtaining programs developed at other schools and running them on a local time-sharing computer system. This makes possible local control over the program, eliminates long-distance phone or network charges, provides a tested program without the expenditure of a lot of development time and money, and affords the option of later tailoring the program to local needs. Fortunately, most all members of the medical CAI community are quite willing to share their programs, particularly with newcomers who are trying to get a start in this field. Comprehensive listings of medical schools which are currently developing and using CAI may be found in Lefever and Johnson (1976) and Kamp (1975). It makes it easier if the programs to be imported are on a computer system similar to the local system. Otherwise, reprogramming to fit the requirements of the local system could take a considerable amount of time and effort.

Currently OMERAD is in the process of implementing a patient simulation program, developed by Dr. Richard B. Friedman (Friedman, 1973), on the CDC 6500 at the MSU Computer Laboratory. As with the use of programs through a network, local use of programs from another institution will require a process of matching them with specific elements of the curriculum. Once Friedman's patient simulation program is fully implemented here, it is hoped we will be able to generate new "patients" tailored to specific needs of our curricula, and in turn make them available to others.

Faculty Interest Survey

As a preliminary step in a national study of the use of simulations in medical education being conducted by OMERAD for the National Library of Medicine, under the direction of Dr. Jack Maatsch and Dr. Dennis Hoban, a survey of MSU's allopathic (CHM), osteopathic (COM), and nursing (RN) faculty was recently completed. The purpose of the survey was to determine their familiarity with and preferences for various types of simulation modes, including computer-controlled simulations, defined primarily as patient simulations. These results, while not necessarily generalizable to other institutions, do provide some interesting information about the views of computer simulations held by 109 faculty members of the health professions schools at MSU.

Initial analysis of the results by Dr. Sarah Sprafka and Barbara Perles showed that 49% of the CHM and COM respondents and 36% of the RN respondents claimed to be familiar with computer-controlled simulation. (Since the CHM and COM responses were quite similar, they were grouped together.) Of those who claimed to be familiar with computer simulation, 68% of the CHM/COM faculty indicated they could see possible applications of it and would use it, if it were made available; while the remaining 32% could not envision applications for computer simulation and would not use it in their current teaching assignment. One hundred percent of the RN faculty familiar with computer simulation said they would use it. Unfortunately the structure of the questionnaire did not allow identification of any who may have answered negatively because their current teaching assignment was of a nature which made use of computer simulations impractical. Of the CHM/COM faculty not familiar with computer simulations, 26% would use it and 44% would not; the remaining 30% did not answer (Sprafka, unpublished data).

When the data were analyzed further, it was found that only 30% of the CHM/COM respondents actually had "hands on" familiarity with computer simulations (i.e., had ever interacted with a computer simulation, used one in a class, or participated in developing one); and only 16% of the RN respondents had similar experience. Of these CHM/COM faculty, 83% said they would use computer simulations if they were made available (S. Sprafka, personal communication).

These results indicate that among medical faculty who are not familiar with computer simulations there is not an overwhelming amount of support for its use; while among those who are familiar with the concept, and particularly among those with first-hand experience, there is a great deal of willingness to use computer simulations. This clearly illustrates the necessity of familiarizing the faculty with the capabilities of instructional applications of computers, as suggested by Casbergue (see Guideline IV, C and E; Chapter 5).

The MIST Project

The last of the OMERAD projects to be discussed is the Medical Information Systems Theory (MIST) Project of Dr. Sui-Wah Chan, of OMERAD, and Dr. John F. Vinsonhaler, of the Department of Educational Psychology in MSU's College of Education. This project has developed a generalized computer simulation of the clinical decision-making process (Chan, 1973b; Chan and Vinsonhaler, 1974; Vinsonhaler *et al.*, 1975; Chan *et al.*, 1977). This computer simulation is a "doctor simulator," or the "mirror image" of the patient simulations discussed previously; here the computer asks for patient information and comes up with the diagnosis.

The primary component of this system is the clinical decision maker, or SIMDOC (SIMulated DOCtor). As can be seen in Figure 3, SIMDOC assumes that a clinical decision is the result of the interaction of a decision theory or approach used by the doctor, and his clinical memory containing information about all types of medical problems and their interrelationships. Briefly, SIMDOC operates as follows. The researcher designs a decision theory or approach, and states it in the formal Decision Simulation Language. A simplified example is seen in the lower left-hand box of Figure 3. The DIAGNOSE command causes the computer to request the chief complaint from the patient. The next step is to associate the cues given in the chief complaint with Problem Data Records (PDRs). The result of this PDR SEARCH is a list of possible diagnoses, or hypotheses, based on the chief complaint. The HISTORY CUE SEARCH and PHYSICAL CUE SEARCH commands cause SIMDOC to collect history and physical (and laboratory) data from the patient, based on the most relevant hypotheses, relevance being determined any of several different ways chosen by the researcher. DIAGNOSIS JUDGMENT causes SIMDOC to attempt a diagnosis; i.e., determine if any single hypothesis has met a specific decision criterion defined by the researcher. The diagnosis of multiple problems is also possible. This basic process, or variations of it, can be repeated until a diagnosis is made; then a treatment and prescription are selected, based on the diagnosis and knowledge of the patient. For instance, SIMDOC will not prescribe aspirin for a patient known to have a peptic ulcer; and if it does not know, it asks.

It should be emphasized that this system is not locked into a particular method of decision-making. It is able to simulate highly complex approaches to problem-solving, and this makes it a unique and powerful tool for research into these critical processes. As an example of SIMDOC's capabilities, an experiment was set up to compare the clinical performances of two stereotypes of the physician. The

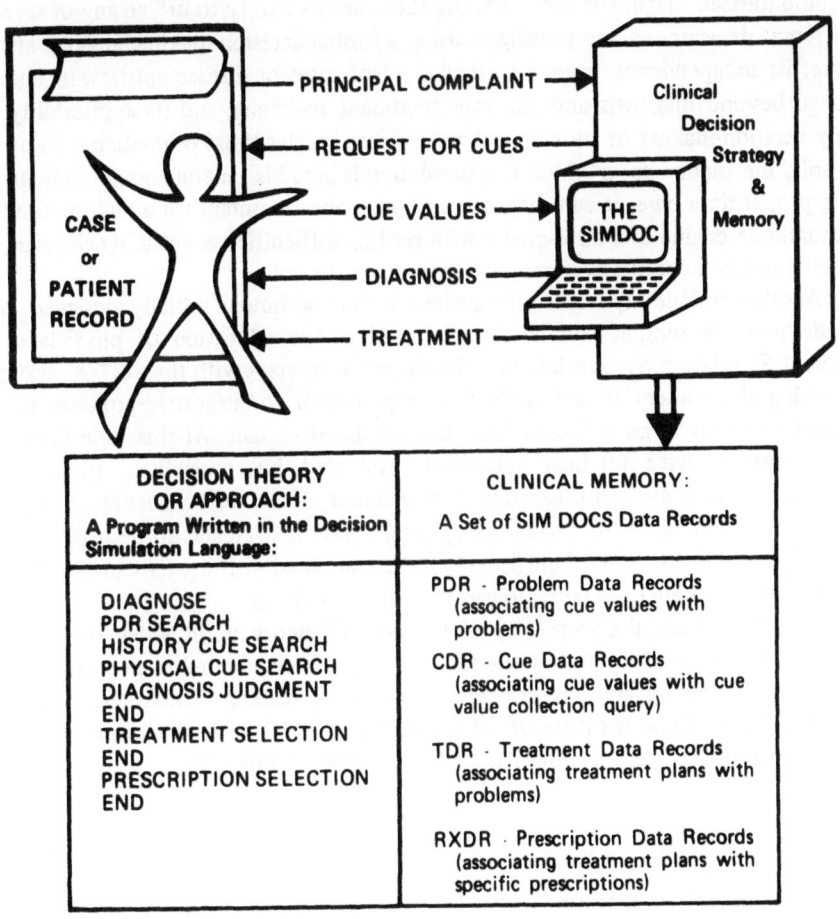

Figure 3. The SIMDOC Concept (from Vinsonhaler *et al.*, 1975).

thorough, precise "academic" physician, who does a careful workup with emphasis on lab studies before diagnosis, was simulated using one decision approach written in the Decision Simulation Language. The "clinic" physician, who strives for good, but efficient, service through rapid identification of the most likely problem with minimum information processing, was simulated using a different decision approach. These two simulated physicians were each presented with two real case records representing patients with identical initial symptoms, one case being mononucleosis and the other viral hepatitis. The results (Vinsonhaler *et al.*, 1975) showed that both simulated physicians diagnosed both cases correctly, but the "clinic" physician required half as many cues and about one-quarter the cost to the patient as did the "academic" physician. It has also been found that SIMDOC can successfully diagnose even when relatively large error rates are introduced in the patient data, such as might occur with inaccurately recalled history data, laboratory errors, or physician fatigue or distraction.

There are many features of this system which make it different from any other "computerized diagnostic aid." Among them are its ability to utilize any of several different decision-making paradigms using a formal decision-making language structure; its independence from a particular set of cases or disease entities; its ability to go beyond diagnosis and generate treatment regimens; and its applicability to any decision-making or problem-solving process besides those of medicine. In other words, the theory upon which this simulation is based is general enough that, given the proper data base, it can diagnose and prescribe treatment for a malfunctioning automobile engine or a third-grader with reading difficulties as well as it can diagnose a patient with hepatitis or hereditary spherocytic anemia.

Another unique aspect of this system is that, although initially designed as a basic research tool, it can be directly used in the education of physicians. A Patient Simulation System has been developed to interact with the SIMDOC system, allowing the student to use SIMDOC as a preceptor to suggest hypotheses to be tested and cues to be collected from the simulated patient. At this time the combined systems have not been completely evaluated, but possibilities for such an educational tool are quite exciting. For instance, it should be possible, using the SIMDOC system alone, to define the optimal decision strategies to be used under a variety of conditions; and then, using SIMDOC combined with the Patient Simulation System, teach these optimal strategies to medical students.

As a final note, the versatility of the general theory upon which the SIMDOC system is based is illustrated by the fact that it has been adapted as an experimental tool for diagnosing and prescribing treatment for reading difficulties. It will be used in the National Institute of Education's new Institute for Research on Teaching, which has just been established at Michigan State University.

Closing Comments

This chapter has discussed some basic aspects of CAI, and the developmental work in computer applications being done at Michigan State University by the

Office of Medical Education Research and Development. There are many applications of CAI in medical education which have not been mentioned here; for instance, possible uses in continuing medical education, such as the placement of CAI terminals in hospital emergency rooms. Hoffer found them to be well accepted by the physicians; and by following the use of certain "tracer" drugs or equipment, it appeared that the CAI programs had a positive effect on physician behavior (Hoffer, 1975). Applications such as this are covered elsewhere in this book.

The primary message the reader should retain from this chapter is that CAI is no panacea for all educational ills, but it has the potential of being an extremely versatile and useful tool *if* it is provided with sound, careful development. CAI is a new educational technique and, as such, it is not completely tested yet; but it is a rapidly developing field which deserves careful consideration for its possible role in medical education. Vinsonhaler (1976) has stated:

> ... the true importance of real-time computing must be kept in mind. In my judgement, real-time systems in instruction and research cannot be dismissed as a "fad," regardless of our ineptitude in applying such systems. Other educational and scientific instruments may come and go, but real-time computers are definitely here to stay. Further, whether implemented on mini-computers, on computer utilities or on both (as is most likely), real-time computing systems are destined to have a major impact upon education and social science. It would be very unwise for the majority of educationists and scientists to continue to ignore these systems. Dealing with the computer revolution is like riding a tiger – it is much, *much* safer to stay on top of the thing.

So CAI should not be just ignored, but neither should it be utilized in a haphazard fashion. All the fancy hardware in the world is completely useless if it doesn't help the student. Our goal in medical education is not the hardware, but producing better medical practitioners, and CAI can be one more useful means of achieving that goal.

ACKNOWLEDGMENT

I would like to thank Dr. John P. Casbergue, Dr. Sui-Wah Chan, Dr. Sarah Sprafka, and Dr. John F. Vinsonhaler for their kind assistance in providing information about their research projects; and Dr. Jack Maatsch and Dr. Ann Olmsted for their helpful comments on the manuscript. Portions of this chapter appeared in a previous paper (Zemper, 1973).

References

Abrahamson, S., Denson, J. S., and Wolf, R. M., 1969. Effectiveness of a simulator in training anesthesiology residents, *J. Med. Educ.* **44**:515.

Association of American Medical Colleges (AAMC) Committee on the Financing of Medical Education, 1974. Financing undergraduate medical education, *J. Med. Educ.* **49**:1087.

Atkinson, R. C., and Fletcher, J. D., 1972. Teaching children to read with a computer, *The Reading Teacher* **25**:319.

Atkinson, R. C., and Hanson, D. N., 1966. Computer-assisted instruction in initial reading: The Stanford project, *Reading Research Quarterly* 2:5.

Bell, N. T., and Sargent, G., 1971. Preliminary Report: Computer Based Instructional Management System, Michigan State University Learning Systems Institute.

Cartwright, G. P., and Cartwright, C. A., 1972. CAI course in the early identification of handicapped children, *Exceptional Children* 38:453.

Cartwright, G. P., and Mitzel, H. E., 1971. Development of a Computer-Assisted Instruction Course in the Identification and Diagnosis of Handicapping Conditions in Children, Final Report USOE Project No. 482129, College of Education, CAI Laboratory, Pennsylvania State University (July, 1971).

Casbergue, J. P., 1974. Computer Assisted Instruction in Health Professions Education: Guidelines for Utilization, Ph.D. thesis, Michigan State University.

Casbergue, J. P., 1975. A study to identify factors influencing the utilization of computer assisted instruction in health professions education, *in Proceedings: Fourteenth Annual Conference on Research in Medical Education*, Association of American Medical Colleges, Washington, D.C. (November, 1975).

Casbergue, J. P., 1978. Computer-assisted instruction in health professions education: Guidelines for utilization, *in* E. C. DeLand (Ed.), *Information Technology in Health Science Education*, Plenum Press, New York.

Chan, S. W. 1973a. The Notion of Generalized Objectives (OCTL) and Individualized Instruction and Learning, Working paper, Office of Medical Education Research and Development, Michigan State University (January, 1973).

Chan, S. W., 1973b. Proposal for a Medical Information Systems Theory, Office of Medical Education Research and Development, Michigan State University.

Chan, S. W., and Vinsonhaler, J. F., 1974. DOCS: A computer based system for diagnosis and treatment, paper read at ACM Conference on Computer Science Education, Detroit (February 1974).

Chan, S. W., Dumas, R., and Dixon, P., 1975. Student Information System Project OCTL Retrieval Program User's Manual, Office of Medical Education Research and Development, Michigan State University (May, 1975).

Chan, S. W., Brown, M., Geiger, M., 1977. DOCS Version III: Doctor Simulation System, MIST Project Technical Memo, Office of Medical Education Research and Development, Michigan State University (March, 1977).

DAVI, 1966. Recommendations for reporting the effectiveness of programmed instruction materials, *AV Communications Review* 14:117 and 243.

Estes, C. A., 1976. The use of computer based instruction in an extended degree program for nurses leading to the Bachelor of Science Degree, paper presented at the 1976 AERA Annual Meeting, San Francisco.

Feurzeig, W., Munter, P., Swets, J., and Breen, M., 1964. Computer-aided teaching in medical diagnosis, *J. Med. Educ.* 39:746.

Friedman, R. B., 1973. A Computer program for simulating the patient–physician encounter, *J. Med. Educ.* 48:92.

Grace, M., Taylor, W. C., Skakun, E. N., and Fincham, S., 1975. Computerized patient management problems: An alternative examination technique, *in: Proceedings: Fourteenth Annual Conference on Research in Medical Education*, American Association of Medical Colleges, Washington, D.C. (November 1975).

Green, B. F., Jr., 1970. Comments on tailored testing, *in* W. Holtzman (Ed.), *Computer-Assisted Instruction, Testing and Guidance*, Harper and Row, New York.

Hall, K. A., 1976. The development and utilization of mobile CAI for the education of nurses in remote areas, paper presented at the 1976 AERA Annual Meeting, San Francisco.

Hanson, D. N., 1969. An investigation of computer-based science testing, *in* R. Atkinson and H. Wilson (Eds.), *Computer-Assisted Instruction*, Academic Press, New York.

Harless, W. G., Drennon, G. G., Marxer, J. J., Root, J. A., and Miller, G. E., 1971. CASE: A computer-aided simulation of the clinical encounter, *J. Med. Educ.* 46:443.

Harless, W. G., Farr, N. A., Zier, M. A., and Gamble, J. R., 1975. MERIT: A model for evaluation and recertification through individualized testing, *in: Proceedings: Fourteenth Annual Conference on Research in Medical Education*, American Association of Medical Colleges, Washington, D.C. (November, 1975).

Harman, H. H., Helm, C. E., and Loye, D., 1968. Computer Assisted Testing, Office of Computational Science, Educational Testing Service, Princeton, New Jersey.

Hartley, J., 1966. Evaluation of programmed instruction: External evaluation, *New Education* 2(1).

Hickey, A. E., 1968. *Computer Assisted Instruction: A Survey of the Literature*, 3rd ed., Entelek, Newburyport, Massachusetts.

Hoffer, E. P., 1975. Computer-aided instruction in community hospital emergency departments: A pilot project, *J. Med. Educ.* 50:84.

Hoffer, E. P., Barnett, G. O., Farquhar, B. B., and Prather, P. A., 1975. Computer-aided instruction in medicine, *Ann. Rev. Biophys. Bioeng.* 4:103.

Jamison, D., Suppes, P., and Wells, S., 1974. The effectiveness of alternative instructional media: A survey, *Review of Educational Research* 44:1.

Jason, H., 1971. Instructional technology in medical education, *in* S. Tickton (Ed.), *To Improve Learning: An Evaluation of Instructional Technology*, Vol. II, R. R. Bowker Co., New York.

Kamp, M., 1975. *Index to Computerized Teaching in the Health Sciences*, Health Sciences Interest Group of the Association for the Development of Computer-based Instructional Systems, Kentfield, Ca.

Kamp, M., and Starkweather, J., 1973. A return to a dedicated machine for computer-assisted instruction, *Comput. Biol. Med.* 3:293.

Kopstein, F. F., and Seidel, R. J., 1968. Computer-administered instruction versus traditionally administered instruction: Economics, *AV Communications Review* 16:147.

Lefever, R. D., and Johnson, J. K., 1976. Survey of the Use of Computers in Instruction, Association of American Medical Colleges, Washington, D.C.

Lord, F. M., 1970. Some test theory for tailored testing, *in* W. Holtzman (Ed.), *Computer-Assisted Instruction, Testing and Guidance*, Harper & Row, New York.

Markle, S. M., 1967. Empirical testing of programs, *in: Programmed Instruction; The 66th NSSE Yearbook*, Part 2, University of Chicago Press, Chicago.

Sackman, H., 1967. *Computers, Systems Science, and Evolving Society*, pp. 254–300, John Wiley and Sons, New York.

Seltzer, R. A., 1971. Computer-assisted instruction – What it can and cannot do, *Am. Psychol.* 26:373.

Skinner, B. F., 1963. Reflections on a decade of teaching machines, *Teachers College Record* 65:168.

Skinner, B. F., 1968. *The Technology of Teaching*, Appleton-Century-Crofts, New York.

Smith, K. V., and Smith, M. F., 1966. *Cybernetic Principles of Learning and Educational Design*, Holt, Rinehart and Winston, New York.

Suppes, P., and Morningstar, M., 1970. Four programs in computer-assisted instruction, *in* W. Holtzman (Ed.), *Computer-Assisted Instruction, Testing and Guidance*, Harper & Row. New York.

Tamowski, H. J., 1976. CMRE: Computer managed review and examination, paper presented at the 1976 AERA Annual Meeting, San Francisco.

Taylor, W. C., Grace, M., Taylor, T. R., Fincham, S. M., and Skakun, E. N., 1976. The use of computerized patient management problems in a certifying examination, *Medical Education* 10(3):179.

Vinsonhaler, J. F., 1976. *Computers in Education and Social Science,* available from College of Education, Michigan State University, East Lansing.

Vinsonhaler, J. F., and Bass, R. K., 1972. Ten major studies of the evaluation of CAI drill and practice, *Educational Technology* 12(7):29.

Vinsonhaler, J. F., Chan, S. W., Wagner, C. C., and Elstein, A. S., 1975. Computer simulation of clinical decision making: A new approach, *in: Proceedings: Fourteenth Annual Conference on Research in Medical Education*, American Association of Medical Colleges, Washington, D.C. (November 1975).

Wilkinson, G. L., 1973. Cost evaluation of instructional strategies, *AV Communications Review* 21:11.

Wilson, H. A., and Fitzgibbons, N. H., 1970. Practice and perfection: A preliminary analysis of achievement data from the CAI elementary English program, *Elementary English* 47:576.

Woods, E. M., 1970. Recent applications of computer technology to school testing programs, *Review of Educational Research* 40:525.

Zemper, E. D., 1973. Computer-Assisted Instruction in Medical Education: Perspectives and Potential at Michigan State University, Office Paper No. 1973-1, Office of Medical Education Research and Development, Michigan State University.

21

Patient Simulations in Clinical Education

Barbara B. Farquhar, Edward P. Hoffer, and G. Octo Barnett

Introduction

Clinical medical education is an intermediate stage between the mastery of basic medical sciences and the practice of medicine; its purpose is to provide students with supervised practice in solving clinical problems so that they will be prepared for independent practice. Ideally, the process of medical education is a well-planned, balanced, ordered sequence of activities designed to produce a physician with competence in solving a variety of clinical problems (Barnett, 1974). In fact, clinical medical education takes place in teaching hospitals where there are often conflicting demands on the time of good teachers and where primary consideration must be given to the welfare of patients rather than to educational effectiveness.

Many medical educators overlook the constraints of hospital-based training and teach as they were taught. Others are searching for ways to supplement traditional clinical education with new educational technologies. Cost is an important factor, and responsible medical educators seek the least expensive form of instruction that will permit students to achieve objectives efficiently. If the objective is to learn facts or procedures, then a book, programmed text, videotape, or slide–tape may suffice; here, there is little justification for more expensive methods of instruction. If, however, the objective is to teach the process of clinical problem-solving, the best method is supervised practice in solving clinical problems. Although for excellent education there is no substitute for the up-to-date, experienced clinician who has the time, interest, and skill to supervise medical students in clinical practicum, computer-based simulations of patient encounters can provide students with valuable additional supervised practice in solving patients' problems.

The purpose of this chapter is to provide an overview of the Massachusetts General Hospital's (MGH) clinical simulations by defining some of the problems encountered in clinical medical education, by highlighting the importance of clinical problem-solving, by demonstrating how computer-based simulations can be used to

Barbara B. Farquhar • Educational Computer Group, Digital Equipment Corporation, Marlboro, Massachusetts. *Edward P. Hoffer* and *G. Octo Barnett* • Massachusetts General Hospital and Harvard Medical School, Boston, Massachusetts. This project was supported in part by Grant No. 5 RO1 HS 00240, awarded by the National Center for Health Services Research, Department of Health, Education, and Welfare, and in part by National Library of Medicine Contract Number NO1-LM-2-4716.

supplement other methods in teaching and testing the process of clinical problem-solving, and by describing the development, content, and instructional strategies used in MGH simulations. The basic description of the MGH simulations given here outlines features that make it well-suited to both authors and users; technical aspects of the system are described in an appendix. This chapter includes a review of uses of the programs in undergraduate medical education, continuing education, self-assessment, and certification of clinical competence. Distribution of programs is considered in Chapter 7.

Clinical Education

Constraints on Hospital-Based Education

Clinical education conducted in hospitals is less than ideal pedagogically (Hoffer *et al.*, 1975) in that factors other than educational goals often play an important role in determining the breadth and depth of a student's clinical experience. The student requires a mix of excellent teaching physicians to serve as role models as well as rich opportunities to observe and solve a wide variety of clinical problems. However, the patient population in the hospital, the variety of clinical problems to be solved, and the simplicity or complexity of those problems can rarely — if ever — be controlled and selected for teaching purposes. Emergency situations provide special teaching problems; some are rare, and all require immediate intervention with little time to discuss alternative actions for the student's educational benefit. In some acute-care hospitals, patients with common illnesses may be scarce, or teaching opportunities may be limited, and a student may encounter only a few patients for whom he is capable of assuming substantial responsibility. Because it is difficult for the student to gain competence in clinical problem-solving merely through observation and reading, he must have opportunities for independent decision-making. However, the amount of responsibility an inexperienced student can be given for independent decision-making is limited since the protection of the patient and his care must take precedence over educational considerations. The practical imperatives of the hospital thus influence both the process and content of clinical medical education.

Medical educators find themselves under continually increasing economic and political pressure to make medical education more efficient and effective. According to a study conducted by the Association of American Medical Colleges, the full cost per year to educate an undergraduate medical student ranges from $16,000 to $26,000 (AAMC, 1973). Students cannot afford to pay these costs, and neither private nor public institutions have the resources to support escalating costs of medical education indefinitely (Lambdin *et al.*, 1975). One of the reasons that medical education is so expensive is that supervised practice in clinical problem-solving requires a very low student/faculty ratio. Whereas in some disciplines it is possible for one instructor to teach many advanced graduate students simultaneously, in clinical settings, one physician may be able to teach only three to five medical students effectively. As demands to decrease costs of medical education and larger classes of medical students have forced some institutions to increase the student/faculty ratio, many students who might have taken an active role in clinical problem-solving with a small group merely watch others in a large group. When as many as a dozen students are working with a single preceptor, the aggressive, articulate student is likely to get the practice and instruction he needs at the expense of others. Medical students are more heterogeneous now than they were several decades ago, and more individualized instruction rather than less is indicated.

The Importance of Problem-Solving

Development of clinical competency demands both knowledge and systematic *application* of that knowledge to solve patients' problems. Feinstein (1967) has called the care of a patient a therapeutic experiment in which the results depend on the clinical judgment used in the design, implementation, and evaluation of the experiment. Clinical practice should be an orderly process, yet clinical educators rarely make systematic, formal attempts to teach explicitly the *process* of clinical problem-solving. Much of clinical education consists of clerkships or apprenticeships, and students are generally expected to learn the process of problem-solving by imitating the behavior of their preceptors. Some students pick up cues about problem-solving quickly and are able to form generalizations; others need explicit instruction in the process of problem-solving to enable them to use their accumulation of the knowledge on which clinical practice rests. It is inefficient, costly, and potentially dangerous to teach *solutions* to problems and expect students to divine the process by which the solutions are reached. The amount of supervision that a student receives decreases as he advances, so it is particularly important that the student receive explicit instruction and develop an appropriate problem-solving style early in his career.

An excellent clinician often finds it difficult to describe to students the process he uses in solving a specific patient's problem, since he has so thoroughly assimilated the elementary steps of clinical problem-solving that he is no longer consciously aware of them. For the experienced clinician, only the unique aspects of a patient's problem require that specialized behavior classified as problem-solving (Travers, 1972). For the medical student who is attempting to solve the identical patient's problem, more attributes of the problem will be unfamiliar, and he will, therefore, require many more problem-solving steps than his preceptor to reach the same solution of the patient's problem.

Computers in Clinical Education

Since computer-based patient simulations can repeat *all* the problem-solving steps in a case indefinitely and patiently with student after student, such simulations offer an excellent means of providing students with individualized practice in developing this important clinical skill. Simulations can thus save time for practicing clinicians and can supplement certain aspects of clinical instruction. Simulations of patient encounters give students practice in the process, the cognitive (Bloom *et al.*, 1956) and affective (Krathwohl *et al.*, 1964) aspects of problem-solving, and the application of facts to the solution of problems. Through these simulations, the student is given practice in solving different clinical problems in a variety of settings. The computer's relatively high cost as an educational tool can probably only be justified when its unique capabilities are used to support clinical simulations.

In a simulation, the computer can serve several functions: it provides information about a simulated patient; it permits the student to interact with the patient, to make decisions, and to take actions to which the patient responds; and it assumes the role of the supervising physician by providing consultation and guidance, and by relating one case to another. The computer can also provide recent, relevant references for a problem. The computer can score the student's performance objectively and compare his performance to that of others, provide him and his instructor with a critique of his performance, and suggest remedial work if that is indicated. The student has responsibility for solving the patient's problem, but the learning process is without risk to real patients and is truly individualized. The student is supervised through the computer by the teaching physician who wrote the medical content and specified the instructional strategy.

Massachusetts General Hospital

Massachusetts General Hospital serves as Harvard Medical School's largest teaching hospital, and approximately 1000 medical students, house officers, and fellows receive clinical education at the hospital each year. The Laboratory of Computer Science is a unit of the Department of Medicine, and the staff of the laboratory shares in the department's teaching responsibilities. The laboratory staff is made up of approximately 30 professionals who have backgrounds in medicine, computer science, and education. The laboratory uses a portion of its unique personnel and computer resources to provide systematic instruction in the process of clinical problem-solving and to develop techniques for assessing clinical competence.

Massachusetts General Hospital devotes three full-time staff equivalents to maintain and improve the simulations, to develop new instructional strategies and simulations, to work with both local and remote authors in the design, development, implementation and evaluation of general- and special-purpose programs, and to support distribution of simulations through the Health Education Network (see Chapter 11, this volume). This staff assists new users of simulations by advising them on a range of issues such as integration of the programs into the curriculum, faculty development, selection and placement of terminals, and demonstration of programs to specialty groups. They set up special protocols for courses, workshops, or conferences, respond to surveys, and participate in national task forces to develop standards for languages as well as standards for review and appraisal of materials. Demands for personnel and hardware exceed resources. The heaviest and most essential commitment of these resources is to support the Health Education Network. Other projects receive attention as time permits.

Patient Simulations

Staff at the Laboratory of Computer Science has developed over 30 computer-based simulations to teach and test clinical problem-solving. Each simulation of a clinical problem includes many cases, but all cases within a simulation share a common instructional strategy and focus on a general problem (e.g., jaundice, abdominal pain, coma). The programs fall within the general classification of computer-assisted instruction (CAI) and share some of the strengths of CAI in general. Although CAI is costlier than donated physician teaching time, CAI may provide some elements that the traditional clinical clerkship does not.

Computer-based simulations can supplement other formal instruction and do offer a number of advantages for students, clinical preceptors, and directors of clinical education. Simulations can be used at each student's pace and convenience since access to the simulation is available continuously and repeatedly. In the simulations, the student has full responsibility for making decisions about a patient's problem and can see the outcomes of his actions without endangering a real patient. The computer keeps an objective record of each student's problem-solving behavior and points out weaknesses or alternative courses of action for the student. The teaching physician can select a simulated patient with the clinical problem(s) and constellation of signs and symptoms that he wishes the student to manage. The computer also gives feedback to the physician responsible for teaching the student; after reviewing the performance of his students, the physician may wish to alter either the content of his course or the instructional techniques he is using.

In addition to providing individual records of performance, the computer can prepare a composite or it can aggregate data for use by a curriculum committee or clinical education director. Objective records of student performance at the clinical level and patterns of behavior common to a class are difficult to obtain with traditional educational methods, but records of many students' actions in identical clinical problems can provide hard data to help evaluate both the students and the clinical education program in which they are participating. A thorough assessment can pinpoint strengths and weaknesses in a clinical training program and permit its director to modify the program until it meets its objectives as measured by student performance (Mankin, unpublished).

Development of Simulations

Determination of Program Users and Objectives

Before an author develops a patient simulation, he should consider many factors and make a number of determinations. He should define the users or target population, describe any prerequisites or behavior the user is expected to be able to demonstrate before he uses the program, describe terminal behavior or what the user should be able to do after he has used the program, define measures of performance, and establish minimum levels of acceptable performance. Instructional objectives should guide the author in developing the program and serve as criteria for its evaluation. Authors who are developing programs to be shared by users at many institutions are encouraged to avoid special procedure-oriented programs and controversial content because procedures and accepted practice vary from institution to institution.

Selecting an Instructional Strategy

After the author has determined whom he is going to teach with the patient simulation, what students should be able to do after they have used the simulation, and what kinds of patient simulations will help the users develop the desired competencies, the author must select an instructional strategy or program format for the simulation. In selecting an instructional strategy, the author should consider the following:

1. The purpose of the program (assessment, problem-solving practice, continuing education)
2. The audience (medical students with limited vocabulary, advanced medical students or house officers with adequate vocabulary, or specialists with extensive vocabulary in limited areas)
3. The user's task (diagnosis or management of a chronic or acute problem)
4. Structure of the task (unstructured, as in the diagnosis of a complex problem, or structured, as in the management of an acute, well-defined problem)
5. Sequence of actions (critical or not important)
6. Timeliness of actions (critical or not important)
7. Reaction of the simulated patient to actions taken by the user (patient static or dynamic)
8. Passage of time (one encounter or multiple encounters)
9. Method of interaction (multiple-choice, vocabulary list, or free text)

If some cues are tolerable, the author may select a multiple choice or prepared vocabulary list for the user to employ during interaction with the program. If cueing is to be avoided, the author may select either an extensive index or free text for user interaction.

The instructional strategy selected will determine, to a great extent, the amount of time required of the author in developing the patient simulation. A program author must specify the content and logic of the program, which means that he must describe how the program and patient should respond to any action that may be taken by the user at any and every point in the simulation. If the author selects a structured, multiple choice instructional strategy, the number of actions available to the user is limited, and the author's job is minimized. If the author chooses an unstructured format in which the user may use free text and type any response to the simulated case, the author must anticipate the responses and describe the actions to be taken by the program and patient as a result of the user's responses. In the latter case, the author's job is complex and time-consuming.

Most authors choose to use one of a number of existing instructional strategies or "drivers." The driver and its associated editor (master programs for existing instructional strategies) collect information about the content and logic of the patient simulation from the author using a predetermined format and thus greatly simplify the writing of the computer program. The author also prepares program documentation for the user's manual, describing the program and including illustrations of interactions and any supplementary visual materials that are needed to operate the program. After the author has a rough draft of his simulation and associated materials, and the program is technically correct and operates the way the author intended, developmental testing begins.

Program Testing and Revision

The cycle of program testing and revision is repeated until the patient simulation consistently produces the instructional objectives established by the author. For the first review, the author invites local experts and members of the target population to use the program individually. The author is present when these users try the patient simulation to observe their interaction with the program and to collect comments and suggestions. He notes nonverbal responses and any apparent content or logic problems. For members of the target population, the author administers measures of performance to establish whether or not the target population meets prerequisites for program use and whether or not the program achieves the instructional objectives set for it. After collecting data and evaluating performance measures, the author modifies the patient simulation accordingly. He may then invite the same or a different group of experts and intended users to take the simulation, and he repeats the processes of data collection and revision.

When the author is satisfied that the program functions properly and meets the standards he has set for it, the program is released or made available within Massachusetts General Hospital for use by its medical students and staff. They comment freely on the content and structure of the program, and their suggestions form the basis for further revision and refinement. Next, the program is released to Countway Medical Library at Harvard Medical School, and additional suggestions are collected. The program is revised frequently at each step. Next, the author may arrange for a field test by inviting target populations at remote institutions to use the program and the performance measures associated with it.

In many instances, a specialty board or nationally recognized panel of experts has been invited to review a new or revised patient simulation. Sometimes, the members of the specialty board or panel review the simulations together at Massachusetts General Hospital or at their headquarters. At other times, individuals review the programs at their home institutions using the Health Education Network.

The programs are revised to conform to recommendations of specialty boards. When national standards are revised, simulations are modified to meet the new standards.

Program Distribution and Maintenance

When the program performs adequately to meet objectives set for it, the program is released to the Health Education Network. Program documentation is sent to all users, and a notice is put on the Network that a new simulation is available. Users are asked to try the new simulation and to comment on it. Comments and suggestions are collected, and the author makes revisions to the simulation. A national network of users helps to keep the author informed of recent research and publications related to his simulation, and users' constructive criticisms are of inestimable worth in refining and updating programs.

As long as the simulation is available on the Massachusetts General Hospital computer systems, the author (or his designee) is responsible for following and maintaining it. He answers users' comments, keeps program content and logic current with generally accepted practice and revised national standards, and keeps references in the program up-to-date. The programs undergo continuous revision as long as they are in use.

Simulation Models

Several different types of simulation have been developed at the Massachusetts General Hospital. The programs cover a wide range of clinical problems, but the simulations represent three basic types of patient models: the static patient, the dynamic patient, and a dynamic simulation of a physiologic system or disease process. Each basic model is described and illustrated.

The Static Patient Model

In the static patient model, the computer has a file of information about a clinical problem and a series of cases. The user interacts with the simulated patient, but the patient's condition does not change as a result of the interaction. This model is used primarily for diagnostic problems. The static patient model can be used with a glossary or numbered vocabulary list in which the student enters the number from the list which corresponds to the action he wants to take. This model may also use free text interaction in which the student enters his actions (history questions, physical examination observations, laboratory test requests, etc.) or diagnoses in English.

One example of the program which uses the static model simulates patients presenting with a chief complaint of abdominal pain. Each patient in this program is defined according to 51 attributes of history, physical examination, and laboratory test data (Figure 1). The general data base for abdominal pain is a probability matrix of 51 patient attributes by 30 possible diagnoses. The matrix (Figure 2) is

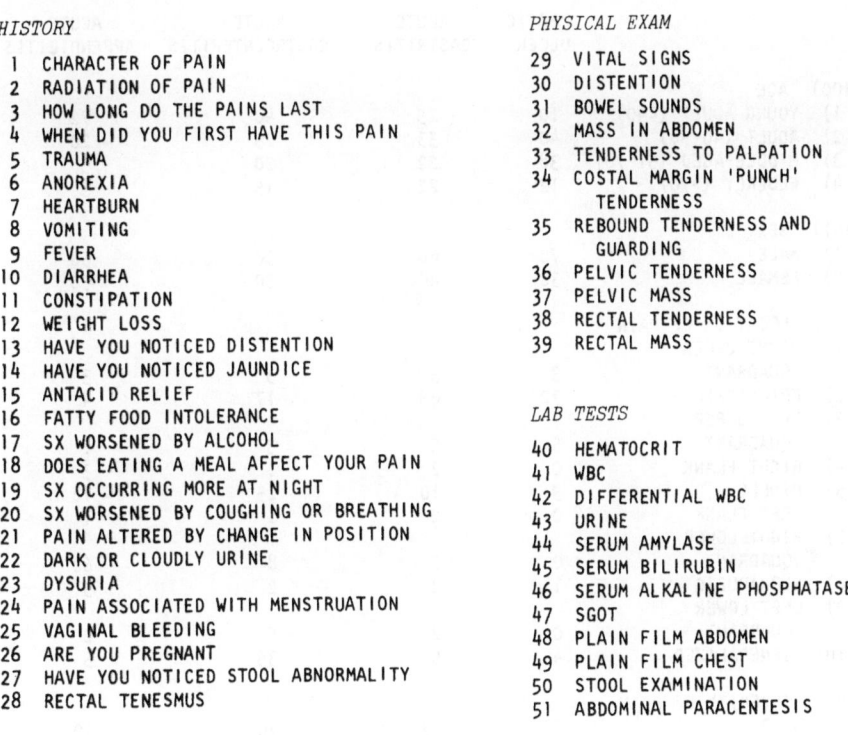

HISTORY

1   CHARACTER OF PAIN
2   RADIATION OF PAIN
3   HOW LONG DO THE PAINS LAST
4   WHEN DID YOU FIRST HAVE THIS PAIN
5   TRAUMA
6   ANOREXIA
7   HEARTBURN
8   VOMITING
9   FEVER
10 DIARRHEA
11 CONSTIPATION
12 WEIGHT LOSS
13 HAVE YOU NOTICED DISTENTION
14 HAVE YOU NOTICED JAUNDICE
15 ANTACID RELIEF
16 FATTY FOOD INTOLERANCE
17 SX WORSENED BY ALCOHOL
18 DOES EATING A MEAL AFFECT YOUR PAIN
19 SX OCCURRING MORE AT NIGHT
20 SX WORSENED BY COUGHING OR BREATHING
21 PAIN ALTERED BY CHANGE IN POSITION
22 DARK OR CLOUDLY URINE
23 DYSURIA
24 PAIN ASSOCIATED WITH MENSTRUATION
25 VAGINAL BLEEDING
26 ARE YOU PREGNANT
27 HAVE YOU NOTICED STOOL ABNORMALITY
28 RECTAL TENESMUS

PHYSICAL EXAM

29 VITAL SIGNS
30 DISTENTION
31 BOWEL SOUNDS
32 MASS IN ABDOMEN
33 TENDERNESS TO PALPATION
34 COSTAL MARGIN 'PUNCH'
        TENDERNESS
35 REBOUND TENDERNESS AND
        GUARDING
36 PELVIC TENDERNESS
37 PELVIC MASS
38 RECTAL TENDERNESS
39 RECTAL MASS

LAB TESTS

40 HEMATOCRIT
41 WBC
42 DIFFERENTIAL WBC
43 URINE
44 SERUM AMYLASE
45 SERUM BILIRUBIN
46 SERUM ALKALINE PHOSPHATASE
47 SGOT
48 PLAIN FILM ABDOMEN
49 PLAIN FILM CHEST
50 STOOL EXAMINATION
51 ABDOMINAL PARACENTESIS

INFORMATION GIVEN IN INITIAL PATIENT DESCRIPTION

100 AGE
101 SEX
102 LOCATION OF PAIN
103 SEVERITY OF PAIN
104 WHEN THIS EPISODE STARTED

Figure 1. Attributes and vocabulary list for each simulated patient in the abdominal pain program.

based on subjective judgments and was developed by medical experts at the American Board of Internal Medicine, the National Board of Medical Examiners, and the Massachusetts General Hospital. For each case of abdominal pain, there is also a different set of 51 responses corresponding to the 51 attributes.

The student's objective is to collect information about the patient and to reach a diagnosis as efficiently as possible. The sequence of actions is important as well as the information collected. To obtain information about the patient, the student enters a number from the vocabulary list, and the computer responds by giving the student information stored for the patient for that item (Figure 3). The student enters his differential and final diagnoses in free text (Figure 4). The computer evaluates each of the student's actions by computing disease probabilities and selecting the next question to ask after *each* action the student takes. The student may request a critique of his entire performance and be told: what action he took;

	PEPTIC ULCER	ACUTE GASTRITIS	ACUTE GASTROENTERITIS	ACUTE APPENDICITIS
100) AGE				
1) YOUNG ADULT (<40)	10	25	40	72
2) ADULT (40-50)	40	33	25	20
3) MIDDLE-AGED (51-70)	38	22	20	5
4) ELDERLY (>70)	12	22	15	3
101) SEX				
1) MALE	70	60	50	50
2) FEMALE	30	40	50	50
102) LOCATION OF PAIN				
1) RIGHT UPPER QUADRANT	9	5	3	3
2) EPIGASTRIC	72	65	17	4
3) LEFT UPPER QUADRANT	5	5	3	1
4) RIGHT FLANK	0	2	1	3
5) MIDDLE	9	10	25	18
6) LEFT FLANK	0	2	1	1
7) RIGHT LOWER QUADRANT	0	2	8	60
8) SUPRAPUBIC	1	2	2	3
9) LEFT LOWER QUADRANT	0	2	5	2
10) GENERALIZED	4	5	35	5
103) SEVERITY OF PAIN				
1) MILD	35	53	70	10
2) MODERATE	50	37	20	70
3) SEVERE, INTENSE	15	10	10	20
104) WHEN THIS EPISODE STARTED				
1) WITHIN LAST 2 DAYS	5	62	60	81
2) A COUPLE OF DAYS AGO	10	32	36	15
3) ABOUT A WEEK AGO	40	5	3	3
4) OVER A MONTH AGO	45	1	1	1
1) CHARACTER OF PAIN				
1) ACHING	25	30	25	39
2) SHARP, STABBING	15	10	15	40
3) BURNING	57	30	10	3
4) CRAMPY, COLIC	3	30	50	18
8) VOMITING				
1) YES	50	80	85	75
2) NO	50	20	15	25

Figure 2. Portion of the probability matrix used by the abdominal pain program for 4 of the 30 diseases.

what action program authors recommend; what diseases are ruled in or out on the basis of the information obtained by the student; what the current probabilities of the diagnoses are; and what action should be taken next to differentiate among the likely diagnoses.

Other simulations that use a static patient model are coma, gastrointestinal

A 45-YEAR-OLD WHITE MALE USED-CAR SALESMAN IS BROUGHT TO THE EW BY HIS ANXIOUS WIFE BECAUSE HE COMPLAINS OF MODERATE EPIGASTRIC PAIN WHICH STARTED ABOUT A WEEK AGO AFTER A NIGHT OUT WITH THE BOYS PLAYING POKER.

At this point, the student begins his interrogation of the "patient."

ITEM #1:   CHARACTER OF PAIN: IT'S A HOT, BURNING PAIN, LIKE MY STOMACH IS ON FIRE.

ITEM #8:   VOMITING: I OFTEN VOMIT, AND THEN THE PAIN IS SOMETIMES BETTER.

ITEM #18:   DOES EATING A MEAL AFFECT YOUR PAIN: I FEEL BEST RIGHT AFTER A MEAL, ESPECIALLY WHEN I HAVE ICE CREAM FOR DESSERT.

ITEM #4:   WHEN DID YOU FIRST HAVE THIS PAIN: I'VE BEEN HAVING PAINS LIKE THIS FOR A NUMBER OF YEARS.   IT SEEMED TO START WHEN I WAS IN KOREA.   IT GETS PARTICULARLY BAD WHEN THE NEW MODEL CARS COME OUT IN THE FALL.

(If the student requests the HELP function at this point, he receives the following information:)

ITEM #HELP

AT THIS POINT

ESTIMATED DISEASE PROBABILITIES
    (3)   PEPTIC ULCER (GASTRIC/DUODENAL)   0.648
    (6)   ACUTE GASTRITIS   0.087
    (7)   ACUTE GASTROENTERITIS (VIRAL OR BACTERIAL)   0.063

WOULD YOU LIKE SUGGESTIONS FOR FUTHER WORKUP?   YES

COMPUTER'S SUGGESTED TESTS

    (4)   WHEN DID YOU FIRST GET THIS PAIN
    (3)   HOW LONG DO THE PAINS LAST
    (33)   TENDERNESS TO PALPATION
    (15)   ANTACID RELIEF

Figure 3. Dialogue between the user and computer in the abdominal pain program (static patient model). *Note*: User's entries are underlined for purposes of illustration.

bleeding, pediatric cough and fever, jaundice, joint pain, and hypertension. Each has a vocabulary of inquiry items or patient attributes, but programs differ in their instructional goals. The abdominal pain program (Barnett *et al.*, 1972) stresses the sequence and logic of diagnosis. The coma and gastrointestinal bleeding simulations (Hoffer, 1974) place less emphasis on the sequence of problem-solving but focus on practical management and differential diagnosis (Figure 5). The jaundice program (Goroll, 1976) provides all the patient data and requires that the student suggest and defend pathophysiological mechanisms responsible for the jaundice.

The Dynamic Patient Model

In other simulations, the simulated patient is dynamic, and his condition changes as a function of the student's actions. The changes are based on a decision tree

WHAT IS YOUR IMPRESSION? GIVEN THE DATA YOU HAVE THUS FAR, WHAT DIAGNOSIS DO
YOU THINK SHOULD BE MOST SERIOUSLY CONSIDERED?

DIAGNOSIS: <u>ULCER</u>
BE MORE SPEC<u>IFIC</u>

DIAGNOSIS: <u>ULCER OF DUDENUM</u>
WHEN YOU TYPED 'DUDENUM,' DID YOU MEAN 'DUODENAL'? <u>YES</u>

>   *(At this point, the computer interrupted to request the student to state*
>   *his leading diagnostic impression. Note that the computer can recognize*
>   *non-specific diagnoses and simple misspellings.)*

YOU MAY NOW COLLECT MORE INFORMATION IF YOU CHOOSE TO DO SO

ITEM #<u>7</u> HEARTBURN: THAT'S WHAT I'VE BEEN TELLING YOU, DOC. I HAVE TERRIBLE
         HEARTBURN, PARTICULARLY WHEN MY WIFE NAGS ME.

>   *(At any time, the student may terminate the interaction by indicating*
>   *that he wishes to make a final diagnosis, i.e. by entering the letter*
>   *"D".)*

ITEM #<u>D</u>
DIAGNOSIS: <u>PEPTIC ULCER OF DUODENUM</u>

AN EXCELLENT CHOICE, BUT PERHAPS A DIAGNOSIS IS SLIGHTLY PREMATURE.
WOULD YOU ADMIT THIS PATIENT TO THE HOSPITAL? <u>YES</u>
WOULD YOU SCHEDULE A LAPAROTOMY FOR THIS PATIENT? <u>NO</u>

Figure 4. Free text entry of differential and final diagnoses in the abdominal pain program.
Note: User's entries are underlined for purposes of illustration.

rather than on a mathematical model, and the changes occur in discrete steps. One
program that uses this model simulates a patient in cardiac arrest (Hoffer *et al.*,
1972). The program uses a branching, multiple choice approach and leads the
student through the sequence of actions required to resuscitate the patient (Figure
6). The student selects actions from a multiple choice list, and the computer reports
how the patient's condition varies as a result of each action the student takes. Other
programs that use this dynamic patient model are hypertensive emergencies, hypertension management, respiratory distress in the newborn, respiratory problems in
the adult, arrhythmias, renal failure, trauma, and orthopedic problems.

Physiologic or Disease Models

Yet another dynamic model is based on underlying mathematical equations to
simulate a physiologic system or disease process. Biological systems are generally
complex, poorly understood, and require vast amounts of computing power if
they are well-described mathematically (Chapter 24, this volume). Once these
models are developed, however, they offer great potential for research, patient
care, and instruction. Students vary parameters and note changes in physiologic
systems or disease processes.

Several dynamic models of effects of drugs, disease processes, and physiological
systems are available on the Massachusetts General Hospital system. One model

THE PATIENT IS A 36-YEAR-OLD WOMAN BROUGHT IN BY HER FRIEND BECAUSE SHE WAS UNCONSCIOUS. ACCORDING TO HER FRIEND, THE PATIENT HAS NOT LOOKED NORMAL ALL DAY. SHE HAS NOT EATEN WELL AND AT TIMES HAS TALKED NONSENSE. TODAY, THE PATIENT WENT INTO THE BATHROOM. WHEN SHE DID NOT COME OUT IN AN HOUR, THE FRIEND PUSHED IN THE DOOR.

ITEM #: 301 BLOOD PRESSURE 80/50
ITEM #: 302 PULSE 87
ITEM #: 303 RESPIRATIONS REGULAR AT 14 PER MINUTE
ITEM #: 304 GENERAL APPEARANCE QUITE OBESE, PT. MOTIONLESS ON STRETCHER
ITEM #: 300 RECTAL TEMPERATURE 101.7
ITEM #: 504 BLOOD SUGAR RESULTS IN 1 HOUR
ITEM #: 700 50 CC BOLUS OF 50% GLUCOSE IV NO OBVIOUS RESPONSE, BUT VERY
             APPROPRIATE TO GIVE THIS THERAPY
ITEM #: 705 HYPOTONIC FLUIDS AT 250 CC/HR INSTITUTED
ITEM #: 531 URINALYSIS RESULTS IN 30 MINUTES
ITEM #: HELP

OPTIONS: 1) CONSULT, 2) INFO, 3) REVIEW, 4) NORMAL VALUE, 5) GO ON
         ANSWER NUMBER? 1
YOUR INITIAL APPROACH TO THE COMATOSE PATIENT SHOULD BE FAIRLY STEREOTYPED. YOU MUST FIRST PAY ATTENTION TO "THE ABC'S": CHECK THE AIRWAY AND RESPIRATIONS, MONITOR THE PULSE AND BP. IF THERE IS THE SLIGHTEST HINT OF RESPIRATORY INSUFFICIENCY, ARTERIAL BLOOD GASES SHOULD BE DRAWN. AN IV SHOULD BE STARTED SO THAT NEEDED DRUGS CAN BE ADMINISTERED. BLOOD SHOULD BE DRAWN FOR GLUCOSE AND OTHER MEASUREMENTS AND A BOLUS OF 50% GLUCOSE ADMINISTERED. YOUR INITIAL PE SHOULD CONCENTRATE ON SEARCH FOR LOCALIZING NEUROLOGIC SIGNS POINTING TO A PRIMARY NEUROLOGIC PROBLEM (THOUGH REMEMBER FOCAL FINDINGS DO NOT RULE OUT A TOXIC-METABOLIC ETIOLOGY), AND ALSO FOR FINDINGS SUGGESTING A SPECIFIC TOXIC-METABOLIC PROBLEM.

WOULD YOU CLASSIFY THE PATIENT'S PROBLEM AS: 1) NEUROLOGIC, 2) TOXIC-METABOLIC 3) PSYCHOGENIC, 4) DO NOT KNOW
         ANSWER NUMBER? 2 RIGHT!!
THIS CLASS CAN BE FURTHER BROKEN DOWN

WOULD YOU CLASSIFY THE PATIENT'S PROBLEM AS: 1) HORMONE EXCESS OR LACK 2) DRUG OVERDOSE OR OTHER EXOGENOUS TOXINS 3) INFECTION 4) ENDOGENOUS TOXINS 5) RESPIRATORY FAILURE 6) DO NOT KNOW
         ANSWER NUMBER 3 RIGHT!!
THIS CLASS CAN BE FURTHER BROKEN DOWN

WOULD YOU CLASSIFY THE PATIENT'S PROBLEM AS: 1) VIRAL (ANTIBIOTICS NOT NEEDED), 2) BACTERIAL (ANTIBIOTICS NEEDED), 3) DO NOT KNOW
         ANSWER NUMBER? 3
A COMATOSE PATIENT WITH EVIDENCE OF SYSTEMIC INFECTION WILL NEED TO BE STARTED ON ANTIBIOTICS AFTER APPROPRIATE CULTURES ARE DRAWN. THE ONLY DIFFICULT DECISION IN THIS CLASS OF PROBLEMS IS AT TIMES DECIDING IF THE PATIENT HAS BACTERIAL MENINGITIS OR VIRAL MENINGO-ENCEPHALITIS. THE FINDING OF LOW SUGAR, HIGH PROTEIN AND/OR MANY POLYS IN THE CSF SHOULD POINT YOU TOWARDS BACTERIAL INFECTION, THE CONVERSE TOWARDS VIRAL. IF THERE IS ANY REAL DOUBT IN YOUR MIND, YOU SHOULD START THE PATIENT ON ANTIBIOTICS AND BE PREPARED TO STOP THEM IF THE CULTURES REMAIN STERILE. IUDR TREATMENT FOR HERPES MENINGO-ENCEPHALITIS IS CONTROVERSIAL, AND NOW THE SUBJECT OF INITIAL AND BADLY NEEDED CONTROLLED TRIALS.

GATHER MORE DATA ABOUT THE PATIENT

Figure 5. Dialogue between the user and computer in the coma simulation (static patient model). *Note*: User's entries are underlined for purposes of illustration.

THE PATIENT IS A 41-YEAR-OLD WOMAN WHO WAS ADMITTED 2 WEEKS AGO WITH SEVERE
BIVENTRICULAR FAILURE. SHE HAD BEEN SLOWLY IMPROVING WITH BED-REST AND
DIURETICS BUT NOW, ACCORDING TO THE AIDE "LOOKS TERRIBLE."
WHAT DO YOU DO FIRST?

1.   TAKE AN EKG
2.   START AN IV
3.   CHECK MAJOR VESSELS FOR PULSES, SEE IF PATIENT IS BREATHING
4.   GIVE A SHOT OF INTRACARDIAC EPINEPHRINE
5.   IMMEDIATE ELECTRICAL CARDIOVERSION
6.   GIVE A SHARP BLOW TO THE PRECORDIUM

>3

THERE ARE NO PALPABLE CAROTID OR FEMORAL PULSES; THE PATIENT IS APNEIC AND
DOES NOT RESPOND TO YOUR SHOUT.
WHAT IS YOUR NEXT MOVE?

1.   START CHEST COMPRESSION
2.   GIVE A SHARP BLOW TO THE PRECORDIUM WITH YOUR FIRST
3.   QUICKLY GO OUT AND YELL FOR HELP
4.   TAKE AN EKG
5.   TILT BACK THE HEAD AND GIVE FOUR BREATHS

>2

THE AMERICAN HEART ASSOCIATION DOES NOT RECOMMEND USE OF THE PRECORDIAL THUMP
IN UN-WITNESSED ARRESTS. THE DANGER IS THAT OF PRODUCING VENTRICULAR
FIBRILLATION IN THE ANOXIC HEART. THERE ARE REPORTS OF SUCCESSFUL USE OF
"THUMP-VERSION" IN SITUATIONS OTHER THAN WITNESSED ARRESTS, BUT THESE ARE
STILL LARGELY ANECDOTAL. THE OFFICIAL POLICY IS THAT PRE-CORDIAL THUMP
SHOULD ONLY BE USED WITHIN THE FIRST MINUTE OF AN ARREST. YOU TILT BACK
THE HEAD AND GIVE FOUR QUICK BREATHS. THE MOST IMPORTANT STEP IS TO ENSURE
AN ADEQUATE AIRWAY AND RESPIRATIONS. THIS ALONE IS SOMETIMES SUFFICIENT TO
RESUSCITATE A PATIENT. NO RESPONSE TO PROVIDING AN AIRWAY AND GIVING SEVERAL
QUICK BREATHS.
WHAT DO YOU DO NOW?

1.   START CHEST COMPRESSION
2.   GIVE A SHARP BLOW TO THE PRECORDIUM
3.   YELL FOR HELP WHILE STARTING EXTERNAL CHEST COMPRESSION
4.   TAKE AN EKG

>3

GOOD. YOU WISH TO INITIATE CPR AS QUICKLY AS POSSIBLE, BUT MUST NOT OVERLOOK
THE FACT THAT CPR IS MORE EFFECTIVELY PERFORMED BY TWO PEOPLE THAN ONE. IN
THE HOSPITAL, TRAINED HELP SHOULD BE JUST A SHOUT AWAY. THE PATIENT REMAINS
PULSELESS. ONE OF THE FLOOR NURSES HAS JOINED YOU
WHAT SHOULD YOU DO. . .

1.   INTUBATE THE PATIENT
2.   TAKE AN EKG
3.   START VENTILATION AND CHEST COMPRESSION
4.   GIVE THE PATIENT AN INJECTION OF INTRACARDIAC EPI

>3

Figure 6. Dialogue between the user and computer in the cardiopulmonary resuscitation
simulation (dynamic patient model). *Note*: User's entries are underlined for purposes of
illustration.

INITIAL CONDITIONS: PT IS DRAINING MATERIAL FROM T-TUBE

CONTROL IS 12.5 SEC

DAY 1 PT IS 12.5 SEC
WARFARIN DOSE: 20 MG

DAY 2 PT IS 14.5 SEC
WARFARIN DOSE: 7.5 MG
PT NOW ON DISULFIRAM

DAY 3 PT IS 22.7 SEC
WARFARIN DOSE: HELP

THE FOLLOWING POINTS MAY BE HELPFUL:
     DISULFIRAM POTENTIATES WARFARIN. IT HAS NOT BEEN WELL-STUDIED BUT IS
     PROBABLY DUE TO INHIBITION OF HEPATIC METABOLISM. A PATIENT WITH A
     BILIARY FISTULA OR T-TUBE DRAINAGE (ESPECIALLY WITH ASSOCIATED PANCREATIC
     DISEASE) IS MORE SENSITIVE TO WARFARIN BECAUSE OF DECREASED VIT K
     ABSORPTION.

WARFARIN DOSE: 7.5 MG

DAY 4 PT IS 31 SEC
WARFARIN DOSE: 5 MG

DAY 5 PT IS 44.3 SEC

HEMORRHAGE HAS OCCURRED BECAUSE OF EXCESSIVE ANTICOAGULATION
...WARFARIN D/C...VIT K GIVEN.

NEW PATIENT

INITIAL CONDITIONS: PATIENT RECEIVING ADRENOCORTICOSTEROIDS

CONTROL IS 13.1 SEC

DAY 1 PT IS 13.1 SEC
WARFARIN DOSE: HELP
DO YOU HAVE A GENERAL IDEA OF DOSES USED? YES

THE FOLLOWING POINTS MAY BE HELPFUL:
     PATIENTS ON ADRENOCORTICOSTEROIDS ARE REPORTED TO REQUIRE A LARGER DOSE OF
     WARFARIN. THE EFFECT IS USUALLY NOT LARGE. THE MECHANISM IS POORLY UNDER-
     STOOD BUT MAY BE RELATED TO THE WELL-KNOWN BUT LITTLE UNDERSTOOD TENDENCY
     OF THE ADRENOCORTICAL STEROIDS TO PRODUCE A 'HYPERCOAGULABLE STATE' BY
     INCREASING CLOTTING FACTOR SYNTHESIS.

WARFARIN DOSE: 35 MG

DAY 2 PT IS 15.4 SEC
WARFARIN DOSE: 0 MG

DAY 3 PT IS 16.7 SEC
WARFARIN DOSE: 10 MG

Figure 7. Dialogue between the user and computer in the anticoagulation simulation (physiologic model). *Note*: User's entries are underlined for purposes of illustration.

simulates the effects of the oral anticoagulant Warfarin on blood clotting time, interaction with other drugs, and the patient's condition (Figure 7). A digoxin dosage adviser uses the same format. Another model simulates a patient with diabetic ketoacidosis. The underlying characteristics of all of these models are empirically derived.

In the diabetes simulation parameters such as blood sugar, acetone, and serum potassium are monitored closely and change as a result of the student's therapy. The diabetes simulation emulates the actual reaction of diabetic patients to dif-

```
THE PATIENT IS A 33-YEAR-OLD FEMALE WHO HAS BEEN BROUGHT IN BY HER HUSBAND
BECAUSE OF EXTREME WEAKNESS OVER THE LAST WEEK.  SHE HAD BEEN UNUSUALLY
THIRSTY FOR THE PRECEDING WEEK.

PE:   MENTAL STATUS OBTUNDED
PE:   VITAL SIGNS BP:85/56 P:121 T:99 PO R:36
PE:   SKIN COLOR NL. TURGOR VERY POOR.
PE:   CHEST NORMAL
PE:   HEART NORMAL
PE:   ABDOMEN BOWEL SOUNDS ABSENT.  NO ENLARGED ORGANS.
PE:   NEUROLOGIC NO FOCAL NEUROLOGIC SIGNS
TEST:  ELECTROLYTES SENT TO LAB
TEST:  BLOOD SUGAR SENT TO LAB
TEST:  UA SP GR: 1.040; SUGAR: 4+; ACETONE: LARGE; MICRO: AMORPH MATERIAL
TEST:  EKG SINUS TACHYCARDIA. NON-SPECIFIC ABNORMALITIES
TEST:  CHEST FILM REQUESTED
TEST:  CALCIUM SENT TO LAB
THERAPY ORDERS FOR NEXT HOUR.

RX:   2 L NORMAL SALINE
RX:   CZI 100U I.V.
RX:   •FACE MASK OXYGEN

***ENDING THERAPY FOR TIME 0***
ONE HOUR WILL NOW PASS

LAB TEST RESULTS FROM PREVIOUS HOUR:
      NA: 138 MEQ/L; K: 3.6 MEQ/L; CO2: 9 MEQ/L
      BLOOD SUGAR 931 MG%
      CHEST FILM NORMAL
      CALCIUM 9.1 MG%

PE:   BP 90/61
PE:   CHEST NORMAL
TEST:  BS SENT TO LAB
TEST:  LYTES SENT TO LAB
TEST:  ELECTROCARDIOGRAM  PROMINENT U WAVES
TEST:  URINE OUTPUT 354 CC PAST HOUR
TEST:  BUN SENT TO LAB
TEST:  SERUM ACETONE +1:4
THERAPY ORDERS FOR NEXT HOUR.

RX:   1L 1/2NS
RX:   KCL 40 MEQ
RX:   CZI 50 U IV

***ENDING THERAPY FOR TIME 1 HOUR***
ONE HOUR WILL NOW PASS.
```

Figure 8. Dialogue between the user and computer in the diabetic ketoacidosis simulation (disease process model). *Note:* User's entries are underlined for purposes of illustration.

ferent management strategies (Figure 8). For example, the student might maintain the patient's fluid volume with appropriate administration of i.v. fluids. If, however, he does not administer insulin, the patient's blood sugar will remain high. Another program using this model is concerned with fluid and electrolyte management. A similar model, developed originally by Dr. C. J. Dickinson, simulates the reflex control mechanisms of the cardiovascular system. The cardiac simulation program sets initial conditions for the simulated patient and runs a short period of simulat-

```
DO YOU WISH TO CHANGE VARIABLES NOW?  YES

INITIAL VALUES ARE . . .
1.  ARTERIAL RESISTANCE= 100% NORMAL
2.  VENOUS RESISTANCE= 100% NORMAL
3.  CARDIAC CONTRACTILITY= 100% NORMAL
4.  INTRATHORACIC PRESSURE= -2 MM HG
5.  CARDIAC LIMIT PRESSURE= 8 MM HG
6.  BLOOD VOLUME= 5000 ML
7.  VENOUS CAPACITANCE= 100% NORMAL
8.  VENOUS FILLING VOLUME= 1400 ML

DO YOU WANT TO CHANGE ANY OF THESE VARIABLES?  IF NO, ENTER 'NO'.
IF YES, ENTER THE # OF THE VARIABLE YOU WANT TO CHANGE.  6

TYPE IN NEW VALUE FOR FACTOR 6 BLOOD VOLUME (ML) 3500

DO YOU WANT TO FREEZE BAROCEPTOR?  YES

BAROCEPTOR FROZEN AT PRESENT LEVEL
  SYSTOLIC (S) AND DIASTOLIC (D) PRESSURES - MM HG HEART RATE (.)
  CARDIAC OUTPUT (C) - DECILITERS/MIN
TIME 0  20  40  60  80  100 120  140  160  180  200  220  240  260  280  300
SECS  .    .    .    .    .         .         .         .         .         .    .    .

0              C    .         S<<<
2         C D      S .
4         C D      S .
6         C D      S.
8         C D      S.
10        C D      S.
12        C D      S.

        I AM VERY TIRED AND EXHAUSTED. . . I DON'T FEEL LIKE DOING ANYTHING.
        I FEEL AS IF I AM GOING TO DIE.  MY EYES ARE GOING DARK. . .

YOUR PATIENT IS PASSING HARDLY ANY URINE

BP SYSTOLIC= +64.25 (+121.92) DIASTOLIC= +40.88 (+76.58)
MEAN BP= +49.00 (+91.69) MM. HG
RIGHT ATRIAL PRES.= +0.10 (+1.79) MM. HG
MEAN CAP. PRES.= +6.01 (+12.66) MM. HG
PRES. ACROSS PULMONARY CAP.= +6.99 (+12.78) MM. HG
CARDIAC OUTPUT= +2.69 (+4.94) L/MIN STROKE VOL.= +37.19 (+68.06) ML
HEART RATE= +72.25 (+72.58)
ART. RESIST.= +16.00 (+16.00) VEN. RESIST.= +2.20 (+2.20) MM. HG/L/MIN
CARDIAC CONTRACTILITY= +1.28 (+1.30) L/MIN/MM HG FILLING PRES.
AVG. VEN. PRES.= +3.06 (+7.22) MM HG
VEN. CAPACITANCE (SLOPE)= +360.00 (+360.00) ML/MM HG
```

Figure 9. Dialogue between the user and computer in the cardiac simulation (physiologic model). *Note*: User's entries are underlined for purposes of illustration.

ing the patient's reaction to the set conditions. Next, the student manipulates patient variables (Figure 9); after changes are specified, the program runs another period of simulating the patient's reaction to conditions. Both the cardiac simulation and a respiratory simulation are designed to illustrate dynamically the interrelationships of physiological parameters.

System Features

There are several features or capabilities of the MGH patient simulation system that permit users to ask for and receive assistance. As the system has developed and become more sophisticated, features which have been found useful have been incorporated into new programs. Not all programs have all features, but some desirable system capabilities are described below.

COMMENT

The patient simulations undergo constant review by their authors and users. Users communicate with authors through a system COMMENT feature; at any point in a program, the user may type the word COMMENT and follow this with a question or suggestion. After he has made the comment, the user returns to his place in the program sequence. Each day, both the comments and the names of individuals making them are printed for program authors. Authors review and respond to comments individually by addressing their answers to the individual users who made them. The next time the user logs on the system, he receives a response to his comment. The COMMENT feature provides authors with continuous feedback from users. The information makes it easy for authors to detect and correct problems with program logic or content, so it accelerates program development. Users find that answers to comments make the simulations a truly individualized, personal experience. Faculty at remote institutions appreciate having the programs maintained and updated by responsible faculty authors at Massachusetts General Hospital.

HELP

During the course of a patient simulation, the user may need assistance; in this case, the user may type the word HELP. The program will ask whether he needs assistance with the format of his answer or if he requires the kind of review and discussion of the patient's problem that a teaching physician or consultant might provide. After the program provides the help requested, it returns the user to his place in the simulation. The user may call the HELP function repeatedly within a single patient simulation.

Each call for assistance and the type of help requested are noted on the daily output for program authors. When authors find many calls for procedural assistance, they know that directions are not clear. If there are numerous calls for medical guidance from the target population or individuals with more advanced training than the target population, the author may reconsider and revise the characteristics or behavior of the simulated patient. Alternatively, the author may enrich the kind of medical guidance the program provides to users when they request advice or consultation.

STOP

Frequently, a user finds it necessary to interrupt a patient simulation. Many users of clinical simulations have responsibility for patients and must terminate interaction with a simulated patient to take care of a real patient. The user may type the word STOP at any point in the simulation, and the program will end and print THANK YOU.

RESTART

At times, there are interruptions in the computer or the communications network, and the user may lose connection with the host computer system. If there is an interruption in the patient simulation either because the user typed STOP or there has been a technical problem, the user may wish to RESTART the simulation at the point at which he left it. A few programs give the user the option to RESTART in the middle of the simulation, to go on to another case, or to go back to the beginning of the interrupted case.

REVIEW

When the patient simulation is long and complex, or in the case of an interruption and RESTART, the user may wish to have a summary of the findings to a given point in the simulation. To get this summary, a few programs allow the user to type the word REVIEW, and the findings are printed so that he can review the data he has collected before he continues the simulation.

MUMPS

Development and maintenance of the computer-based patient simulations are facilitated by a powerful yet simple programming language, MUMPS (Massachusetts General Hospital Utility Multi-Programming System). Program authors do not need special training in mathematics, electrical engineering, computer science, or computer programming to create patient simulation in MUMPS (Greenes *et al.*, 1969). The language is easy to learn and use; people with no previous training are able to write and debug a basic MUMPS program in less than a week with no other aid than a MUMPS programming manual. Learning to use the full intricate capabilities of MUMPS, however, and to use its associated global file structure optimally takes time and practice.

MUMPS is well-suited to creating medical education programs because it is an interpretive system which provides program flexibility. All programming is done on-line, and it is easy to detect and correct errors. The corrected version can be run immediately and tested. Medical education programs undergo changes continuously in the process of their development and refinement, and MUMPS allows these changes and additions to be made easily in operating programs without hampering their use. Technical details of the MUMPS system are given in an appendix to this chapter.

Many physicians do not want to learn about computers or computer programming but do want to create patient simulations. MUMPS driver programs permit authors to create and modify complex simulations without writing MUMPS program code by using a program format or instructional strategy that already exists in the form of a driver program. A driver is a set of special-purpose utility programs designed to execute a repetitive task. Definition of the task is independent of the data, but the data "drive" or control the execution of the program. Drivers reduce the amount of program code that must be available on the system; one copy of a driver can be shared simultaneously by many users. A driver is slower on execution than a specially coded program, but it is more economical than a custom-made program in terms of reduced storage and a shorter time to create a new simulation. The driver includes definition of options, format, branching, and file structure of the data on which it operates. An author who is not a programmer can develop content and logic, specify branching, and enter his data base for a driver using an editor program. An editor is an on-line author aid which elicits the data base and logic from the author, checks syntax, and verifies that new data or modifications are consistent with the structure of the driver. The specifics of the computer and the language it uses are transparent to the author.

Currently, all of the Massachusetts General Hospital simulations are written in the MGH dialect of the MUMPS language (Barnett and Greenes, 1970). A Standard MUMPS language has been specified (O'Neill, 1976), and MGH plans to convert its simulations to Standard MUMPS. Versions of MUMPS also run on Burroughs, IBM, Artronix, and Data General equipment as well as on many models of Digital Equipment Corporation computers. A MUMPS Users' Group and a MUMPS Development Committee exist to facilitate communications among users and to promote language commonality for program interchange.

Program Use

The programs are used in a wide variety of ways. In undergraduate medical education, some students use the simulations to fulfill course requirements; others use them for independent study. They use the programs both for practice in clinical problem-solving and for self-assessment. In graduate medical education, practicing physicians use the simulations for private self-assessment, for continuing medical education, and for certification and recertification.

Medical Student Use

The programs were designed for individualized instruction, but students may consult books, journals, other students, or teaching physicians during the course of a simulation. In most simulations, they also have the option of typing the word HELP or CONSULT to get the kind of medical advice they seek. Sometimes a group of students and perhaps a preceptor will use a program jointly. At each point in the simulation requiring user action, the group discusses alternative actions, reasons for them, and their likely outcomes. Students working on a single clinical simulation are likely to force one another to say not only what action they would take at any particular moment but also why they would select that action over others, what they are trying to rule in or out, what disease process they are seeking, what impact the action will have on the patient, what information will be gained as a result of the action, and, depending on the result of the proposed action, what likely sequence of actions will be taken next.

Not only can the students go through a particular simulation once with one strategy or series of actions, they can go through the same simulation with a different series of actions and observe the results of their actions in the condition of the patient. No two real patients are identical, and practice of hindsight is not possible in the real world; in the world of simulation, a student does have a chance to see what happens when he has the opportunity to revise his handling of the same case from the beginning. Typically, medical students repeat a simulation until they are confident that they can solve all cases available for each clinical problem.

Some general clinical problems may be considered in several different clinical clerkships. Coma is a case in point. A coma simulation exists on the Massachusetts General Hospital computer system, and it is possible to set up a series of cases of coma with either neurologic or metabolic bases. The faculty member in neurology can request one series for his students, and his colleague in internal medicine can request another series of cases for his students. A single student who goes through both rotations could use the same simulation but with different cases appropriate to the different clerkships.

The programs take into account the user's clinical background and his performance on previous simulations, and the program the student uses is tailored to these factors. For example, the emergency phases of some clinical problems tend to be similar. The basic life support phase of cardiopulmonary resuscitation (CPR) is similar for all patients. Once a student has demonstrated proficiency in handling a subset of a problem, the computer will permit him to skip over that subset and work on other aspects in which he has not yet had experience or demonstrated competence.

Continuing Education

Computer-based educational materials in the field of continuing education have perhaps the greatest promise, yet to date have shown the least impact. Continuing education for physicians has been growing rapidly in recent years. In

1973–74 the A.M.A. listed 2441 continuing education courses available for physicians (J.A.M.A., 1973); by 1975–76 there were 4862 courses offered (J.A.M.A., 1975). In a growing number of states, continuing medical education activities are mandatory for maintaining licensure and/or membership in state medical societies. Some specialty societies have instituted similar requirements. Thus, there is considerable incentive for physicians to participate in continuing education activities beyond their inherent desire to keep current.

Computer-based education is generally cost competitive with more traditional forms of continuing education. Programs certified for AMA Category I credit by the Harvard Department of Continuing Education are currently offered via computer from the Massachusetts General Hospital. Costs range from $4 to $10 per hour of use depending on volume; this is similar to, or less than, most traditional course offerings. Computer-based continuing education also offers the advantage of bringing the educational medium to the user via telephone. Terminals can be placed in any hospital or even in the physician's home or office. This eliminates the very large indirect cost of leaving a practice to attend a postgraduate course.

The experience to date with physician use of programs for continuing education has been limited, and the literature is therefore fairly scanty (Harless *et al.*, 1969; Weinberg, 1973; Morrison *et al.*, 1973). MGH has had several experiences with computer-based continuing education. In 1971 and 1972 terminals were placed in three community hospitals in eastern Massachusetts with access to the MGH computer via telephone hookup. Despite enthusiastic support from the directors of medical education in these hospitals, very little physician use occurred. Retrospective analysis of this experience indicated that the single greatest factor inhibiting physician use was the need for them to seek out the computer terminal in order to use the programs. Most simply did not take the initiative to do this. Those who did were discouraged from returning if any problems were encountered in using the terminal.

Three times each year, the Unit of Medical Education at the Massachusetts General Hospital offers an intensive 2-week course to prepare graduate physicians who will work full-time in the emergency departments of hospitals or clinics. Physicians in this course spend 6 to 9 hours using the computer as an instructional tool. They find the programs on cardiopulmonary resuscitation, coma, diabetic ketoacidosis, and hypertensive emergencies most useful. The computer-based simulations provide private self-assessment as well as instruction (Farquhar, 1976). Physicians evaluate the entire course after completing it, and they consistently rate the use of the computer-based simulations among the most valuable portions of the course.

During 1973 and 1974 MGH placed terminals in four community hospitals. The physicians in these hospitals used the terminals over the Experimental CAI Network funded by the Lister Hill Center of the National Library of Medicine (Chapter 8, this volume). Patterns of use at the four different hospitals varied considerably. At one hospital there was very little physician use, but very heavy use by nurses and paramedical personnel, while at another the five emergency physicians completed almost thirty simulated cases each. (Hoffer, 1975).

Some conclusions can be reached from the MGH experience to date. The first is that there is a great deal of competition for the continuing education dollar. Physicians have a wide choice of locale and methodology for meeting their continuing education needs. In many cases, the computer programs have to compete with a week at a pleasant resort area. This would suggest that continuing education uses must offer other appealing advantages to overcome the disadvantage of not giving any of the side benefits offered by traditional continuing education courses. A second important factor is that physicians in general have a fairly low tolerance of technical problems. The simplest terminal is the best, and the service offered must be of a high order of reliability to encourage repeated use. Finally, since there is a major hurdle to be overcome in sparking initial user interest, a dedicated and forceful individual should be present at each site where terminals are placed. The single largest factor in promoting success seems to have been the presence of an individual who was convinced of the merits of computer-based educational materials, who could show other people how to use them, and who could encourage continued use.

Assessment of Clinical Competence

The future of the computer as a device for testing clinical competence is promising, and the Massachusetts General Hospital has collaborated with the National Board of Medical Examiners in developing the prototype of the computer-based examination (CBX) (Farquhar *et al.*, 1973) and in devising subsequent models for testing. The American Board of Internal Medicine and the National Board of Medical Examiners are also developing plans for a computer-based certification mechansim which might be used for recertification as well (Harless, 1976). The American Academy of Orthopaedic Surgeons has long been a pioneer in education and evaluation of both residents and practicing orthopedists (Mankin, 1971). The MGH staff in the Laboratory of Computer Science worked with the Academy to design, develop, implement, and evaluate a computer-based Orthopaedic In-Training Examination for residents. Once a battery of such examinations has been developed and validated, it could be used not only to evaluate residents in training but also for self-assessment and continuing education for those in practice (Mankin, 1976).

Summary

One of the most important goals of clinical medical education is the teaching of the problem-solving process. The process is best taught in clinical settings, yet the constraints imposed by patient care and the unpredictability of the clinical problems that will be available for study may limit the effectiveness of such educational experiences. Computer-based patient simulations can serve as a valuable adjunct to education in clinical settings. Simulated clinical problems allow medical students to receive uniform instruction by computer and to learn from their mistakes in clinical judgment in a variety of cases without risk of harm or harassment to real patients, without undue repetition of materials by their clinical preceptors, and without regard to the vagaries in clinical problems presented by a particular patient population. Patient simulations can also be used by graduate physicians for continuing education, self-assessment, and for certification and recertification.

The Massachusetts General Hospital Laboratory of Computer Science has developed a series of computer-based simulations that stress the process of decision-making and that supplement practice in clinical problem-solving. Programs are written in MUMPS, a language well-suited to clinical simulations. The programs, which are carefully tested and continually revised, are available locally and throughout the United States via the Health Education Network.

Appendix: MUMPS Technical Characteristics

The text-processing capabilities and file structure of MUMPS make it especially suitable for patient simulations. The language provides elaborate string or text-processing features in addition to standard arithmetic and Boolean capabilities. MUMPS handles string data in symbolic form and performs syntax checking by pattern matching to determine whether a string contains a predetermined sequence of numerics, alphabetics, punctuation, or combination of these. Strings can be assembled, disassembled, modified, or searched easily. MUMPS uses a common, random-access file structure. Data files are stored in dynamic tree-structured form. Nodes of the tree are referenced symbolically using N-dimensional subscripts. Files are created and manipulated dynamically, and space is allocated as it is needed. A datum in the file can be changed without disturbing other data in the array. Together, these features provide capabilities which make it possible to write sophisticated simulations that are easy to modify on a relatively inexpensive computer system.

An experienced computer programmer who is creating a patient simulation may elect to use a driver but insert MUMPS code or call other programs to perform certain special functions. Most computer languages distinguish between programs (executable code) and data. They permit programs to create, reference, change, and exchange data but do not allow programs to modify their own or other program's code. In MUMPS, a program may create, modify, or expunge part or all of its own executable code. A driver usually interprets data and executes the option indicated. When a driver finds MUMPS statements, it creates a program and executes commands.

MUMPS simulations run at Massachusetts General Hospital on any of five Digital PDP-9 and PDP-15 computers. Each computer has a minimum of 32K of core, a 3-million-character fixed-head disk, and two 30-million-character movable-head disks. The interpreter uses 12K of core, and the remainder is divided into 20, 1K user partitions. Programs are core-resident, and they are interpreted rather than compiled. Extended core supports more than 20 simultaneous users on a single computer. The system supports ASCII terminals at the rate of up to 2400 baud in-house. Systems are half-duplex and asynchronous. Average response time is 0.5 seconds, but response time varies as a function of the task to be performed, particularly as a function of disk activity and of the number of other users of the system. Response time may be as long as 2–5 seconds when the system is loaded heavily.

References

AAMC (Association of American Medical Colleges), 1973. Undergraduate Medical Education: Elements, Objectives, Costs, Report of the Committee on the Financing of Medical Education, Association of American Medical Colleges, Washington, D.C.

Barnett, G. O., 1974. The use of a computer-based system to teach clinical problem solving, *in* B. Waxman and R. Stacy (Eds.), *Computers in Biomedical Research*, Vol. 4, pp. 301–319, Academic Press, New York.

Barnett, G. O., and Greenes, R. A., 1970. High level programming languages, *Comput. Biomed. Res.* 3:488–494.

Barnett, G. O., Baillieul, J. B., and Farquhar, B. B., 1972. The testing of clinical judgment – An experimental computer-based measurement of sequential problem-solving ability, *in* J. Jacquez (Ed.), *Proceedings of 1970 University of Michigan Conference*, pp. 191–202, Charles C Thomas, Springfield, Illinois.

Bloom, B. S., Engelhart, M. D., Furst, E. J., Hill, W. H., and Krathwohl, D. R., 1956. *Taxonomy of Educational Objectives, Handbook I: Cognitive Domain*, David McKay Company, New York.

Farquhar, B. B., 1976. Computers and the education of health personnel, *in: Medical Data Processing*, Taylor and Francis, Ltd., London.

Farquhar, B. B., Barnett, G. O., Goldfinger, S. E., and Dinnen, J. J., 1973. Computer-based examination: A technique to evaluate clinical competence, *in* J. P. Lysaught (Ed.), *Instructional Technology in Medical Education*, pp. 91–99, University of Rochester, Rochester, N.Y.

Feinstein, A. R., 1967. *Clinical Judgment*, Williams and Wilkins, Baltimore, Maryland.

Goroll, A. H., Barnett, G. O., Bowie, J. E., and Prather, P. A., (submitted for publication), A pathophysiological approach to teaching differential diagnosis using a computer-based program.

Greenes, R. A., Pappalardo, A. N., Marble, C. W., and Barnett, G. O., 1969. Design and implementation of a clinical data mangement system, *Comput. Biomed. Res.* 2:469–485.

Harless, W. G., 1976. MERIT, presentation at the Association for the Development of Computer-based Instructional Systems, January, 1976, Santa Barbara, California.

Harless, W. G., Lucas, N. C., Cutter, J. A., Duncan, R. C., White, J. M., and Brandt, E. W., 1969. Computer-assisted instruction in continuing medical education, *J. Med. Educ.* 44:670–674.

Hoffer, E. P., 1974. Ask the computer; problem: G. I. bleeding, *Emergency Medicine* (November, 1974): 193.

Hoffer, E. P., 1975. Computer-aided instruction in community hospital emergency departments: A pilot project, *J. Med. Educ.* 50:84–86.

Hoffer, E. P., Barnett, G. O., and Farquhar, B. B., 1972. Computer simulation model for teaching cardipulmonary resuscitation, *J. Med. Educ.* 47:343–348.

Hoffer, E. P., Barnett, G. O., Farquhar, B. B., and Prather, P. A., 1975. Computer-aided instruction in medicine, *Ann. Rev. Biophys. Bioeng.* 4:103–118.

J.A.M.A., 1973. Medical education in the United States 1972–1973, Section 4, Continuing medical education, 1973, *J.A.M.A.* 266:893–995.

J.A.M.A., 1975. Continuing education courses for physicians, 1975, *J.A.M.A.*, *(Supplement*, August 11, 1975), 233:6.

Krathwohl, D. R., Bloom, B. S., and Masia, B. B., 1964. *Taxonomy of Educational Objectives. Handbook II: Affective Domain*, David McKay Company, New York.

Lambdin, J. A., Johnson, D. G., and Kurtz, G., 1975. Survey of How Medical Students Finance Their Education, Association of American Medical Colleges, Washington, D.C.

Mankin, H. J., 1971. The orthopaedic in-training examination, *Clinical Orthopaedics*, 75:108–116.

Mankin, H. J., unpublished, Development of educational characteristics for orthopaedics, Massachusetts General Hospital, Boston, Massachusetts.

Mankin, H. J., 1976. The MARK programs for the American Academy of Orthopaedic Surgeons, presentation to the Advisory Committee on Continuing Education, April 2, 1976, Boston, Massachusetts.

Morrison, C. C., Boswick, G., Hassan, R., and Belknap, S., 1973. The computer and office practice, *Journal of the Maine Medical Association* 64:266–270.

O'Neill, J. T. (Ed.), 1976, *MUMPS Language Standard*, Systems and Software Division, Institute for Computer Sciences and Technology, National Bureau of Standards, Washington, D.C.

Travers, J. F., 1972. Types of learning III – problem solving, *in Learning: Analysis and Application*, 2nd ed., pp. 128–151, David McKay Company, New York.

Weinberg, A. D., 1973. CAI at The Ohio State University College of Medicine, *Comput. Biol. Med.* 3:299–305.

22

Management of Clinical Problems by Physician–Computer Dialogue

Howard L. Bleich

Introduction

In recent years hospitals have begun using a computer program designed to help physicians manage patients with electrolyte and acid–base disorders. The program directs a dialogue during which the physician supplies clinical and laboratory information. When requested data are unavailable, the program proceeds with incomplete information. On the basis of the abnormalities detected, it then asks further questions as needed to characterize the electrolyte and acid–base disturbances. Upon completion of the interchange, the program produces an evaluation note that resembles a remotely located consultant's discussion of the problem presented. The note includes a list of diagnostic possibilities, an explanation of the pathophysiology, therapeutic recommendations, suggestions for additional laboratory studies, precautionary measures required by the illness or the treatment, and references to the medical literature. Since additional hospitals are scheduled to begin using the program shortly, and additional computer consultation programs are under various stages of development, it seems appropriate to compare computerized and human consultation, and to consider some of the implications of this adjunct to patient care.

The Computer Compared with the Brain

The computer differs from the human consultant in many important ways. It is immune from fatigue and carelessness: it works day and night, weekends and holidays, without coffee breaks, overtime, fringe benefits, or human courtesy. It requires occasional repair, but even in the absence of an extra machine, it is more

Howard L. Bleich · Thorndike Memorial Laboratory and Department of Medicine, Harvard Medical School and Beth Israel Hospital, Boston, Massachusetts. Supported by a grant from the John A. Hartford Foundation and by a grant (HS 00188) from the U.S. Public Health Service. Adapted, with permission, from "The Computer as a Consultant," *New England Journal of Medicine* 284:141–147 (1971).

likely than its human counterpart to be available at the moment of need. On the other hand, current computer programs do not discuss the patient's condition with members of his family. They cannot perform their own physical examination or verify a laboratory technician's questionable finding; their output is critically dependent upon the accuracy of the information supplied by the referring physician.

Of greater importance than these considerations may be the difference in the class of problems that the computer and the brain solve best. This difference can be appreciated by comparison of some of the characteristics of the PDP-15 computer (Digital Equipment Corporation, Maynard, Massachusetts) on which the Electrolyte and Acid–Base Program is currently used with those of the human brain (Table 1).

Information storage in the brain is poorly understood, but von Neumann has estimated its memory capacity at approximately 10^{20} bits, where a bit (a contraction of "binary digit"), the standard unit of information, corresponds to a single binary alternative such as YES–NO, ON–OFF, ZERO–ONE, or TRUE–FALSE (von Neumann, 1958). By contrast, information stored in the computer can be located precisely. Under control of the program, it may be moved from less expensive areas of storage, such as disk or magnetic tape, to areas of more rapid recall, such as ferrite core. By devoting 6 bits to each character, the computer can represent up to 2^6 or 64 different characters. In this way, it can store letters and punctuation marks as well as numbers. Memory capacity of the computer, including its peripheral disk storage, is approximately 10^7 bits.

Construction of a device that consumes so much power, that has a comparatively small memory, and that contains one-tenth as many circuits as the brain of an ant is justified by the accuracy and speed with which the computer operates. Although internal mistakes are made, checking procedures shield virtually all mistakes from the user; during 10 years of work, we have occasionally encountered garbled messages due to noisy telephone circuits, but have yet to encounter a single erroneous character that could be traced to the computer. With respect to speed, electronic circuits conduct 10,000,000 impulses per second; neurons conduct 100. The computer can subtract serial 7s 1,000,000 times faster than the brain. In other words, the computer has a small number of exceedingly reliable and fast circuits, and is designed to perform many simple tasks, one, or perhaps a few, at a time: the

Table 1. The PDP-15 Computer Compared with the Human Brain

Agent	Circuits	Weight (lb)	Size (ft)	Power (watts)	Memory (bits)	Conduction rate (impulses/ sec)	Time to subtract serial 7s from 100 (sec)
PDP-15 computer	10^4 transistors	2300	225	6000	7×10^8	10^7	30×10^{-6}
Human brain	10^{10} neurons	3	1/20	10	10^{20}	10^2	30

brain has a huge number of relatively slow circuits, and is therefore better equipped to cope with large amounts of information presented and processed simultaneously.

The importance of matching the presentation of data to the processing device can be appreciated from Figure 1, the results of a hypothetical research study in which serum sodium concentration was measured twice a day for 15 weeks. An effective and compact way to present these data to a computer would be as a series of fifteen strings of numbers, each consisting of the determinations performed during one week. The computer could assimilate the data, identify the abnormal values and perform other routine calculations almost instantaneously, but this serial presentation is ineffective and confusing for the brain. Figure 2 presents the same data in parallel; it is now immediately apparent that serum sodium concentration decreased transiently from normal to hyponatremic levels during the eighth week of the study.

Just as the brain does poorly with serial information, the computer does poorly with recognition of patterns. A child easily identifies a letter or number, regardless of its size, position, color or spatial orientation; on the other hand, the information required to recognize even such simple patterns is too much for a computer to ingest simultaneously. The computer must scan the pattern and translate the result into a stream of binary digits that can be assimilated serially. To program the computer to interpret this stream of data is a difficult task that, so far, has been only partially accomplished, although it would be useful for identifying postal zip codes and other purposes. Attempts to program computers to interpret medical patterns such as electrocardiographic arrhythmias and Papanicolaou smears have also been only partially successful, despite widely recognized need and intense efforts by competent investigators.

WEEK OF STUDY	SERUM SODIUM CONCENTRATION (MEQ/L)
1	140 137 142 137 138 139 138 137 137 140 140 141 137 142
2	139 141 140 140 142 138 140 139 137 138 141 138 142 139
3	141 137 138 141 142 139 141 142 141 137 139 139 139 138
4	137 137 139 139 137 142 140 107 140 140 142 141 140 142
5	140 138 137 139 140 139 142 138 141 142 141 140 138 141
6	137 142 141 142 138 139 138 137 137 137 141 141 138 137
7	140 142 140 141 137 142 140 138 138 138 140 140 142 141
8	137 137 135 130 127 126 123 127 129 134 134 133 136 142
9	139 140 137 141 139 141 142 139 139 141 138 141 140 138
10	138 139 139 140 138 142 141 139 140 141 140 138 138 142
11	142 142 142 139 142 140 138 141 137 142 139 142 139 139
12	140 142 139 141 137 141 137 141 141 141 138 142 137 137
13	141 141 139 139 140 137 141 142 141 141 139 138 141 141
14	141 141 137 141 142 139 139 137 137 137 142 138 141 138
15	141 142 139 138 139 141 142 139 140 142 138 139 138 137

Figure 1. Serum sodium concentration, measured twice a day for 15 weeks, and presented serially. This is an effective presentation to the computer, but a torturous presentation to the brain.

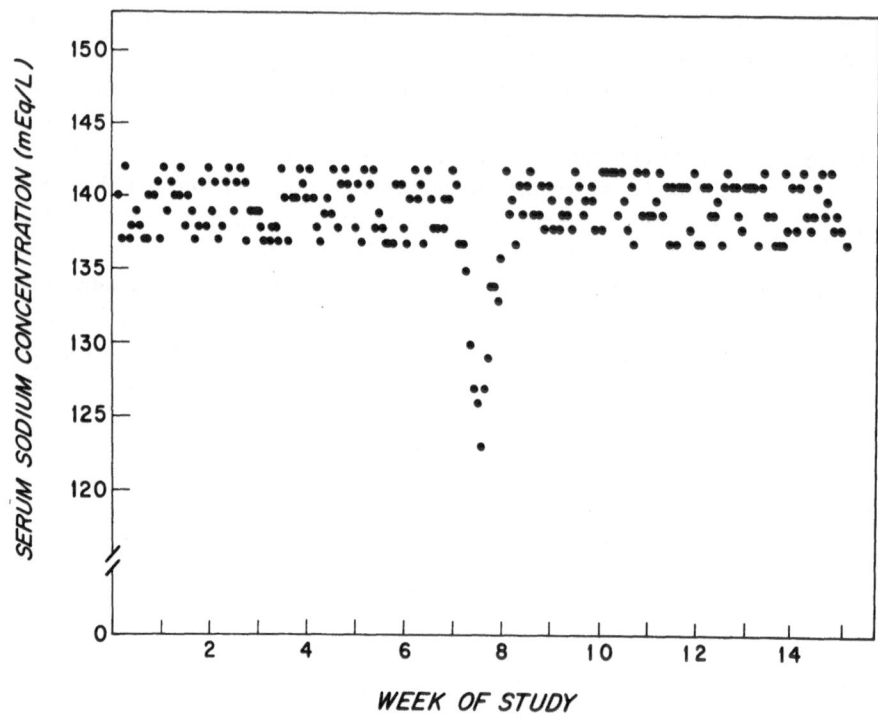

Figure 2. Data in Figure 1 presented in parallel.

If the recognizing of myxedematous facies, Parkinsonian gait, and abnormal shadows on a chest film are, at least for the moment, primarily human tasks, other medical problems are largely serial, and these seem to be particulary amenable to solution by computer. In recent years, two important developments have made it practical to use the computer to assist the physician with medical decisions. One is the advent of programming languages that can manipulate strings of text according to rules of syntax, just as the more widely used languages manipulate numbers according to rules of arithmetic. The other is the development of interactive or conversational computer programs that communicate with the user not via a batch of punched cards, but via a suitable terminal such as a teletypewriter or cathode ray display, which exchanges messages with the computer over ordinary telephone lines.

The PDP-15 computer is programmed for time-sharing; it cycles from one telephone line to the next, and works on each problem either until it is complete or until 16 msec have elapsed, when the unfinished portion of the problem is preserved for completion during a subsequent time slice. In this way, the computer can serve as many as 22 remotely located terminals simultaneously, and any terminal may be used either to write a new program or to run a program previously developed. Although the time-sharing computer works for many users and appears to perform many different tasks simultaneously, in fact it goes from task to task seriatim, capitalizing on the enormous speed of the computer in comparison with the slower speed of the terminal, and providing the user with a nearly continuous stream of typeout. Having many users share a central computer fractionates the cost. More important, however, it permits a single copy of a program to be updated by committee, and the resulting revision to be instantaneously available throughout the geographic area that it serves.

The Electrolyte and Acid—Base Program

If medical decision-making is to be amenable to computer programming, it must be possible either to measure or to verbalize the data on which each decision is based. The data need not be numerical; it is possible, for example, to program answers to YES—NO or multiple choice questions, but not alterations of facial expression unless the changes can be measured or described in words. Electrolyte and acid—base equilibrium was selected for the computer-based consultation program because virtually all the required data could be measured or verbalized. Furthermore, clinical problems in this area are relatively common, and the numerical calculations required to solve these problems may be cumbersome for the physician.

A flow diagram depicting some of the pathways used by the Electrolyte and Acid—Base Program is shown in Figure 3. To write the program (that is, to translate the logical pathways into instructions for the computer) is a uniquely delightful task since each quantum of knowledge needs to be transmitted precisely once. On the other hand, the computer does exactly what it is told, which is not necessarily what the programmer wants. If, for example, a 4-year-old boy is asked to put on his shoes and socks, there is a finite chance that he will obey. If the same instruction could be given to a computer, it would invariably return an error comment explaining that the socks will not fit over the shoes.

Some of the instructions serve to select and arrange strings of separately stored English text that ultimately comprise the evaluation note. Distributed throughout the text are the names of variables; when, while printing text, the program encounters the name of a variable, it types the value of the variable before continuing with the remainder of the text. In this way, the program inserts given or calculated numbers that modify the evaluation note for the particular patient. The insertion of words such as "relatively" and "probably" may shade the meaning in a borderline conclusion; other insertions may substantially alter or completely reverse the meaning of a text string. The program acts as a personalized textbook that presents to the physician only the excerpts from the medical literature that pertain to his patient, and it potentiates the usefulness of this information by interweaving it with given or derived information from the data base.

When the program is called, it directs a dialogue as shown in Figure 4. The computer transmits the electrolyte and acid—base evaluation, the date, and the time, and then asks for the serum electrolytes in milliequivalents per liter. After typing "Na =" the terminal pauses until the physician makes a response. To enter a

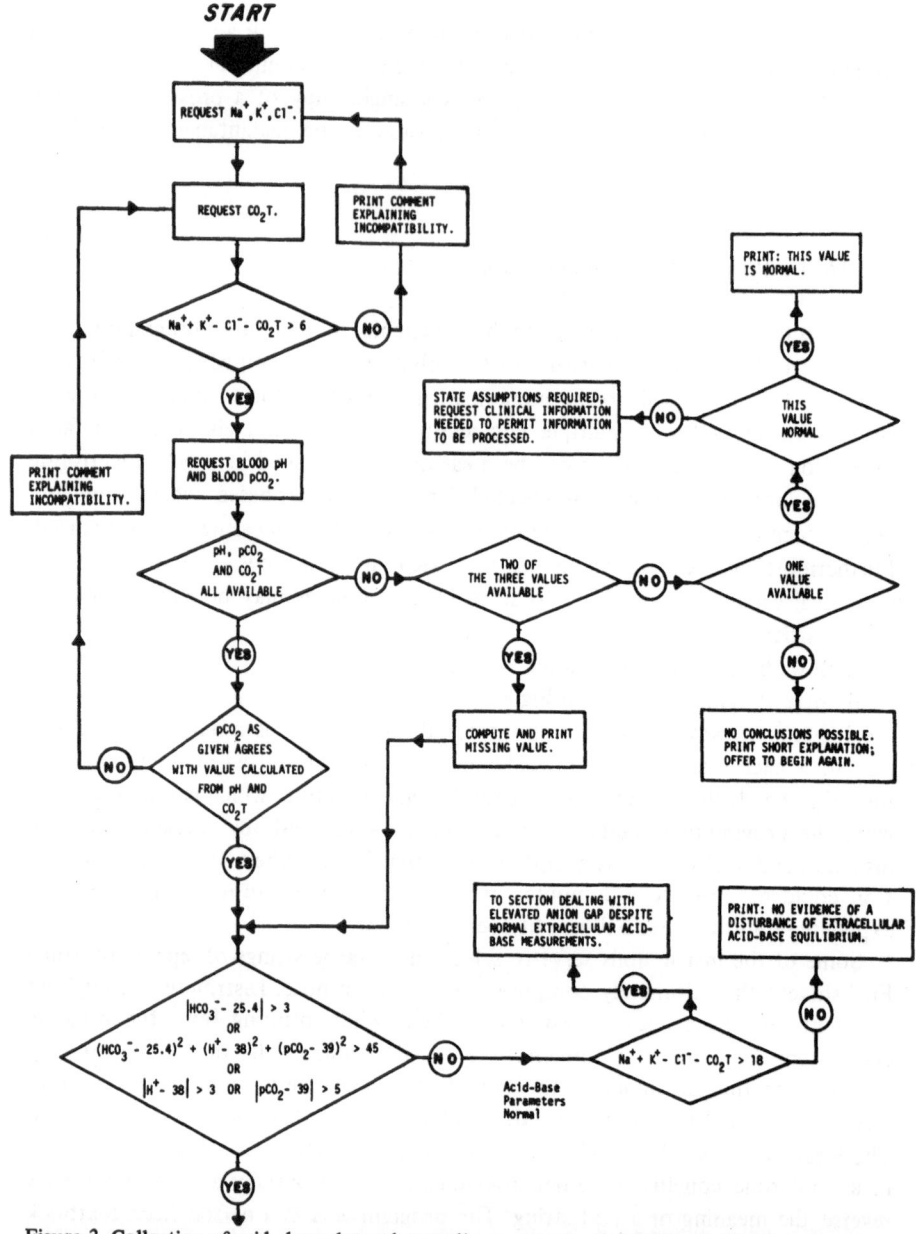

Figure 3. Collection of acid—base data when sodium, potassium, and chloride have been provided (adapted from Bleich, 1969, and reproduced with permission from the publisher). Serum electrolytes are expressed as milliequivalents per liter, carbon dioxide tension as millimeters of mercury, and hydrogen ion activity as nanoequivalents per liter. Only principal pathways are shown in the figure (for example, additional pathways that check each entry for proper syntax and compatibility with life have been omitted). The program checks each entry for compatibility with all previous entries, and, where possible, calculates values that were not supplied. The terminating arrow at the bottom leads to pathways that deal with acid—base abnormalities; after completing the acid—base sections, the program considers abnormalities of the other electrolytes.

value, the physician can type a number and then press an ENTER button. Mistakes can be erased with a RUBOUT button; values that violate required syntax or that are incompatible with life are requested again. Any entry may be left blank. Upon completion of the dialogue, the program generates an evaluation note as shown in Figure 5.

This program may be used from any teletype-compatible terminal connected to the Bell Telephone System. The program is written in MUMPS, a special, text-manipulating language developed at the Massachusetts General Hospital (Greenes *et al.*, 1969). Earlier versions of the program were translated into BASIC, COURSE-WRITER and FORTRAN, and in these forms it was available at the Dartmouth Medical School, in hospitals served by the Ohio State Regional Medical Program and at the University of California, Davis. In most cases, however, we have discouraged efforts to translate the program; translation into the more familiar languages that lack many of the text-manipulating features required by the program involves considerable effort, and to run the program in such languages has always proved more costly than to run it in MUMPS. More important than cost, however, is the fact that improvements, which are continually made in the MUMPS version as a result of new data in the literature and suggestions from users, do not immediately become available in the translated versions.

Experience with the program in our hospital reveals a number of cases in which patient care was favorably influenced. On one occasion, physicians had decided to administer hypertonic saline to a hyponatremic patient until advised by the program to restrict fluids instead. Consultation was requested, and the latter course adopted. The renal service has received numerous consultations after the program revealed a problem not previously appreciated by the physicians. At times the program outperforms its inventor; it was, after all, written during his lucid intervals, while relevant literature was on his desk, and while physicians more knowledgeable than he were nearby.

Although the program has now been used several times, repeated usage cannot be taken as evidence of a positive contribution to patient care. Like sales of a textbook, use of a program may be an important measurement for its vendor, but it is not necessarily relevant to the health of the community. Similarly, peer review may be a satisfactory means of evaluating accuracy of content, but the peer who already understands a subject may not be able to judge how effectively the information is being communicated to the user. Perhaps a more useful test would be to compare charts in hospitals with and without the program and to determine the percentage of patients reached, and whether or not patient care was favorably influenced.

Even if the program could be shown to be perfect, it is possible that a patient could be harmed through its use. For example, a brief burst of noise on the telephone line or a subtle defect in the teletypewriter could lead to the printing of an erroneous, but otherwise plausible number that could cause the administration of an incorrect dose. The probability of error can be reduced by the addition of redundant equipment, but to reduce it to zero would require infinite cost. On the

ELECTROLYTE AND ACID-BASE EVALUATION   AUG 2, 1976   12:39 PM

SERUM ELECTROLYTES (MEQ/L):

    NA   = 142
    K   = 2.8
    CL   = 92
    CO2T = 35

ARTERIAL PH = 7.48   (H+ = 33 NEQ/L)

BLOOD PCO2 = 47 (CALCULATED FROM CO2T AND PH)

PATIENT'S WEIGHT (IN POUNDS)   = 150

DOES A RECENT CHEST X-RAY SHOW CONGESTIVE HEART FAILURE, OR
IS THERE CLINICAL EVIDENCE OF CONGESTIVE HEART FAILURE AT THE
PRESENT TIME?...   NO

IS THERE PITTING EDEMA THAT CANNOT BE ATTRIBUTED TO LOCAL
FACTORS SUCH AS VARICOSE VEINS, VENOUS OR LYMPHATIC OBSTRUCTION,
PHLEBITIS, OR CELLULITIS?...   NO

IS THERE EVIDENCE OF DEPLETION OF EXTRACELLULAR FLUID VOLUME?... NO

SERUM CREATININE (MG%) =   1.1

BLOOD SUGAR (MG%) = 100

24 HOUR URINARY POTASSIUM EXCRETION (MEQ/DAY) = 56

HAS HYPOKALEMIA BEEN PRESENT FOR LONGER THAN 2 WEEKS?...   YES

DOES THE PATIENT HAVE SEVERE LIVER DISEASE?...   NO

                         EVALUATION NOTE

     THE PCO2 OF 47 MM HG AND ARTERIAL PH OF 7.48 UNITS ARE
COMPATIBLE WITH UNCOMPLICATED METABOLIC ALKALOSIS. THE MOST COMMON
CAUSES OF METABOLIC ALKALOSIS ARE:
     1) VOMITING OR GASTRIC ASPIRATION
     2) DIURETIC THERAPY (THIAZIDES, MERCURIALS, ETHACRYNIC ACID, OR
        FUROSEMIDE)
     3) HYPERADRENALISM (CUSHINGS SYNDROME, PRIMARY OR SECONDARY
        ALDOSTERONISM, ADRENAL STEROID THERAPY) OR LICORICE
        INGESTION
     4) EXCESSIVE ALKALI INTAKE (ALKALOSIS USUALLY TRANSIENT)
     5) POST HYPERCAPNIA (PARTICULARLY IF CHLORIDE INTAKE IS SMALL)
     6) HYPERCALCEMIA (POSSIBLE--LITERATURE NOT CLEAR)
     7) BARTTER'S SYNDROME (A RARE DISORDER CHARACTERIZED BY
        HYPOKALEMIA, HYPOCHLOREMIA, METABOLIC ALKALOSIS, AND, IN
        SOME INSTANCES, HYPONATREMIA, SHORT STATURE, AND MENTAL
        RETARDATION)

Figure 4. Entry of patient's data and first portion of evaluation note. (Underlined information was typed by the physician, everything else by the computer.)

IF HYPERADRENALISM IS ABSENT IT SHOULD BE POSSIBLE TO CORRECT THE METABOLIC ALKALOSIS BY ADMINISTERING SUFFICIENT CHLORIDE TO REPLACE PREVIOUS LOSSES AND TO ALLOW A URINARY CHLORIDE EXCRETION OF AT LEAST 10 TO 20 MEQ PER DAY. IN AN EFFORT TO ACHIEVE THIS GOAL IT IS SUGGESTED THAT, IN ADDITION TO REPLACING KNOWN CHLORIDE LOSSES, 140 MEQ OF SODIUM, POTASSIUM, OR AMMONIUM CHLORIDE BE GIVEN DURING THE NEXT 24 HOURS, AND THAT SERUM ELECTROLYTES AND BLOOD PH BE MEASURED AT LEAST DAILY UNTIL SIGNIFICANT IMPROVEMENT IN THE ACID-BASE ABNORMALITY OCCURS.

THE FINDING OF A LOW SERUM POTASSIUM CONCENTRATION (K = 2.8 MEQ/L) INDICATES THAT BODY POTASSIUM STORES HAVE BEEN SIGNIFICANTLY DEPLETED. FURTHERMORE, THE FINDING OF SIGNIFICANT URINARY POTASSIUM EXCRETION (56 MEQ/DAY) IN A PATIENT WHOSE POTASSIUM DEPLETION HAS BEEN PRESENT FOR AT LEAST 2 WEEKS INDICATES THAT RENAL POTASSIUM CONSERVATION IS IMPAIRED. COMMON CAUSES OF RENAL POTASSIUM WASTING INCLUDE, IN ADDITION TO THE CAUSES OF METABOLIC ALKALOSIS, OUTDATED TETRACYCLINE, RENAL TUBULAR ACIDOSIS (NOT PRESENT HERE), AND THE DIURETIC PHASE OF ACUTE TUBULAR NECROSIS.

IN AN EFFORT TO REPAIR THE POTASSIUM DEFICIT SIMULTANEOUSLY WITH THE METABOLIC ALKALOSIS IT IS SUGGESTED THAT, IN ADDITION TO REPLACING ANTICIPATED POTASSIUM LOSSES AT LEAST 60 MEQ OF THE CHLORIDE RECOMMENDED ABOVE BE ADMINISTERED AS POTASSIUM CHLORIDE. BECAUSE OF THE SEVERITY OF THE HYPOKALEMIA (K = 2.8 MEQ/L), THIS SHOULD PROBABLY BE DONE WITHIN THE NEXT 12 HOURS AND SERUM ELECTROLYTES MEASURED AGAIN AT THAT TIME.

THANK YOU FOR REFERRING THIS INTERESTING PROBLEM TO US.

REFERENCES:

1) SHEAR, L. AND BRANDMAN, I.S.
HYPOXIA AND HYPERCAPNIA CAUSED BY RESPIRATORY COMPENSATION
FOR METABOLIC ALKALOSIS
AMER. REV. OF RESP. DIS., 107:836,1973.
2) BEESON, P.B. AND MCDERMOTT, W.
CECIL-LOEB TEXTBOOK OF MEDICINE.
14TH EDITION (1975), P.1579.
3) GARELLA, S., CHAZAN, J.A., AND COHEN, J.J.
SALINE-RESISTANT METABOLIC ALKALOSIS OR "CHLORIDE-WASTING
NEPHROPATHY."
ANN. INT. MED., 73:31,1970.
4) SCHWARTZ, W.B.
POTASSIUM AND THE KIDNEY
NEW ENG. J. MED., 253:601,1955.

Figure 5. Remainder of evaluation note generated by the program immediately after the last entry was made in Figure 4.

other hand, decision-making can never be entirely free of error, and the real question is probably whether a new device makes a positive or negative contribution. At present, both the patient and the law look to the physician as the source of medical decisions. The physician may choose to employ laboratory tests, textbooks, articles in the literature, conversations with colleagues and computer programs, but these aids are rarely to blame if a decision proves unsatisfactory; it is the doctor who is responsible for assessing the applicability of what each can offer a particular patient. The extent to which physicians will choose to employ computer programs and their motivations for doing so remain unknown. Our preliminary experience suggests that they welcome the intellectual challenge of mastering a new device that responds in a helpful manner, that accurately performs tedious numerical calculations and that submits its product to their complete control. To the extent that computer programs broaden the range of decisions that can be delegated to paramedical personnel, they seem to amplify the responsibility and importance of the supervising physician.

It also seems likely that use of such a program can contribute to the education of physicians. Several have told us that they no longer need the program for certain disorders since they can predict its typeout. In addition, many of the phrases and logical conclusions that appear in the typeout have begun to appear in physicians' progress notes.

In conclusion, it is of interest to recall that when Copernicus proved that the earth was not the center of the universe, but rather a tiny speck, he injured man's pride. When Darwin suggested that we are not specially created, but rather an extension of the animal world, he salted this wounded pride. When Freud taught that we are not the master of our own house, but that we must be content with tiny vignettes of the events in our minds, he seared our salted wound. Finally, in a paper entitled "The Fourth Discontinuity," Mazlish (1967) suggested that the computer constitutes yet another blow to man's ego, for, in a sense, it places him on a continuous spectrum with the machines that he builds. If so, let us now swallow our pride like those who preceded us, comfort ourselves with the reminder that we can always pull out the plug, and set about the task of developing humanitarian uses for this machinery.

References

Bleich, H. L., 1969. Computer evaluation of acid–base disorders, *J. Clin. Invest.* 48:1689–1696.

Bostrom, R. C., Sawyer, H. S., Tolles, W. E., 1959. Instrumentation for automatically pre-screening cytological smears, *Proc. I.R.E.* 47:1893–1900.

Caceres, C. A., Steinberg, C. A., Gorman, P. A., *et al.*, 1964. Computer aids in electrocardiography, *Ann. N.Y. Acad. Sci.* 118:85–102.

Greenes, R. A., Pappalardo, A. N., Marble, C. W., and Barnett, G. D., 1969. Design·and implementation of a clinical data management system, *Comput. Biomed. Res.* 2:469–485.

Mazlish, B., 1967. The fourth discontinuity, *Technology and Culture* 8:1–15 (Winter, 1967).

Pipberger, H. V., Freis, E. D., Taback, L., *et al.*, 1960. Preparation of electrocardiographic data for analysis by digital electronic computer, *Circulation* 21:413–418.

Rosenberg, S. A., Ledeen, K. S., Kline, T., 1969. Automatic identification and measurement of cells by computer, *Science* 163:1065–1067.

von Neumann, J., 1958. *The Computer and the Brain*, pp. 63–64, Yale University Press, New Haven.

23

Clinical Simulation in Medical Education: The Wisconsin Experience

Richard B. Friedman

The past 5-years have seen a dramatic increase in the enrollment in the nation's medical schools. This, unfortunately, has not been coupled with a concomitant increase in faculty size. It has, however, coincided with a decrease in ward service populations, the traditional source of "teaching" patients. These events have put a considerable strain on existing medical school clinical teaching facilities. In response to this medical educators have begun to investigate the use of alternate training techniques. One area that has come under close scrutiny has been the use of computers in medical education.

Computer-assisted instruction has been examined in a number of pilot medical school teaching programs (Griesen *et al.*, 1971; Harless, 1967; Weinberg, 1973; Williams *et al.*, 1971), interdisciplinary symposiums (Griesen, 1970; Starkweather, 1967; Stolurow *et al.*, 1970), and individual research projects. In most cases it is the computer-assisted didactic instruction that has found its way into the medical school. This type of instruction has been particularly useful during the first 2 years of basic science didactic training. Computer programs to develop the clinical skills of medical students by permitting them to interact with computer-based simulated patients have to date been less widespread in their general application.

The clinical teaching programs developed to date have varied in purpose and scope. Some allow the physician to query the patient in free-text form (Harless *et al.*, 1971), while others require the user to enter code names or numbers obtained from the directory (DeDombal *et al.*, 1969; Entwisle and Entwisle, 1963; Feurzeig *et al.*, 1964; Hoffer, 1973; Schneiderman and Muller, 1972; Stolurow, 1955). Several permit the user to query the patient in detail about his illness (Harless *et al.*, 1971; Hoffer, 1973) but most simply allow him to request information by test name. A few systems provide for maximum teaching during the case presentation (Feurzeig *et al.*, 1964; Hoffer, 1973; Stolurow, 1955), while most attempt to simulate the entire patient–physician encounter. One existing system manipulates a predefined set of test results using the interaction of random numbers and symptom probabilities to develop a large number of unique case

Richard B. Friedman · Department of Medicine, University of Wisconsin Medical School, Madison, Wisconsin.

histories (Hoffer, 1973; DeDombal *et al.*, 1971). Most programs present cases extracted from actual patient records.

In practically all cases the purpose of the computer-based clinical simulation is to give the student the opportunity to experience the direct interaction with a patient. It gives them an opportunity to make diagnostic and therapeutic decisions and to see the results of these decisions. It permits the user to make decisions and take actions in a noninvasive fashion so that one has the opportunity to develop essential medical skills without jeopardizing the health of a "real" patient.

The Hospital Encounter Simulation

The University of Wisconsin has utilized a computer program for simulating the patient–physician encounter as part of its third-year medical student teaching program for the past $3\frac{1}{2}$ years. This program simulates the patient–physician encounter in a hospital setting. It has been utilized both in individual and group sessions: for teaching and self-evaluation. The program has met with widespread student acceptance, and preliminary data indicate that it has resulted in a definite increase in student factual data retention in those method areas in which it has been utilized.

The Hospital Encounter Simulation (HECS) session begins with the presentation of a brief introductory statement describing the patient. The student is then informed of the time, day of the week, and is asked to request any tests or consultations necessary to determine the diagnosis. The following will serve as an example:

> BACKGROUND INTRODUCTORY REMARKS:
>   A 20-YEAR OLD MAN WAS ADMITTED TO THE HOSPITAL BECAUSE OF FEVER. IT IS CURRENTLY 7:00 A.M. ON THURSDAY DAY 1 OF HOSPITALIZATION. THE PATIENT HAS NOW BEEN PLACED IN THE CARE OF DR. SMITH.

The physician is then free to request any tests he desires in any order he desires. All tests or consultations available at a good general hospital are included. The user may make a diagnosis at any time during the encounter. The user requests information either by typing into the computer the actual text of his request (for example, "spinal tap") or, if he is unable to type, by entering the code number designation for the test (for example, "111" for spinal tap). The physician may request tests individually or in groups, and after each test request he is informed whether the test is available, how long it will take, and how much it will cost. He may then decide either to request the test or to reject it without penalty. In the example given above, the dialogue might continue in this manner:

> REQUEST?
>   <u>HISTORY</u>
>
> HISTORY $9.00

PROCEDURE REQUIRES 0.2 HOURS   RESULTS DUE THURSDAY AT 7:12 A.M.
ORDER THIS PROCEDURE?
    YES

The physician is charged the stated amount for each test ordered and once the results of the tests are requested the time sequence ("clock") is moved ahead to the time the test would be available. If the user decides to order a number of tests at one time the system will "stack" these requests and return the results when the "clock" reaches the date and hour the test would normally be completed. Test results are only available during that period of the day those tests would normally be available in a functioning general hospital. If the user wishes to obtain a result on an emergency basis he may order the test or consultations as a STAT. All tests that can be ordered STAT are obtained in a shorter period of time, but at an additional cost. To illustrate, the sample program might resume as follows:

IT IS CURRENTLY 7:00 A.M. ON THURSDAY DAY 1 OF HOSPITALIZATION

REQUEST?
    VITAL SIGNS

VITAL SIGNS $.00
PROCEDURE REQUIRES 0.1 HOURS   RESULTS DUE THURSDAY AT
ORDER THIS PROCEDURE?   7:06 A.M.
    YES

REQUEST?
    RESULTS

IT IS CURRENTLY 7:06 A.M. ON THURSDAY DAY 1 OF HOSPITALIZATION

RESULTS OF VITAL SIGNS $.00
T-41.2 C.   R-50/MIN.   P-110.   BP 90/55

REQUEST?
    CBC

COMPLETE BLOOD COUNT $7.00
RESULTS DUE THURSDAY AT 5:00 P.M.
ORDER THIS LAB. TEST?
    NO

REQUEST?
    STAT CBC

EMERGENCY COMPLETE BLOOD COUNT $7.00
LAB. TEST REQUIRES 0.5 HOURS   RESULTS THURSDAY AT
ORDER THIS LAB. TEST?   7:36 A.M.
    YES

Any time there is a change in the patient's condition the model automatically generates "Nurse's Notes." These notes appear spontaneously when the clock passes the time when the patient's condition would be altered. A "Nurse's Note" automatically stops the movement of the clock so the physician is free to reassess his test requests in light of this new development in the patient's condition.

IT IS CURRENTLY 11:30 A.M. ON THURSDAY DAY 1 OF HOSPITALIZATION

REQUEST?
    STAT CHEST XRAY

EMERGENCY CHEST XRAY $22.00
PROCEDURE REQUIRES 0.5 HOURS   RESULTS DUE THURSDAY AT
ORDER THIS PROCEDURE?   12:00 P.M.
    YES

REQUEST?
    RESULTS

IT IS CURRENTLY 12:00 P.M. ON THURSDAY DAY 1 OF HOSPITALIZATION

NURSE'S NOTES:
T-41.1 C. TACHYPNEIC PLACED ON AMPICILLIN, CODEINE, ASPIRIN

IT IS CURRENTLY 12:00 P.M. ON THURSDAY DAY 1 OF HOSPITALIZATION

RESULTS OF EMERGENCY CHEST XRAY
PULMONARY VASCULAR CONGESTION AND A DIFFUSE INCREASE IN
DENSITY THROUGHOUT THE LUNGS WITH A SOMEWHAT NODULAR
APPEARANCE. THE RIGHT LEAF OF THE DIAPHRAGM WAS OBSCURED
BY A PLEURAL EFFUSION.

REQUEST?

The results of all tests in the system can vary daily as a result of changes in the patient's condition or because of the effects of the medication prescribed by the house staff. Once the user feels that he has enough information to make the correct diagnosis, he types the text of that diagnosis (or its code number) into the computer. If the user makes an incorrect diagnosis, he is penalized in time and money, an amount corresponding to how serious that misdiagnosis would be in this particular case. If he is correct, he is given the total cost of the workup as well as the amount of time the patient has been in the hospital. The computer–physician dialogue for the sample case might be as follows:

DO YOU WISH TO MAKE A DIAGNOSIS?
    YES
    DIAGNOSIS = ACUTE BACTERIAL ENDOCARDITIS

    CORRECT DIAGNOSIS

        THIS YOUNG MAN SUFFERED FROM ACUTE BACTERIAL ENDO-
CARDITIS. BLOOD CULTURES ON THE SECOND AND ALL SUBSEQUENT
DAYS GREW OUT STAPH. AUREUS. HE HAD SEVERE MITRAL VALVE
INVOLVEMENT WITH CONCOMITANT MITRAL INSUFFICIENCY.
        MANY OF HIS PROBLEMS WERE SECONDARY TO THE LEFT SIDED
HEART FAILURE THAT RESULTED FROM THE LESION. HE ALSO
DEVELOPED DISSEMINATED INTRAVASCULAR COAGULATION PROB-
LEMS DUE TO THE OVERWHELMING SEPTICEMIA.
        ACUTE BACTERIAL ENDOCARDITIS IS ALL TOO FREQUENTLY
SEEN IN YOUNG MEN WITH DRUG ADDICTION.

NUMBER OF DAYS IN HOSPITAL	7
COST OF DIAGNOSTIC WORKUP	$ 723.00
COST OF THE HOSPITAL ROOM ($90/DAY)	$ 630.00
TOTAL COST OF HOSPITALIZATION	$1,353.00

The student is then asked if he wishes to have his workup evaluated. If he answers affirmatively his entire workup is processed by an evaluation program.

Data for the evaluation program are generated by a committee of clinicians with recognized expertise in the area covered by the case material. This committee goes over the case and, for each of the over 400 possible tests, procedures, or consultations in the model, assigns each of them scores. These scores range from +3 (a test which is essential to do) to −3 (a test which is essential to avoid). (See Figure 1.) When a student requests an evaluation the program first goes through its file and prints all tests not ordered by the user which were essential (+3) or important to do (+2). It next prints out a list of all tests ordered by the candidate which were essential (−3) or important to avoid (−2). The program then computes an Efficiency, Proficiency, Errors of Omission, Errors of Commission, and Competency Index (see Figure 2) based on these previously assigned scores. An evaluation of the above case might be as follows:

EVALUATION FOR SCRIPT NUMBER 15

TESTS ORDERED WHICH WERE ESSENTIAL TO AVOID
    THORACOTOMY

TESTS ORDERED WHICH WERE HARMFUL TO THE PATIENT
    NONE

TESTS NOT ORDERED WHICH WERE ESSENTIAL TO DO
    BLOOD CULTURE
    PHYSICAL EXAMINATION
    URINE ANALYSIS
    BLOOD UREA NITROGEN
    ELECTROLYTES

TESTS NOT ORDERED WHICH WERE IMPORTANT TO DO
    GRAM STAIN OF SPUTUM
    FECES GUAIAC

EFFICIENCY	80
PROFICIENCY	26
ERRORS OF OMISSION	80
ERRORS OF COMMISSION	5
COMPETENCE INDEX	21

The program can be used in conjunction with a wide range of audiovisual source materials. If the script writer wishes to incorporate such material into his case he constructs it so that instead of printing the results (or the interpretation of these results) at the terminal the program informs the user which X-ray, EKG, biopsy slide, or other material he is to take from the nearby files and examine. In this way

+3   = Test or procedure which is essential to do in this case.

+2   = Test or procedure which is important to do in this case.

+1   = Test or procedure which is useful to do in this case.

 0   = Test or procedure which is optional to do in this case.

-1   = Test or procedure which is useless to do in this case.

-2   = Test or procedure which is harmful to do in this case.

-3   = Test or procedure which is essential to avoid in this case.

Figure 1. Scoring for simulated encounter.

the program can still control the cost, availability, and results of each test, and yet permit the physician to view the source material and make his own interpretation.

Cases are entered into the system via a special script-writing program. This program operates in an interactive mode so that the script writer need have no knowledge of computers or computer programming. Script writing is simplified by the fact that the model itself contains all information on test costs and test availability as well as the normal results for each test. The script writer need only enter the results for those tests that are abnormal. For each case this usually represents a subset of 20 to 50 tests of the over 400 available tests.

The system is programmed using the MIIS dialect of MUMPS. MUMPS (Massachusetts Utility Multi-Programming System) was developed at the Massachusetts General Hospital under the direction of Dr. Octo Barnett. It is an interpretive high-level time-shared computer language. Our programs operate on a time-sharing Digital Equipment Computer PDP-15 located at the University of Wisconsin. The computer can handle up to 28 users simultaneously and interaction with the computer requires no peripheral devices other than a standard computer terminal connected to the computer via telephone lines. The programs have been adapted by schools around the country for their teaching programs. The model has been reprogrammed in CPS/PL–I, FORTRAN IV and BASIC computer

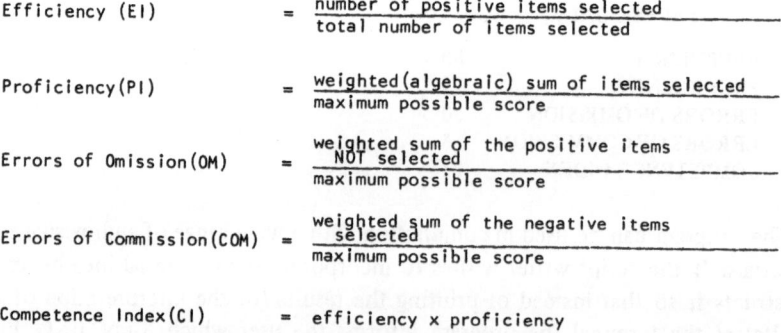

Figure 2. Clinical encounter scoring parameters.

languages. The average case encounter lasts 30–45 minutes, and requires less than 10 seconds of central processing time.

Results

During the past 4 years over 3000 individual simulated encounters have been completed by over 500 medical students, house staff officers, academic faculty, and practicing physicians at the University of Wisconsin. Overall acceptance of the clinical simulation has been excellent and it is now an integral part of the medical student and house staff training programs.

Acceptance

In an attempt to elicit those computer-related factors that enhance or decrease user acceptance of the model, a study was conducted during a one-year period in which 130 medical students were required to complete three simulated encounters as part of their third-year medicine rotation. After completing the three required cases the students were given the opportunity to do additional cases on their own during the remainder of their medicine clerkship. During the three initial cases, a number of computer-related factors were varied for subgroups of the students to determine if they impacted on the student's acceptance of the model (as reflected in the number of additional cases voluntarily attempted by those students). Since students were randomly assigned to the various medicine rotations and all students were members of the same medical school class at the University of Wisconsin it was felt the subgroups represented reasonably matched control entities. The following factors were studied.

1. Latency of Response Time

If the computer response time between the student's entry of a request and the computer's answer remained below 3 seconds, the students undertook substantially more additional cases than if response time was greater than 3 seconds. When "response" time was less than 3 seconds, no additional increase in the number of cases attempted occurred. When "response" time increased past 3 seconds, user dissatisfaction (as reflected in additional cases) increased so that by the time an average 10-second "response" time was reached almost no additional cases were attempted.

2. Speed of Printing

If the computer terminal printout occurred at 10 characters per second, the students undertook substantially fewer additional cases than if it occurred at 30 characters per second. Increasing printing speed beyond 30 characters per second had no appreciable effect on the number of additional cases completed by the students.

3. Use of Special Sign-On Codes

The use of special complex sign-on codes decreased user satisfaction. One group of students, could start the program hitting a break key and typing in two three-letter codes. The other group was required to enter a one-line JOB card which consisted of five long (up to ten letters and characters) codes, some special characters ("@"), and the requirement that placement of all codes, characters, and commas be in an exact sequence. Student satisfaction with the model was noticeably decreased by the use of more detailed entry procedures.

4. Computer Breakdown

One group of students experienced no computer failures (interruptions), while the other group experienced one, two, or three interruptions. An "interruption" was defined as a computer failure that required the student to reinitiate his connection with the computer and restart his current case (having lost all previous data on that case). We found that one interruption during the initial three cases was tolerated by the students and resulted in high user acceptance (additional optional cases). Two or more interruptions during the initial session resulted in poor user acceptance and frequently resulted in a termination of the initial session.

5. Scheduling Cases

One group of students was permitted to go to the computer terminal on an *ad hoc* basis to do the additional cases while the other group was required to sign up for a particular block of time at least one day in advance. We found the sign-up group showed greater user satisfaction than the *ad hoc* group. The *ad hoc* group, often arrived at the terminal when it was in use, became frustrated and did not return.

6. Free Text vs. Numerical Codes

One group of students was required to enter test requests as free text and the other group was required to look up the test name in a book positioned next to the computer and then enter the appropriate numerical code. We found no significant difference in student acceptance between the groups. However, when subdivided by prior typing ability, we found typists preferred the free-text option and the non-typists the code number plan.

7. Location of Computer Terminal

For one group of students the terminal was located in the hospital where the students were taking their third-year medicine rotation while the other group's terminal was located in the medical library, a 4-minute walk from the hospital (connected by a tunnel). Student acceptance was greater when the terminal was located in the hospital.

8. Orientation to the Model

One group of students had a member of our staff instruct them on the use of the model and then sit with them as they did the first case. A second group was required to complete an interactive computer-based teaching session, and the third group was given printed instructions on the use of the model. On the average, the group instructed by a member of our staff took the longest time from the start of the session until they completed the three mandatory cases and the group with the written instructions the least time. However, the staff-oriented group showed the greatest satisfaction with the model, the computer-oriented group the next highest, and the group given the written instructions the least.

9. Difficulty of Cases

One group of students was given three difficult (as judged by two faculty members) encounters as their required cases and the other group was given three easier cases. The group given the easier cases showed greater use satisfaction.

10. Program Errors

For one group of students the cases (inadvertently) contained one or more factual errors (incorrect X-ray reports or lab values) while for the other group the errors were eliminated. User satisfaction markedly decreased if even one factual error occurred.

It was also observed that while each of these mechanical factors impacted on student satisfaction with the model, they also appeared to impact on the student's performance on the initial cases. We found factors that tended to prolong the encounters unnecessarily (i.e., slower response time, slow typing speed, need to use complicated entrance codes, computer breakdowns, etc.) all caused the students to shorten their case workup in a manner that resulted in a lower competency score. The importance of these mechanical factors cannot be over-emphasized as they can severely and artificially impact on all evaluation parameters and markedly affect user satisfaction with the models. In many cases, these factors appeared to play a much more significant role in student acceptance of the model than the realism or teaching value of the model.

Evaluation

During a 3-year period from July, 1972 through July, 1975, all third-year medical students at the University of Wisconsin were required to complete at least three simulated encounters while on their 3-month Medicine rotation. At the end of their Medicine rotation they were sent a one-page questionnaire to complete and return (unsigned) indicating their reaction to the encounters. During this period, 360 questionnaires were sent out and 110 questionnaires were returned. The students were asked to rate the encounter with regard to enjoyment, ability to use the model, how useful they found the encounter, and how helpful it was for self-evaluation. In addition, they were asked to indicate how accurately performance on the model reflected their medical knowledge or their performance on the ward. Finally, they were asked if they would be interested in using the simulation model for self-evaluation, gaining experience, or testing. The results of the questionnaire (see Figure 3) clearly reflect a high degree of user enjoyment, a general consensus that the model was easy to use, and a belief that the simulated encounter sessions were useful. The results also demonstrated a general agreement that the model would be helpful for self-evaluation. There did, however, appear to be some belief

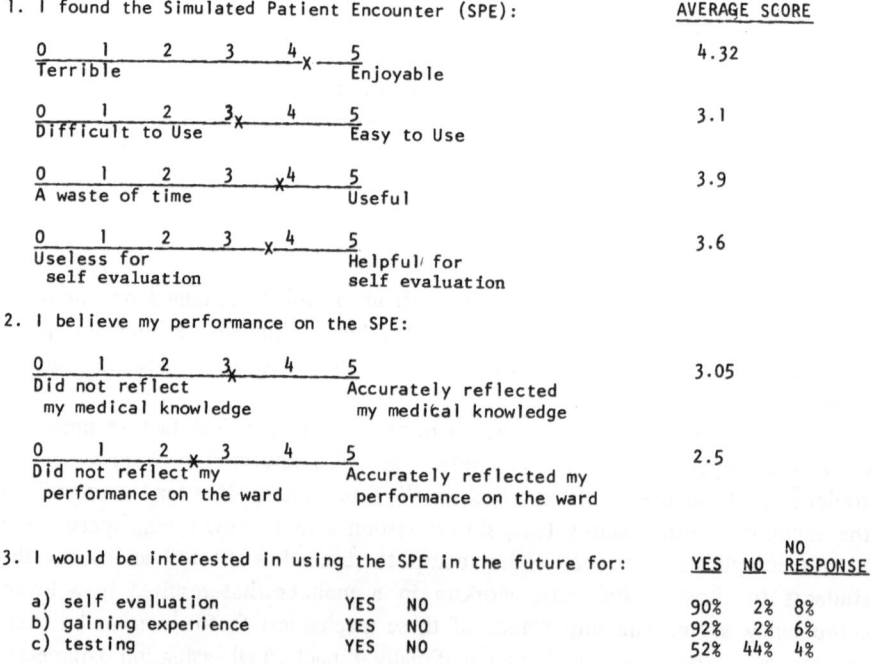

Figure 3. Student evaluation of clinical encounter simulation (110 students responding).

on the part of the students that their performances on the model did not reflect either their medical knowledge or their performances on the wards. Finally, there were substantial reservations about using the model as a testing device.

Teaching

At the University of Wisconsin the computer-based clinical simulation has been used as an integral part of the third-year medical student teaching program for the past $3\frac{1}{2}$ years. The model has been incorporated into the teaching program in the following manner.

1. To Permit Students to Gain Clinical Experience

All third-year students are told of the availability of the computer-based clinical simulation at the start of their Medicine rotation. A computer terminal is available at each of the major teaching hospitals in the program. The students are given the opportunity to complete simulated encounters on their own as a means of gaining experience in case workups and diagnosis. Between 20 and 30% of the students avail themselves of this option each quarter.

2. As Part of a Series of Structural Conferences

Each week during the 3-month Medicine rotation, a $1\frac{1}{2}$-hour topic-oriented conference is held in which one area of medicine is considered in some detail (i.e., hypertension, anemia, abdominal pain, etc.). For each session two students serve as the conference organizers, and they are responsible for planning the conference, developing handouts, and inviting a faculty expert to attend the conference. These conferences have met with high student acceptance and attendance is excellent.

Each group of students can plan the conference as they wish, utilizing lectures, audiovisual materials, paper-and-pencil case simulations, computer simulation, etc. Each quarter these student leaders elect to utilize computer simulations for about five (30%) of the conferences. The simulations are utilized in two different ways. In one format the students are each requested to complete a simulated case encounter on the week's topic prior to the conference. The case is then discussed at the conference by the faculty expert. In the second format, a terminal is brought to the conference and a case dealing with that week's topic is worked on by the group. The group orders each test after a consensus is reached and the expert serves as a consultant.

The use of the simulated encounter as part of the conference serves the following objectives:

1. The students all have the opportunity to work up a patient with the disease entity being discussed. This "peaks" their interest in that entity and permits them to conceptualize that disease in the context of an actual "patient."

2. The students gain experience in test ordering under the guidance of a faculty expert. They see how test availability and the amount of time it takes for a test result to return can affect test selection.

3. The model always responds with the cost of the test when it is ordered. Therefore, the students gain knowledge of test costs and learn to consider cost as a factor when ordering tests. They learn to balance test costs vs. room rates in considering the availability and length of time until the results are returned.

4. The students have the opportunity (through group interaction) to see that there is often more than one way to work up a case. Preliminary data have shown that students completing a simulated clinical encounter and then given factual material (lectures) on a topic have a greater recall of factual material on that subject than students presented only with the factual material.

3. As Part of a Testing Program

All third-year students are given three unknown clinical simulations as part of their final examinations in Medicine. They are given 2 hours to complete the three cases. They are informed that their performance on these cases will remain confidential, that it will not be placed in their records and will not be used to determine their grades. The student's performance on each case is recorded with respect to (a) whether the correct diagnosis was obtained; (b) the number of "simulated" days until correct diagnosis; (c) the total patient hospital bill; (d) the total "actual" time spent by the student on each case; and (e) the student's performance on each of the following parameters:

> Proficiency
> Efficiency
> Errors of omission
> Errors of commission
> Competency index

During the past 3 years, all student scores have been recorded and compared (using a T-test correlation) with the student's:

1. Grades on the Medicine rotation
2. Score on the Medicine final examination
3. Score on the Medicine part of the National Board Examination
4. Evaluation of the student's ward performance by the physician attending on the ward
5. Overall 3-year medical school class standing.

In no case could a statistically significant correlation between any of the parameters defined for the encounter be demonstrated with any of the traditional scoring modalities. In addition, no clear intercase correlation for an individual student could be made using any of the clinical-encounter parameters. The absence of a significant correlation can be interpreted in one of five ways:

1. The simulated encounter measures a competency not evaluated using the

conventional testing methods. Standard testing methods are heavily dependent on factual recall (i.e., National Board Examination, Medicine final) or the ability to get along with others, present cases, cooperate, etc. (i.e., ward attending physician's evaluation).

2. Sufficient simulated encounters were not given to each student to accurately measure their overall competency. Since inter-case reliability for individual students could not be demonstrated, it is clear that this is at least a partial factor.

3. Mechanical impediments of the system and the student's relative newness in using computers had a marked influence on their performances.

4. The parameters used to gauge student performance in the simulated encounter were deficient.

5. Clinical simulations do not measure clinical competency but rather test one's ability to do a specific type of interaction on a specific computer terminal.

Attempts to discriminate between heterogeneous groups (medical students, house staff and faculty) using the previously stated clinical-encounter parameters also did not prove significant statistically. However, significant discriminatory power was evidenced when only difficult cases were used and the scoring parameter was the student's ability to make the correct diagnosis. The ability of a very difficult case to discriminate between grossly dissimilar groups has been previously noted (Hubbard *et al.*, 1970; Farquhar *et al.*, 1973) and most likely stems from the fact that grossly dissimilar groups have different factual knowledge bases from which to do the clinical simulation. If the case is sufficiently difficult the less-experienced groups will have little or no familiarity with the disease entity, while the more highly trained group will be more familiar. Thus, if one uses very difficult cases for evaluation, one is not testing clinical competency as much as familiarity with the disease entity (factual knowledge).

Conclusion

The use of clinical simulation in medical school teaching has proven effective because of the following reasons.

1. It gives the student the opportunity to personally direct a patient workup. The student can gain experience making important diagnostic decisions about what tests are to be ordered, when they are to be ordered, and how the data gathered is to be used, without subjecting a real patient to any risk.

2. It gives the student the opportunity to witness the important effect of time on test ordering and diagnosis. Most current medical student clinical-teaching techniques are unidimensional. The student learns what tests are important, how to interpret abnormal values, and how to synthesize this information in making a diagnosis; however, he never is given the opportunity to see the important interaction of time on this process. The fact that some tests are not available at all times of the day or on weekends, that some tests take longer than others, or that some results are different for a STAT vs. a standard procedure is never emphasized. The

simulated model gives the user an opportunity to see these interactions as they occur and to face the realities of the time axis.

3. The model gives the student some experience with the costs involved in a diagnostic workup. It is becoming increasingly apparent that few physicians have any formal training in the costs of the test or therapy modalities they order. Consequently, little consideration is ever given to this monetary factor when tests are ordered. No one is taught to consider whether there are equally effective but less costly diagnostic or therapeutic modalities available. No training is given in cost-effective strategies for workup planning. The traditional teaching has always been not to consider costs, but to do whatever is necessary for the patient. While this is laudable, it has resulted in the ordering of costly tests or procedures when equally effective, but less-expensive modalities are available. Experience gained on the model makes the student more aware of the realities of the cost axis.

4. Self-evaluation gives the student an opportunity to evaluate his own ability to utilize his factual knowledge in a clinical setting. In the past this evaluation has not come until the student has completed his medical training and been placed in a "real" patient situation. He is often asked to make important clinical judgments for the first time when a patient's health is at stake. The simulated encounter gives him an opportunity to face these decisions earlier in his training and to see the effect of his own weaknesses or deficiencies. The student then has the time to take the necessary remedial actions.

References

DeDombal, F. T., Hartley, J. R., and Sleeman, D. H., 1969. A computer-assisted system for learning clinical diagnosis, *Lancet* i:145.

DeDombal, F. T., Horrocks, J. C., Staniland, J. R., and Guillou, P. J., 1971. Production of artificial 'case histories' by using a small computer, *Brit. Med. J.* 2:578.

Entwisle, G., and Entwisle, D. R., 1963. The use of a digital computer as a teaching machine, *J. Med. Educ.* 38:803.

Farquhar, B. B., Barnett, G. O., Goldfinger, S. E., and Dinnen, J. J., 1973. Computer-based examination: A technique to evaluate clinical competence, *in* J. P. Lysaught (Ed.), *Self-Instruction in Medical Education* pp. 91–94, University of Rochester, Rochester, N.Y.

Feurzeig, W., Munter, P., Swets, J. A., and Breen, M., 1964. Computer Aided Teaching in Medical Diagnosis, *J. Med. Educ.* 39:746.

Griesen, J. V., 1970. Computer assisted independent study, *in: Proceedings of the Conference on Information Systems for Health Sciences Centers*, Health Sciences Center, State University of New York, Stony-Brook.

Griesen, J. V., Beran, R. L., Folk, R. L., and Prior, J. A., 1971. A pilot program for independent study in medical education, *in* J. P. Lysaught (Ed.), *Self-Instruction in Medical Education*, pp. 3–27, University of Rochester, Rochester N.Y.

Harless, W. G., 1967. The development of a computer-assisted instruction program in a medical center environment, *J. Med. Educ.* 42:139.

Harless, W. G., Drennon, G. G., Marxer, J. J., Root, J. A., and Miller, G. E., 1971. CASE: A computer-aided simulation of the clinical encounter, *J. Med. Educ.* 46:443.

Hoffer, E. P., 1973. Experience with the use of computer simulation models in medical education, *Comput. Biol. Med.* 3:269.

Hubbard, J. P., Levit, E. J., Barnett, G. O., Goldfinger, S. E., Dinnen, J. J., Farquhar, B. B., and Schumacher, C. F., 1970. Computer-based evaluation of clinical competence, *ACP Bull.*, 502–505.

Schneiderman, H., and Muller, R., 1972. The diagnosis game: A computer-based exercise in clinical problem solving, *J.A.M.A.* 219:333.

Starkweather, J. A., 1967. Educational use of computer-assisted instruction, *in Proceedings of the 8th IBM Medical Symposium*, pp. 141–142, IBM, Pough Keepsie, N.Y.

Stolurow, L. M., 1955. Socrates, in *Proceedings of the 17th Annual Industrial Engineering Institute*, University of California, Berkeley and Los Angeles.

Stolurow, L. M., Peterson, T. I., and Cunningham, A. C. (Eds.), 1970. *Computer-Assisted Instruction in Health Professions*, Entelek, Newburyport, Mass.

Weinberg, A. D., 1973. CAI at the Ohio State University of Medicine (1973), *Comput. Biol. Med.* 3:299.

Williams, T. E., Jr., Beran, R. L., Folk, R. L., Prior, J. A., and Zollinger, R. M., 1971. The Ohio State University Pilot Medical School, *Surgery* 70(1):47.

24

Simulation and Research Models as Teaching Tools

Edward C. DeLand, R. B. Dell, and R. Ramakrishnan

Introduction

The most challenging task for an author of a computer-assisted instruction program is to capture and hold the student user's attention. A system designed for elective education — where student motivation can neither be coerced or assumed — can and should have distinct, even dramatic advantages over classical methods. Thoughtfully organized, computer-based programs can be intrinsically compelling and can bring a quality of excitement to learning that is possible no other way.

The challenge is to introduce characteristics such as flexibility and credibility but also in a literal sense to bring the process of learning into an interactive, dynamic mode where the student is involved and intellectually stimulated by the process. One attribute of a system that is of immeasurable assistance in this regard is to arrange matters so that the program appears to be smarter and more knowledgeable than the prospective student, as a real-time professor usually is. Suppose, for example, that the program can "see" the patient but the student user cannot. That is, the student can ask any question of the history and physical or chemical attributes of the patient and the program is bound to reply truthfully, as though it were an introspective patient or a clinical laboratory. This might be sufficient for the student user to become engaged in the problem of forming a diagnosis.

Now, in addition, suppose the student could institute a course of treatment, interactively following the patient over a period of days and modifying the treatment appropriately until the patient is ready for discharge. This program would now have the potential for being attractive or even compelling depending only upon its credibility and upon the system's transparency, a technical term meaning that the system itself does not divert the user's attention from the problem.

Edward C. DeLand · Division of Thoracic Surgery, Health Science Center, University of California, Los Angeles, California. *R. B. Dell* and *R. Ramakrishnan* · Columbia College of Physicians and Surgeons, Babies Hospital, New York, New York. Portions of this chapter appeared in a symposium presentation at the International Conference on Computing in Medicine, MEDCOMP '77, Berlin, 1977, AMK Berlin Company for Exhibitions, Fairs & Congresses Ltd. This work was supported by grants-in-aid from the Gilmore Foundation and the ORPIC/T. K. White Foundation, and by U.S. Public Health Service Grant No. GM-15320.

Credibility is required on two levels; the first is that the simulated patient must exhibit the characteristics of a real patient as judged by expert clinical opinion, and the second is that at any point in the therapeutic course the user should be able to ask the system for more clinical details, and these, too, should be accurate.

In this chapter we wish to describe a computer-assisted instructional system called FLUIDMOD that has been designed according to the above prescription. At the core of FLUIDMOD is an abstract but credible model of the human system to be studied. The student may be required to accomplish a variety of tasks. For example, he may be required only to understand the mechanism of the model, and for this purpose he will be presented with mathematical equations or flow diagrams or physiological principles.

In another instance he may wish only to investigate the overall function, the input/output relationships of the model, and perhaps to experiment with a new therapeutic fluid or a Fick diffusion parameter. In another session the model may be used as above in a clinical simulation of the characteristics of a human patient.

A general abstract model can at various times serve many of these purposes. A general abstract model is a model that embodies the intrinsic mechanism of the physiological system rather than the behavioral simulation of that system. Thus, a general model of a physiological system will respond to an arbitrary stress according to and limited by the basic principles and assumptions designed into the model.

Such a model is a natural teaching tool on an interactive computer and also, for limited classes of disease states, can be used to pretest and evaluate a proposed course of fluid therapy. In FLUIDMOD a mathematical model of the patient's particular acid—base biochemistry is constructed from the normal model and from available history and clinical data of a particular patient. This model is then used to simulate the responses of the patient to the student's proposed course of therapy for acid—base and fluid balance problems. Our experience has been that students find this approach to learning intellectually challenging and absorbing.

Background

The development of FLUIDMOD was begun in 1970, and the program was first reported in 1972 (DeLand *et al.*), when it was being tested for its applicability as a computer-assisted instruction tool for undergraduate medical students. At that time, a basic model for the simulation of the human biochemistry relevant to acid—base problems had been evolved. The basic model was the kernel of an interactive computer program with which the student could compute steady-state, or time-independent, responses to discrete therapeutic inputs. Subsequent development has emphasized the kinetic, or time-dependent, aspects of the model such as the kidney (Deland and Dell, 1974), validation of the abstract mathematical model (DeLand, 1975), improved methods for modeling particular physiological subsystems (Lindberg *et al.*, 1973), and extensive work in smoothing the interactive interface and improving the verisimilitude of the clinical environment.

The kernel is a mechanistic mathematical model that might be described heuristically as a set of biochemical equations subdivided into groups that represent the various rapidly exchanging fluid spaces of the human body. It is a general model in the sense that its default parameter values are set to those of a normal human adult male, but these parameter values can be reset to those appropriate for a specific application. Similar models have been used for animal and physiological laboratory research (Villamil *et al.*, 1975) where they are useful in dealing with problems of acid–base balance and fluid and electrolyte distribution in the rapidly exchanging spaces. In FLUIDMOD we have adapted a human model for interactive computer evaluation of acid–base disorders. Other computer programs have also been written for this purpose, notably those of Bleich (1969), Barnett (Memm *et al.*, 1967), and Garfinkel (Goldberg *et al.*, 1973). Generally, however, these other models do not have the generality of the kernel model of FLUIDMOD, nor do they contain a kidney model; therefore, it is difficult to achieve a detailed clinical simulation with any of these.

FLUIDMOD is being used regularly as a teaching tool for medical students where interest is primarily centered on the response of the physiological system to various electrolyte and metabolic loads. In this paper, we focus on recent developments that indicate that FLUIDMOD may also be useful as a teaching tool in the clinic, or even as a device to support physician decisions.

Our objectives have been to create a computer-based simulation having sufficient clinical verisimilitude that say, a member of the teaching staff experienced in electrolyte and fluid problems would find credible, and then to explore the parameters required to simulate real patients. The amounts, distributions, and concentrations of water and electrolytes in the body are normally closely controlled by a variety of homeostatic mechanisms, but critical disparities may frequently occur in acutely ill patients. Because of the potentially serious consequences of water and electrolyte imbalance, the attending physician must be able to quickly form a hypothesis about the nature of such an imbalance and, particularly with the very young patient, begin therapy immediately. Treatment generally consists of either withholding or giving various combinations of therapeutic fluids, along with the administration of drugs designed to affect one or more of the homeostatic subsystems. FLUIDMOD does not yet explicitly contain mechanisms to reflect the administration of drugs, although the kidney submodel necessarily is designed to function as though normotensive hormones may be present.

System Components

The components of the FLUIDMOD computer system have been previously discussed in detail (DeLand *et al.*, 1972; DeLand and Dell, 1974; DeLand, 1975). Here, the emphasis is upon how these components function together to create a unique and valid simulation of a specific patient. The system may be regarded as having three major subdivisions: the kernel biochemical model, peripheral metabolic and kidney functions, and a user interface that allows the user interactively to request data and to issue orders as though he were managing a patient. The bio-chemical model computes the electrolyte and fluid distribution over four fluid spaces of the body (plasma, red cells, interstitial space, and "intracellular compartments") at a point in time, given the total molar amounts of each species, the conservation-of-mass equations, and the chemical reactions thought to be important in each compartment. These calculations necessarily take into account osmotic equilibria, consequences of the cation pumps, electrical charge constraints, and the several buffering reactions and other reactions of proteins. The current model is similar in structure to a related model reported in DeLand (1971), where the principles for the construction of a model of blood biochemistry are described, and DeLand and Bradham (1966), where an application was made in conjunction with a dog laboratory. Figure 1 illustrates a partial result of a particular calculation

		GAS PHASE	PLASMA	RED CELLS	INTERSTITIAL	INTRACELL
X-BAR		1.00000D 06	2.07852D 01	1.05106D 01	9.54251D 01	1.96977D 02
PH		-0.0	7.40152D 00	7.30268D 00	7.42390D 00	6.83649D 00
O2	M/LH2O	1.18792D 02	1.29398D-04	2.11218D-04	1.29398D-04	1.29398D-04
CO2	M/LH2O	4.75151D 01	1.26879D-03	1.35299D-03	1.26879D-03	1.26879D-03
N2	M/LH2O	6.81372D 02	4.15558D-04	6.85139D-04	4.15558D-04	4.15558D-04
H2O	M/LH2O	5.51370D 01	5.51370D 01	5.51370D 01	5.51370D 01	5.51370D 01
H+	M/LH2O	-0.0	3.96292D-08	4.97571D-08	3.76391D-08	1.45564D-07
OH-	M/LH2O	-0.0	6.03235D-07	4.80448D-07	6.35130D-07	1.64230D-07
NA+	M/LH2O	-0.0	1.54427D-01	1.33390D-01	1.46672D-01	2.04001D-02
K+	M/LH2O	-0.0	4.80101D-03	9.78654D-03	4.55991D-03	1.61889D-01
CA++	M/LH2O	-0.0	1.48565D-03	1.65070D-03	1.34018D-03	1.01467D-03
MG++	M/LH2O	-0.0	2.21632D-04	5.79752D-04	1.99931D-04	1.31547D-02
CL-	M/LH2O	-0.0	1.12734D-01	8.97875D-02	1.18695D-01	2.98385D-03
ORGAN-	M/LH2O	-0.0	1.90948D-03	1.52082D-03	2.01045D-03	5.05403D-05
HCO3-	M/LH2O	-0.0	2.54317D-02	2.15991D-02	2.67764D-02	6.92169D-03
H2CO3	M/LH2O	-0.0	1.77557D-06	1.91243D-06	1.77557D-06	1.77557D-06
CO3=	M/LH2O	-0.0	3.64874D-05	2.46814D-05	4.04479D-05	2.70440D-06
H2PO4-	M/LH2O	-0.0	4.30188D-04	3.42625D-04	4.52934D-04	1.17028D-04
HPO4=	M/LH2O	-0.0	7.01660D-04	4.45089D-04	7.77821D-04	5.05216D-06
SO4=	M/LH2O	-0.0	3.27296D-04	2.07616D-04	3.62822D-04	1.01703D-02
NH4+	M/LH2O	-0.0	2.21530D-05	2.78145D-05	2.10405D-05	8.36970D-04
NH3	M/LH2O	-0.0	7.38002D-07	7.38002D-07	7.38002D-07	7.59106D-06
UREA	M/LH2O	-0.0	3.67687D-03	3.67687D-03	3.67687D-03	3.67687D-03
GLUCOS	M/LH2O	-0.0	5.30871D-03	5.30871D-03	5.30871D-03	5.30871D-03
PROTN	M/LH2O	-0.0	8.02878D-04	-0.0	1.31665D-04	2.28028D-03
X-MISC	M/LH2O	-0.0	1.00045D-03	3.77074D-02	2.29140D-03	2.53961D-02
HB4	M/LH2O	-0.0	-0.0	1.86920D-05	-0.0	-0.0
HB4O2	M/LH2O	-0.0	-0.0	4.38240D-05	-0.0	-0.0
HB4O4	M/LH2O	-0.0	-0.0	2.09259D-04	-0.0	-0.0
HB4O6	M/LH2O	-0.0	-0.0	9.13363D-05	-0.0	-0.0
HB4O8	M/LH2O	-0.0	-0.0	6.46376D-03	-0.0	-0.0
PHOSX-	M/LH2O	-0.0	-0.0	-0.0	-0.0	3.20003D-02
PHOSX=	M/LH2O	-0.0	-0.0	-0.0	-0.0	1.66456D-02
MCARB-	M/LH2O	-0.0	-0.0	-0.0	-0.0	1.04564D-02

Figure 1. Computed distribution of principal electrolytes for normal man (partial solution in moles per liter of H_2O).

showing the distribution of a variety of components over five conceptual compartments of the body, including the gas phase at a particular instant of time. There are considerably more data in Figure 1 than are normally considered by the physician, but this amount of detail and more (e.g., the buffering reactions) is required to create a general simulation with sufficient accuracy over the range of physiologic variables.

The essence of this model is a procedure to find a mathematical solution satisfying many simultaneous chemical reactions under the conditions presumed to exist within and among the fluid compartments. Administration of a therapeutic fluid in the model amounts to recalculation of the distribution, including the new molar amounts introduced by the fluid. Similarly, losses through the kidney, skin, or lungs or contributions from metabolism merely increment the species involved in the new distribution. An increment in any component affects the distribution of every other; for example, a change in carbon dioxide component in the gas will be reflected through the hydrogen ion to affect every species, e.g., the oxygenation of hemogloblin or the distribution of water.

FLUIDMOD is a steady-state model, and yet the most interesting aspects of biological systems occur as functions of time. In order to move this model in time, kidney and metabolic function submodels are designed to be time-dependent. The kidney and metabolic function models are essentially different from the biochemical model in another important way in that they are behavioral or phenomenological models rather than mechanistic ones. The kidney and metabolic models are designed to behave like the real organs and functions, although their structure does not reflect and will not map onto or explain the function of the components of the real system. A behavioral model is, instead, a mathematical embodiment of observational data such as the clearance curves for various electrolytes by the kidney under specified conditions. Clearance curves are available in the literature for a variety of species that depend upon the plasma levels for these same species, and in addition considerable theoretical work has been done on the kidney to elucidate the cross-coupling effects of one species upon another. The task of model building, then, is to describe the observational data in functional equation form, which may be called the transfer functions for the kidney, incorporating the cross-coupling effects as parameters in these functions. The parameters of the functions must then be adjusted to fit the observational data. We thus have both a system-identification and a parameter-identification problem in a model that is not unique in the sense that there is no reason to prefer one model over another if each produces within observational error the same result.

Figure 2 illustrates one such model of the kidney that has been described in more detail by DeLand and Dell (1974). The essence of this model is that the clearance of each chemical species from the body by the kidney is first considered as a function of the composition of the plasma, extracellular fluid volume, and glomerular filtration rate. Cross-coupling is then considered, including the necessary conservation of charge, and finally output volume is adjusted to be compatible with both the current composition of the body and the capabilities of the kidney. Meta-

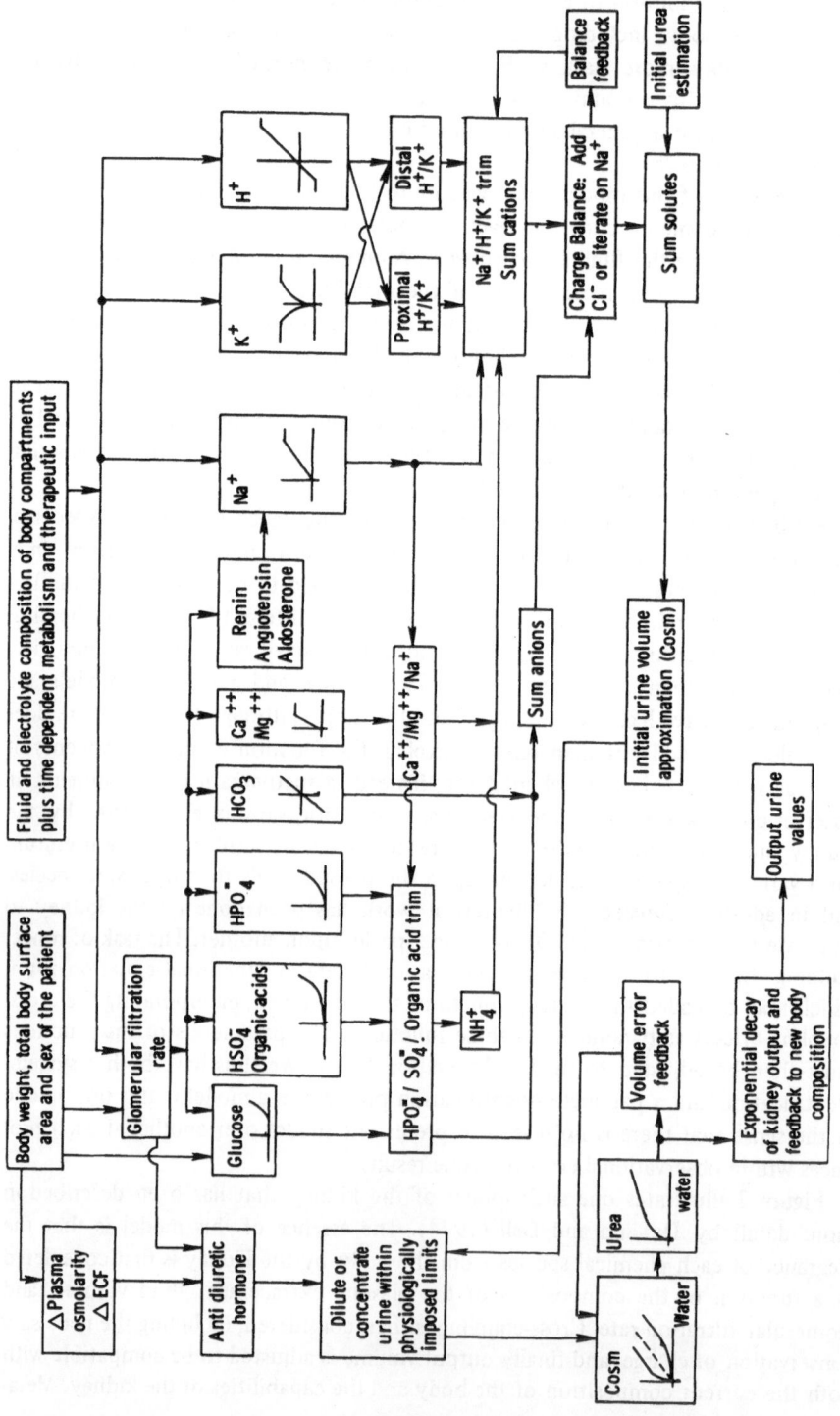

Figure 2. Generalized signal flow diagrams, behavioral kidney model.

bolic functions and skin and lung losses are similarly constructed from behavioral equations. In particular, the model contains only simplified metabolic equations following relationships discussed in Winters (1973). Primary data for the kidney were obtained from Wesson (1969).

Finally, an interface program is written around these functional models in such a way that none of the mathematical activities show at the surface; rather, the user interacts with the system in natural language — the language he would normally use for patient management in the clinic. He may issue orders from a menu which includes orders for physical workup, laboratory chemical analysis, and the common therapeutic procedures. Since the problems for which this system was designed are specifically electrolyte and fluid imbalance, therapeutic procedures are currently limited to intravenous infusion of electrolytes, allowance of oral fluids, and transfusion. It would be useful in the future to incorporate the effects of specific drugs, for example, those that affect kidney function, vascular pressure and volume, or blood composition (e.g., the fluids of hyperalimentation).

The system changes with time as a consequence of kidney amd metabolic functions and the administration of therapeutic fluids. At the end of each period of time, a new calculation is made using the kernel model for the current distribution of electrolytes and fluids. However, the user does not receive a report unless he specifically requests one. No more information is volunteered to the user than would normally be available to him in the clinic. Therefore, the model has been designed to predict kidney function over the long periods of time (say, 8 to 12 hours) thay may occur between visits by the physician. This is handled in a manner similar to variable-step-size methods for integration, that is, in this multiple-boundary-value problem step-size is sequentially reduced until error conditions are satisfied at the second boundary.

The course of a patient may be followed over several days if necessary, and the data accumulated may be reviewed at any time. The user also has the option of going back to a previous point in the treatment course to test an alternative therapeutic hypothesis.

Each patient simulation is referred to as a case, and at the present time cases are cataloged for recall by the user. A new case is constructed in two steps. First, the normal weight, height, and age of the patient are used along with normal height, weight, and body composition tables to scale the normal model compartments to the mean normal size for that patient. Second, using the medical history of the patient, estimates are made of the losses or gains of electrolytes and fluids that may be contributing to his current imbalance. These estimates may reflect considerations of the diagnosed disease state and possibly the influence of prior drugs if their effects on electrolyte balance are well known. An initial test of the model is made by computing the current distribution of fluid and electrolytes and the current function of the kidney, then comparing results with those from the patient. In practice, the data available for creating a model of the patient are far from ideal. An "exact" model of the patient would require additional data, including total body electrolytes as well as plasma electrolytes, intracellular protein content as well as plasma protein, estimates of kidney or lung pathology if any, and estimates of possible hormonal dysfunction. DeLand *et al.* (1970) illustrate the detailed procedure on a smaller model where, using available red cell data, it was shown that patient blood could be modeled with a precision limited only by the precision of the chemical analyses. In practice, a history may be very sketchy, and the only available data on the patient other than those revealed in the physical exam may be plasma electrolytes and gases. Therefore, a credible model of the patient may require two or even three iterations on the original estimates of electrolyte gains and losses.

Given a satisfactory initial model of the patient, a second test of the model may then be exercised: determining whether the dynamic responses of the model follow those of the patient under similar circumstances. This added dimension, time, characteristically is used to determine the validity of the model. Theoretically, it is possible to obtain a given distribution of electrolytes and fluids at a given point in time by an infinite variety of model structures. Presumably, though it has not yet been proved, only one of these models — or at least a much smaller set — will then proceed to simulate the dynamic behavior of the system. There are two fundamental reasons why this conjecture has not yet been demonstrated: First, observational data against which the hypothesis may be tested are contaminated with biological variation and by imprecision of chemical analyses. Second, and more importantly, any practical mathematical model that is tractable on current computing machinery is necessarily only an approximation of the much more complex biological chemistry of the real system. It can be shown that the current model that forms the kernel of FLUIDMOD is the minimum model necessary for biological credibility; the size of a larger model necessary to capture perhaps critical subtleties of the system is not yet known.

Results

An interactive session at the terminal is reproduced below. It has been edited and truncated to show only the most significant aspects pertinent to the subsequent discussion. Responses by the user are indicated by an arrow.

THIS PROGRAM USES A MATHEMATICAL MODEL TO SIMULATE FLUID AND ELECTROLYTE PHYSIOLOGY IN PATIENTS.

CHOOSE A CASE AND PROVIDE FLUID THERAPY TO BRING THE PATIENT
  BACK TO NORMAL.
YOU MAY VISIT THE PATIENT AS OFTEN AS EVERY HOUR.
(CLINICAL DATA ARE PROVIDED ONLY IF ORDERED.
YOU CAN TYPE MULTIPLE ORDERS ON THE SAME LINE.
RESPONSES MAY BE SHORTENED FOR CONVENIENCE.)

IF YOU DON'T UNDERSTAND A QUESTION, TYPE "HELP" OR "?"

CASE NUMBER?
→ 4
CASE NO. 4
CASE RECORD BEING PULLED

HISTORY ON ADMISSION

THE PATIENT IS A ONE YEAR OLD INFANT WHO PRESENTED WITH A FOUR DAY HISTORY OF PROFUSE DIARRHEA, PASSING FOUR TO EIGHT EXPLOSIVE, WATERY STOOLS PER DAY. INTAKE OF STANDARD EVA-PORATED MILK HAD DIMINISHED IN THE PRECEDING TWO DAYS. THE 24 HOURS PRIOR TO ADMISSION, THE INFANT VOMITED ALL LIQUIDS OFFERED. A STOOL CULTURE HAS BEEN OBTAINED.

PHYSICAL EXAMINATION

TIME	TEMP	PULSE	RESP	B.P.
0	37.4	154	42	73/51

GENERAL: LETHARGIC, EYES SUNKEN, ACUTELY ILL
SKIN: GRAY, MODERATELY DECREASED TURGOR
MUCUS MEMBRANES: VERY DRY
HEENT: NORMAL
CHEST: NORMAL BREATH SOUNDS, NO RALES, NO MURMURS
ABDOMEN: NO TENDERNESS, MASSES OR ORGANOMEGALY
NEUROLOGICAL: DTR'S NORMAL AND SYMMETRIC

TIME	WEIGHT	HEIGHT
0	8.4	75.0

YOU ARE AT HOUR 0
ENTER ORDERS
→ ?

PE	= PHYSICAL EXAMINATION	WT	= WEIGHT
HB	= HEMOGLOBIN AND HCT	UA	= ROUTINE URINALYSIS
ECG	= ELECTROCARDIOGRAM	LYTE	= SERUM LYTES AND BUN
AB	= ACID BASE STUDY	URI	= URINE ELECTROLYTES
IO	= INTAKE AND OUTPUT	VS	= VITAL SIGNS
IV	= I. V. FLUIDS	PO	= P. O. FLUIDS
TX	= TRANSFUSION	REV	= REVIEW THE CASE
CAN	= CANCEL AN ORDER	NUM	= NO. OF ORDERS ISSUED
STOP	= TERMINATE THIS CASE	DIS	= DISCHARGE THE PATIENT
WAIT	= LOOK AT PT IN A WHILE		

TO GET RESULTS OF YOUR ORDERS: NONE OR DONE OR O.

NEXT ORDER?
→ UA, LYTES, AB, HB
ROUTINE URINALYSIS
SERUM LYTES AND BUN

ACID BASE STUDY
HEMOGLOBIN AND HCT

NEXT ORDER?
→ IO 4
INTAKE & OUTPUT EVERY 4 HOURS

NEXT ORDER?
→ IV
ENTER THE IV'S IN THE INFUSION ONE BY ONE
→ HELP
SELECT FLUIDS BY NUMBER
NONE OR DONE OR 0 = SELECTIONS COMPLETED

1 = KCL 1 MEQ/ML	2 = NACL 1 MEQ/ML
3 = NAHCO3 1 MEQ/ML	4 = D3W
5 = D10W	6 = NORMAL SALINE
7 = NS – D2.5W	8 = NS – D5W
9 = NS – D10W	10 = $\frac{1}{2}$ NS
11 = $\frac{1}{2}$ NS – D2.5W	12 = $\frac{1}{2}$ NS – D5W
13 = $\frac{1}{4}$ NS – D5W	14 = 5 PERCENT NAHC03
15 = 1/6 M LACTATE	16 = NORMOSOL-M D5W
17 = NORMOSOL-R	18 = NORMOSOL-R D5W
19 = RINGER'S LACTATE	20 = RING LACT – D5W
21 = RINGER'S	22 = RINGER'S – D5W

NEXT IV SOLUTION?
→ 8 300
NS – D5W
    300ML
NEXT IV SOLUTION?
→ NONE
ENTER DURATION IN HOURS OR RATE IN ML/HR
→ 150 ML
AT 150 ML/HR
NEXT ORDER?
→ DONE

                    HEMATOLOGY
TIME   HGB   HCG
  0   18.3   49%
                    URINALYSIS
TIME   SP. GRAV.   PH   GLUC   ACET   PROT
  0   1.046   6.0   NEG   NEG   NEG
BLOOD DRAWN FOR ELECTROLYTES – RESULTS IN 1 HR
BLOOD DRAWN FOR ACID BASE – RESULTS IN 1 HR
ENTER ORDERS

→ 0

PATIENT UPDATE BEGINNING

SERUM CHEMISTRY

TIME	NA	K	CL	HC03	GAP	BUN
0	156	4.9	133	5.2	23	74

ACID-BASE DATA

TIME	PH	PC02	HC03	BE	P02	SAT
0	7.206	13	5.2	−21.6	100	99

YOU ARE AT HOUR 1

ENTER ORDERS

→ NONE

PATIENT UPDATE BEGINNING

THE IV SOLUTION HAS BEEN USED UP AT HOUR 2

YOU ARE AT HOUR 2

ENTER ORDERS

→ NONE

PATIENT UPDATE BEGINNING

INTAKE AND OUTPUT

TIME	WT	URINE	I.V.	P.O.
4	8.6	58	300	0

YOU ARE AT HOUR 4

ENTER ORDERS

→ WAIT

HOW MANY HOURS DO YOU WANT TO WAIT?

→ FOUR

PATIENT UPDATE BEGINNING

INTAKE AND OUTPUT

TIME	WT	URINE	I.V.	P.O.
4	8.6	58	300	0
8	8.5	64	0	0
DAY TOTAL		122	300	0

YOU ARE AT HOUR 8

ENTER ORDERS

It is evident that we can accumulate a time history of several parameters of the patient which may then be plotted, and that this could be done automatically. Each species, therefore, has a time course which can be compared with that accumulated for the patient. Here we present for illustration two cases, the first of which is drawn from the literature (to facilitate perusal by the reader) and the second from the emergency room (Case No. 092–17–35) at UCLA. Maxwell and

Keeman (1962) cite the first case on page 464. It is a simple case of pure isotonic dehydration resulting from a 4-day history of diarrhea and an intake of evaporated milk. The patient's skin had lost its turgor and its color was ashen and mottled. From the history and the physical findings, the loss of isotonic fluid was estimated at 50 to 70 ml/kg of extracellular fluid. Therapy consisted of rapid infusion of 20 ml/kg Ringer's lactate solution to restore circulation. Thereafter, the patient received 100 ml/kg of 5% glucose solution and 100 ml/kg of Ringer's lactate solution as a continuous iv infusion for the next 24 hours.

Table 1 shows the calculated result of the simulation of this case compared with the data presented in the literature. The case simulation begins by recognizing that the history and physical together imply isotonic dehydration. However, the inference must be carried one step further. The diarrhea loss combined with severe acidosis, and at the same time elevated potassium and normal chloride, indicate that the principal loss to the patient was that of sodium bicarbonate. Accordingly, the model is scaled to a 10-kg male, sodium bicarbonate is deducted isotonically at the rate of 70 ml/kg and HCl is deducted up to 5 mEq/kg. The results are as shown in Table 1.

The second case is a 25-year-old white female with a 6-day history of mid-epigastric abdominal pain, nausea, and projectile vomiting. She had dry oral mucosa, sunken eyes, decreased skin turgor, midabdominal tenderness, and absent bowel sounds. She was diagnosed as having upper bowel obstruction, but for reasons not relevant here surgery was postponed. Simulation of the case proceeded as follows: Water loss was estimated at 5–7 liters or approximately 10% of her body weight of 60 kg. From the clinical data of Table 2, she was dangerously hypotonic. She was alkalotic with normal potassium and therefore there was very little potassium loss. Accordingly, 5 liters of water were deducted containing 155 mEq/liter naCl, 34 mEq/liter KCl, and 1 mEq/liter HCl, and 190 mEq/liter Cl. Table 2 shows the results of this experiment. Therapy in both of the actual and simulated cases consisted of 5% dextrose/normal saline, 800 cm^3 over 40 minutes, followed by the same solution at 175 cm^3/hour for 8 hours, followed by the same solution plus 10 mEq of potassium/liter at the rate of 220 cm^3/hour for 24 hours. Note that in both cases potassium initially rises with the expansion in volume but then falls until potassium administration is begun at the tenth hour.

Table 1. Computed Results (C) versus Clinical Results (P) for Case No. 1 Described in Text)

Time	Na		K		Cl		HCO$_3$	
(hours)	C	P	C	P	C	P	C	P
0	139	137	5.7	6	106	106	5.0	3.2
6	139		5.3		106		7.4	
12	141		4.2		104		12.1	
24	142	140	3.9	3.5	103	103	18.0	16.2

Table 2. Computed Results (C) versus Clinical Results (P) for Case #2
Described in Text

Time	Na		K		Cl		HCO$_3$	
(hours)	C	P	C	P	C	P	C	P
0	132	129	3.2	3.4	70	63	36	39
2	131	128	3.4	4.0	69	62	35	36
6	135	130	3.2	3.1	71	74	30	30
10	139		3.4		81		28	
24	141		3.2		92		26	
34	148	143	3.6	3.2	105	103	24	29

Discussion

It is evident that reasonable simulations of the sparse data normally encountered in the clinic can be achieved using the procedures of FLUIDMOD, but because the data are sparse two important questions remain to be answered: Is the simulation unique? Are the results of the simulation credible? The answer to the first of these questions is certainly no, while the answer to the second is a qualified yes.

A strict interpretation of the word unique with regard to the mathematical model implies that any other mathematical model of the same system would necessarily carry less validity, whereas we know that many other models, particularly behavioral models of the kidney and metabolism, could be designed that would perform as well. Neither the kernel mechanistic biochemical model nor the peripheral behavioral models can approach the complexity of the real system, and there is room to evolve a more realistic, i.e., valid, model. Models of this type grow both by adding detail and by adding new system components, such as another body organ or tissue. The goal in either case is to improve the validity of the simulation results *vis-à-vis* observational data. Thus, this simulation would not work as well without, say, the metabolic equations, but its results would be closer to reality if hormone systems were incorporated.

Validity of the system is also improved by the gradual replacement of behavioral equations with mechanistic hypotheses. If the mechanisms by which the kidney performs its variety of functions were well known a model incorporating these mechanisms would, no doubt, be superior to the current behavioral model. Also, if the mechanistic hypotheses prove to be correct, then the uniqueness of the model is also improved, since no other model is correct. Thus, the validity of the model is a technical matter and can be measured by the goodness of fit to observational data.

The validity of the kernel model is a research tool has been tested many times and its shortcomings are well known (see, for example, DeLand, 1975; DeLand and Bradham, 1966). The behavioral models are not yet well investigated, since they have been tested only within this system, and the wide variety of circumstances under which they may be expected to perform have not yet been encountered. The kidney model has been tested separately (DeLand and Dell, 1974), but in this context test results continue to accumulate, some of which may indicate changes that should be made in the model. Patient simulation, such as that shown in Tables 1 and 2, is by no means exact, and continual attention must be paid to improving the model.

The credibility of this large model is not necessarily related to its validity. A user may believe a result that is invalid, and conversely. In particular, the user of this simulation is far removed from the basic data and calculations of the system and he sees only the derived data that we choose to display in response to his questions. Since he knows nothing of the internal functions of the model, his notion of credibility necessarily depends upon whether the course of the patient in response to his orders is believable — that is, whether the responses jibe with his experience and expectations. Although it might appear intuitively that each added layer of simulation — removing the user further from the basic biochemistry — would decrease the credibility of the simulation, experience has shown that just the reverse is true. A researcher using the entire patient simulator views the result quite differently from a result he might obtain using, say, the isolated blood model. In the latter case he expects detailed, basic science fidelity; in the former his expectations are not as precise and the standards he brings to bear are more relaxed, perhaps because it is more difficult to judge whether or not the result is valid. Confidence is derived from observational tests over a period of time comparing results of the simulation to corresponding results in individual patients. The user of this system is more frequently a clinician than a researcher, so that the functions of the model must only be consistent with the presumptions of expert opinion.

Because of biological variations and because the exact conditions in the clinic are not well known, exact or deterministic tests of FLUIDMOD are usually difficult to design. Neither is it possible to repeat the same tests over and over on the same patients in order to accumulate data for statistical evaluation of the model. Rather, credibility in the eyes of the user must derive from using the model in a wide variety of circumstances over a period of time. At the same time, each of these circumstances is a challenge to the model builder to test the validity of the model and perhaps to improve its function.

Finally, the utility of FLUIDMOD as a functioning tool in the clinical environment remains to be evaluated, but the protocols for this process are not yet well defined. As mentioned above, with sufficient data an acceptable model of fluid and electrolyte imbalance can always be constructed. However, more frequently, the data are either very sparse or simply inaccurate, and iterations of the model may be required to achieve an adequate simulation. Automatic procedures have been designed for creating a patient model from patient data; however, manual procedures are currently used to improve the model of an ill-defined patient. Vomitus and diarrheal fluids of standard composition have been designed, and procedures exist in the interface of FLUIDMOD for incorporating losses of those fluids or for specifying the composition of fluids that may be gained or lost in a particular case. Automatic procedures can be invoked to increment a standard fluid, while a manual procedure is still necessary to specify the design of a particular fluid. As illustrated in Tables 1 and 2, during this procedure it is not necessary to match the patient exactly; measurement errors in the observational data do not justify great precision. However, because of continuity in the system function, similar patients behave similarly, and a valid model will produce responses essentially parallel to those of the patient it simulates. Current work on this system is concerned with shifting more of the patient simulation technique to automatic procedures, and with accumulating data to improve credibility and to further quantify modeling results *vis-à-vis* the clinic.

Our experience has been that student users become engrossed in their "patient's" problem, and also that they improve their performance with practice. We believe they are practicing clinical principles, since the course of their patient's progress tends to improve and to approach a course developed by faculty members. The success of this research model-turned-teaching tool encourages us to proselytize the use of general models to teach principles and to engage the students' intellectual interest.

References

Bleich, H. L., 1969. Computer evaluation of acid–base disorders, *J. Clin. Invest.* 48:1689–1696.

DeLand, E. C., 1971. The classical structure of blood chemistry, presented at Alfred Benzon Foundation Symposium IV. Oxygen Affinity of Hemoglobin and the Red Cell Acid–Base Status, Munksgaard, Copenhagen, 1971.

Deland, E. C., 1975. Validation of very large simulations of human biochemistry, *in Proceedings of the Summer Computer Simulation Conference, San Francisco, July, 1975,* Society of Computer Simulation, 16 pp.

DeLand, E. C., and Bradham, G. B., 1966. Fluid balance and electrolyte distribution in the human body, *Ann. N.Y. Acad. Sci.* 128:795–809.

DeLand, E. C., and Dell, R. B., 1974. A behavioral model of kidney function, *in Proceedings of the Society for Computer Simulation, Burlington, Vt., October, 1974.*

DeLand, E. C., Magnier, E., and Maloney, J. V., Jr., 1970. Unique Models of Individual Blood, The Rand Corporation, RM-5396, 94 pp. (May, 1970).

DeLand, E. C., Winters, R. W., Dell, R. B., and Zuckerman, A., 1972. FLUIDMOD, a versatile CAI system for medical students, *in Proceedings of the USA–Japan Computer Conference, Tokyo, October, 1972,* American Federation of Information Processors' Society.

Goldberg, M., Green, S. B., Moss, M. L., Marbach, C. B., and Garfinkel, D., 1973. Computer-Based Instruction and Diagnosis of Acid–Base: A Systemic Approach, *J.A.M.A.* 223: 269–275.

Lindberg, D. A. B., Garten, S., Kingsland, L. C., and DeLand, E. C., 1973. Experimental Use of a Thermodynamic Model of Human Blood for Detection of Errors in Clinical Laboratory Determinations, Technical Report MOU-IS-TR-10, University of Missouri, Columbia (August, 1973).

Maxwell, M. H., and Keeman, C. R., 1962. *Clinical Disorders of Fluid and Electrolyte Metabolism,* McGraw-Hill, New York.

Memm, S. J., Barnett, G. O., Schmechel, D., Owens, W. D., and Pontoppidan, H., 1967. A Computer Program to Assist Acute Respiratory Care, Request reprints from G. O. Barnett, Laboratory Computer Sciences, Massachusetts General Hospital, Boston, Mass, 02114.

Villamil, M. F., DeLand, E. C., Heney, R. P., and Maloney, J. V., Jr., 1975. Anion effects on cation movements during correction of potassium depletion, *Am. J. Physiol.* **229**:161–166.

Wesson, L. G., 1969. *Physiology of the Human Kidney*, Grune & Stratton, New York.

Winters, R. W., 1973. *The Body Fluids in Pediatrics*, Little-Brown, Boston.

25

Evaluation of Computer-Assisted Instruction (CAI) by Analytic Appraisal

Leo L. Leveridge

Evaluation deserves special consideration in this volume because it frequently influences the selection of methods and media to use for producing educational programs and is needed for refining production and for selecting materials after they are completed.

Although rigorous evaluation of methods, media, and materials is the *sine qua non* of any educational program worthy of support, there is no universally accepted definition for educational evaluation. Abrahamson (1971) noted this situation in stating:

> Evaluation is a deceptively simple term which over the years has tended to become an Alice-Through-The-Looking-Glass kind of word meaning exactly what the speaker wants it to mean. Different authors have provided different definitions, each one suggesting that his is the 'true' definition. But one does not find serious quarrel with the major concept of (1) determining what is of value, (2) judging the attainments of these values, and (3) reflecting on the newly collected information.

Usage of "evaluation" in the literature of medical education indicates that it is best considered to be a general term that encompasses four subcategories. These can be listed and described in this chapter according to the degree of rigor of scientific method used, as follows:

1. Use tallying: enumeration of the number of times a vehicle is used
2. User polling: "happiness indices" or "subjective evaluation," as elicited by questionnaires
3. Analytic appraisal: criteria-based evaluation which "constitutes a limited prediction of the likely usefulness of teaching/learning materials, based upon judgment of the quality, rather than measurement of effects upon learners" (World Health Study Group, 1973)
4. Measurement of educational quality: based upon an attempt to quantify learning achieved by students following exposure to the materials

Leo L. Leveridge • Department of Continuing Medical Education, American Medical Association, Chicago, Illinois.

Use Tallying

Computer-assisted instruction (CAI) lends itself more easily to determinations of amount of use than any other form of education because the computer can automatically tally the number of times a program is used, and for how long, at the same time as it is put to use. The computer can be further programmed to obtain demographic data about those who elect to participate in each program, and it can determine how much of a program each participant selects. The computer can also provide statistical analyses and printouts of the data so obtained, in the course of the study and/or at its conclusion.

However, while CAI is the kind of instruction most easily and completely evaluated in terms of amount of use (and this information does have limited utility as a measure of acceptability, for preparing budgetary projections, for reporting progress of programs, and for obtaining administrative and financial support), statistics so obtained are merely indicators of popularity – and perhaps of commercial success. They cannot be used alone as a measure of true educational value.

Actually, the amount of use of a program depends also upon such factors as the effectiveness of promotion by the providers and by word of mouth among users, the attractiveness of the topic (whether or not there is a genuine need to learn the material), the location of terminals and their ready availability to participants, and the absence of conflict with other attractive activities. All such extraneous factors make enumerative findings of more apparent than real significance, and all must be taken into account in analyzing and interpreting such data.

User Polling

Like any other form of educational offering, computer-assisted instruction can be evaluated by paper-and-pencil questionnaires, or the computer itself can be programmed to pose the questions, receive, store, analyze, and report the responses. Of course, if this function is added, the computer will be tied up longer than when it is used merely for teaching and this may cause participants and/or other users to wait longer to use the computer.

When computer and terminal are fast, they certainly provide the most efficient means for the participant to receive questions and to respond to them. Moreover, it is the quickest and most efficient way for teachers to obtain data. Furthermore, use of the computer in polling can improve upon the paper-and-pencil form of questionnaire in two important ways: (1) by using the computer's facility for interacting and branching – whereby the computer poses new questions depending upon how previous questions were answered – and (2) by using the flexibility of the computer to easily improve wording whenever any questions are found to be misunderstood, or to add questions based upon experience with the initial responses or as a consequence of further thought. Nevertheless, whether or not they are presented with a computer terminal, questionnaires have innate serious limitations as tools for any kind of evaluation.

One prime drawback is that special skills are required for formulating questions that are not ambiguous or otherwise inadequate. Although this expertise can be and sometimes is acquired, it is not as prevalent among medical school faculty members as among, say, professional political pollsters, who nevertheless have had some notorious failures despite use of costly, one-to-one, in-person interviewing technics. Nor do educators have the costly resources of the political pollster to facilitate gathering the more numerous and complex data necessary for evaluating educational materials.

Ideally, questionnaires should be individualized for each item so studied, but the extra time and effort this would require is not customarily given to the preparation of questionnaire forms.

Even when questionnaires are formulated with great care by experts, responses are too often inconsistent, which probably reflects inadequate care in reading by the responder as well as careless formulation of the response. When off-the-cuff handwritten comments are invited, responses frequently are illogical or inappropriate, showing little critical judgment or understanding of the objectives of the materials, and even less thought and/or skill in communicating the responses.

Nevertheless, some useful information has been gained from well-structured questionnaires. Also, internal inconsistencies of response or seemingly invalid comments have been useful when they flagged unsuspected strengths or weaknesses in the presentation.

Analytic Appraisal

Just as observation, experience, logic, and judgment are a useful basis for both the science of biology and the practice of medicine, so can observation, critical analysis, logic, and judgment in well-structured appraisal processes serve as the basis for the design, production, selection, and utilization of educational materials.

Although little or no analytic appraisal has been applied to CAI on a large scale, there has been considerable appraisal of audiovisual materials in recent years. These appraisal activities have taken several forms. One kind, frankly termed "subjective appraisal" is conducted by the Department of Audio-Visual Communication of the British Medical Association (An International Working Party, 1973). Films are sent to "review panel organizers" who, as volunteers, are "not asked to devote (their) time to this activity on more than four or five occasions in any one year" so none has a concentrated experience with which to develop expertise.

The National Library of Medicine sponsors the Educational Materials Project (Jones *et al.*, 1976) conducted for it by the Association of American Medical Colleges, the National Medical Audiovisual Center, and, initially, the American Association of Dental Schools. This project is funded mainly for identifying available materials and judging which are good enough for entry into the AVLINE computer information service. This data base, which is accessible to all U.S. MEDLINE users since January, 1976, is limited to descriptions of "recommended" and "highly recommended" materials. Because it is required that a large volume of materials be appraised in a few years, most review panels cannot view each item in its entirety within the time allotted to their convening. (During the first 2 years there were 29 sessions to appraise over 3000 items out of a list of approximately 22,000 items that could be subjected to national review panels. An average of more than 100 items, viewed in the usual 2-day period for which the panels convened, permitted an average of less than 10 minutes per item. Obviously, in most instances only the first few minutes of each offering could be sampled and any discussion among members of the panel was necessarily very brief.)

Superficial appraisals can be misleading to the potential user and, when negative, can also be unfair to conscientious producers and distributors who have a financial stake in seeing their materials used more widely.

Analytic appraisal was first developed on a national scale in medicine by the Medical Film Institute of the Association of American Medical Colleges more than 25 years ago when it was called "Critical Cataloging" (Nichtenhauser and Ruhe, 1951). What is described and advocated here, therefore, is critical cataloging modified for computer-assisted instruction and updated through the experience of the intervening years to meet today's needs.

The Needs for and Uses of Analytic Appraisal

With the rapid advance in educational technology which has occurred in recent years there has been a steady accumulation of computerized programs for medical education. This increase deserves encouragement, but not at the expense of educational quality. Analytic appraisal is the most practical tool for improving quality because it is directed specifically at those elements of educational design which are responsible for teaching effectiveness and efficiency, because it identifies specific strengths and weaknesses and because it gives reasons for each opinion while pointing out better alternatives that could have been followed.

Appraisal is needed to identify programs that use the computer in narrow ways that do not exploit its full educational potential. Published reviews can, for instance, object to programs which merely automate a simple question-and-answer-type tutoring session and praise others which use carefully conceived simulated or real patients' records and sophisticated programs skillfully to provide training and experience in solving challenging medical diagnosis and patient management problems. Similarly, reviews based upon appraisal will serve to identify programs which use CAI exclusively when other methods and/or media would be better suited to meeting portions of the objectives.

Authors and producers of inadequate programs need, and some would welcome, the objective analytic appraisal that recommends ways to improve existing programs, or, at least, suggests how to do better next time. Beginners can avoid the mistakes of others and emulate successes after studying analytic reviews. Those teachers and programmers who have used the medium efficiently and effectively deserve the encouragement and rewards of favorable reviews based upon conscientious analytic appraisal.

Improvement of Production Quality. When a list of appraised programs is published, its dissemination helps to avoid unnecessary duplication in production and identifies gaps which need to be filled with effective new programs. Analytic criticism aids all those who are actively involved in the design and production of programs by identifying worthwhile technics to be copied and by warning against unsatisfactory approaches. It will motivate improvement in production if recognition is given dedicated teachers who have produced educational offerings of superior merit. Recognition will motivate the pursuit of excellence and help gain the support it needs.

Facilitation of Selection. The utilization of programs unworthy of the learner's time should be discouraged. Worthy materials need and deserve the help of favorable appraisal in promoting their wider use. A well done appraisal reported as a detailed review provides information which is specific enough to enable teachers to match content with the students' educational needs and to enable the potential user to make a preliminary decision of its usefulness as a whole or in part.

It has long been advocated that teachers preview all materials they plan to use in teaching or which they advocate for self-instruction. But to select CAI programs simply for preview can be a difficult, unrewarding step. Teachers often do not have easy access to the needed terminals or the time available for making their own appraisals. Mere listing in catalogues and uncritical description or superficial appraisals are of little help, and unjustifiably laudatory promotional literature is misleading. Consequently, some institutions and state organizations conduct their own appraisal programs. Of necessity, these must be superficial. Only a national or international program can command the resources for conducting the kind of detailed analytic appraisal program described here. Nevertheless, while the procedure can be simplified for local use, the same principles can and should be followed if meaningful findings are to be obtained.

Reviews based upon processes more casual than those of analytic appraisal tend to be idiosyncratic. They often praise or condemn in a sentence or two of broad, sweeping generalizations which inspire little confidence and neither serve the production team with specific criticism that can be made use of in its subsequent efforts nor help users make independent judgments regarding the utility of part or all of the productions for meeting their individual needs.

Improvement of Use. An analytic description of goals and objectives and the manner in which they have been realized assists teachers in the integration of these programs into their courses. Such analysis reduces educationally inappropriate and wasteful uses of computers and advances the effective integration of the CAI with other forms of medical teaching.

Use in Educational Measurement. Studies which purport to compare CAI with other forms of education – or even to identify the value of CAI in education –

should always include appraisal of the representative items studied in order to support whatever conclusions are reported.

The Elements of Analytic Appraisal

Identification of Goals and Objectives. Before evaluating any educational offering the appraiser must first know its goals and objectives in order to relate them to the CAI and understand why certain production decisions were made. One measurement of success of a CAI program is the degree to which the author(s) have achieved the stated objectives.

The better CAI offerings provide students with a stated goal and list of objectives to give focus to their study. But if not stated, the educational intent can be clearly and easily inferred from well-produced materials. Conversely, ill-defined objectives are usually associated with poor educational design and production.

On the other hand, the recent much-needed emphasis upon a clear definition of goals and objectives has been at the expense of attention to skillful and appropriate uses of the educational media. Goals and objectives are essential, but by themselves do not guarantee the production of worthwhile materials. It is equally important to pitch the program to the level of intended learners, to select the most appropriate medium or media, to use the full educational potential of the technology selected, to produce with care and skill, and to provide solid, authentic content and organize it well, so that it all adds up to an effective, efficient and useful production.

Identification of Learners. A solitary, clearly defined educational level, personified as one participant — the primary target of the educational offering — is essential to the proper instructional design of a program and should be explicitly identified or be readily ascertained by inference. How accurately the production is aimed at this target is one measure of its quality. Additionally, other participants for whom the material is educationally suitable should also be identified for consideration in its utilization.

Consideration of the Appropriateness of CAI for Purposes. In appraisal, both under- and overutilization of the computer should be noted. A program should skillfully exploit the special capabilities of the computer: its potential for time-saving, for sophisticated branching and interaction with participants, its rapid, detailed feedback, and the like. But the computer should not be used to carry the entire educational burden when part of the content could be more efficiently and effectively presented with another medium — especially the oft-neglected, simpler audiovisual media. For example, photographs, rather than words alone, should be used to communicate medical visual information, and motion pictures or videotapes should be used whenever motion is an integral part of the subject to be taught, or when motion would facilitate communication of static information, as when motion provides a three-dimensional effect.

Estimation of Quality. All elements of the appraisal process are focused upon educational quality (efficiency and effectiveness). In addition special attention is directed to the quality of the programming and the degree of refinement of the production. When the subject matter is complex it requires analytic treatment and careful organization to achieve clarity. Time-saving as well as time-wasting formats and devices deserve particular attention, as do ease of use of the system and the frequency of programming and keypunching errors.

Content Description. Even in less rigorous kinds of appraisal, and always with analytic appraisal, the primary concern is with the content or substance of an educational communication — its technical accuracy, appropriateness, and importance in medicine. No educational presentation can be any better than its content.

Published analytic reviews are important to potential users to obviate the necessity of obtaining the program itself and a terminal for personally previewing it. When use of CAI is being considered, more often than not the necessary equipment is not yet available because lease or purchase usually follows the decision to use the programs. Therefore, it is essential that a content description provide in sufficient detail all that the teacher or other user needs to know in order to ascertain whether a given program presents the specific information sought and how comprehensively it does so.

The suitability of the content and its complexity are considered in terms of the targeted participant and, when the program is part of a curriculum, the relevancy to the courses for which the CAI is designed is also appraised. Medical errors, omissions, incorrect terminology and the like must be identified. The content should be appropriate to the intended participant's level of competence as a result of his prior education and experience. When bias is excessive or unreasonable, this, too, must be noted. When necessary, the staff also refers to the published medical literature to check on the content.

Consideration of Treatment of Subject. Treatment of the content is considered in terms of implementation of the objectives. Is there evidence of care in preparation and in programming? Is the scope of the content appropriate to the objectives? Is the content complete or is essential material missing? Does the program contain extraneous elements? Are the emphases correct and clear? Is the material developed logically and in the ideal sequence for understanding? Is basic science integrated with its clinical applications? Is the coding–decoding required of the participant excessive? (Some systems require that participants look up code numbers to type as a response. The same or other computer systems print out code numbers which must be looked up in order to obtain the full message.) Must he do much typing, spend undue time and effort in learning to operate the equipment? All these details and those in the criteria checklist which follows are essential elements to consider in appraising the treatment.

Criteria Checklist. As discussed above, questionnaires have been shown to be unsatisfactory tools for obtaining useful opinions of the value of educational materials. The following list is suggested, therefore, not as the basis for the formulation of questionnaires, but as a means of communicating more completely and more specifically, criteria for use in appraisal of CAI by the processes described in this chapter.

Content

1. Validity
2. Scientific accuracy
   a. Medical authenticity of models used in simulation
   b. Absence of internal inconsistencies
3. In case presentations, availability of all medical information pertinent to cases, including visual information, such as roentgenograms and photographs
   a. Provision of normal laboratory values in tests wherever participant is not expected to have memorized them
4. Provision of pertinent literature references
   a. Keying of references to the item (as for self-assessment questions)

Presentation

1. Evidence of care in preparation; minimum of errors; refinement of communication
2. Clarity of directions to participants and of scenarios, when used
3. General organization
4. Simplicity of system
5. Appropriateness of sequence when the steps are in a fixed order (Provision of medical information in customary sequence for case histories)
6. Provision of a system for altering sequences in keeping with responses
7. Automatic individualization to the needs of the participant
8. Design for predominantly *active* learning through interaction
9. Exploitation of all reasonable opportunities for teaching/learning and of full teaching potential of the computer medium (This criterion is not met, for example, by CAI which offers no more than automated tutorials or similar conventional forms of teaching or testing, when patient management problems would be more effective.)
   a. Educational strategies (e.g., use of clinical correlation)
   b. Feedback to learner (at appropriate points during the program and at its end)
   c. Feedback to author and program developers for use in refining program
10. Provision of all reasonable options in patient management problems (simulations)
    a. Appropriateness of consequences to following each option
11. Capacity of program for handling data from a real patient
12. Minimal amount of encoding and decoding required of participant
13. Natural language capability
14. Minimal coaching with clues in tests (as can occur from lists of options or from wording of items)
15. Professional character, precision, economy, and quality of language
    a. Appropriateness of level of language to the intended participant
16. Appropriateness of size of steps for intended learner

17. Adequate use of branching
18. Skill in use of branching technics
19. Quality of computer-generated images
20. Supplemental use of other media when content indicates their need
    a. Appraisal of the supplemental materials using criteria appropriate to their media
    b. Effective integration of the supplemental materials with the CAI
21. Uniqueness of systems with enhanced efficiency and effectiveness or broadened utility (e.g., PLATO and TICCIT)
22. Time-saving features of system, of equipment, and of instructional design:
    a. Simplicity of logging-in procedure
    b. Provision of a touch-response panel
    c. Minimal requirements for typing by participant
    d. Provision of cathode ray tube (CRT) terminals, to save participant time, whenever the instructional design does not require use of printouts
    e. Adequate character-transmission rate
    f. Ease of operation of terminals
    g. Accessibility of terminals

Programming

1. Provision for verification of entries
2. Provision for recognition of words entered by participant, despite misspellings
3. Ease of encoding, noting especially whether there is provision for the teacher to do his own programming and, if so, the average duration of teacher training required
4. Ease of correcting, editing, and updating
5. Adequacy of debugging
6. Absence of loops
7. Provision for modifying program automatically to suit participants' educational level and/or prior experience
8. Means for recording responses and analyzing the data for the author, teacher, and others
9. Scoring
    a. Provision of immediate scores
    b. Provision of norms of scores for comparisons with peers
    d. Error analyses
10. Transplantability (availability to users in other institutions through compatibility of equipment)
11. Cost effectiveness
    a. Absence of cost-saving steps at the expense of learner time

Estimation of Effectiveness. Answers are sought to the questions: "What can be learned?" "Who can learn?" "How well can one learn?" Once thought is given to these questions some answers are perfectly obvious; other conclusions are purely educated guesses that would require rigorous educational measurement to substantiate.

Consideration of Utilization. How a CAI program may best be utilized will, in part, become obvious by the time the appraisal is completed. Note should also be made of whether or not the CAI, as offered is suitable for self-instruction, or whether it can easily be made suitable. When CAI is designed for self-assessment only, this too is noted. Whether or not the CAI can serve for group use and discussion is also stated. It is useful to further identify which programs should be used for introduction, which for review, and which can serve for the main teaching task. When appropriate, suggestions are made for integrating CAI into entire courses.

The utilization of portions of a program may be recommended as preferable to use in its entirety, and these portions are identified. Accompanying study guides (user's manuals) and other supplemental materials are examined for their intended value, for their correlation with the CAI, and for their role when the CAI is used.

The Procedure for Analytic Appraisal

Summary of Procedure

1. Obtaining information from producer or distributor
2. Previewing, preliminary analysis by staff and preparation of questions to pose to review panels
3. Identification of persons needed and recruitment of members for one or more review panels composed of authorities on and teachers of the topic, and one or more panels representative of the intended learners
4. Presentation of the program to members of review panels individually
5. Convenings of each panel for discussion of the program and to answer the prepared questions
6. Preparation of a critical review by staff, identifying each strength and weakness of the offering, the reasons for these judgments, and appropriate recommendations
7. Sending of draft review to the author(s) and others responsible for the production, inviting comments
8. Revision of review to accommodate valid comments
9. Publication of review

Information Gathering. A form is sent to the source of a program (the "host" in the case of a computer network) to obtain as much pertinent information as possible. This includes such items as series name, program title, order number, full production credits including authorship, estimated or average length of time required to participate, year produced, copyright ownership, availability, distribution arrangements and charges; goals, objectives, target learners and others for whom the program is intended and/or useful; bibliography of related scientific papers; computer language used, equipment needed, core storage, system performance, transplantability, and complete printout or transcript of the program. Other helpful documents are requested, such as promotional items, study guides, teacher manuals, supplemental materials, and reprints of cited references.

Preliminary Preparation. The form is checked for completeness of information supplied and an attempt is made to have any important gaps filled. Whenever a printout is not provided on request, one is made with a teletypewriter terminal, if feasible, or a transcript is prepared either photographically or by a typist.

The staff appraiser first interacts with the program, putting himself or herself in the place of the learner, then, after recording initial impressions, critically goes over the printout and other materials submitted, frame-by-frame and several times if necessary in order to prepare a content description and analyze the strengths and weaknesses of the presentation in terms of the criteria. While so doing, questions to be answered by the review panels are prepared, and the kinds of experts needed for answering these questions authoritatively and the kinds of students who will be representative of participants are identified as the basis for recruiting panel members.

Reviewing by Panels. Authoritative, knowledgeable, and experienced subject matter experts must be recruited. A large part of staff time goes into preparing to make intelligent use of panel members and into incorporating their comments and answers in the final published reviews.

After the program has been experienced in its entirety by each panel member, discussions of the CAI by authorities on and teachers of the subject matter are conducted in groups of preferably three to six members, led by the staff appraiser. The discussion is at first unstructured and informal. It may wander from the program, but gradually the appraiser guides it in order to focus on the CAI to elicit specific comments on the program's strengths, weaknesses, and unique qualities. Interplay of opinions is encouraged. Biased comments are identified for what they are, sometimes by adroit questioning. Answers are obtained to the prepared list of questions, ensuring that all important aspects of the analysis are covered.

Preferably the group discussion is recorded on audiotape and later transcribed, or the tape is used directly in the preparation of the review. If it seems important to know who said what, a videotape with sound is made instead of audiotape alone. The names of the reviewers are kept on file but are not published so that freedom of discussion will not be inhibited by attribution.

The above procedure is repeated with a small but representative sample of those for whom the program is intended. Here the focus is on clarity and effectiveness of presentation. An attempt is made to estimate these qualities by judging areas in which members of the group seem to have learned from the CAI, those in which the CAI seems to have failed and why. Again, answers to prepared questions are sought.

Panel reviews with additional groups are conducted when it is felt that important questions, including those raised by the panel members, remain unanswered, until the point of diminishing returns seems reached. In conducting discussions of groups in which the members differ in seniority, it is essential to encourage the junior members to speak first in order to prevent their comments from being influenced by those of their seniors.

As is apparent from the responsibilities outlined above, the staff appraiser must know the analytic procedure, be familiar with the criteria for excellence of CAI, have a working knowledge of CAI in medical education generally (preferably from having designed such programs), have some experience or knowledge of medical practice in order to be able to judge relevance of materials and to be able to communicate on a par with members of the review panels, be fair and impartial, and have leadership qualities without being domineering.

Writing of Reviews. A review is written by the staff from all the data accumulated. It is intended to help users identify appropriate and best programs and to offer guidance to producers that will help them improve the educational quality of their offerings. It contains the following:

1. Subject matter classification
2. Title; data: average duration of participation; computer language used; kinds of equipment usable, transferability; names and addresses of sources; network, if any
3. Summary statement
4. Potential users (primary target and others)
5. Content description
6. Detailed appraisal of goal, objectives, treatment of subject, use of medium, quality of content, quality of presentation
7. General appraisal of a program: A program may be judged to be exemplary for its content, for use of the computer for teaching, for displaying innovative and skillful uses of the medium, or for otherwise advancing the state of the art, or a program may be said to provide inadequate learning opportunities and be badly produced, excessively time-consuming for the amount of learning obtainable, significantly inaccurate, obsolete, or grossly biased.
8. List of supplemental materials
9. Utilization recommendations; also, existing programs which may serve the same purposes equally well or better than the program being reviewed are mentioned.

Measurement of Educational Quality

The true endpoint for any experiment in education is the learning achieved, but whenever there is a serious discussion of the matter there seems to be little agreement on how to measure learning. Techniques such as pre- and posttesting are commonly used. Occasionally attempts are made to measure changes in clinical performance. Neither approach is entirely satisfactory.

The tests that are easiest to score are the multiple-choice, true-false types. But these are, by their nature, limited to measuring the recall of isolated facts. What we really want to know is whether a student understands and can make use of the facts that were taught. Since the object of education in medicine is to enable a physician to practice medicine, it is not until the clinical phase that we can examine a student's real use of basic science learning, as well as of clinical knowledge and skills. The ability to solve patient management problems comes closer to proving the acquisition of skills, but the problem of scoring such tests acceptably has not been surmounted. Some educational research has been based on observations of changes in practice performance. These studies, however, are difficult and time-consuming to conduct and the question of whether the changes in performance have benefited the patient sometimes remains.

Both efficiency and effectiveness are major attributes of educational quality. Yet reports of research in medical education often fail to consider *efficiency*, despite the well-known high cost of medical education to the learner, to universities and to society — a cost which, in continuing medical education, is augmented by the value of time away from income-producing work while patients are deprived of physician services. However, this is not an intrinsic or unavoidable weakness of educational measurement — on the contrary it simply derives from a general lack of appreciation of the importance of efficiency in education. It could easily be remedied by keeping records of the time spent by teachers and learners, then analyzing and reporting measurements of time expended, along with the other findings. Time measurements are essential when evaluating educational technology because much of its advantage fails to show up in comparisons that do not bring out the efficiency of technological approaches. CAI is especially vulnerable in this respect because its ability to save time for teacher and student alike (through automation and rapid response systems) is one of its most valuable characteristics and, unless time is measured, the advantage of a program may not be revealed. In fact, in simpler forms of CAI which merely mimic other kinds of instruction but present it quicker, the only difference between the CAI and the other kinds of instruction is the efficiency of CAI. When time-saving is not included in comparisons between media it is no wonder that the frustrating "no significant difference" is reported.

For educational measurement, it is convenient to use the same computer that is used for teaching to do the pre- and posttesting, and also to gather, store, analyze, and report the data concurrently and/or at the conclusion of the participation. The computer can also be used for measuring the time consumed in participation, storing these data, and reporting them.

Most evaluations by means of measurement of educational quality use rigorous behavioral-research kinds of studies. Carefully selected control groups and impeccable complex statistical analyses are used; but no chain is stronger than its weakest link. Thus it is often concluded, incorrectly, that a given medium is less effective than another, or no more effective than traditional methods, when actually that medium is inappropriate for communicating the topic chosen or was used poorly.

For instance, there is a study in which a dynamic visual medium was used merely to record a lecture on a nonvisual subject. It was reported that the same learning was achieved by the group attending the classroom lecture as was achieved by the group that was exposed to the identical lecture via a motion picture with sound. The author then solemnly concluded that there is "no significant difference" between motion pictures and lectures for teaching.

Although it is not customary to include analytic appraisals of instructional instruments used in educational measurement studies, such appraisals are essential to any meaningful conclusions. From the appraisals the reader can judge whether or not the instruments used are representative of the best which that medium has to offer for education. Therefore, the reports of the appraisals should be included in the research report to substantiate the findings and to help in their interpretation.

Concluding Comments

Each kind of evaluation has its place, and, like the media, when used appropriately, each is of value. But the results of none can be accepted as gospel. It is necessary to look behind the conclusions to discover how they were reached. And it does a disservice to medical education to quote conclusions of evaluations without qualifying them. Otherwise, faulty deductions regarding the comparative value of the media are spread and, when negative, these reports become tools of those who automatically discourage anything new in teaching, including CAI.

Similarly, insistence upon evaluation is also used as a weapon against the introduction of new methods and media. Yet, the advantages of some new systems are self-evident to the open mind, and it is wasteful to have to prove the obvious. Moreover, the behavioral sciences have not reached the accuracy and reliability of the physical and pure biological sciences, partly because there are too many uncontrollable variables, so it is impractical to have all judgments in education based upon scientific studies and unfair to demand it.

For most definitive studies it would be desirable to employ all four kinds of evaluation: use tallying to measure popularity, user polling to estimate acceptability, educational measurement to determine learning achieved, and analytic appraisal to identify the elements of a production responsible for its successes and failures. Just as we use several different laboratory tests for arriving at a diagnosis, used together the several kinds of evaluation can build up a more complete picture and also serve as a partial check, one upon the other. A study should employ all four kinds of evaluation most especially when making comparisons between the various educational media and methods. Even then, at best, the results will be valid only for the conditions of the study and generalizations can be made only with clearly indicated qualifications.

Appropriately designed educational measurements can be used to help validate systems of analytic appraisal, to improve them and to contribute to their acceptance. As a guide to production and utilization, analytic appraisal provides specific information which is more helpful to producers and users than what is obtainable from the other kinds of evaluation. Analytic appraisal has been accomplished effectively for motion pictures (Nichtenhauser and Ruhe, 1951) and, with small modifications to adapt the process to a different medium, can be used equally well for CAI. The development and wider use of analytic appraisal of current CAI output will aid both producers and users in recognizing the more valuable special capabilities of CAI for medical education. Standards of production and utilization will rise as learners begin to demand better education, as understanding of the potential roles of this newer medium becomes more general, and as exemplary quality receives recognition through publication of laudatory, critical reviews based upon painstaking analytic appraisal.

References

Abrahamson, S., 1971. Aims of Evaluation, *in* J. A. L. Gilbert (Ed.), *Proceedings of Conference on Evaluation in Medical Education*, pp. 18–25, Bulletin-Commercial Printers Ltd., Publications Division, Edmonton, Canada.

An International Working Party established by the Audio Visual Communication Panel, Board of Science and Education, British Medical Association, with the Medical Committee, British Industrial and Scientific Film Association, 1973. *Film in Medical Education – Production and Use*, Council for Educational Technology and the Department of Audio Visual Communication, British Life Assurance Trust for Health Education with the British Medical Association, London, England.

Jones, N. A., Swanson, A., and Johnson, J., 1976. Educational materials reviewed for AVLINE, *J. Med. Educ.* **51**: 299.

Nichtenhauser, A., and Ruhe, D. S., 1951. The critical cataloging of medical films, *J. Med. Educ.* **26** (Part Two): 3.

World Health Study Group, 1973. The Selection of Teaching/Learning Materials in Health Sciences Education, Report (April, 1973), Geneva, Switzerland.

26

Transferability of Computer-Based Learning Materials: Guidelines and Limitations

Richard F. Walters

Introduction

Computer-assisted instruction (CAI) has only recently been accepted as a viable method for instruction in the health professions. Its acceptance is based on a number of successful programs developed at a few institutions and, for the most part, available only at those institutions or remotely though some network. Only limited experience has been accumulated thus far on the appropriate mechanisms for transfer of those learning materials to other systems.

Those few instances in which program transfer has been attempted have not been entirely trouble-free (Walters, 1974). In fact, the general process of transfer of CAI materials has to date been thorny, despite a sincere desire on the part of originator and recipient to effect a change (Denk, 1972; Anastasio *et al.*, 1972; Weeg *et al.*, 1973).

In this chapter we will discuss the problems associated with effective exchange of CAI material, not as prophets of gloom predicting that transfer cannot be achieved, but rather to provide guidelines that should aid those sincere in their desire to accomplish program exchange. Despite all the problems encountered in such exchanges, experience has shown that materials can and are being shared when people of good faith and mutual trust will commit their energies to the process. This important fact should be borne in mind when reading the rest of this chapter.

In general, three types of problems have hampered effective program transfer. The first type relates to technical considerations having to do with hardware or software differences between institutions. To individuals who have worked with computer-supported instruction, most of these problems are familiar either by direct experience or by legend. Second, the problems associated with effective documentation have proved a major stumbling block. These difficulties include documentation of the actual programs, their educational content and objectives and, in addition, systems and other computer-related documentation essential to the execution of the learning materials. Finally, a series of problems can be identified

Richard F. Walters · Medical Learning Resources, School of Medicine, University of California, Davis, California.

which, for lack of a better term, are referred to as political, relating to funding, the authorization for distribution of materials, incentives for cooperation and exchange, and uncertainties as to the degrees of freedom associated with physical transfer of a program that may well undergo subsequent modifications at the originator or recipient site. It is hard to say which of these three categories is the most troublesome; each has led to failure or near failure in otherwise well-intentioned efforts at program transfer or exchange.

Anyone genuinely desiring to share CAI should therefore study in depth the technical, documentation, and political problems described here so that he can devise procedures which minimize or eliminate as many of these pitfalls as possible. In this chapter we will consider guidelines for effective program exchange by separating in a temporal sequence those problems most likely to arise before, during, or after a program is offered for transfer. In addition, we will explore some less direct factors that might help in creating a favorable climate for the exchange of programs. These guidelines should contribute to some successful experiments in transferability over the next few years.

Conditions Necessary Prior to Consideration of Program Transfer or Storage

Political Conditions

Some of the most important problems inherent in exchange of programs arise long before the program may even be considered a candidate for that process. Of these problems, the most fundamental relate to so-called political factors, independent of the manner in which the material is implemented or documented.

Perhaps the most important first step is to establish the potential benefits for such transfer. There must be benefits for each participant in a potential program transfer. Quite evidently, unless the originating individual or institution is willing and anxious to assist in a program transfer, no such exchange will occur. Similarly, despite the eagerness of an individual to offer his programs to the world at large, if there are no takers, no effective transfer can be expected. The experience involving one-sided transfers has all too often been disappointing.

It might be appropriate to explore the types of incentives that would induce a program originator to devote his time and energy to program exportation. Effective inducements might include improvement of the product through broader review, monetary reward, fulfillment of contractual obligations associated with the creation of the material (an indirect monetary incentive), a form of barter involving exchange of complementary program materials, or professional recognition aiding academic promotion, tenure, or other professional credit. Amplification of these incentives would require more space than is available; suffice to say, however, that the academic incentive is one factor that appears to require the most careful attention in the short-term future to rectify shortcomings of the past several years.

The recipient requires a different set of incentives which might include self-education in a new process, cost benefits in accepting available materials, enhancement of his course or curriculum, application of the materials to optional or even required continuing education (implying both monetary and associated public relations benefits), or other indirect factors such as using the new material or low-cost entry exposure to justify improvements in local CAI facilities. There must also be safeguards against negative factors, such as hidden costs that threaten the credibility of the instructor, lack of success of the program attributed in part to the individual ordering the material, or perhaps even improper interpretation of the reliance on "foreign" materials in terms of questioning the instructor's personal effectiveness or creativity.

All of these political considerations can be effectively resolved, particularly if the underlying principle of mutual self-interest is respected and encouraged. In light of the real need for increased program transfer, it might be well at the outset of design of new CAI materials to address the potential merits and requirements of eventual program export, so that the road will be smoother when the program is ready for distribution.

Technical Considerations

Once the proper conditions have been developed to ensure a real motivation for both offering and receiving computerized learning materials, then the process can begin in earnest. It is advisable, prior to program exchange, to consider a number of technical considerations that may have political or other ramifications.

The hardware for which a computer exercise is developed may have some unique capabilities; these unique features may render transfer difficult, or at least uneconomical, in many situations. A system that draws on capabilities of special terminals (e.g., PILOT), peripheral devices such as tapes or plotters, or other non-standard equipment may be considerably more difficult to export than one designed to operate on standard systems. This is not to say that the special equipment is undesirable, but only to point out that program exchange is limited by the degree to which special devices or supporting features are incorporated.

There are a number of CAI languages, many of them in use in medical education around the country. Some languages are only available through one manufacturer; others are available on several systems, even different sizes of systems. The same language may be different on different machines (BASIC is a prime example), so that seemingly compatible programs may in fact prove to be incompatible, at least in part. In minicomputers especially, it is tempting to add new capabilities to operating systems, languages, or other supporting features and then to use these new features in learning packages developed for those machines. This increased strength in computing will almost invariably add to the transfer or exchange problem, usually in a subtle way, because, once implemented, the users become unaware of the existence of these features and assume that their system is similar to others available around the country.

If an institution recognizes that it is likely to serve as an originator (or a recipient) of educational programs, then it is incumbent on that institution to lay the groundwork for effective exchange by excluding use of special local features or by providing documentation and support for those locally developed elements which are felt to be essential for effective computer-based learning. Similarly, the author should also endeavor to limit his use of unconventional techniques and systems.

Documentation Considerations

There is a vast difference between preparing materials to supplement one's own course and authorizing those same materials for use by another institution. Quite naturally, most learning materials are developed for an individual instructor's use; they augment his other local resources, including his own lectures and discussions. They may even refer to auxiliary materials or discussion sessions. As such, they are not yet stand-alone resources and hence are not ready for export.

If an instructor plans to make his materials available for transfer he is faced with preparing somewhat different and more complete documentation and support than is needed for local use. It becomes essential, for example, to define the learning objectives of the materials (he may or may not have taken this step when he first prepared and tested the original package). The entry points of target audiences should be specified. There should be information for the prospective instructor, the prospective student, and the prospective technical implementer of the materials. The latter may be generated by technical staff at the originating institution, but it should accompany each package and be sufficiently explicit to document all problems anticipated in transferring the program from one system to another.

Since it often happens that the principal exportable item is the pedagogy employed by the instructor (the technical implementation can often be more cheaply rewritten than adapted [Weeg, *et al.*, 1973]), it is especially important for the instructor to take the time to document the educational strategy that he has employed, if possible giving sufficient detail so that the program can be in large measure replicated by qualified individuals at another location. The instructor who provides this additional level of support protects the recipient from many technical problems of transfer. In addition, he creates a record that allows his colleagues to relate the educational strategy to the effectiveness of the course, thereby promoting subsequent program revisions and improvements at his own and recipient institutions.

Conditions Necessary at the Time of Program Transfer

Political Guidelines

Somehow, it seems so easy to the willing requester of a program. All he has to do is write or telephone Professor A. asking for a copy of "XYZ" program that he heard about at the most recent CAI conference, so that he can use it in his course at the U. of X. Not so, unfortunately. Anyone who has attempted to embark on this route will soon learn that a few minutes or hours spent in defining the details of the transfer will help to avoid many common problems of exchange.

First, there are considerations relative to the economics of program transfer. Is the program in the public domain (i.e., now-proprietary)? What is the cost, and what does the cost cover? What are the restrictions for sale or duplication? Are there any continuing usage royalties? Is the program available for lease or preview in any form? What costs and commitments are involved in such leases?

Next, one should ask if there are any legal implications in the use of these materials. For example, if the program includes clinical consultation recommendations, is there any potential for liability in the event that a patient makes unsatisfactory progress in a case in which the program was used? Are there restricted materials imbedded in the learning package, such as a proprietary data base describing dangerous drug interactions in proposed medications?

When the groundwork for program exchange is established and all preliminary legal and associated hurdles overcome, the questions of specifics arise. What will be furnished by the originator in terms of program materials and supporting documentation, including extra copies? How much consultation, training, and other support for technical transfer are included or separately available? Many institutions, having become hardened by repeated abuse of favors to the problems of the requester, simply refuse to provide any follow-up help. The demands on originator are often not understood or appreciated by receivers, who may feel that they have invested good money in a product, only to receive inadequate assistance in implementation. These guidelines are equally important to originator and to recipient; it is essential that all parties concerned be fully aware of exactly what is to transpire when a program is to be exchanged.

The matter of payment often causes problems. It is easier to acquire equipment in many institutions than it is to acquire software ("Why can't you write it yourself?"). Sometimes the originating institution is not able to receive funds for duplication costs, and sometimes an author's legitimate requirement for royalties raises unforeseen complications.

Finally, individuals responsible for shipment, receipt, approval, and troubleshooting should be designated. If, upon receipt, the program is incomplete or incorrect, procedures should be established to provide for the correction of the real problem or definition of the misunderstanding that led to the supposed error. At the other end, responsibility for program receipt and verification should be spelled out, so that the originating institution does not receive a call months or years later attempting to resolve complications.

These guidelines point out potential sources of irritation or conflict that can be avoided, if only a few precautionary steps are taken early in the game.

Technical Guidelines

Today's technology has created a wondrous array of machine-readable forms of data storage devices. Usually, however, any given computer installation is likely to have at most a very few different types of these devices. When it comes to preparing a set of machine-readable data for export, certain systems are more versatile than others.

The worst solution, from a humanistic point of view, is the delivery of a printout of the formerly machine-readable information. This approach requires that programs and data be reentered in machine-readable form at the recipient site, with all the concomitant potential for error, some of it difficult for the novice to recognize (especially when the printer ribbon is faint). An alternate solution that is only slightly better is to provide paper tape. This mode requires teletype entry unless the receiving institution has a high-speed tape reader.

Unfortunately, many minicomputers use storage devices that are not "industry compatible." DECtapes, cassettes, and certain disk formats are by no means standardized at this time. Transmission of medium-sized files by direct, on-line communication is a distinctly viable option, but it requires compatibility of communications that is not always readily available.

Solutions to these incompatibility problems involve a little planning. At most institutions today it is possible to find some way of transferring computer files to a 9-track magnetic tape. Currently, this form of storage represents the most universally acceptable machine-readable medium for exchange (a medium density of 800 bits per inch is the most common form of data storage on minicomputers with 9-track tapes). In most medical institutions there will be at least one system on which 9-track tapes can be created. The prudent exporter will investigate this option well before the question of a specific transfer is raised, and similarly, the institution planning to receive CAI material should know whether, and under what circumstances, 9-track tapes may be read and converted to the medium most suitable to the target system. An alternate solution lies in developing a communication compatibility with a system known to include one or more machine-readable data forms likely to be used by originating institutions, such as tapes or disks. Such communications, even at medium or slow speeds, may prove to be the most economical means for obtaining programs and data files.

Software considerations are equally or perhaps even more important. A program written in a language for which there is no locally available compiler or interpreter is of limited value, requiring careful translation and verification. Even when the language is ostensibly the same, however, there are often major differences in job control language, core restrictions, overlay or linking options and, most frequently, special supporting subroutines written to handle concatenation, input/output from interactive terminals, random disk access, and other features not standardized in many higher-level languages. *Caveat emptor!*

A consideration often overlooked in program transfers is the reliance on CRT terminals (i.e., programs with direct cursor control) that cannot be easily installed on a printer device.

In summary, it is wise to agree beforehand exactly what form of machine-readable material is to be delivered and if possible to test any questionable aspects with a subset of the data before acceptance of a complete package is attempted.

Documentation Considerations

The need for preparation of adequate documentation prior to offering a program for export has been stressed before. This documentation should be available at the time of delivery of programs and data. It should be accompanied by any systems-specific routine documentation that the teaching package utilizes (something that the developer may not even be aware of). The documentation should include a description of the format in which the data exist with a listing that matches the programs and data that were shipped. It should have installation instructions based on anticipated problems of machine-to-machine conversion. It should also include description of the number and nature of files and ways in which they should be installed and linked. If possible, the documentation should include descriptions of any link or overlay structure used, the size of core and random-access storage required, and other system requirements that might affect the receiving installation.

One item frequently neglected is the procedure for validation and verification of the program as received. Careful attention should be given to this aspect of the deliverability of a working program. In cases where it is necessary to embark on translation or modification of components of the delivered package, it is particularly important to have such a validation routine available for the recipient's peace of mind, and, in the case of legal requirements, for actual documented verification that the delivered program is functioning according to specifications. This portion of the documentation should include not only the routines used for validation but also descriptions of the manner in which they are to be used and, if possible, sample output from a certified run.

Postdelivery Conditions for Transfer

When a book, a record, a film, or a baby is delivered to the recipient, the product is not subject to recall for revisions, nor is it expected that the recipient will himself suggest or even insist on revisions as a part of the acceptance procedure. When a computer-based learning module is delivered to the user, it is not only desirable, it may even be mandatory that provisions be made for the periodic revision of the product. This revision process may become necessary as the content is updated to reflect current changes in understanding of the topic and also in order to improve the educational strategies used in the system. In order for the latter process to be effective, it is necessary for the originator to obtain feedback from the receiver institutions. The need for two-way communication arises whenever it is appropriate that the package is to be revised at periodic intervals (the usual case). Each revision creates problems involving political, technical, and documentation aspects of the system. In this setting, however, the problem is more complex than during initial transfer, since now a two-way communication is required, offering opportunities for new levels of inconsistency to cause difficulties.

Political Aspects of Program Revision

Consider the following situation: An institution has acquired a learning package designed for instruction of third-year medical students, with the prior understanding that the program would be tested for use in a school of nursing. An agreement is reached whereby the recipient institution will continue to provide feedback about the use of the program. In addition, the recipients indicate that they plan to modify the program in certain segments in order to adapt those sections to the new target population (i.e., nursing students).

Consider the consequences if (a) the parent institution revises a fundamental concept in the original program to adapt it to new concepts in clinical management; (b) the recipient institution suggests changes based on its use that are not acceptable to the originating institution; (c) the originating institution wants to receive the modified version, subject to still more of its own changes, to target their own nursing school students; or (d) a new school requests copies of the revised version, possibly because the recipient's policies are more lenient with regard to costs of duplication and distribution. We do not pretend to have answers to these problems. We merely raise them to point out that an infinite series of complexities can and almost surely will arise, and, since medical practice is involved, legal components will also contribute to the confusion.

Identification of these problems is not tantamount to disavowal of the process of exchange. It does, however, suggest that a clearly worded contract of agreement must be established to cover not only the initial installation of the program but also its future life, including limitations with respect to further modifications and transferability.

Technical Considerations

It is tempting, at the successful conclusion of an initial program transfer to say, "I'm glad *that's* over." Don't believe it! If acceptance includes an agreement for continued modification and feedback to the originating institution, then the problems are nearly doubled. Some means for providing response from users at recipient sites must be devised to return information to the originator. If it is sufficient to provide listings, the problem is minimal, and requires only consistent collection procedures and regular mailing of the accumulated information. If, however, the returns are to be in machine-readable form (as may be appropriate in some cases of tracing pathways through programs or offering modifications to program logic), then it is necessary to solve in reverse the problem addressed in the previous section. Data feedback may be made considerably more difficult by the degree of translation effort required to adapt the learning package to the recipient hardware.

Almost certainly the most acceptable format for data transfer would be through on-line communications. Such links may not be feasible in many settings; where they are practical, however, they should be encouraged, especially when supported by printed verification. A system that might solve both political and technical problems of program revision and feedback for program originators would be to mail revised copies of the program on formats such as disk or cassette, subject to the requirement that the earlier version, or the accumulated feedback, be returned prior to receipt of the revisions.

Documentation Considerations

The matter of revising documentation – providing replacement sheets for individual pages or sections of appropriate documentation or listings – appears to be among the more readily accomplished elements in program maintenance. A procedure that identifies recipients of the programs and sends them listings at the same time they are distributed locally should be sufficient for programmatic changes. For changes in systems support, it may be necessary to exercise more caution, making sure that any changes that affect a given package are identified and provided to all recipients. These problems appear relatively minor, however, when compared with some of the difficulties cited above.

Similarly, the needs for feedback in documentation on a continuing basis are also relatively minor and straightforward. If an originating institution accepts responsibility for distribution of versions running on several systems, then it is important that the same care is exercised at the originating institution and recipient sites in terms of systems-support documentation. Other requirements appear for the most part to be relatively straightforward, except perhaps when recipients document major program changes that were effected, presumably with the originator's permission.

Creation of an Environment Conducive to Program Exchange

The casual reader of this chapter may be convinced by this time that under no circumstances will he embark on program exchange in the foreseeable future. If the pitfalls loom so large, then perhaps it is time to offer some encouraging words for the fainthearted. There are indeed ways in which the process can be simplified. Some of the suggestions listed below have already been implemented; others remain to be investigated, and it is to be hoped that their time will come soon.

Networks for Education

The existence of networks is essential for the promotion of transfer and exchange of computer programs. For the novice, they offer exposure to available programs so that the potential recipient can test them without having to invest in installing them on his own system. At the point of actual transfer, they offer opportunities for direct communication that may prove to be the best mode of program exchange. Networks can provide continued assistance by offering ways in which systems can be modified, providing two-way communications for revision and feedback, and they may even open the door for a reciprocal exchange if a receiver institution contributes new material of general value.

Chapter 10 of this volume deals with the potential and requirements of networks for education. One of the most important considerations of networks, however, relates to the transferability of the experience of one institution to another, whether or not that experience includes physical transfer of programs or learning packages.

Sponsored Efforts at Standardization

The mere mention of centralization tendencies, controls, standards, rules of exchange, or penalties for noncompliance smacks of excessive bureaucracy and restrictive measures. In the context of program exchange in the health sciences, however, it may very well be necessary to consider such measures seriously. The satisfaction of legal requirements may be the principal reason for program control. The need for certified program execution, update, verification, and subsequent modification may benefit from control by a central group, whether that agency is a user-dominated or government-dominated one.

In the context of standard languages, the desirability of such efforts is more obvious. The MUMPS standardization effort was a success in part because the community involved recognized a need to achieve such standard definitions.

Acceptance of some standards in operating systems support will come much more slowly, partly because the impetus will come from users, not from manufacturers, and partly because the state of the art in understanding macro elements in operating systems is not yet as far advanced as is the case for programming languages.

Standards in machine-readable media and in communications disciplines will also aid significantly in program exchange. Work is proceeding in these fields independent of medical education, and it is to be hoped that the progress will be rational and reasonably rapid.

Incentives for Exchange

Early in this chapter, reference was made to the creation of adequate incentives for faculty involvement in creation and use of effective learning materials mediated by computer. This problem is a sensitive one, since it touches on questions of academic review processes, most of them conducted in secret. However, there exists a real need to convince academicians that the sacred concept of "contact hours" is not an adequate measure of teaching effectiveness. Acceptance of the concept of a teacher as a facilitator of learning will go a long way toward solving this dilemma. Further advances will be made when it is recognized that computer-mediated instruction can itself be evaluated in terms of learning achieved, longevity, distribution to other institutions, or acceptance in certification or continuing education procedures. A great deal of work remains in the reeducation of senior faculty in this domain.

The question of royalties and credits for CAI materials is uncertain at present, but it offers some possibility for institutional or individual incentives that might provide benefits over current informal exchange.

The Role of Mediating Groups in Facilitating Program Exchange

A unique characteristic of medical education in contrast to other professional and higher education programs is the existence of groups variously referred to as medical learning resources, offices of medical education, etc. These groups are distinguished from campus wide, computer-based instructional centers in that they are oriented toward the improvement of medical education (not all branches of higher education), and they are not confined to computer-based forms of learning. Instead they contain branches concerned with other media and with educational methodology, evaluation, and other forms of support for the medical education process.

The existence of such groups often serves to promote more effective use of technology in instruction. These groups are also highly effective in promoting exchange of resources, including computer-based learning materials. Their effectiveness comes from their overall mission – the improvement of the overall learning process. As units concerned more with process than with content, they are able to devote their attention to getting programs to run, evaluating their effectiveness in terms of student acceptance and improved performance, and providing a technically competent base for communication with other institutions.

Medical education resource groups are also effective in promoting the distribution of materials. They have less personal identification with the individual programs and have a broader overview of the problems and opportunities associated with groups of programs. They are thus in a better position to evaluate the exportability of programs and to work cooperatively with the content specialist to prepare a program for export. As media specialists they can be on the lookout for new advances in technology, regardless of the discipline in which it originated. In short, they have the opportunity to serve as catalysts in the exchange process. Health sciences education is fortunate in this respect, and it is, therefore, important that health science educators provide support for the activities of these groups. The government should also provide support in promoting exchange, through support of those components difficult to negotiate by individuals or single institutions (e.g., national communication networks), by serving as the repository for certain forms of standard materials and languages, by sponsoring professional exchanges (meetings, workshops, and publications) in which progress in this field is publicized, or by other supportive means suggested elsewhere in this chapter and volume.

In summary, the opportunities for exchange of computer programs remain for the most part ahead of us, owing to the relatively small number of existing programs, and the difficulties in establishing a sound political, technical, or supportive base for exchange. This chapter has outlined some of the considerations important in such a program exchange, and it has pointed in particular to those pitfalls associated with adequate safeguards for both originator and recipient in the continuing process of program acceptance, revision, and documentation.

References

Anastasio, E. J., and Morgan, J. S., 1972. *Factors Inhibiting the Use of Computers in Instruction*, EDUCOM Interuniversity Communications Council, Inc., Princeton, N.J.

Denk, J. R., 1972. "CONDUIT – A concrete pipeline for software-starved little people, *in Proceedings, Third Conference on Computers in Undergraduate Curricula*, Atlanta, June, 1972, pp. 547–554.

Walters, R. F., 1974. Exchange of MUMPS programs: Methods and realities, *in Proceedings, 1974 MUMPS' Users' Group Meetings*, pp. 29–34, St. Louis, Mo.

Weeg, G. P., Anderson, R. E., Boynton, G. R., Denk, J., and Dunnagan, T., 1973. Panel: Disseminating computer-based curriculum materials in the social sciences, *in Proceedings, Fourth Conference on Computers in Undergraduate Curricula*, Claremont, June, 1973, pp. 443–453, National Science Foundation, Washington, D.C.

27

Programming Languages

Christopher R. Brigham

Introduction

A variety of computer languages have been used to program computer-assisted instruction (CAI) material. The languages differ in their technical and functional characteristics and in their suitability for certain applications and users. Incompatabilities have made transferring of course material from one computer to another difficult.

This chapter focuses on the software used to prepare computerized health sciences instruction. Functional and technical characteristics are reviewed, the 15 most significant programming languages which have been used for CAI are discussed, and factors influencing the suitability and compatability of languages are presented. The chapter is based upon a study performed in 1973 for the Lister Hill National Center for Biomedical Communications of the National Library of Medicine (Brigham, 1973). It is based upon a report that was prepared with the support of the Lister Hill National Center for Biomedical Communications, National Library of Medicine. The report was written at the Laboratory of Computer Science, Massachusetts General Hospital. Related studies have been performed by Karl L. Zinn (1969, 1970, 1973), Charles Frye (1968), and Edward N. Adams (1972).

Significance of Software

Studies of factors influencing the use of CAI have shown that difficulty in sharing software is a major obstacle. The need for new and more appropriate and powerful CAI languages is thought by some to be comparatively unimportant, since programming represents only a small portion of the task of preparing computer-based instructional material. Several of the recommendations made by these studies, however, relate to language capabilities and use. Lack of proven CAI effectiveness is felt by many educators not to be due to the medium being inherabtly ineffective, but rather to its capabilities not being fully utilized. The difficulty and time required to prepare computerized instruction material by conventional means has contributed to the shortage of quality teaching programs.

Christopher R. Brigham • Family Practice Center, Eastern Maine Medical Center, Bangor, Maine.

A study of factors inhibiting the use of computers in instruction performed by EDUCOM in 1972 concluded that the educational dimension, i.e., the problems related to the availability of adequate materials and the lack of CAI effectiveness, were more crucial than the technical limitations (Anastasio and Morgan, 1972). There was uncertainty about the importance of natural-language processing and artificial intelligence techniques. This was a reflection of different concepts of the ultimate role of CAI. Six of the first eight recommendations made by the participants in this study relate to the capabilities and use of programming languages:

1. Concentrate curriculum development efforts on utilization of the computer's unique capabilities, e.g., in problem-solving, simulation, and gaming.
2. Develop systems that allow more learner control of the material and the style of teaching.
3. Organize a team of industrial designers, engineers, teachers, and students to develop one or several educationally oriented computer terminals.
4. Develop a foundation of theories of learning and experimental data which would enable the computer to be maximally flexible and effective in teaching, as opposed to being a page-turning and response-recording device.
5. Establish a format for the production of software that will make CAI usable in a variety of hardware systems.
6. Develop programs in which the student questions the computer rather than the reverse (cooperative rather than competitive use of the computer in a learning situation).

These recommendations impose technical requirements which cannot be met, or can be met only with considerable difficulty, by many CAI languages. The EDUCOM participants felt that general-purpose languages are often more appropriate and useful for specific tasks, such as simulation, since many CAI languages are trivial and do not handle all the problems encountered in preparation of a program. Many of the participants felt that the proper production of CAI material should be by an author working solely on content and a technical-support team performing the programming. With this arrangement there is no need for a simple authoring language.

A study performed by Bernard Luskin (1972) of the Coast Community College District in California yielded similar results. The inability to share educational software among institutions due to language and hardware restrictions, was viewed as a considerable problem by administrators and industry and as a crucial problem by educators. The study also concluded that the limiting factors of a language would become important only when faculty were experienced in its use. Although the limitations of the language may become evident to a faculty member only after he has used it, these limitations may initially restrict authors and block their awareness of the full potential scope of the medium so that they do not effectively utilize it.

Status of Software

Types of Languages

A "programming language" has been defined by Jean Sammet to be a set of characters and rules for combining them so that it has the following characteristics: machine code knowledge by the programmer is unnecessary, good potential for conversion to other computers, instruction explosion (from one high-level instruction to many machine-language instructions), and notation which is closer to the original problem than assembly language would be (Sammet, 1969).

There are two schemes for classifying languages used to develop course material. The first, adopted by Zinn, categorizes the languages by their capability to perform certain instructional tasks (Zinn, 1970). He has specified four categories: (1) presentation of successive frames or items, (2) conversation within a limited context, (3) presentation of a curriculum file by a standard procedure, and (4) data analysis and revision of materials. These categories are more useful for discussion than for classification, since most languages are capable of performing more than one function.

An alternative method of classification is by the level and orientation of a language. The higher the level of the language the closer it is to the user's needs, and the further it is from a machine orientation. The following classification scheme will be used:

> Low-level languages
> High-level languages
>   Procedural languages
>   Procedural languages modified for CAI
>   CAI languages
> Very-high-level approaches

Low-level languages are machine-oriented. Machine language is the native language of the computer and is different for each type of machine. It consists of precoded binary bits representing hardware operations. Because of the tedious programming involved and difficulty in modifying a program, only a few CAI courses have been coded in it. Symbolic assembly language permits symbolic representation of instructions and storage locations and is therefore slightly easier to use and modify.

High-level languages allow a programmer to represent his problem in a manner more closely related to his application area. General-purpose programming languages are procedure-oriented and permit a programmer to identify the operations and sequencing necessary to perform a task. Some commonly used procedural languages have been modified to provide functions necessary for CAI, such as answer matching and student-performance recording. Within the past ten years several languages have been created specifically for computerized instruction. Some of these languages, although they were developed specifically to overcome deficiencies in preexisting languages, have resulted in only slightly different outcomes.

Very-high-level approaches (generative techniques and drivers) separate instructional content from strategy and divide the process of course production into separate tasks for the programmer and the subject area expert. These approaches involve the use of preprogrammed content-free instructional strategies and separately stored data files containing content material. Generative systems use content material to code an instructional program in a prespecified language which is later automatically translated and executed. Drivers are content-free presentation procedures which access content files to directly produce an instructional interaction.

Usage

Three hundred and sixty-two health sciences CAI programs, written in 23 programming languages, were identified in a survey performed in 1973 (Brigham and Kamp, 1974). Thirty-five programming languages were available among the health science institutions using CAI. Not all languages available for CAI have yet been used to prepare course material in the health sciences. The programming languages used for course development and the extent of their usage is shown in Table 1. Those most commonly employed were: COURSEWRITER (146 courses), TUTOR (45), FORTRAN (43), and MUMPS (22). Sixty-three percent of the programs were written in CAI authoring language, 26% in a procedural language, 8% in a low-level language, and 2% in a modified procedural language.

The majority of the courseware was prepared by only a few schools. Forty-four percent of the computerized teaching material in clinical medicine was

Table 1. Programming Languages Used for Health Sciences CAI — Extent of Usage as of 1973

Language	Number of courses written
COURSEWRITER	146
TUTOR	45
FORTRAN	43
LOW-LEVEL LANGUAGES	30
MUMPS	22
PILOT	12
BASIC	10
ATS	9
FOIL	7
PL/1	6
APL	4
FOCAL	4
LINGO	4
CAISYS-8	3
ALGOL	2
FORTWRITER	2
MIL	2
Other	

developed by a single institution, The Ohio State University College of Medicine, using the COURSEWRITER language. Seventy-four percent of the 129 clinical teaching programs were written by only three institutions, Ohio State University College of Medicine, the Massachusetts General Hospital, and the Washington/ Alaska Regional Medical Program. Although many courses have been written in TUTOR and MUMPS, these languages are being used on only a few computers. APL is available at several institutions, even though few instructional programs have been written in it.

Only four languages (COURSEWRITER, FORTRAN, APL, and BASIC) are common to more than 12 of the 94 institutions. These languages account for 203 (56%) of the instructional programs. Fifty-four percent of the languages cited were available only at a single institution; 17 programs were written in these languages.

Language Suitability

A language used to program CAI should permit convenient preparation of programs, make effective use of the computer hardware and its overlying systems software, allow full use of the computer's capabilities, and be machine-independent. Programming logics, tasks, users, and the process of course production are discussed in this section.

Programming Logic

Program logic can be classified as frame-oriented, conversational, or generated.

Frame-oriented systems are the most common application of computers for instruction and appear to be an extension of programmed instruction; depending on the extent of branching and feedback, little use of the computer's capabilities may be made. For each question or frame presented to the student, there are defined, anticipated answers; the student is expected to respond with one of these answers and the program acts to deal with these anticipated or other unanticipated answers by including the presentation of text or branching to another portion of the program. The question—answer units are referred to as "frames." The actions the system takes are predefined by the author to occur under certain conditions and consist of a finite set of alternatives; the student responds only to direct questions.

Conversational logic allows for dialogue between the student and the program such that a student can assert an answer or ask a question at any point in time. An extensive branching network is normally defined. Application of this logic becomes most practical when the field of inquiry and the format for questioning have been carefully defined.

Programming for free-text input can be difficult. Syntax and context can be considered, a wide variety of responses may be anticipated, and responses which are unanticipated should be acknowledged appropriately. Most CAI authoring languages and a few procedural languages have facilities for matching strings of characters (keywords) in the student's input. Text manipulation is generally limited to characters and words. Sophisticated natural-language analysis involving semantic processing is difficult and has been applied only to a limited degree in CAI.

Generating systems manipulate a data base to produce a student interaction. Actions are not predefined, as with frame-oriented logic, but are rather the sum result of the interaction between the student and the system. Such systems have been employed primarily in simulation of the clinical encounter.

Tasks

The instructional tasks of a language can include drill-and-practice, tutorials, self-evaluation, clinical encounter simulation, modeling, numerical problem-solving, graphic display, audiovisual presentation, and data retrieval, to name a few.

Drill-and-practice, tutorials, and self-evaluation applications, especially when multiple choice questions are used, make the least demands of a CAI system and can be programmed in nearly all languages. Most CAI programs employing frame-oriented logic are used for these tasks.

The computer is particularly well-suited for simulating the role of a patient in a physician–patient encounter. In clinical encounter simulation, the user typically assumes the role of a health care professional, e.g., a physician, dentist, or nurse. On the basis of computer-produced results of history questions, physical examination, and laboratory tests, the student diagnoses and prescribes treatment for the simulated patient. Simulations provide students with an opportunity to deal with a variety of clinical simulations in which they can independently exercise clinical judgment without the risk involved if real patients were used. The programming is usually difficult, hence it is worthwhile to prepare generalized procedures which can access data particular to a case or a clinical area. Programming language requirements are determined by the logic of the simulations. The system may be based on a branching network, where contingencies are developed (e.g., the CASE system developed by the University of Illinois Medical Center), or on a statistical or mathematical model of a disease process (e.g., the simulations developed by the Massachusetts General Hospital).

Modeling, numerical problem-solving, and some simulations require substantial numerical processing capabilities. Most of the CAI authoring languages are limited in this, hence numerically oriented procedural languages have been more commonly employed.

Data retrieval, graphic display, and peripherals under computer control and other audiovisual support are additional functions which may be required in preparing an instructional package. Most CAI systems, with the exception of PLATO–TUTOR, have limited facilities for carrying out these operations.

Users

Faculty authors, programmers, and students are three principal users of CAI languages; each requires different capabilities and conveniences.

The faculty member is concerned with the content of the program and should not be unnecessarily distracted by the computer programming. This can sometimes be accomplished by interfacing faculty members with a programmer or by providing them with some simplified procedures for preparing course material. It is desirable to minimize the manpower used in preparing a course, both on the part of the faculty author and the programmer, while maximizing the effectiveness of the course and the use of all the potentials of the technology. Faculty time is perhaps more of a limiting factor in the health sciences than in other fields because of the other responsibilities of faculty, e.g., patient care and research.

Simple authoring languages intended for use by faculty unaided by programmers have typically failed to make full use of the technology. Direct coding in procedure-oriented languages by programmers has been time-consuming. A promising alternative is the use by faculty of preprogrammed and validated instructional strategies (drivers) and generative systems which have been coded by programmers. These programs can be prepared using procedural languages and directed toward specific applications and strategies. Their design could be by a team of faculty authors, educational technologists, computer scientists, and programmers; the team approach is best exemplified by the TICCIT Project (Stetten, 1972).

The programmer requires a language which allows maximum access to the facilities of the computer system with minimum effort. The language should not be limited to one instructional strategy nor should it sacrifice operating efficiency. Strategy depends on the content, the simulated environment, and the student's task. The language should permit convenient preparation and revision of instructional programs.

Students require a system which is simple to use, responds quickly, is easily accessible, makes available information about its operation and status, provides information processing capability, and is nondistracting. They need to know whether the system is operating, and whether an answer can be accepted or if it has been. Procedures need to be available for correcting and canceling student input, entering student comments, and permitting students to request assistance. Problems imposed by the man—machine interface, which interfere with the learning situation, should be minimized.

Course Production

Course production has been separated into the processes of organizing content, preparing procedure, and filing substance (Zinn, 1970). Collaboration among subject area specialists (content writers) and computer specialists (programmers) is required to prepare good instructional modules.

Defining objectives and organizing the content of instruction in a manner appropriate for computer presentation is the task of the author and does not require a programming language, although the author must be aware of and work within its constraints. This first process is the most time-consuming and the most crucial.

The second stage, preparing the procedure, can be performed by the author, using a CAI authoring language, or by a programmer. A programmer, using a procedure-writing language capable of performing CAI, can prepare a procedure for presenting the author's content material. A less effective, but more commonly employed, method is one in which the author or an instructional programmer codes the content and the procedure together.

As regards presentation procedures, there is a third part to course production: entering the subject material into the necessary files. Convenience and execution efficiency must be considered by curriculum writers and computer experts. Procedural languages are generally well suited for developing presentation procedures.

Before computerized instructional units are ready for use by students, they must have their operation thoroughly checked, and any errors must be corrected. Testing and revision must be repeated until the program meets its objectives.

Technical Characteristics

The technical characteristics of languages used for CAI can be discussed in terms of the taxonomy developed by Zinn. The classification scheme was published as an EDUCOM document and was used for comparing a number of CAI languages in 1969 (Zinn, 1969). The scheme has been used by Steven Lower of Simon Fraser University to evaluate the COURSEWRITER language (Lower, 1973), and it serves as the basis for the specifications of a standard CAI programming language being proposed by the National Research Council of Canada. The taxonomy is divided into the following eleven topics.

Displaying Information

Display information can be prestored, either in the internal storage of the computer or in a computer-controlled external device, or generated by a predefined algorithm. Graphics, other visual display, and audio information are often necessary in health sciences instruction.

Display devices are characterized by the information they display and their ability to coordinate modes of display, define spatial position of material displayed, time display, define special characters, modify existing display, combine displays, define motion, and assemble material at time of display.

Accepting User Input

The ability to accept user input can also be discussed in terms of the information handled and the facilities provided. Input can consist of characters, graphics, or audio signals. Audio input is rarely employed because of technical difficulties. Tasks in accepting user input include defining a limit on the time or characters permitted, allowing user alteration during input, permitting communication between users, accepting special requests, measuring elapsed time of user input, and interrupting input when some processing rule has been satisfied. Advantage of the facilities offered by special input devices should be provided by the system without the user being burdened by detailed equipment-handling routines.

Processing User Input

The ability to process user input determines to a large extent the capabilities of a CAI system. It involves delimiting fields, editing strings, and processing characters, numerics, algebraics, graphics, unrecognized input, and student questions. A programmer should be able to invoke these capabilities without having to resort to complex and time-consuming programming.

Delimiting fields involves identifying or defining segments of input strings on the basis of delimiters, determining the location of a given character or substring in the input, and counting the number of times a given character or substring appears in a student input string. Editing strings can entail deleting specified characters, changing a character or string into another, providing binary flags for specified substrings or patterns in student response, transforming strings when a substring is embedded in text, encoding student input strings in phonetically reduced form, and extracting only numeric or only alphabetic characters from input. Functions for processing characters are provided most effectively in string-handled procedural languages (e.g., SNOBOL) and, to varying degrees these capabilities are present in CAI authoring languages. Numerical processing languages (e.g., FORTRAN) generally are not strong on these features.

Identifying Locations in Programs

Locations in a program are identified either by label or by condition. A label serves as an identifying point to which a branch may be made. In some languages, alphanumeric labels may be treated as variables. Identifying by condition means identifying an aspect which may be true of more than one statement, e.g., the statement type, a tag or other descriptor, the initial characters of text, or any transformation applied to the text. The identification of locations is important in establishing a restart point at which execution will begin again if a disconnection occurs before a sequence is completed, whether by accident or intention.

Sequencing Execution

Languages used for CAI must be capable of extensive and flexible branching in order to permit the programming of individualized instruction. Several types of branching have been identified by Zinn: branching to a specified location, branching to a location defined in relation to a present condition, branching to a subroutine and saving the location of the return point, returning from a subroutine to the location saved, iterating to a specified or calculated limit, branching based on the condition of a logical expression, branching on a computed value, branching on restart of execution, and predefined implicit branching. Implicit branching is especially useful in frame-oriented CAI and is typically provided by only those languages designed for CAI.

Recording and Manipulating Data

A wide range of data generated by and necessary to the operation of an instructional program must be handled by the programming language. The ability to record and manipulate data is characterized by the type of data handled and how they are processed. Capabilities may be provided for storing data on student use of the program and on student performance for later summary and evaluation, for defining data analysis, for executing computations using variables and matrices, and for processing characters, expressions, words, strings, lists, or other symbol structures. In simulation it is especially important that the language be able to manipulate numeric data. Self-modification of a program is possible if program-use data are made available to the program logic.

User Tools

It is desirable to provide the students access to a simple computational facility and to other languages which may be available within the computer system, if they are required to solve computational problems.

Coding Convenience

Zinn discusses coding convenience in terms of the facilities for: abbreviation of text and statements, automatic modification preliminary to execution and at execution time, assigning identification attributes to data items in the program, predefining data collection and summary, precoding procedures for standard logic or patterns, defining modal conventions for interpretation of code, accessing other languages or subroutines, and making comments or remarks in the program. If the language is to be used directly by nonprogrammers, i.e., faculty authors, all possible coding conveniences must be provided. However, these same conveniences should not interfere with access to sophisticated facilities of the system by the advanced programmer.

Programmer Operations and Utility Routines

Programmer operations deal not only with the language but with the environment in which the language is used. Factors to be considered include: mode of preparation of computer copy of interactive program; format characteristics of statements, programs, and data bases; translation of program and pretranslation assembly or automatic editing; diagnostic and test features; on-line consultation;

storage of program and data; programmer editing mode and features; and test features. Provisions for testing the program during and following execution can include tracing execution, interrupting on specified conditions, examining values, variables, or log of interaction, modifying values or the program itself, and resuming execution at any desired location.

Supervisor Operations

Some CAI systems provide facilities for a supervisory user, although this is not necessary. The supervisor may register users, restrict use of the system, provide on-line assistance, initiate record handling, and identify errors in operations through checking routines and test programs.

Systems Operations

Systems operations encompasses the operating system, the translator (interpreter or compiler), the processor and storage, terminals and communication lines or modems, provisions for automatic recovery from system failure, and routines for automatic retrieval of material and records of the status of the system and the students.

Compatibility, Conversion, and Standardization

Difficulty in sharing computerized instructional material is often due to software and hardware incompatibilities. Even though a teaching program dealing with a particular topic may be technically compatible, significant differences in content, opinion, and emphasis could make it inappropriate for the curriculum at another school.

Compatability

The availability of a language is dependent on the constraints imposed by the specific technical configuration of the hardware and systems software. There may be difficulty in sharing software between computers even of the same model if the configurations are different; languages may have the same name but be differing versions. High-level languages are supposedly characterized by their ability to be machine-independent. Although this is true to some degree of many procedural languages, this is not true of most instructional programming languages; machine dependence of CAI languages may be due in part to smaller user groups and the use of special hardware.

Most CAI languages are dependent to some degree on a particular machine or class of machines. This is exemplified by the COURSEWRITER III language which is supported only on IBM System 360 and 370 computers. Machine dependence can also occur when there is use of hardware features specific to a machine, e.g., the TUTOR language requires PLATO hardware and plasma display panel terminals. Typically the more elaborate languages require sophisticated hardware and are therefore not available for use on simpler machines.

The development of language dialects introduces additional compatability problems. Modifications are the result of individual attempts to improve on a language or to adapt it to a specific application. The modification may lead to extension of the language rather than to a change in it. COURSEWRITER is perhaps the most modified CAI language; it has been modified by Ohio State University, Simon Fraser University and other institutions, and has been adapted for specific applications, e.g., data retrieval.

Subsets imply an incomplete implementation of a language. Upward compatibility is usually permitted but downward compatibility is not, i.e., a program written in the subset will run on a system supporting the full language, but a program utilizing the features of the full language will not typically run on the subset implementation. Languages available on large machines, e.g., the COURSEWRITER and PILOT languages, have been subsetted for minicomputers.

Extent of compatibility determines the ease by which users of the "same" language can share software. Languages tend to change when implemented on different machines. If the change is major, conversion necessary to run a program on the different machine will be time-consuming. The utility of an automatic translator is determined by the number of different "dialects" in use, the extent of their differences, and by the time required to construct the translator.

Conversion between Languages

A more difficult conversion problem is translating from one language to another. This task is simplest when the languages are similar and support identical logic. If the languages are different, but support the same type of logic and have similar capabilities, it is possible to recode programs from one language to the other. The automatic conversion on a statement-by-statement basis of a less powerful language to a more powerful one is not efficient and the conversion of a more powerful one to a less powerful is not feasible. Hence, translation (automatic or otherwise) between languages is most useful for languages which are similar and at the same level.

The more closely two languages are related, the greater are the similarities and the easier is the task of converting instructional programs between them. Many of the CAI author languages were motivated by deficiencies in COURSEWRITER. It is generally possible to convert from COURSEWRITER to PILOT, TUTOR, or PLANIT. However, because of the additions made to these languages, it may be difficult to go back from them to COURSEWRITER. FORTRAN IV provides a common link to many of the procedural and modified procedural languages; conversion among these languages is usually feasible. Manual conversion from a CAI language to a procedural language which supports text processing is frequently possible, but may require additional programming if the program is coded directly in the language; an alternative is to construct an interpreter in the procedural language for the CAI language programs. If a program written in one language requires features that are not present in another language, then it is not possible to rewrite that program in the other language, i.e., numerically based programs written in a procedural language cannot be rewritten in COURSEWRITER because of its limitations in arithmetic capability and storage of variables.

Interlanguage conversion is often facilitated by higher-level approaches to courseware development and their separation of content material from strategy code. Once a strategy procedure has been implemented in another language, content material utilizing that strategy is made accessible to that system. Data files may be translated to meet minor specification differences or entered manually into the computer system by clerical staff.

Standardization

The purpose of standardizing programming languages is to improve transferability of programs. Languages for CAI can be standardized individually or a universal CAI language could be developed.

Standardization has been inhibited by conceptual, technical, procedural, and political problems (Sammet, 1969). There are two major conceptual problems: timing for early impact on programming activity and risk of stifling technical progress. The optimal time for standardization is once all objectives of the language have been well-defined operationally, but before much effort has been wasted in preparing incompatible languages or variations. A language that is standardized too soon or is not open-ended will limit the potential of the applications using it. Technical problems evolve around how the language should be defined and at what level. If a complex version is defined, few groups will be capable of implementing the standard. If the standards are designed for the smallest machine, the value of the standard is lowered. A solution is to include provision for controlled subsetting and modularity of features. Most standards of a language are adaptations or reworkings of existing practices, *de facto* standards. There may be standardization by industry (e.g., the FORTRAN language), by government (e.g., COBOL), by international organization (e.g., ALGOL), or by user groups (e.g., MUMPS and PILOT).

It is clear that individual languages should be standardized, but it is not as evident that a universal CAI programming language should be developed at this time. The advantage of transportability has prompted the National Research Council of Canada to develop specifications for a Canadian national standard. IBM of Canada has been contracted to prepare detailed specifications for the language. It will be implemented initially on the National Research Council's PDP-10. Recognized subsets of the language will be defined and use of the language will be voluntary. There are several factors to be considered prior to deciding on a standard; there are also alternatives.

A single language does not presently exist which fulfills the requirements for all purposes and procedures of computerized instruction. Imposing the use of a standard would be difficult. Users of existing languages would be slow in converting to it and at some institutions where a general-purpose programming language was used both for CAI and other tasks it could be difficult to implement or justify a language used strictly for CAI. Although allocation of federal funds could be contingent on the use of the standard, funds would continue to be available from other sources.

Zinn recommends a more viable approach; a few computer languages, justified by different requirements, should be recognized as standards for CAI development (Zinn, 1970). These languages would be individually standardized, and among languages of similar purpose there would be provisions for automatic and manual translation. The use of presentation procedures and other very-high-level approaches, such as program-code-generating systems, based on sophisticated procedural programming languages, would tend to reduce the need for specific CAI authoring languages.

Language Descriptions

The 15 most significant programming languages used for health sciences computerized instruction are presented in this section. Technical and functional characteristics are discussed.

Low-Level Languages

Low-level languages are of limited use in CAI development because of the tedious programming involved. The languages are machine-dependent and usually developed by the hardware manufacturer. Although 30 courses have used low-level languages, very little, if any, course development presently involves their direct use. Most of the courses that were developed were in pharmacology and involved the use of drivers written in assembly language by the University of Kansas Medical Center.

Machine and symbolic assembly languages are not restricted in their information-processing capabilities, since they have direct access to hardware facilities, but are severely limited by the difficulty in coding; their use should be restricted to tasks which cannot be performed effectively by higher-level languages.

Procedural Languages

Procedure-oriented languages are machine-independent languages which describe the process by which a problem is to be solved. Several procedural languages which were developed for other applications have been found useful for preparing CAI material. The languages can be used for directly coding course material or for preparing presentation procedures. The following procedural languages will be discussed: FORTRAN, BASIC, FOCAL, PL/1, APL, and MUMPS.

FORTRAN

FORTRAN, BASIC, and FOCAL are procedural languages designed for scientific numerical problem-solving. FORTRAN (**FOR**mula **TRAN**slator) was the first widely-used compiler language designed for solving numerical problems. It was originally designed by IBM for the IBM 740 computer and is presently available on most computers. There are two standards of the language: FORTRAN II and FORTRAN IV (USA Standards Institute, 1966).

The availability of FORTRAN has contributed substantially to its use for CAI. A recent survey showed that FORTRAN has been used to prepare 43 health sciences courses and is in use for instruction at 26 health sciences institutions. Many of the FORTRAN programs were developed by the Washington/Alaska Regional Medical Program.

FORTRAN has extensive numerical processing capabilities, but is awkward in handling text. There are format difficulties in displaying information and accepting input. Locations can be identified in the program by assigning statement numbers and elaborate branching is possible; subroutines can be defined; however, the language lacks block structure. Programming directly in the language is difficult, as all actions must be explicitly defined and the coding is bulky. With time-sharing versions of FORTRAN, programs are prepared on-line and extensive diagnostics and editing features typically are provided.

FORTRAN is suitable for instructional applications requiring numerical processing and logical capabilities, but is poorly suited for text processing. It is useful mainly for preparing presentation procedures.

BASIC

BASIC (**B**eginner's **A**ll-purpose **S**ymbolic **I**nstruction **C**ode) was designed on a GE 225 by Dartmouth College in 1965 as a simple language for on-line numerical problem-solving (Kemeny, 1967). BASIC is supported by many computers and is frequently used on minicomputer systems. Many versions of the language exist and there are significant compatibility problems. On large systems BASIC is usually a compiler language, while on small systems it is most often an interpreter. As of 1973 ten health sciences courses had been written in BASIC and it had been used for computerized instruction at 13 medical institutions.

The language is similar to FORTRAN and the general remarks made concerning FORTRAN apply also to BASIC. Extensions of BASIC, e.g., BASIC–PLUS developed by the Digital Equipment Corporation, add text-processing capabilities to the language. An example of a multiple choice question frame coded in BASIC is shown in Figure 1.

FOCAL

FOCAL (**FO**rmula **CAL**culator) was initially designed by the Digital Equipment Corporation as an interpretive language for the PDP-8 computer. The language is

EXAMPLE OF BASIC CODE

```
 100 print   'THE PRIMARY PACEMAKER OF THE HEART IS A PIECE OF SPECIALIZED'
 200 print   'MYOCARDIAL TISSUE CALLED THE -'
 300 print   'A.  ATRIAL-VENTRICULAR NODE'
 400 print   'B.  SINO-ATRIAL NODE'
 400 print   'C.  NONE OF THE ABOVE'
 600 input   x$
 700 if x$ = 'a' then 1200
 800 if x$ = 'b' then 1600
 900 if x$ = 'c' then 1400
1000 print 'PLEASE TYPE ONLY a, b, OR c'
1100 goto 600
1200 print 'NO, THE AV NODE IS NOT THE PRIMARY PACEMAKER'
1300 goto 1700
1400 print 'NO, IT IS ONE OF THE TWO - TRY AGAIN'
1500 goto 600
1600 print 'CORRECT'
1700
```

EXAMPLE OF STUDENT INTERACTION

```
THE PRIMARY PACEMAKER OF THE HEART IS A PIECE OF SPECIALIZED
MYOCARDIAL TISSUE CALLED THE-
A.  ATRIAL-VENTRICULAR NODE
B.  SINO-ATRIAL NODE
C.  NONE OF THE ABOVE
? c
NO, IT IS ONE OF THE TWO -TRY AGAIN
? b
CORRECT
```

Figure 1. Example of BASIC code.

somewhat supported by DEC and more so by some enthusiastic users of DEC equipment. FOCAL has been implemented on PDP-8, PDP-11, PDP-12, and PDP-15 minicomputers; more than a dozen versions of the language have been produced. The language has been extended by the George Washington University Medical Center where teaching programs have been developed.

Although FOCAL resembles BASIC and FORTRAN somewhat, the coding is more streamlined and the language is easily modified.

PL/1

PL/1 (Programming Language/One) was designed by IBM to be a successor to FORTRAN and to have an extremely wide application area, encompassing both numerical scientific computing and business data processing (Bates and Douglas, 1967). The language has been implemented in a time-sharing mode on IBM System 360 and 370 computers. PL/1 has been used to construct clinical encounter simulations and is being used for instructional purposes at a few health sciences institutions.

The language is powerful, complex, and can process text well. Mathematical capabilities, coding convenience, authoring capabilities, and functional characteristics are similar to FORTRAN. The language does have block structure which is useful in organizing the flow of conversational programs. Unfortunately, as with FORTRAN, procedures coded directly in PL/1 must be explicitly defined. PL/1 is suitable for coding course material when the services of a programmer are available and is very useful for developing very-high-level programs.

APL

APL (A Programming Language) is an interpretive language characterized by exceptional power and flexibility (Iverson, 1962). It was developed by K. Iverson of IBM and has been implemented on IBM System 360 and 370 computers.

Although not designed for CAI, it has been found useful for this task. Four health sciences teaching programs have been coded in it and it has been used by eleven medical institutions. APL can be used either directly or as defined functions that constitute the elements of an authoring language. This second approach has been taken by the Cornell University Medical College to develop ATS (A Tutorial System). An interesting discussion of the potential of APL for building a CAI system is provided by Lower (Lower, 1973).

The APL language is based upon 80+ primitive numerical operators. The language handles numerics well, but is unable to handle character string data and implicit branching in a straightforward and efficient manner. Since the notation of the language can be complex, it is desirable to define a series of APL functions with arguments for author use.

The interpretive nature of the language can cause it to be slow when extensive computations are involved. Despite these disadvantages, the power of APL offers considerable potential for the construction of a CAI system.

MUMPS

In 1967 the Laboratory of Computer Science of the Massachusetts General Hospital (LCS-MGH) began the development of MUMPS, the MGH Utility Multi-Programming System. MUMPS is a procedural interpretive language capable of manipulating large amounts of text data efficiently in a time-sharing environment (Sheretz 1972). It was designed specifically for medical information processing, but has been used in other areas; it has been implemented on several Digital Equipment minicomputers (PDP-9, PDP-15, and PDP-11) using a variety of different sizes of core and disk systems. A language standard was prepared in April, 1974 with support of the National Bureau of Standards and the National Center for Health Sciences Research and Development.

LCS-MGH has prepared several teaching programs in clinical subjects which have been made available to other medical schools through the Lister Hill National Center Biomedical Communications Network. Most of these programs are simulations of clinical encounters and are not directly coded in the MUMPS language, but rather employ general-purpose macros or driver programs written in MUMPS which use data bases containing the subject material (Hoffer, 1973).

The MUMPS language is characterized by its string-processing features, its unique disk file structure, and by being interpretive. Handling string data in a symbolic fashion, MUMPS can do simple syntax checking by means of a pattern-matching operator, determining if a string contains a predetermined sequence of numerics, alphabetics, and/or punctuation. Strings can also be disassembled, modified, and concatenated. Boolean and limited arithmetic capabilities are provided. Fixed-point numbers have a limited range and only two decimal places of accuracy; floating-point numbers can also be used. The language is flexible in displaying and accepting information. Random-access files are stored in a common, dynamic tree-structure form. The nodes in the tree are referenced symbolically using N-dimensional subscripting and space is allocated only as needed.

A major advantage of an interpretive language is that the user's program is never compiled into machine code but kept only in symbolic form; program debugging is simplified and program storage is compact. However, relatively slow execution may be a disadvantage. With a typical MUMPS system, however, disk-accessing time is the limiting factor, rather than execution time. Since the source language is concise, the amount of core required for a program is smaller than for a compiled program. It is therefore possible to have time-sharing on a relatively modest-sized computer by partitioning core, rather than by repeated swapping of programs from disk to core. Restrictions imposed by the small partition size are handled by overlaying program segments. Coding directly in the language requires a programmer; adequate editing and extensive test features are provided. A subject material expert can develop a program directly without learning to program if an appropriate driver is provided.

MUMPS has been shown to be useful for applications involving string manipulation and for preparing presentation procedures; however, it is handicapped by relatively slow numerical processing capabilities, lack of an implicit restart capability, and storage limitations imposed by the partitioning of core.

Modified Procedural Languages

Modified procedure-oriented languages represent an attempt to make conventional procedural languages more useful for preparing instructional material. Routines for answer-matching, test-outputting, and record-handling are typically added to simplify the programmer's task. MIL (an extension of FORTRAN) and MENTOR (an extension of LISP) are examples of this approach.

MIL

MIL (Minnesota Instructional Language) was developed by the Programmed Learning Center of the University of Minnesota and has been implemented on the MERITSS (CDC 6400) time-sharing system. The language has been used by the school to prepare courses in hematology and ophthalmology.

The language was designed to provide a "shorthand" for CAI programs, to make efficient use of the time-sharing system it is running on, and to allow full use of the computer's potential. It permits segmenting courses into small units which can be accessed individually. This permits lengthy CAI courses to be subdivided and thus keeps the amount of computer memory devoted to the course at a minimum. Convenient operations for the formatting and output of text and for the processing and analysis of student responses are featured. FORTRAN statements can be inserted within the program at any point.

MENTOR

In 1963 Bolt Beranek and Newman, Inc. developed the MENTOR language, an extension of LISP, on a Digital Equipment Corporation PDP-1. In subsequent work, use was made of the Xerox SDS-940. MENTOR has served as the basis for an early simulation of a clinical encounter (Feurzeig, 1964).

The MENTOR language was designed for programming complex case studies in the form of Socratic tutorial dialogues. The basic constructs of the language are statements of the form: If the student makes the following input, then if the following conditions (describing some state of the student's previous actions) are satisfied, take the following actions (actions can include typing a message, recording a condition, and changing the context of the discourse).

The MENTOR system was well-suited for the tasks for which it was designed; however, it has not been used at health science institutions because interactive LISP is not commonly available.

CAI Languages

Several languages have been developed specifically for the task of computerized instruction and include capabilities for building and administering instructional strategies. COURSEWRITER, PILOT, PLANIT, TUTOR, ATS, FOIL, and CAISYS-8 are presented.

COURSEWRITER

COURSEWRITER, a proprietary product of IBM (COURSEWRITER III Applications Description Manual, 1971), was available first in 1964 and is the most widely used programming system for preparing instructional materials. Its ancestor is TIP (Teacher Interpretive Program), developed to facilitate the preparation of computerized programmed instruction. The system has gone through three major stages: COURSEWRITER I for the IBM 1400 in 1964, COURSEWRITER II for the IBM 1500 in 1966, and, most recently, COURSEWRITER III in 1969 for the IBM System 360 and 370. Despite its evolution, the language encourages a frame-oriented approach to CAI. Effective use of the system requires adding user-written function routines. A functional evaluation of COURSEWRITER, prepared by Lower (1973), serves as the framework for this discussion.

Forty percent of the computerized instructional programs in the health sciences have been written in COURSEWRITER. The language is used by more institutions for health sciences CAI than is any other language. The Ohio State University College of Medicine has authored over 75 courses in the health sciences using COURSEWRITER.

The COURSEWRITER III system operates in a multiprocessing and teleprocessing environment under control of the IBM System 360 or 370 operating system. The minimum core partition required is 70–100K. The system consists of four elements: the language, used in presenting the course material, administering the course, and recording student responses and progress; the processor, which consists of control, author, student, monitor, and supervisor routines; and input/output control program, which maintains the current status of the telecommunications lines; and the student response processor, which prints and extracts specified student records.

COURSEWRITER III statement consist of simple two-character operation codes, followed in most cases by up to 100 characters of text. These operation codes are divided into problem, major, and minor hierarchies. Instructional frames are defined by the problem codes, which may specify a question (qu) or a problem (pr), await a student response, or call a macro. Major codes specify anticipated answers (ca, wa, aa) and the text for anticipated and unanticipated (ua) answers. Minor codes designate several functions, including typing a message (ty), doing simple arithmetic, and branching (br). Minor operation codes are executed whenever they follow a problem code or a major operation code that has been executed. Successive minor codes are executed up to next major or problem code. Thus a type (ty) statement which is a minor code will be executed following a match of a major-code-anticipated answer. An example of a COURSEWRITER frame and its use by a student is shown in Figure 2. Operation code modifiers more than double the 31 available operation codes. Statement numbering is automatic and labels may be inserted at any point. In COURSEWRITER III a sophisticated macro facility is provided.

Although COURSEWRITER offers many features useful for preparing CAI, the language has several deficiencies. It lacks the facility to handle decimal and floating point variables and does not have block structure. The language is oriented to frame-by-frame processing, although this may not be apparent to the student user. It would be useful if there were assignable character string variables, improved calculation capabilities, tests for numerical results within a specified range, and improved natural-language capabilities. Although one can quickly learn the basics of COURSEWRITER, sophisticated programming can only be performed by an experienced programmer. This statement is also true of many other languages.

COURSEWRITER is supported only on IBM computers. It has been modified and subsetted by several institutions to permit the implementation of COURSE-WRITER instructional programs on other hardware.

The COURSEWRITER system is useful, but the language is dated in its philosophy

EXAMPLE OF COURSEWRITER CODE

```
QU  THE PRIMARY PACEMAKER OF THE HEART IS A PIECE OF SPECIALIZED
    MYOCARDIAL TISSUE CALLED THE _____ _____ _____.
CA(L)  SIN&ATRIAL&NODE&
TY  CORRECT.  IT IS SITUATED IN THE UPPER PART OF THE RIGHT ATRIUM,
    CLOSE TO ITS JUNCTION WITH THE SUPERIOR VENA CAVA AND CLOSE TO THE
    SULCUS TERMINALIS.
AA(L)  S&A&
TY  SINO-ATRIAL WHAT?
AA(L)  S&A&N
TY  IT LOOKS LIKE YOU MAY HAVE IT, HOWEVER, I AM NOT TOO SURE OF YOUR
    SPELLING OR PERHAPS THE TERMINOLOGY YOU HAVE USED.  PLEASE TRY AGAIN.
WA  ATRIAL&VENTRIC&
WB  A&V̄&
TY  NO.  THE ATRIAL-VENTRICULAR NODE IS INVOLVED IN THE CONDUCTION
    SYSTEM, HOWEVER IT IS NOT THE PRIMARY PACEMAKER.
WA  PACEMAKER
TY  WAKE UP AND TRY AGAIN!
UN  YOUR ANSWER WAS INCORRECT.  PLEASE TRY AGAIN.
UN  YOU DID NOT GET IT THAT TIME EITHER.  THE ANSWER CONSISTS OF THREE
    WORDS:  S... -A..... N...  TRY AGAIN.
UN  PLEASE TYPE:  SINO-ATRIAL NODE
```

EXAMPLE OF STUDENT INTERACTION

```
THE PRIMARY PACEMAKER OF THE HEART IS A PIECE OF SPECIALIZED
MYOCARDIAL TISSUE CALLED THE _____ _____ _____.
atrial-ventricular node
NO.  THE ATRIAL-VENTRICULAR NODE IS INVOLVED IN THE CONDUCTION
SYSTEM, HOWEVER IT IS NOT THE PRIMARY PACEMAKER.
sino-atrial
SINO-ATRIAL WHAT?
sino-atrial node
CORRECT.  IT IS SITUATED IN THE UPPER PART OF THE RIGHT ATRIUM,
CLOSE TO ITS JUNCTION WITH THE SUPERIOR VENA CAVA AND CLOSE TO THE
SULCUS TERMINALIS.
```

Figure 2. Example of COURSEWRITER code.

and capabilities, and it only becomes useful when it is extended by user-written functions. The use of the language will decrease significantly in the next 10 years, if a more powerful CAI language is offered by IBM.

PILOT

PILOT (Programmed Inquiry, Learning Or Teaching) is a programming system written in PL/1 developed for the IBM/360 computer by the Office of Information Systems of the University of California at San Francisco (PILOT 1.6 Guide, 1971). It has been used for a variety of instructional activities in the health sciences. Its predecessor system is COMPUTEST, which operated on an IBM 1620 computer. PILOT has been translated to run on an SDS 940 computer and rewritten in BASIC for a GE 635. Dialects of PILOT (PYLON, NYLON) have been written in BASIC for a number of Digital Equipment Corporation and Hewlett-Packard computers. A user's group has defined a standard set of core instructions called PILOT 73 and implementation is in progress on a variety of computers, including a Datapoint 220 intelligent terminal.

A PILOT program consists of a series of statements identified by a single-letter operation code. There are nine operation codes: "t," type a message; "a," accept an answer; "r," recognize specified keywords in the answer; "g," good match, a keyword has been matched and the specified text will be typed; "b," bad match, no keyword was matched, the specified text will be typed; "n," note data and save for later use by an external program; "f," frame, permits an author to use several "r" statements in succession; "c," control, specifies the strategy and flow of the program; and "e," end of program. A simple example of PILOT is given in Figure 3. Although the language is quite simple, it has sufficient language-recognition and response capability to allow translation and operation of instructional material written in other CAI languages.

When an author or programmer has written a PILOT program, it is compiled by a program written in PL/1 and then placed as object code on a direct-access data set. The users access the compiled course via a PILOT monitor and the execution is performed in real-time by a PILOT execution routine, a reentrant PL/1 main procedure which uses an assembly language interface to a teleprocessing monitor. Core requirements are high for the IBM 360 implementation; for a four-terminal configuration 140,000 bytes of core storage are required.

The most attractive feature of PILOT is its ease in initial use and readability for program authors. It lacks on-line program-authoring and -editing capability, and also sophisticated numerical capability; some newer versions will be more flexible. PILOT is simpler than most languages used for CAI, but still allows flexible text-handling and -recognition strategies.

EXAMPLE OF PILOT CODE

```
T:   ARE YOU OVERWEIGHT?;
A:   ;
R:   NO, NOT;
G:   GOOD FOR YOU.;
B:   YOU NEED TO DIET.;
```

EXAMPLE OF STUDENT INTERACTION

```
ARE YOU OVERWEIGHT?
no, I'm skinny
GOOD FOR YOU.
```

Figure 3. Example of PILOT code.

PLANIT

PLANIT (Programmed LANguage for Interaction and Teaching) is a language designed by the Systems Development Corporation for man-machine interaction (Feingold, 1968). The language is the outgrowth of efforts to prepare a computerized instruction course in statistics. The initial design started in January 1966, was written in JOVIAL, and used a time-shared IBM AN/FSQ-32V computer. The language was rewritten in FORTRAN to make it transportable and has been implemented on IBM System 360 computers, RCA Spectra 70/45 computers, and the CDC 6000 series computers. The implementations are not efficient; inefficiency typically occurs when a language is written in a commonly available language in order to be readily transportable. PLANIT has not yet been used in the health sciences.

The PLANIT system operates in four modes: lesson building, editing, execution, and calculation. Most of the features found in other CAI languages are also present in PLANIT. In addition, sophisticated calculator capabilities, criterion branching, and service routines are provided. Student answers may be evaluated in terms of a keyword match, phonetic comparison, or, in the case of mathematics, formula equivalents.

TUTOR

TUTOR is the programming language of the large-scale PLATO IV CAI system created by the University of Illinois at Urbana (Blomme, no date). Forty-five health sciences instructional programs have been written in it; this is second only to COURSEWRITER. TUTOR is used by seven health sciences institutions.

The TUTOR language is an integral component of the PLATO (Programmed Logic for Automated Teaching Operations) system (Alpert and Bitzer, 1970). The TUTOR language was first used in 1967, with its predecessor being CATO (Compiler for Automatic Teaching Operations) on the PLATO III system. The PLATO IV hardware consists of a large computer (CDC 6000 series) and a large number of terminals utilizing plasma display panels for graphic output. The terminals and computer are interfaced to commerical communication lines by specially designed controllers. User input can be keypress or similar activity, and the computer output can consist of text or graphics on the display panel, rear projection of a photograph on the panel, or other computer-controlled output.

TUTOR is the most sophisticated CAI language presently being used; this is largely a function of its elaborate hardware. Some of the distinguishing features of TUTOR are: a large repertoire of powerful graphic display and answer-judging commands; shared pure procedure lessons in core, not on disk, permitting complex subroutines and branching structures; and full calculational capabilities. TUTOR is capable of transmitting special character patterns to the display screen and handling input and output for any digital device attached to the external input/output connectors of the PLATO IV terminal. Production and revision of lessons are facilitated by a wide range of editing aids. Student and lesson performance may be automatically recorded and evaluated by the computer.

The PLATO system offers much potential for CAI; unfortunately the TUTOR language is utilizable only with this system and its unique student terminals. Optimally used by 4000 terminals, predicted cost per student contact hour would be approximately 50 cents. The system has been shown to be effective in instruction; however it has not yet been determined if the system will actually support the very large number of terminals necessary to achieve a low cost.

ATS

ATS (A Tutorial System) is a system designed to prepare computer-mediated tutorials which permit students to respond in free language and to ask questions (Weber and Hagamen, 1972). ATS was created by the Department of Anatomy of Cornell University Medical College and is based on APL. The language can be implemented on any system supporting APL, e.g., an IBM System 360 or 370, in a 32K workspace. It is being used routinely in the teaching of anatomy at Cornell, and the method and course content have been shown to be pedagogically effective and competitive in cost to other teaching methods.

The system is composed of an author-interrogation program, a tutorial supervisor with author feedback, and automatically produced tutorials. Input to the system, e.g., words, phrases, sentences, and paragraphs, are encoded as single numbers and on output are decoded back into text. This encoding and decoding scheme reduces storage requirements and permits convenient comparison of responses.

In creating a course, the author defines questions to be asked of the student and actions to be taken for anticipated answers. Typically these actions consist of giving a comment and indicating another question to be presented. Keywords are scanned for in the student's response and their proper relationship and content are checked. Pronouns are handled by keeping track of the subject material under discussion. Authoring is eased by having the teacher converse with an author-interrogation program in ordinary English. Facilities for copying blocks of text, finding selected text, and tracing a student's path through a tutorial are provided.

Several artificial-intelligence concepts have been incorporated. After the author has defined keywords to recognize student answers, ATS will select appropriate branches for students to follow to reason out any concepts with which they are having difficulty. The system is unique in being able to handle student questions. The questions must be clear in order to be answered. They may be answered directly, if for example a definition is asked, or indirectly, by asking the student a series of simpler questions designed to show him how to reason through the answer to the question he just asked. The system does not generate the questions nor does the author have their sequence planned, rather the system looks at all the questions the author has provided and selects the most logical route for the student to follow.

ATS is one of the few systems used for CAI which attempts to make any extensive use of the computer's logic capabilities. It is not a general-purpose CAI language but is designed specifically for computer-generated tutorials. As could be expected, response time, processing requirements, and core allocation are significantly greater than for other similar languages.

FOIL

FOIL (File-Oriented Interpretive Language) was developed by the Center for Research on Learning and Teaching of the University of Michigan (Barnett, 1971; Hesselbart *et al.*, 1969). The language has been implemented on the IBM 360/67 Michigan Terminal System. It has been used by the University of Michigan and Wayne State University to develop teaching programs in the medical area.

The predecessor to FOIL simply added to FORTRAN features for recording student performance and searching for keywords, and has made accepting text input, branching, typing messages, and testing of logical expressions more convenient. FOIL is constructed as an interpeter with a similar set of capabilities. The added features make the language more convenient for a programmer to prepare instructional programs.

CAISYS-8

CAISYS-8 is an example of a software system developed specifically for a minicomputer-based system (Holm, 1973). It was created by the University of Texas Medical Branch at Galveston for a Digital Equipment Corporation PDP-8-E with 8000 words of core storage. Course material has been developed in renal problem-solving, acid—base balance, and orthopedic patient management simulation.

The problem of the limited core size and shorter work length of the minicomputer was dealt with by storing only the logic and control instructions specific to the program on the computer. Course text material is stored in computer-controlled peripheral devices, e.g., slide projectors, or, eventually, video disks. The language specifies the logic and controls and peripheral devices. Minimal facilities are provided for specifying display, accepting responses, scanning for keywords, and conditional branching.

The CAISYS system is an innovative approach to medical instruction; however, it is limited in its computational and text-processing capabilities.

Very-High-Level Approaches

In the future less CAI course material will be coded directly in a programming language; content will be separated from strategy, and generative programs and drivers, written in general-purpose programming languages, will be used to facilitate course development.

Generative Systems

With generative systems, authors specify an established instructional strategy they would like to use and supply only content material. The generative system uses this material to code a program in a prespecified language.

The Stony Brook Authoring System, developed by the State University of New York at Stony Brook, is a generator written in PL/1 which can code CAI programs either in BASIC or COURSEWRITER (Siegel, 1972). Display and response-processing— feedback strategies are coded in content-free macro form with text as a variable. The text for each lesson and specification parameters are input for a PL/1 program which assembles a series of calls to appropriate macros. This output is fed to a macro expander which outputs a tape containing the final code in the desired programming language.

Hewlett-Packard has developed a generative system called IDF (Instructional Dialogue Facility) to assist authors in preparing CAI programs coded in BASIC. The system is being used on an HP 2000 computer by The Ohio State University College of Pharmacy.

At the University of Illinois Medical Center in Chicago, a semiautomatic generative system, GENESYS, is being used to prepare a library of CASEs (Computer Aided Simulations of the clinical Encounter) (Harless, 1973). A COURSEWRITER III program, called MREC (Medical Record Entry Course) interrogates an author interactively to gather information, and this is subsequently processed by a series of PL/1 programs to form a CASE coded in COURSEWRITER.

Drivers

Drivers are reentrant content-free strategy programs which access separately stored content files to produce an instructional interaction. They are especially useful as a framework for producing clinical encounter simulations.

At the Laboratory of Computer Science of the Massachusetts General Hospital several drivers have been written in the MUMPS language to offer different structures to format program data in the preparation of teaching programs (Prather, 1973). Drivers exist for multiple choice frame-oriented applications, text material presentation, and simulation. Drivers for simulation of clinical encounters have also been developed at the University of Wisconsin, in CPS, and at the Sate University of New York — Upstate Medical Center, in BASIC, FORTRAN, and PL/1.

Strategy and content are also separated in the minicomputer-based TICCIT (Time-shared, Interactive Computer-Controlled Information Television) system, which is being developed by The Mitre Corporation in collaboration with Brigham Young University (Stetten, 1972). Software is divided into a courseware-processing system, an application system, and an operating system. The course content is packaged into prespecified and validated instructional strategies, coded in an extended version of ALGOL 60, for delivery to students by the application and operating systems.

QUEST is a frame-oriented teaching program driver developed in 1976 at the Washington University School of Medicine and written in MUMPS (Zimmerman and Brigham, 1976; Brigham *et al.*, 1976). It permits efficient authoring and editing of computer-based tutorials, teaching and testing students by means of these tutorials, and processing and display of responses entered by students. Multiple-choice, yes/no, and sophisticated key-phrase answers are allowed. All interaction with the system is done in simple English. QUEST has been successfully employed in the preparation of tutorials in surgery and a course on the Standard MUMPS language.

ACKNOWLEDGEMENTS

This chapter is based upon a report prepared for the Lister Hill National Center for Biomedical Communications of the National Library of Medicine (Brigham, 1973). The author gratefully acknowledges the assistance provided by the Lister Hill National Center and the Laboratory of Computer Sciences of the Massachusetts General Hospital. The author would also like to thank the following individuals for critically reviewing the original report: Barbara B. Farquhar, Edward P. Hoffer, Craig J. Richardson, Penny A. Prather, and Harvey Botman, of the Laboratory of Computer Science, Massachusetts General Hospital; Harold Wooster of the Lister Hill National Center for Biomedical Communications; Karl L. Zinn, of the Center for Research on Learning and Teaching, University of Michigan; Martin Kamp, of the Office of Information Systems, University of California at San Francisco; Jean Bonney, of the Center for Computer and Information Services, Rutgers University; Edward N. Adams, of the International Business Machines Corporation; and Charles Tidball, of the Department of Physiology of the George Washington University Medical Center.

The opinions and recommendations in this chapter are those of the author and not necessarily those of the National Library of Medicine.

References

Adams, E. N., Technical considerations in the design of a CAI system, *Programmed Learning.* 9(5):256–271.

Alpert, D., and Bitzer, D. L., 1970. Advances in computer-based education, *Science,* 167: 1582–1590.

Anastasio, E. J., and Morgan, J. S., 1972. *Study of Factors that have Inhibited a More Widespread Use of Computers in the Instructional Process,* EDUCOM, Interuniversity Communications Council, Inc., Princeton, New Jersey.

Barnett, M., 1971. *An Introduction to FOIL Programming in MTS,* Center for Research on Learning and Teaching, University of Michigan, Ann Arbor, Michigan.

Bates, F., and Douglas, M. L., 1967. *Programming Language/One,* Prentice-Hall, Englewood Cliffs, New Jersey.

Blomme, R., Parry, J., Sherwood, B., and Tenczar, P., *PLATO IV System Software,* Computer-Based Education Research Laboratory, University of Illinois, Urbana, Illinois.

Brigham, C. R., 1973. *Programming Languages Used for Health Sciences Computer-Assisted Instruction*, Report No. PB-224421/AS, National Technical Information Service, U.S. Department of Commerce, Springfield, Virginia.

Brigham, C. R., and Kamp, M., 1974. The current status of computer-assisted instruction in the health sciences, *J. Med. Educ.* **49**(3):278–279.

Brigham, C. R., Kamp, M., and Cross, R. J., 1973. *A Guide to Computer Assisted Instruction in the Health Sciences*, National Technical Information Service, U.S. Department of Commerce, Springfield, Virginia.

Brigham, C. R., Halverson, J. D., and Zimmerman, J., 1976. QUEST: A teaching program driver, *J. Comp. Based Inst.* **3**(2):42–50.

COURSEWRITER III, Version 3 Application Description Manual, GH20-0987-2, International Business Machines Corporation, White Plains, New York, 1971.

Feingold, S. L., 1968. PLANIT – A Language for CAI, *Datamation* **14**(9):41–47.

Feurzeig, W., Munter, P., Swets, J., and Breen, M., 1964. Computer-aided teaching in medical diagnosis, *J. Med. Educ.* **39**(8):746–754.

Frye, C. H., 1968. CAI languages: Capabilities and applications, *Datamation* **14**(9):34–37.

A Functional Specification for a Programming Language for Computer-Aided Learning Applications, Associate Committee on Instructional Technology, National Research Council of Canada, Ottawa, Ontario, July 1972.

Harless, W. G., Drennon, G. G., Marxer, J. J., Root, J. A., Wilson, L. L., and Miller, G. E., 1973. GENESYS – A generating system for the CASE natural language model, *Comp. Bio. Med.* **3**(3):247–268.

Hesselbart, J. C., D'Arms, T., and Zinn, K. L., 1969. *A Manual for FOIL in Two Volumes*, Center for Research on Learning and Teaching, University of Michigan, Ann Arbor, Michigan.

Hoffer, E. P., 1973. Experience with the use of computer simulation models in medical education, *Comp. Bio. Med.* **3**(3) 269–280.

Holm, C., Thompson, W. M., Wilber, M. C., and Wells, C. H., 1973. CAISYS-8 – A CAI language developed for a minicomputer, *Comp. Bio. Med.*, **3**(3):281–292.

Iverson, K. E., 1962. *A Programming Language*, John Wiley and Sons, New York.

Kemeny, J. G., and Kurtz, T. E., 1967. *BASIC Programming*, John Wiley and Sons, New York.

Lower, S., *A CAI System Based on APL*, Simon Fraser University, Burnaby, British Columbia.

Lower, S. K., and Arsenault, G., *A Functional Evaluation of COURSEWRITER III*, Simon Fraser University, Burnaby, British Columbia.

Luskin, B. J., Gripp, T. H., Clark, J. R., and Christianson, D. A., 1972. Sharing programs and selecting a language, *in Everything You Always Wanted to Know About CAI*, Computer Uses in Education, Huntington Beach, California.

PILOT 1.6 guide, 1971. Office of Information Systems, University of California, San Francisco.

Prather, P., 1973. *Teaching Program Drivers*, Laboratory of Computer-Science, Massachusetts General Hospital, Boston, Massachusetts.

Sammet, J. E., 1969. *Programming Languages: History and Fundamentals*, Prentice-Hall, Englewood Cliffs, New Jersey.

Sammet, J. E., 1972. Programming languages: History and future, *Communications of the A.C.M.* **15**(7):601–610.

Sheretz, D. D., *MUMPS Reference Manual*, Laboratory of Computer Science, Massachusetts General Hospital, Boston, Massachusetts.

Siegel, B., 1972. The Stony Brook authoring system – How it facilitates curriculum development, *ACS SIGCUE Bulletin* **6**(4):25–26.

Stetten, K. J. 1972. *Toward a Market Success for CAI – An Overview of the TICCIT Program*, MITRE Corporation, Washington, D.C.

USA Standard FORTRAN, *USAS X3.9–1966*, United States of America Standards Institute, New York, March 1966.

Weber, J. C., and Hagamen, W. D., 1972. ATS: A new system for computer-mediated tutorials in medical education, *J. Med. Educ.* 47:637–644.

Zimmerman, J., and Brigham, C. R., 1976. *QUEST Design Manual*, Biomedical Computer Laboratory, Washington University School of Medicine, St. Louis.

Zinn, K. L., 1969. *A Comparative Study of Languages for Programming Interactive Use of Computers in Instruction*, EDUCOM, Boston, Massachusetts.

Zinn, K. L., 1976. *Requirements for Programming Languages in Computer-Based Instructional Systems, Technical Report CERI/CT/70.62*, Center for Educational Development, Paris.

Zinn, K. L., 1973. Instructional Software, *in* K. Zinn, M. Refice, and A. Romano (Eds.), *Computers in the Instructional Process: Report of an International School*, Elsevier, New York.

28

Writing Computer-Aided Instruction Lessons: Some Practical Considerations

Alan B. Forsythe and James R. Freed

Introduction

Computer-aided instruction has some absolute advantages over other modes of teaching. The computer can be utilized as an amplifier of a teacher's effort since it can take an initial teaching program and apply it over and over again, reorganizing the text individually to meet the unique needs of each student. Another important advantage of CAI is that it can allow students to proceed at their own rates of speed, rather than one which is either convenient for the administration or designed for the "average" student. Given the educational advantages, it would appear that teachers would be active in utilizing this technology in their courses. However, this is not the case. Very little good material is available for use by today's student, or to serve as a model for future lessons.

Why is this true? Our view is that a major factor limiting the growth of CAI is the reluctance of many faculty members to work with a new and unfamiliar technology. The goal of this chapter, therefore, is to demonstrate an author language for writing CAI lessons so that faculty and administrators will gain some familiarity with actually developing course materials. We hope that through this process, educators will better understand an author's task so that those directly responsible for writing CAI lessons and those responsible for determining the use of institutional resources can make a more informed decision regarding the use of CAI in health science education.

There are two other impediments to a greater involvement of faculty in CAI which, though no solutions are offered, should be noted. The first of these is the faculty review and evaluation procedures of most major universities. A teacher faced with the decision whether to put effort into CAI or some other endeavor soon sees that CAI may be of doubtful personal reward. A year of effort in CAI may reduce the amount of research or number of publications with a consequent loss of recognition and promotions. There will be no royalties from a new textbook. Will the dean or department chairman give release time from other teaching responsibilities

---

Alan B. Forsythe and *James R. Freed* • Health Sciences Computing Facility and Department of Biomathemetics, and School of Dentistry, University of California, Los Angeles, California.

and community service? How long will the school support CAI? Will the effort have been wasted because interest and funds disappear within a year or two?

Working on CAI material is essentially a teaching function, so the general issues related to the methods of rewarding faculty for teaching ability must be faced if CAI is to be promoted. CAI, however, poses additional problems since existing criteria for evaluating teaching effectiveness may not be flexible enough for innovations such as CAI but may rely on such standard measures as direct student contact hours. Once the faculty members believe that they will be recognized and rewarded for the time devoted to developing new teaching methods, efficient and effective new instructional modes such as CAI are likely to expand more rapidly.

The other inhibiting factor is the cost of CAI (Williams and Milner, 1975). Cost is certain to be an issue in the development of teaching methods and cost–benefit analyses of various programs are often used to help determine the desirability of taking certain actions. However, the use of a standard cost–benefit analysis to assess the desirability of CAI, or perhaps any new educational method, may be inappropriate or misleading. Certain costs can be measured such as machine time, cost of terminals, and maintenance of the computer program. The major costs, however, are in the personnel time required to develop the materials, and these costs may be less obvious than the expenses of computer time and terminals.

In addition to the problem of calculating costs, it may be extremely difficult to assign a dollar value to the benefits. For example, if CAI raises the quality of what a student learns or how fast he or she learns it, how is this measured and what value can be assigned to such benefits? How is it possible to determine the worth of a faculty member having more hours to devote to research if this results from using CAI? Or if the teaching time stays the same but more hours are devoted to advanced seminars, how are the benefits to be measured in relation to the obvious dollar costs of the program? A traditional cost–benefit analysis, therefore, is difficult to apply since qualitative as well as quantitative issues must be considered when evaluating both the costs and benefits of CAI in an educational program.

Background

The author language is a key element in CAI since this is the point at which the faculty member who is actually writing the course material is likely to interface with the computer technology. Author languages should be convenient and natural for an instructor and should be designed to allow the instructor to prepare materials directly for the students (Computer Applications, 1971). To achieve these goals, Programmed Instruction Nucleus (PIN) was developed. This is an author language which should enable educators to write lessons with a minimum of assistance from computer programmers.

PIN is only one example of an author-oriented language and several extensions would be desirable if it were to become a major language for CAI (which is not being advocated). Other author languages can certainly be developed. PIN, for example, went from conception to a working version in less than the equivalent of one month. The point here is that developing languages is not the problem: writing the course material is.

The approach taken in developing PIN was to use as a model the interaction that would take place in a student—faculty conversation. In most cases, the faculty member would ask a question. If a student was way off the mark in the answer, the faculty member might indicate that the question required a certain type of answer, thus narrowing the scope of possible responses. For example, if a student gave the answer "addition" to the question "How much is 2 plus 2?" the faculty member might simply indicate that the student's answer should be a number.

Once the student was answering in the general context required by the question, several alternatives could occur. First, the student could give the right answer. If the question was difficult and required the understanding of several concepts, the instructor might decide that the student knew the material and move on to new topics. If the question was not complex, the instructor might want to ask more questions to make certain that the student understood the individual concepts.

The student could give a wrong answer to the question. Certain wrong answers would indicate that a student had an incomplete understanding of the material or had made a commonly occurring error. In such cases, the instructor might wish to provide some commentary on the answer and then either ask a different question or give the student another chance to answer the same question. For a particular question, there may be several incorrect answers of this type.

Other wrong answers, however, would be totally unexpected. In these cases, the instructor might have several other responses which would provide some information or would simply tell the student that the answer was wrong and that he or she should rethink the question and try again. If several wrong answers were given, the instructor would give up and go to another question of the same type or back track and ask more remedial questions.

PIN is designed to facilitate writing CAI lessons in the manner just described. An author writes a text in which questions are asked; certan types of responses are required; right and wrong answers are specified; and other responses can be included. The author's text is then either punched onto IBM cards or is entered into the computer via a terminal.

Construction of CAI Lessons

The following series of illustrations are designed to demonstrate the use of the PIN author language and should enable an author to write CAI material for a course. Most of the illustrations are taken from CAI material prepared for an introductory statistics class given to first-year dental students at UCLA School of Dentistry. This material has been used by a total of 125 students over a period of 3 years with a total student exposure time of 1500 hours.

A detailed description of PIN has been published (Forsythe *et al.*, 1975). We have sought to simplify the requirements for an author by developing forms which can be used for: (1) questions which require a numerical response; (2) multiple choice questions; (3) true—false questions; and (4) fill-in type questions. Relatively simple changes would be required to prepare the lessons to be entered into the computer. These modifications could be added by the teacher or an assistant once the lesson had been composed.

An illustration of each of the four types of questions will be presented: each example will show a completed form as written by the author. So that the various elements can be described more easily in this discussion, numbers of each line are given in parentheses in the left-hand margin.

Much of what is written by the author is not displayed to the typical student at a computer terminal. Instructors with no experience in CAI may find it useful to examine sample student interactions which could occur with each of these lessons before proceeding. These interactions are given at the end of the chapter.

The first example (Figure 1b) is a question requiring a numerical answer. The question is designed to check the student's understanding of the definition of a mean by asking the student to calculate the mean of five observations. On line 1, the number of the question is given. The number should be convenient for the author, such as CH3Q3, which could indicate chapter 3, question number 3. In PIN, the question number must begin with an alphabetic character and can consist of a maximum of 6 characters.

The question posed to the student is given on line 2. The question is displayed and the indication for the student's response is a question mark given at the beginning of the next line. This is produced automatically by the PIN system. After a student has entered a response, he or she strikes the carriage return key which prompts the computer to continue with the program.

The fact that this question requires a numerical response is indicated by the name of the form. The question is entered into the computer so that any response other than a number will automatically cause NUMERICAL ANSWER PLEASE to be displayed when the student strikes the carriage return.

At this point, the question to be posed to the student and the general type of response (a numerical answer) have been specified. The author would next indicate the answer or answers that are considered to be correct, any comments on the correct answer, and the number of the question which is to be executed next. These are illustrated on lines 10 and 11. In this example, if the student enters 8 and strikes the carriage return, the message, GOOD. THE MEAN IN THIS CASE IS EQUAL TO 40 DIVIDED BY 5. will be displayed and the program will then proceed to the next question which in this example is CH3Q6.

Next an author could list the incorrect response which he or she anticipates a student might make. The author can comment on the mistake by a message and then direct the student what to do next. It is possible to allow the student to make another response to the same question, or the program can move to another question.

In this example, a common mistake is to confuse the mean and median so the author has listed the value for the median as an incorrect answer. If the student enters a 7, as shown on line 13, the word WRONG is not displayed: only the message

NUMERICAL QUESTION

(1) Question Number: _____

(2) Question: _____

(3) _____

(4) _____

(5) _____

(6) _____

(7) _____

	Check <u>one</u>			Number of next
(8)				
(9) Choice	Right	Wrong	Message to Student	Question
(10) __	__	__	_____	_____
(11)			_____	
(12)			_____	
(13) __	__	__	_____	
(14)			_____	
(15)			_____	
(16) __	__	__	_____	_____
(17)			_____	
(18)			_____	
(19) __	__	__	_____	_____
(20)			_____	
(21)			_____	
(22) __	__	__	_____	_____
(23)			_____	
(24)			_____	
(25) __	__	__	_____	_____
(26)			_____	
(27)			_____	

Figure 1a. Author text for a numerical question.

NUMERICAL QUESTION

(1) Question Number: ___CH3Q3_____

(2) Question: What is the mean of the observations 3, 4, 7, 12 and 14?

(3) _____

(4) _____

(5) _____

(6) _____

(7) _____

(8)		Check **one**			Number of next
(9)	Choice	Right	Wrong	Message to Student	Question
(10)	8	X	___	Good. The mean in this case is equal to 40	CH3Q6
(11)				divided by 5.	
(12)					
(13)	7	___	X	You must have the mean and median confused. 7	
(14)				is the median or middle observation. Try again.	
(15)					
(16)	10	___	X	The mean is the sum of the observations divided	CH3Q5
(17)				by the number of observations. In this case, 40	
(18)				divided by 5. The mean is 8.	
(19)	Other 1	___	X	I am not sure if your math is in error or you	
(20)				are not clear on how to calculate the mean.	
(21)				Try again.	
(22)	Other 2	___	X	That is still not the correct answer. The first	
(23)				step in solving this problem is to add together	
(24)				all of the observations.	
(25)	Other 3	___	X	No, you are still missing it. The sum of the 5	CH3Q4
(26)				observations is 40. The mean is 40 divided by 5.	
(27)				It is 8. Review the definition on page 22.	

Figure 1b. Author text for a numerical question – answers.

is seen by the student. Note in this example that the number of the next question is not given. This means that the program does not move to a new question but that another question mark is automatically displayed to indicate that the student should respond again.

Another mistake a student might possibly make would be to divide the sum of the observations by 4 instead of 5, and conclude that the answer was 10 as shown on line 16. This could occur if the student used as the divisor the number of observations minus 1, which might indicate some confusion with the computation of the variance, which does use $N - 1$ as the divisor. In this case, the teacher decided to supply the answer to the question and routed the student to another question for further review.

Other incorrect answers besides 7 and 10 might be given by the student. The author can list these as "other" and should also label them as 1, 2, etc. These numbers indicate the number of times a student has attempted to answer this particular question. When a student enters a response, it is checked against each of the answers which have been specified. If the response matches the number, the message for that answer is displayed. If the response matches none of these, the message corresponding to the number of times the student has answered the question is triggered.

In this example, if a student entered any number other than 8, 7, or 10 on the first attempt at answering the question, the "Other 1" message would be displayed. Another similar mistake would trigger the "Other 2," and a third attempt without indicating 8, 7, or 10 would execute "Other 3." If a student entered the incorrect answer 7 and then another incorrect answer besides 10, the "Other 2" message would be displayed since this was the second attempt by the student to answer the question. Note that no question number is given after "Other 1" and "Other 2" so that a question mark will be displayed, asking the student to answer the same question again. After "Other 3," the answer is given and question CH3Q4 is displayed next.

The question number is the basis for the branching capability of PIN. If the student answers the question correctly as shown on lines 10–11, the program can skip ahead to more advanced material presented in the question CH3Q6. On the other hand, a student making enough incorrect responses to trigger "Other 3" would be routed to CH3Q4 which could ask a more remedial question designed to help the student understand the concept of the statistical mean. Finally, if a student gave the incorrect response on line 16, question CH3Q5 would be executed next, which might ask a question requiring the student to calculate another mean similar to the one just performed.

Figure 2 is an illustration of a multiple choice question. Incorrect answers are anticipated most easily by teachers in this type of question. A finite number of incorrect answers illustrative of certain concepts can be listed and the student must select an answer from the list provided. For this reason it may be easiest and most logical for an instructor to begin writing CAI lessons using multiple choice questions. Also, it is usually unnecessary to use "other" answers since it is possible to list all the possible answers.

MULTIPLE-CHOICE QUESTION

(5 CHOICES)

Question Number: _____

Question: _____

_____

_____

_____

_____

_____

_____

_____

a. _____

b. _____

c. _____

d. _____

e. _____

_____

_____

Choice	Check **one** Right	Wrong	Message to Student	Number of next Question
a	—	—		—
b	—	—		—
c	—	—		—
d	—	—		—
e	—	—		—

Figure 2a. Author text for a multiple-choice question.

MULTIPLE-CHOICE QUESTION
(5 CHOICES)

(1) Question Number: ____CH1Q2____

(2) Question: The laws of which of the following have their proof in statistical facts:

(3) _____

(4) _____

(5) _____

(6) _____

(7) _____

(8) _____

(9) _____

(10) a. Physical science

(11) b. Biological science

(12) c. Social science

(13) d. All of the above

(14) e. A and B only

(15) _____

(16) _____

	Check **one**			Number of next Question
(17)				
(18) Choice	Right	Wrong	Message to Student	
(19) a	___	X	This is the truth, but not the whole truth.	_____
(20)			Try again.	
(21) b	___	X	Statistics is useful in other sciences besides	_____
(22)			biology. Enter another choice.	
(23) c	___	X	Statistical proofs are used in the "hard sciences"	_____
(24)			as well as the social sciences. Try again.	
(25) d	X	___	Correct. We use statistics whenever we wish to	CH1Q3
(26)			make statements about the real world.	
(27) e	___	X	You should have chosen d since statistics is a tool	CH1O3
(28)			of all three scientific areas.	

Figure 2b. Author text for a multiple-choice question – answers.

The question number on line 1 and the question on line 2 are the same as in the numerical questions. The question space on lines 2 through 16 can be thought of in three parts. First, there is space for the question leading to the choices. Next, on lines 6 through 9, come the choices themselves. Finally, lines 15 and 16 can be used to supply the closing part of the question. The spacing presented here, as is true for all the forms, is illustrative and is not a rigid requirement.

Note that it is not necessary to write a specific response for each incorrect answer. For every answer except "d," for example, the author could simply write, "There are still more, try again." These nonspecific responses to incorrect answers are often not desirable from a teaching standpoint since the student is not provided with an informative response.

Of course, these approaches are not exclusive. An author might wish to write a specific response for one or more of the incorrect answers and "No, try again," for others. Also, the author can have a student try the same question again by leaving the number of the next question blank as shown on lines 19, 21, and 23. However, the student can be allowed to proceed to the next question even if an incorrect answer is given, as on line 27.

Figure 3 illustrates a true–false question. These are quite straightforward. If a student gives the correct answer, a message can be given and then the number of the next question, as on line 20. If the student enters the incorrect answer, a message and the number of the next question could also be given. For incorrect answers, the author could require that the correct response be entered so that the message written for that response would be displayed. As stated above, this would be accomplished by leaving blank the number of the next question, as shown on line 14.

Once again, questions can be constructed depending on the goals of the faculty member. The messages given in this example could simply have been "No. The answer is false." and "You are correct." followed by the number of the next question for each.

Questions requiring a fill-in response, shown in Figure 4, may be the most difficult to develop. Since the possible answers a student might enter are much greater than an instructor's ability to anticipate, fewer informative responses are generally provided.

For fill-in questions, a student can enter any string of characters. In this example the author has elected to specify two correct words shown on lines 10 and 13. If a student enters an acceptable word other than the two specified such as "increased" or "enlarged," or if the student uses the words "larger" or "bigger" or mispells a word, the answer would be treated as incorrect and an "other" response would be triggered. A similar situation exists for the words specified as wrong on lines 16 and 19.

The message provided in "Other 1" is designed to help direct the student to a word which has been specified. If the student still enters some other word, the "Other 2" response will be executed and the student routed to the next question.

TRUE-FALSE QUESTION

(1)   Question Number: _____

(2)   Question: _____

(3)   _____

(4)   _____

(5)   _____

(6)   _____

(7)   _____

(8)   _____

(9)   _____

(10) _____

(11) _____

	Check one				Number of next
(12)					
(13) Choice	Right	Wrong		Message to Student	Question
(14) True	__	__		_____	_____
(15)				_____	
(16)				_____	
(17)				_____	
(18)				_____	
(19)				_____	
(20) False	__	__		_____	_____
(21)				_____	
(22)				_____	
(23)				_____	
(24)				_____	
(25)				_____	

Figure 3a. Author text for a true–false question.

TRUE-FALSE QUESTION

(1) Question Number: ___CH4Q10___

(2) Question: All universes (or populations) are infinite. True or false?

(3) _____

(4) _____

(5) _____

(6) _____

(7) _____

(8) _____

(9) _____

(10) _____

(11) _____

	Check one		Message to Student	Number of next Question
(13) Choice	Right	Wrong		
(14) True	___	X	No. The answer is false. If we wanted to know	___
(15)			the distribution of blood pressure of men cur-	
(16)			rently living in Los Angeles, for example, we	
(17)			would be working with a population that is quite	
(18)			large but is finite. Please enter the correct	
(19)			response.	
(20) False	X	___	You are correct. In most cases, however, the	CH4Q11
(21)			universe is large enough to let us consider it	
(22)			infinite and use the simpler formulas that result.	
(23)			_____	
(24)			_____	
(25)			_____	

(12) Check **one**

Figure 3b. Author text for a true—false question — answers.

FILL-IN QUESTION

(1) Question Number: _____

(2) Question: _____

(3) _____

(4) _____

(5) _____

(6) _____

(7) _____

		Check <u>one</u>		Message to Student	Number of next Question
(8)					
(9)	Choice	Right	Wrong	Message to Student	Question
(10)	__	__	__	_____	____
(11)				_____	
(12)				_____	
(13)	__	__	__	_____	____
(14)				_____	
(15)				_____	
(16)	__	__	__	_____	____
(17)				_____	
(18)				_____	
(19)	__	__	__	_____	____
(20)				_____	
(21)				_____	
(22)	__	__	__	_____	____
(23)				_____	
(24)				_____	
(25)	__	__	__	_____	____
(26)				_____	
(27)				_____	

Figure 4a. Author text for a fill-in question.

FILL-IN QUESTION

(1) Question Number: ___CH3Q13___

(2) Question: _Measures of dispersion will usually be ... if the observations_

(3) _____ _are distant from the mean._

(4) _____

(5) _____

(6) _____

(7) _____

(8)	Check one			Number of next Question
(9) Choice	Right	Wrong	Message to Student	
(10) Large	X	___	Correct answer.	CH3Q15
(11)				
(12)				
(13) Big	X	___	Correct answer.	CH3Q15
(14)				
(15)				
(16) Small	___	X	You seem to have things turned around. Try again.	
(17)				
(18)				
(19) Little	___	X	You seem to have things turned around. Try again.	
(20)				
(21)				
(22) Other 1	___	X	I am interested in the relative size. Enter	
(23)			another word.	
(24)				
(25) Other 2	___	X	The answer is large. Review section 3.2 in the	CH3Q15
(26)			text.	
(27)				

Figure 4b. Author text for a fill-in question – answers.

Conclusion

Until recently, a major consideration in the development of CAI has been hardware. The major issue now is the development of a repertoire of quality curriculum materials. Simply stated, more faculty members must become active in authoring CAI lessons if CAI is to play a more significant role in the future of medical education.

In our view, many authors are reluctant to become involved with CAI because of the problems they believe are associated with translating curriculum materials into a language that can be understood by the computer. The necessity to learn detailed terms, notation, and rules or to work with computer programmers can have a dampening effect on an instructor's enthusiasm. Our goal in this chapter has been to describe one author language which we feel is easily comprehensible and provides the capability of writing fairly complex curriculum materials.

We believe that PIN (and other author-oriented languages) illustrates that CAI lesson construction is basically a teaching function that need not be complicated with computer-programming considerations. It takes time and effort to prepare materials that will respond to the students' needs. Subject matter knowledge and an awareness of students are the keys to good materials. The ability to design multiple paths through the same materials can be cultivated in the good teacher once the technical details are removed as an obstacle. CAI is hard work, and it is the work of a teacher, not a computer programmer.

Finally, blank forms for each of the four types of questions described above have been included. To complete this chapter, those with little or no experience in writing CAI lessons are encouraged to prepare questions of each type. We believe that if educators have some actual experience in preparing lessons, much of the mystique that may accompany CAI can be overcome.

Typical Interactions

Some authors may find it difficult to visualize the interaction that could occur between the student and computer when these CAI lessons are used. The following examples are included to demonstrate what is displayed on a terminal in a typical transaction with a student. Recall that the prompt for a student response is a question mark displayed at the beginning of a line. When the student has entered a response, he or she strikes the carriage return key to continue with the program.

Each question begins with the listing of the question number so that student inquiries or comments can be quickly located. The teacher may also supply a list referring the student to further information for each question.

Typical Interaction of Figure 1

CH3Q3

WHAT IS THE MEAN OF THE OBSERVATIONS 3, 4, 7, 12 AND 14.

?6

I AM NOT SURE IF YOUR MATH IS IN ERROR OR YOU ARE NOT CLEAR ON HOW TO CALCULATE THE MEAN. TRY AGAIN.

?7

YOU MUST HAVE THE MEAN AND MEDIAN CONFUSED. 7 IS THE MEDIAN OR MIDDLE OBSERVATION. TRY AGAIN.

?8

GOOD. THE MEAN IN THIS CASE IS EQUAL TO 40 DIVIDED BY 5.

CH3Q6

(The next question is automatically displayed.)

Typical Interaction of Figure 2

CH1Q2

THE LAWS OF WHICH OF THE FOLLOWING HAVE THEIR PROOF IN STATISTICAL FACTS: (A) PHYSICAL SCIENCE; (B) BIOLOGICAL SCIENCE; (C) SOCIAL SCIENCE; (D) ALL OF THE ABOVE: (E) A AND B ONLY

?B

STATISTICS IS USEFUL IN OTHER SCIENCES BESIDES BIOLOGY. ENTER ANOTHER CHOICE

?A AND B

A THROUGH E PLEASE

?E

YOU SHOULD HAVE CHOSEN D SINCE STATISTICS IS A TOOL OF ALL THREE SCIENTIFIC AREAS.

CH1Q3

(The next question is automatically displayed.)

Typical Interaction of Figure 3

CH4Q10

ALL UNIVERSES (OR POPULATIONS) ARE INFINITE. TRUE OR FALSE.

?NO

TRUE OR FALSE PLEASE.

?FALSE

YOU ARE CORRECT. IN MOST CASES, HOWEVER, THE UNIVERSE IS LARGE ENOUGH TO LET US CONSIDER IT INFINITE AND USE THE SIMPLER FORMULAS THAT RESULT.

CH4Q11

(The next question is automatically displayed.)

Typical Interaction of Figure 4

CH3Q13

MEASURES OF DISPERSION WILL USUALLY BE . . . IF THE OBSERVATIONS ARE DISTANT FROM THE MEAN.

?LOW

I AM INTERESTED IN THE RELATIVE SIZE. ENTER ANOTHER WORD.

?SMALL

YOU SEEM TO HAVE THINGS TURNED AROUND. TRY AGAIN.

?LARGE

CORRECT ANSWER.

CH3Q15

(The next question is automatically displayed.)

References

Computer Applications in Dental Education, 1971. Department of Health, Education, and Welfare, San Francisco.

Forsythe, A. B., Freed, J. R., and Frey, H. S., 1975. Programmed instruction nucleus (PIN): A simplified author-language for computer-aided instruction, *Comput. Biol. Med.* 5:77–88 (June).

Williams, M. C., and Milner, S. D., 1975. The attitudes of medical school administrators toward cost factors relating to computer-assisted instruction, Paper presented at the Association for the Development of Computer-Based Instructional Systems, Winter meeting, Charleston, South Carolina, January 28–30, 1975, Educational Resources Information Center (ERIC), Washington, D.C., ED 110072.

29

Audiovisuals and Computer-Based Learning

Gary S. Kahn

Overview

Educational technology has been defined as "the systematic process of learning and teaching in terms of specific objectives based on research in human learning and communications and employing a combination of human and non-human resources to bring about a more effective instruction" (McMurran, 1970).

The past decade has seen many attempts – some successful, some abortive – to bring educational technology into the mainstream of medical education. From the successes and especially from the failures, there is much to be learned about the nature of the technology itself and the process of introducing it into health professions education.

The discussion of the complementary nature of audiovisual and computer technologies for medical education will begin against the backdrop. But first, a couple of definitions: When used in this chapter as a noun, the term *audiovisual* or *AV* will generally refer to an instructional unit or package, e.g., a film, a slide—tape package, a videotape. When used as an adjective, the term will refer to those instructional methods that rely on electronic and/or optical hardware to display visual images and reproduce audio signals. The term *instructional media*, or just *media*, overlaps with audiovisual except it is more inclusive, subsuming printed materials (texts, handouts, etc.) as well as audiovisuals and the more established nonprint instructional vehicles (blackboards, flip-charts, etc.). To set the stage, we will begin by discussing the common legacy of computers and audiovisuals and the lessons learned from the early days of technological innovation in medical education. We will then try to show how audiovisual technology can be integrated with computer-based learning systems within the less-than-ideal realities of present hardware, institutional priorities, and faculty expertise. We will end with a fanciful look at future prospects for these powerful new educational tools.

The Legacy and the Lessons

The following section obviously oversimplifies a rather complex situation. However, in the author's opinion it represents the prevailing view of the events leading up to the present situation and some of the lessons learned from these events.

Gary S Kahn · Educational Research and Evaluation Branch, National Medical Audiovisual Center, Atlanta, Georgia.

Until somewhere in the early 1960s, the standard list of audiovisual equipment in a typical medical school included a 16 mm projector, a lantern slide projector, and perhaps a microscope slide projector. Then, as federal dollars began to flow into the medical schools at an unprecedented rate, a rapid succession of audio-visual media and devices made their appearance: synchronous slide—tape and film-strip devices, film-loop projectors, videotape recorders, closed-circuit television systems (CCTV), dial-access retrieval systems, microfiche readers, individual multi-media learning stations, etc.

Each of these new delivery vehicles captured the imaginations of enthusiastic educators who perceived in them a real opportunity to improve teaching efficiency. However, extravagant claims were common, and it was often difficult to separate what was truly innovative and valid from what was merely novel. The literature fairly blossomed with excited reports of "new approaches" using this or that new device. Anecdotal reports or naively designed studies compared traditional approaches to the newer methods. These reports and studies frequently cited the advantages accruing from automating education: freeing the professor from needless repetition of the annual lecture; extending the audience reached by particularly brilliant or outstanding teachers; permitting students to use materials at their convenience and at their own pace; etc. However, many of these studies, which often purported to demonstrate the superiority of one medium (e.g., slide—tape) over another (e.g., lecture), were, in fact, trying to compare apples and oranges. Most such studies, when controlled properly, usually fail to demonstrate a signifi-cant difference attributable to the delivery vehicle itself.

The problem here probably resulted from the fact that many individuals engaged in innovative efforts in medical education tended to oversimplify the educational process. They operated as if there were only two elements to consider in their educational planning: (1) content (e.g., coronary artery disease, the countercurrent mechanism) and (2) method (e.g., lecture, film, lab, small-group discussion). They selected content on the basis of what the professor knew the most about, what had been taught before, and how much time was available. Similarly, they chose the method on the basis of how the content had been presented before or, in the case of mediated instruction, which new device captured their imagination or was in vogue at the time. Little or no attention was given to such factors as how the information would ultimately be used, how it should be organized to insure learn-ing, what method would provide the most compatible vehicle for the kind of information involved, how the learning environment might be arranged to optimize learning, or how the faculty member would know if he were successful in promoting the desired learning outcomes.

In short, in spite of their recognition of the virtues of instructional media, many of these educators in their enthusiasm for the new hardware unwittingly lost sight of the fact that educational technology, properly applied, must encompass much more than the use of automated techniques and electromechanical devices. As the definition of the President's Commission suggests, it embodies a number of systematic processes that lead to more effective and efficient learning programs. These processes are involved in the design and evaluation of instruction as well as overall curriculum planning.

After the initial excitement over the new techniques began to wane, the problems related to producing course material utilizing the new hardware began to emerge. Recognizing that producing quality AV or computer programs is an expensive and time-consuming process, previously enthusiastic department chairmen and faculty found it necessary to fall back upon more traditional instructional approaches. Students, too, eagerly responded to the new materials and hardware – until the novelty wore off. Gradually, the new devices were relegated to the status of showpieces or to collect dust in equipment closets, and this eventually led to disenchantment on the part of funders.

Some educationally unsophisticated materials are still being developed. However, more and more faculty are directing their efforts toward the application of educational technology in its broadest sense. They are considering such factors as the need to establish the validity of their objectives, the appropriateness and cost effectiveness of the instructional method, and measurement of learning outcomes resulting from the instruction.

Here are some other lessons learned from early experience with audiovisual instruction and CAI:

1. Authorship – The best approach to developing instructional materials for these new technologies resembles more the process of making a movie than of a textbook. That is, it utilizes in a systematic manner the expertise of specialists in a team approach (Brooke *et al.*, 1974). As a minimum, the following skills should be represented on the team:

   a. Content expertise
   b. Instructional design and evaluation expertise
   c. Relevant technical expertise (artist, computer programmer, media specialist, systems analyst, etc.)

2. Curriculum integration – Mediated instructional materials should be meaningfully integrated into the overall curriculum, and this should be planned systematically prior to production. AV or CAI programs which have been produced largely as a result of faculty fascination with hardware rather than to meet specific curricular needs and offered to students as optional resources have achieved a notorious history of disuse.

3. Developmental testing – all instructional materials should undergo rigorous student testing and faculty peer review at several points during the developmental stages of production to assure the effectiveness and acceptability of the final product.

4. Continuing usefulness – Periodic update and revision should be planned in advance of release of any new material to insure its continued usefulness to the target audience.

Audiovisuals and Computers — When to Use Them

The lessons learned from these early experiences have been embodied in various systematic instructional development and curriculum-planning models. At a minimum, these models all include steps for (1) defining goals and objectives of instruction, (2) selecting and planning instructional strategies, and (3) planning and developing evaluation techniques. Many books and manuals have been written at various levels of sophistication which divide these steps into component processes (Gagné and Briggs, 1974; Kempe, 1971; Gentry and Saches, 1976).

It is beyond the scope of this chapter to elaborate on the processes involved in defining curricular goals, instructional objectives, and evaluation strategies. However, it is germane to our discussion to say a bit more about selection of instructional strategies and a component of this process, selection of media.

Learning psychologists have developed many varied taxonomies and constructs in their attempts to classify types of learning (Bloom, 1956; Krathwohl *et al*, 1964; Gagné, 1963). The classification most commonly used by educators in the health professions involves three general areas: (1) cognitive (dealing with knowledge), (2) affective (dealing with feelings or values), and (3) psychomotor (dealing generally with manipulative skills). Of course, these can be broken down much further. For example, cognitive learning can be looked at on various levels from simple recall learning to complex problem solving.

The point is that the kind of learning that is supposed to occur as the result of instruction has important implications for the choice of a particular teaching strategy or method. To take an obvious example, if one wishes a learner to be able to distinguish various heart sounds, he must be provided an opportunity to make the discriminations involved, perhaps using a heart-sound simulator. A student could hardly be expected to do this after merely hearing a series of lectures. Thus, it becomes incumbent on the teacher, before deciding to use computers or AV devices, to analyze the nature of the desired learning outcome so he can make an informed judgment as to the way the material should be presented.

Of course, there are other factors besides the nature of the content and kind of learning that must be taken into account before deciding to use CAI or a particular audiovisual method. These include the availability and reliability of the hardware; the cost of development and utilization; the ease of revision; the need for motion, sound, color; the degree of image resolution required, etc.

Consider, for example, a faculty member who is going to prepare a pathology lesson on cirrhosis of the liver. Let us presume he wants a unit that can be used in a self-instructional format, and he has a choice of 16 mm film, videotape, 35 mm filmstrip, or 35 mm slides as visual presentation media. He could rule out videotape because the television screen might not give a high enough resolution to see details on the microscopic specimen he wishes to use. He could rule out both film and videotape on the basis that the learning objectives of his unit would not require motion and thus these media would be too expensive. This leaves him with filmstrip or slides. Because he might want to change some portion of the lesson at a later date, he would select slides because filmstrip, although cheaper, is not as flexible. This example is an oversimplification, but it points out the kinds of questions that must be addressed in making decisions to use particular instructional media.

In general, audiovisuals, as a class of media, are optimally used when the information to be learned can be most effectively communicated through visual (graphic) and/or aural channels. This need may be inherent in the nature of the information itself or it may relate to the learning style of the individual.

The obvious need for a mechanism to display graphic images to accompany verbal information is well established. Whether the image can be in the form of a stick drawing on a sandy beach, a picture in a printed book, a lecture with illustrations on a blackboard, a slide—tape unit, or a cathode ray tube (CRT) display, it has long been recognized that many concepts are difficult if not impossible to communicate simply through the spoken or printed word. Making discriminations on the basis of visual information is important in most areas of the medical curriculum but is especially critical in highly visual disciplines such as anatomy, pathology, radiology, and dermatology. Here, there is an obvious need to augment traditional or computer-based instruction with visual devices capable of displaying images with photographic-quality resolution. Imagine, if you will, trying to teach or learn the pathology of the liver, the anatomy of the cerebral circulation, or the physiological concept of the countercurrent mechanism without the benefit of schematic or pictorial representations. Graphic illustrations of such complex principles make it easier for the student to conceptualize the spatial, temporal, or qualitative relationships involved.

The need for devices to teach auditory discrimination is much less frequent. However, in disciplines related to cardiovascular, pulmonary, and gastrointestinal systems the development of auditory skills is of critical importance, particularly in learning the discriminations required in auscultation (using the stethoscope), such as when listening for heart sounds, vascular bruits, breath sounds, and bowel sounds. It is important to note that in using audio devices to reproduce or simulate these sounds one focuses the attention of the learner only on the auditory component of what is often a composite skill. The skill might actually require tactile and visual as well as aural input. However, by eliminating distracting variables, auditory learning can often be accomplished more efficiently.

Similarly, the use of audio media might also be valuable in psychiatry and the teaching of interpersonal communications skills. Oral elements of the communications process can be isolated to enable the learner to pick up subtle changes in intonation, rhythm, etc., that may signal specific emotional overlay. It is conceivable that "empathy training" drills, which use such techniques, could be adapted for computer delivery, minimizing the need for trained faculty, who are in short supply.

Considerations of individual learning styles and motivation can sometimes justify the use of an audiovisual approach even when this might seem equivocal from the perspective of aural and visual learning requirements. Some students find that they can learn better through well-designed AVs than through the printed word whether in a textbook or on a CRT display. Among these individuals, listening and visual comprehension (visual literacy) skills seem to be more highly developed and thus more effective as learning channels than traditional reading skills. Although the proportion of such individuals in a given class may be relatively small at present, it is widely believed that the number of such learners may grow as the present generation enters the classroom with a background in which television has replaced reading as a primary source of information and entertainment.

The computer as an instructional delivery vehicle may be selected as the most appropriate medium to teach concepts in which a high level of branching or simulation is needed. High-level branching refers to the process of selecting the next instructional event to be presented from a wide variety of possibilities based on a particular student response or response pattern. Simulation refers to the process of capturing selective models of reality and making them available for student manipulation. The computer's ability to individualize via high-level branching and simulation of complex systems is unique among instructional media. This feature will make the computer increasingly valuable as faculty recognize the necessity for teaching problem-solving and applications skills rather than the rote learning that has characterized so much of the medical school curriculum.

Of course, computers have not yet begun to approach their full potential as instructional resources. The future will surely see the evolution of more and more computer-based educational systems in which the computer will fulfill many administrative and instructional management functions as well as directly mediating instructional encounters with the student. When this feature becomes a reality, the efficiency and effectiveness of many instructional techniques will be enhanced. As the computer is more widely used as a manager of education and as the cost of the hardware continues to plummet, the decision-making process of media selection will alter considerably. Under these circumstances, the cost—benefit of using the computer as the instructional delivery medium may often make CAI the medium of choice, whereas before it would have been totally unjustifiable.

For example, under usual circumstances today, it would be hard to justify using a computer to present a unit of programmed instruction with little or no branching. This could generally be provided to a student much more economically in a printed format. A computer might be justified, however, if the unit were a part of an overall instructional system where it was prescribed (maybe even custom-edited) on the basis of computer-stored response records, or where the student's responses were to be stored for future computer decision-making.

Achieving Synergy with Media and Computers

Ideally, decisions regarding media selection should be made in the context of planning an overall curriculum and using accepted principles of instructional development. But most faculty do not have the luxury of controlling the overall curriculum nor do they have the time or technical expertise to assume these tasks. Thus, with such notable exceptions as Ohio State (Griesen *et al.*, 1971), the University of Illinois at Urbana (Hody, 1974), and a few others, most medical CAI is presently being developed at the level of the individual course or lesson.

In the context of this less-than-ideal situation, many medical school faculty find that they have both computer and audiovisual support available in their institutional setting but are not using either resource to its fullest advantage. Without having elaborate computer-based evaluation, administration, and management systems, it is still possible to achieve a synergistic effect by combining the two types of resources to take advantage of the unique properties of each.

For purposes of discussion, we will think of the relationship between CAI and AV instructional systems as occurring along a continuum with one end being called "computer-enhanced media" and the other "media-enhanced CAI." Although we will focus our discussions on the ends of this spectrum, many applications fall somewhere toward the center.

Computer-Enhanced Media

In this section we will show how the computer can be used to increase the learning effectiveness of what might otherwise be considered as self-contained, non-computer-based learning resources. This concept is often referred to as computer-managed instruction or CMI.

There are two main ways that come to mind for using the computer to enhance planned or existing AV programs — prescription and evaluation. At these levels, the computer can, in some measure, function as the instructor might in an optimum learning setting employing AVs.

Prescription

Functioning as a manager of instruction, the computer can be used to prescribe non-computer-based learning activities such as AVs. At the present time, many existing AVs are unused or are used at a time that is not necessarily best for the individual learner. The computer, while keeping track of the student's progress through the curriculum and other factors that affect his learning, could store information about existing AVs (titles, specific objectives, audience level, etc.). This information could be retrieved in the form of an educational prescription at the time when a given AV would be optimally useful for the individual learner. Thus, the value of the existing audiovisual unit would be substantially enhanced.

Even in the context of a general CAI encounter when there is no elaborate management or record-keeping system, the CAI lesson can be planned to integrate existing off-line AV modules for primary learning or in-depth exploration. At specific response nodes, the student might be directed, in either a forced or optional mode, to sign off temporarily and study an instructional unit that was originally designed as a self-contained package.

Let us consider the example of a hypothetical CAI course on the diagnosis and treatment of congestive heart failure. Most of this hypothetical unit utilizes the computer to mediate instruction consisting of simulations, interactive tutorials, and programmed instruction. Assume that during the course of the CAI unit the student is asked to interpret an X-ray and does so incorrectly. Now, the computer might assess his ability to read radiographs and on the basis of this assessment might prescribe a remedial AV unit on "Interpreting the Chest Film." Depending on the level of the learner and whether he had previously mastered the objectives of the remedial AV unit, he might be directed to complete it before being allowed to proceed with the main instruction on the computer; or given the option of reviewing the AV unit or some specific segments of it.

Some of the possible advantages accruing from the use of the computer-prescribed AV in this situation include: (1) releasing the terminal for other students while the AV is being used; (2) allowing the instructor to focus his developmental efforts on those instructional modalities best handled by the computer, e.g., simulation; and (3) providing a basic instructional resource that fills a curriculum gap (with the understanding that it can later be brought on-line when time and hardware capabilities permit). The AV module becomes significantly more meaningful when prescribed in the context of the curriculum at a time when the learner is likely to be most receptive. At the same time, this use of the AV can provide a mechanism for conserving costly developmental resources.

Evaluation

The computer can further augment the educational value of off-line resources, such as AVs at the level of evaluation. It can be used both for evaluating learner performance and for evaluating the effectiveness of the instructional materials themselves.

In evaluation of learner performance, the computer can be used to give the student intraunit diagnostic feedback so he can determine whether he has grasped a particular point or concept before continuing with the rest of the presentation. The ability of the computer to store and retrieve specific feedback for a wide variety of responses or patterns of responses gives it a significant advantage over a printed evaluation instrument. To accomplish such complex analysis with appropriate feedback with a printed format would be cumbersome at best.

The computer can also be used to perform final or certifying examinations at the end of an AV unit to document satisfactory performance. Its record-keeping function allows the computer to administer and collect evaluation data, whereas its ability to handle complex branching and simulations makes it possible to evaluate high-level learning outcomes such as problem solving.

Use of the computer to evaluate learner performance on AV materials can also provide the author with data on errors and misconceptions. Given feedback on the specific way students respond incorrectly, the author can pinpoint the cause of the erroneous responses and revise the material to increase its effectiveness. In other words, exploiting this formative evaluation potential makes it relatively easy for authors to monitor and "debug" AV materials continuously both during and after developmental testing stages.

Depending on the logistics of AV resources and computer terminals, a number of approaches are possible to interface the off-line AV learning experience with the computer for purposes of evaluation. The easiest way is to have the evaluation of these off-line resources administered by the computer. If there are financial or logistical reasons for not doing this, evaluation data can be collected on paper and later entered into the computer by the student or a clerk. Another approach that is particularly useful for large numbers of students or when batch processing is desired, is to use machine-readable recording formats. These include OpScan form, mark-sense cards, or the outputs (punched tape, punched cards, digitally encoded magnetic tape cassettes, etc.) of the variety of response units that are a part of some of the automated teaching devices with limited response capabilities often referred to as "teaching machines."

Media-Enhanced CAI

Now that we have seen how computers can be used to enhance the educational value of audiovisual-based learning through the prescription and evaluation functions, let us move to the other side of the continuum and see how visual and audio technologies can be used to enhance instruction mediated primarily by the computer.

In this section, we shall iterate the educational rationale for the use of these aural and visual communication channels, take a look at a state-of-the-art computer terminal, and suggest some practical strategies for combining them within the constraints of most existing institutional settings.

Although the term is inexact, we will use the term CAI (computer-assisted instruction) to mean instruction in which the main delivery vehicle is the computer via a CRT or teletype terminal. Such is the case with most computer-based instruction developed in the health sciences to date.

As we discussed earlier, it is all but impossible to teach certain concepts and skills purely through printed messages. Since we cannot learn to distinguish heart sounds or dermatologic lesions simply by reading or listening to verbal descriptions, the developer of a CAI program intended to teach these skills must employ the necessary auxiliary media to accomplish this.

Media-enhanced CAI has great potential for teaching clinical skills requiring aural and visual discrimination. Without audio and visual media as storage and presentation vehicles, learning such skills would have to depend upon laboratory and clinical approaches that are usually too expensive, inefficient, or cumbersome to give every student a systematic experience in making important discriminative judgments. However, the availability of audio and visual media alone is no assurance of systematic coverage. It is in this area that the computer is most valuable. By keeping track of what the student has mastered and using these data to determine subsequent learning experiences, the computer can insure complete coverage in spite of the fact that the various discriminations might have to be practiced through a wide assortment of temporally separate lessons and learning activities.

There are other factors besides the requirements of specific kinds of learning that should lead one to consider using audiovisual media to complement CAI. One such factor, to which we previously alluded, is individual learning style. For example, a "visual learner" might learn much more efficiently if a concept were presented in a pictorial or graphic form instead of a printed page. Another factor is attention span. For example, after 40 minutes of straight CAI on a CRT/keyboard terminal, a 10-minute segment of instruction via AV media may provide sufficient new stimuli to relieve fatigue and eliminate the need for a 10- to 20-minute study break.

Now, let us address the question of how to implement these visual and auditory enhancements for CAI. Ideally, there should be a cheap computer terminal designed specifically for educational use that would be able to access and display at random visual and audio information stored in a central computer or in the terminal itself. Probably the closest thing to this sort of terminal now available is the PLATO IV developed at the University of Illinois under the leadership of Dr. Don Bitzer (Hyatt *et al.*, 1972; Johnson *et al.*, 1971). This terminal uses a device called a plasma screen, which consists of an array of gas-filled cells that emit light when electric voltage is applied. This technology, which has achieved a high quality of resolution with up to 1600 cells per square inch, makes possible a unique kind of display screen. The plasma screen is essentially transparent except where the gas is ignited to form the alphanumeric or graphic display and, when mounted over a rear-projection screen, the plasma screen messages and images can be superimposed over images from a computer-controlled microfiche projector built into the terminal. To date, however, the technology for producing high-resolution fiche images has kept this feature of the terminal from being fully exploited, especially in medical teaching programs.

Another advanced feature of the PLATO terminal is a touchpanel that allows the computer to sense any point on the display that is touched. Other available terminals permit interaction with and manipulation of screen displays by using light pens and joy-sticks, etc. However, PLATO's touchpanel, which uses a photocell array around the periphery of the screen face, is much cheaper, and screen displays can be manipulated merely by the user's finger.

Making use of this capability, the School of Veterinary Medicine at the University of Illinois has projected the picture of a dog on the screen and asked the student to touch the area on the dog where he would like to listen to the heart. The computer senses the area touched by the student and signals an experimental random-access magnetic disk device to play the heart sound from that area. With this sort of terminal available, one can see the possibilities of truly interactive audiovisual learning. The potential educational uses for such a system are limited only by the imagination.

Although the PLATO IV terminal is a remarkable achievement, it still has limitations. It is relatively expensive – five to six thousand dollars per unit – and there are still some technical bugs in the plasma screen and the microfiche system. It also depends upon a rather large and elaborate computer system for support.

It is not necessary, however, to wait until the day when there are inexpensive terminals capable of PLATO's feats and more. There are many approaches, easily within the capacity of most developers of CAI, for the audio and visual enhancement of existing CAI. These approaches vary somewhat depending on the need for random access and on the requirements for such things as static or motion visual display, for audio, or for some combination of these. Since computer-generated speech and graphics are not yet practical for the average developer, they will be considered when we discuss future prospects.

Beginning with the static visual media, one simple approach is to place the AV hardware, such as a slide projector, next to the terminal so that the student may be directed by the computer to a particular visual segment. This requires no special terminal for interfacing equipment. It does have the disadvantage of forcing the student to shift his attention from the lesson material to manipulating equipment. This is made easier if the audiovisual device is equipped with a random-access control, like the Kodak RA 960 carousel slide projector. These machines, however, sell for four to six times the cost of a simple projector. If expense is not a factor, the problem of equipment manipulation can be further simplified if the random-access projector device is directly interfaced with the computer. Commercially available terminals, such as the IBM 1050, do just this and have been used successfully by Harvard Medical School in several applications including histology, pathology, and simulated patient-management problems (Hellerstein, 1972) and by Ohio State as a part of their computer-based evaluation programs in an experimental independent study project (Evans *et al.*, 1972). Students still have to mount the slide trays, etc., but the system works well. Another static visual medium that has been used quite successfully to enhance CAI is the microfiche card reader/projector. This allows the storage of 60 to 100 individual photographs on a single 4 X 6 card and provides good-quality resolution. Thus, a shoebox-sized file can store the same number of slides that would require literally thousands of standard 2 X 2 slide trays. Furthermore, if it is desirable for students to have copies of the microfiche for independent study, they can be made available for around fifty cents each as opposed to 10 or 20 dollars for a comparable set of standard slides.

Microfiche readers are simple to operate, relatively trouble-free, and permit rapid manual random access. Computer-controlled readers are also available and are being used successfully at the University of Washington in Seattle, where several programs have been developed in urology, cardiology, ob-gyn, and other areas using a CRT terminal with a random-access microfiche projector (Lekan, 1970). And, mentioned previously, a computer-controlled microfiche projection system is built into the PLATO terminal. However, although the cards used hold up to 256 images — more than twice the capacity of the standard format — highly specialized and still experimental equipment is required to make and duplicate the microfiche cards, and for many medical applications, the resolution still leaves much to be desired.

In our consideration of static visual media used to enhance CAI, we would be remiss if we did not consider the "paper-based" media, i.e., teaching aids such as actual photographs, X-rays, charts, etc. These can be assembled according to the required content, placed in folders or loose-leaf binders, and stored within easy access of the terminal. This is a convenient, relatively low-cost way of enhancing CAI or tests with visual materials without additional equipment. This works well in low-use situations in which only a few copies are required and random-access and branching requirements are minimal. This method has been used successfully by Ohio State in conjunction with the computer-based testing of their independent study modules. Anatomical and pathological specimens or models may also be used in this manner to provide additional visual or even tactile experiences.

It is particularly advantageous to use these "paper-based" materials in this way during the developmental stages of preparing media-enhanced CAI whose support-ing visuals will ultimately be displayed via electronic or optically projected media. In this flexible form, visuals can be tested with the instruction and then easily rearranged or revised before a final commitment is made to an exact format that may require expensive production. In fact, if the visuals needed to enhance the CAI materials should turn out to be only diagrams, charts, graphs, line illustrations, or black-and-white low-resolution photographic items, it might be well to consider reproducing these on paper (mimeograph, offset, Xerox, etc.) to be used as part of a take-home study guide. Perhaps in this way the need for additional AV hardware at the terminal with all the attendant hassles could be avoided completely and the student provided with a take-home study resource as a bonus.

Enhancing CAI with motion media presents more difficulties given present technologies. Videocassette players offer a somewhat workable solution if not too many segments are involved and random-access requirements are not great. The problem is that because individual segments on the tape are keyed by the counter which measures revolutions of the spool and not the tape footage, starting points are somewhat unreliable. The same is true even with the add-on automatic random-accessing devices used with these machines. This is not the case, however, with conventional open-reel videotape players whose counters indicate footage; these can be relied upon to locate a particular segment of tape more or less exactly.

Let us look at an example of the addition of motion to a CAI program. The student needs experience in analyzing doctor—patient interaction. To provide this experience, several dozen segments are recorded on videotape showing examples of good and poor interviewing techniques.

(Assume this is a natural language, interactive program like CASE — Computer-Assisted Simulation of the Patient Encounter — developed by Harless *et al.*, 1971.)

COMPUTER: NOW WATCH THE FIRST SEGMENT ON THE VIDEOTAPE BEGINNING AT 005. BASED ON THE INTERVIEWING PRINCIPLES YOU HAVE JUST LEARNED, DETERMINE WHAT MAJOR ERROR(S) ARE BEING MADE. WHEN THE SEGMENT IS OVER, STOP THE TAPE AND PRESS "NEXT."

Student views videotape segment illustrating a physician's failure to begin with an open-ended question when interviewing a patient with vague somatic complaints.

STUDENT: "NEXT"
COMPUTER: WHAT WAS WRONG?
STUDENT: PHYSICIAN FAILED TO ESTABLISH RAPPORT WITH PATIENT.
COMPUTER: PERHAPS, BUT THE PROBLEM ILLUSTRATED HERE CAN BE DES-
              CRIBED MORE SPECIFICALLY. TYPE "A" TO TRY ANOTHER
              EXAMPLE OR "B" TO REVIEW THE CHECKLIST OF INTERVIEWING
              PRINCIPLES.
STUDENT: "A"
COMPUTER: VIEW TAPE BEGINNING AT 235. PRESS "NEXT" WHEN READY TO
              MAKE YOUR ANALYSIS.

Student views a second segment similar to the first (beginning at 005).

STUDENT: "NEXT"
COMPUTER: NOW, WHAT DO YOU THINK?
STUDENT: FAILURE TO BEGIN WITH AN OPEN-ENDED QUESTION.
COMPUTER: VERY GOOD! LET'S CONTINUE –

Another kind of motion hardware that lends itself to this application is the 8 mm (or Super 8) film-loop projector. The loop cartridge offers a convenient, relatively inexpensive mechanism for enhancing CAI with individual 5- to 10-minute single-concept motion segments. These would be particularly useful to display short techniques or physical findings requiring motion. However, loop projectors would not be as efficient as videotape, if the instructional branching required random accesses to many short segments. In addition, many of the film-loop systems on the market have had a rather poor track record with regard to equipment failures.

Thus far, we have been discussing visual enhancement of CAI and have considered ways to use various still and motion media, including printed materials. Now we will consider some approaches and problems with using the audio component of AVs with CAI.

One may approach the use of audio playback equipment in much the same way as video devices. For example, an audiocassette player can be placed next to the terminal and the specific segments accessed under the direction of the computer:

COMPUTER: NOW ADVANCE THE TAPE TO 132 ON THE COUNTER AND LISTEN
              TO THE PATIENT'S HEART SOUNDS. THE ANNOUNCER WILL IDEN-
              TIFY THE AREA ON THE CHEST WALL WHICH IS BEING LISTENED
              TO. WHEN YOU'VE COMPLETED THIS SEGMENT (1 AND 2 ON THE
              COUNTER) PRESS "NEXT" TO CONTINUE.

In some circumstances it may be desirable to use computer-directed display of visual elements along with the audio, such as with a synchronous slide–tape program as in this example: The student has completed an off-line, computer-prescribed slide–tape unit on "Pathology of Alcoholic Liver Disease" and has returned to the CAI lesson to continue a clinical simulation.

COMPUTER: THE SLIDE ON THE SCREEN REPRESENTS A SECTION PREPARED
            FROM THIS PATIENT'S LIVER BIOPSY. NAME THE LESION TO WHICH
            THE ARROW IS POINTING.
STUDENT: A BALOON CELL.
COMPUTER: INCORRECT. YOU MAY WANT TO REVIEW SEGMENT II OF S/T UNIT
            #4 ON "PATHOLOGY OF ALCOHOLIC LIVER DISEASE." IF SO, LOAD
            THE UNIT, BRING UP SLIDE #18 AND FASTFORWARD THE CASSETTE
            UNTIL THE COUNTER READS "318."

The student can thus be directed to various segments within such an AV unit by
the computer.

As is the case with motion media, perhaps the biggest stumbling block to the
efficient use of audio with today's AV equipment to enhance CAI is the lack of
rapid random-access capability. This sharply limits the capacity to take advantage
of the computer's branching ability. Virtually all of the media with audiotracks
physically linked to the visual (videotape, sound film) are in linear formats and
cannot be physically manipulated fast enough to make random access really practical. This also applies to audiotape, whether cassette or open reel. And thus, when
used in conjunction with physically separate visuals, such as slide—tape, filmstrip—
tape, or microfiche—tape programs, the limiting factor is not the visual format
but the linear audiotape.

There are some relatively expensive devices on the market that are attempting
to solve this problem. One such device, which solves this problem in a limited way,
is 3M's Sound-On-Slide system in which a circular magnetic tract surrounds a
35 mm slide mounted in the center of a plastic disk. These disks, containing both
the visual and the accompanying audio, can be loaded into a "slide" tray. In effect,
the flexibility of slides is retained while the addition of audio is permitted without
a separate audio device. Drawbacks to this system are its cost and the fact that
only 30 seconds of audio per slide can be accommodated. In addition, there is
no manual control or computer interface for random access to permit easy
retrieval of the individual slide/sound disks for use with branching CAI.

Future Trends

Thus far we have discussed AVs and computer-based learning systems and how,
with present technology, they can be used synergistically for more effective learning. Now, we will look into the future of audio and visual enhancement of CAI.

Admittedly, it is somewhat artificial from an educational point of view to
separate audiovisuals from other instructional resources and methods — that
include standard and programmed texts, three-dimensional anatomical models
and other simulation devices, even lectures and small-group discussions. All of
these media share common characteristics in relation to the computer, which is
evolving not merely as an instructional delivery vehicle but as a manager of all the
various educational processes.

With the rapidly changing technology, the day can be envisioned in the not-too-distant future when many of the issues we have just been discussing will no longer be problems. Decreasing costs and increasing user simplicity of computers and other electronic media may soon obviate the need for peripheral or off-line audio-visual display devices. One of the main elements that has been handicapping the use of computers for instruction is the lack of availability of an inexpensive computer terminal specifically designed for educational use. When all necessary audiovisual images can be stored and retrieved in electronic form, this will do much to facilitate the development of a self-contained electronic educational computer terminal.

There are many signs that point in the direction of this becoming a reality. As microprocessor applications which are rapidly unfolding come into general use, we will continue to see the evolution of standard AV display devices into more sophisticated "teaching machines" until the lines between instruction with these stand-alone devices and computer-based instruction on larger machines become blurred. For some years now there have been on the market AV devices capable of some degree of logical control and branching. These have been largely confined to the still-framed visual media. One example is the Autotutor which uses an optically encoded 35 mm filmstrip and is capable of multiple branching responses. This device, however, is limited by the linear format of the medium and the problems of wear and maintenance associated with mechanical transports and 35 mm film.

A new device recently on the market makes response-controlled random access of motion segments possible. This "teaching machine" by Videonics uses micro-processor technology with a U-matic videocassette machine to allow branching programmed instruction. Again, the limitation of the linear format and the mechanical transport characteristics of the videocassette machine restrict its application.

Although many companies are developing mini and microcomputer stand-alone terminals specifically for instructional purposes, it seems that the incorporation of audiovisuals is lagging behind. The problem has been in finding an efficient and economical way to store and retrieve audio and visual information. The evolution of videodisk technology may help obviate this problem. However, it may be several years before a practical application is realized. At present, the main developers of videodisk technology are planning systems for software mastering and distribution mainly for mass audiences. This will make it difficult, if not impossible, for medical users with limited software needs to tie into these systems.

Other systems under development may eliminate some of the problems related to reproduction costs. One such system uses laser-encoded photographic sheet film that can theoretically be reproduced by conventional photographic techniques. It is said that a 4 X 5 sheet of black-and-white film can be laser-scanned to play back 30 minutes of color-video programming. Hundreds or thousands of these might be stored within an educational terminal or stand-alone device and accessed jukebox style. Holographic cubes, capable of high-density storage, are also being touted as a possibility. Systems like this would make it possible for the computer to use large volumes of stored AV information to select and edit a customized AV program that is based upon individual learner needs and characteristics.

There are still other aspects of the future of computer-based instruction that will broaden our existing concepts of what is possible in the educational experience. There is already on the market a variety of sophisticated (albeit, expensive) graphic terminals capable of feats, such as three-dimensional color display, allowing the manipulation of physical objects stored in memory. These objects can be rotated in space, directed, and viewed from any angle or at any magnification.

It is easy to imagine the medical student of the future peering through his computer terminal window on a "Fantastic Voyage," as in the film by that name. In that movie, scientists in a submarine-like vehicle were shrunk and injected into the bloodstream of a human being. They were then in a position to gain a bacterium's eyeview of the structure and function of various body organs. With an almost limitless degree of freedom a student of the future could move down the alimentary tract, stopping to examine microscopic structure in healthy and diseased tissue, using special-function keys to retrieve labels and didactic instruction, increase magnification, etc.

The learning of basic science concepts could be greatly facilitated by allowing students to interact with dynamic biological models; the student receiving instantaneous graphic feedback (even in three dimensions and color) as he manipulated the variables in a biologic system would achieve a far better understanding of the concepts involved than he would using existing approaches. For example, consider how much more meaningful the concept of bioavailability of drugs might be if a student could see a graphic representation of the bioavailability curves as he manipulated dosages, routes of administration, the introduction of other drugs, the time of day, etc.

There are also some very exciting prospects on the audio side of the technology. Progress is being made with voice-interaction capabilities of the computer. Work at Bell Labs, the University of Florida, and elsewhere is making speech analysis and speech synthesis less and less of a futuristic notion. The day is probably not too far away when the student will be able to conduct a computer-simulated patient interview in natural-language speech while looking at a holographic three-dimensional image of a patient who would appear as if he were actually sitting across the table.

Even sooner, the learner will probably be able to have his choice of the kind of verbal representation he wishes to receive at the terminal: computer-generated speech, or alphanumeric display (electronic or hard copy), or some combination thereof. And with the speech compression/extension technology already available, any voice output could be individually paced by the computer for maximum learning efficiency.

Summary

Within the dramatic growth and development of educational technology in medical education over the past two decades, computers and audiovisual media have weathered some similar maturational storms. In the process, some lessons have been learned about the importance of such things as proper educational planning, curricular integration, and the team approach. And although the diligent application of these lessons may be an end to be devoutly wished for, this may for the moment be somewhat impractical. However, in the context of present realities, it is quite possible for developers of both computer-based education and audiovisual resources to use these companion technologies synergistically, taking advantage of the unique qualities of each. And hopefully, this experience will provide a springboard for these faculty to begin to make some of the conceptual leaps in teaching and learning strategies that will become increasingly necessary to exploit the mind-boggling potential of computer-based education in the future.

References

Bloom, B. (Ed)., 1956. *Taxonomy of Educational Objectives, Handbook 1: Cognitive Domain*, David McKay, New York.

Brooke, M. L., Bell, R. W., and Oppenheimer, M. J., 1974. A team approach to developing an audiovisual, single-concept instructional unit, *The Physiology Teacher* 3(3): 8–13.

Evans, L., Ingersal, R., and Griesen, J. V., 1972. CAI at Ohio State *in* L. Stolurow, T. Peterson, A. Cunningham (Eds.), *Computer Assisted Instruction in the Health Professions*, pp. 31–44, Entelek, Newburyport, Mass.

Gagné. R. M., 1963. *The Conditions of Learning*, Holt, Reinhart and Winston, New York.

Gagné, R. M., and Briggs, L. J., 1974. *Principles of Instructional Design*, Holt, Rinehart and Winston, New York.

Gentry, C. G., and Sachs, S. G., 1976. Michigan State University's new instructional development models, paper presented at the Association for Educational Communications Technology (AECT), Anaheim, Ca.

Greisen, J. V., Beran, R. L., Folk, R. L., and Prior, J. A., 1971. A pilot program for independent study in medical education *in* J. P. Lysaught (Ed.), *Self-Instruction in Medical Education*, University of Rochester, Rochester, N.Y.

Harless, W. G., Drennon, G. C., Marxer, J. J., Root, J. A., and Miller, G. E., 1971. CASE: A computer-aided simulation of the clinical encounter. *J. Med. Educ.* 46: 443–558.

Hellerstein, E. E., 1972. CAI at Harvard *in* L. Stolurow, T. Peterson, A. Cunningham (Eds.), *Computer-Assisted Instruction in the Health Professions*, pp. 21–44, Entelek, Newburyport, Mass.

Hody, G., 1974. A basic science PLATO IV network for medicine and allied health instruction *in Proceedings of the Association for Development of Computer-Based Instructional Systems (ADCIS) Summer Meeting, Billingham, Washington*, ADCIS, Washington, D.C.

Hyatt, G., Eades, D. C., and Tenczar, P., 1972. Computer-based education in biology, *Bio-Science* 22: 401–408.

Johnson, R. L., Bitzer, D. L., Slottow, G. H., 1971. The device characteristics of the plasma display element, *FEEE Transactions on Electronic Devices* 18: 642–649.

Kempe, J. E., 1971. Instructional Design, Fearon Publishers, Belmont, Ca.

Krathwohl, D. R., Bloom, B. S., and Masia, B. B. (Eds.), 1964. *A Taxonomy of Educational Objectives, Handbook II, Affective Domain*, David McKay, New York.

Lekan, H. A. (Ed.), 1970. *Index to Computer-Assisted Instruction*, pp. 83–102, Harcourt Brace Jovanovich, New York.

McMurran, Sterling (Chairman), 1970. *To Improve Learning*, President's Commission on Instructional Technology.

30

Some Nostalgic Reflections on Computer-Assisted Instruction

Charles W. Slack, Douglas Porter, and Warner V. Slack

There is no question that what Norbert Wiener called the "cybernetic revolution" has begun to hit full stride. The computer is now used routinely in many organizations to perform tasks that are difficult and time consuming for its human inventors, and automated data-processing is having an impact on our thought processes analogous to the impact of industrial power tools on our work habits. Although computers have not created unemployment, as many people once feared, there are lingering concerns that humanity will be depersonalized by dependence upon machines.

It is generally true that the less direct experience people have had with any machine the more they tend toward both fear and unreasonable admiration. At one time, many people feared that household appliances would destroy the moral fiber of the housewife, while, in reality, they have helped her achieve new freedom and dignity. In like fashion, admirers of the computer have predicted that it would replace the classroom teacher. In reality, computers will not replace the teacher any more than the power mower has replaced fatherhood.

On the other hand, every machine replaces a human or animal function. Once people dragged their belongings on sticks that slid along the ground. The wheel replaced dragging. Before the invention of dragging sticks, people carried their belongings on their backs. Before the invention of the computer, people performed its functions by hand. There is nothing the computer does that cannot, in principle, be done by human beings. The computer may do it much faster and more reliably, thus allowing for greater — sometimes inestimably greater — total accomplishment, but these accomplishments are made by people assisted by computers, not by computers alone.

The demonstrated usefulness of this remarkably fast and efficient machinery suggests that it has many potential applications. Since computers can solve problems, perhaps they can also teach problem solving. Perhaps the computer, which is

Charles W. Slack, Douglas Porter, and *Warner V. Slack* • Thorndike Laboratory, Department of Medicine, Harvard Medical School and Beth Israel Hospital, Boston, Massachusetts. Supported in part by a grant (HS 00188) from the National Center for Health Services Research, United States Public Health Service. This chapter was freely adapted, in part, from C. W. Slack, 1967b and W. V. Slack and C. W. Slack, 1972.

such a good learner, can also become a good teacher, can help learning become less of a drag, and keep students off the teacher's back.

Can Computers Teach?

To answer this question, bearing in mind that computers and other machines perform human functions, we must first answer the question, can people teach? At first glance, the question seems frivolous, but further investigation reveals one piece of information that is obscured by the pedagogue; it is not the teacher who really does the teaching: it is the information itself, some of which is conveyed by the teacher. Students, on the other hand, are not taught; they learn, on the basis of whatever materials are available (Scheffler, 1965).

Certainly, the presence of another human body is unnecessary to learning as long as the educational content is delivered in some effective manner. We can learn from Plato and Aristotle even though they are dead. Much of the time, in fact, we can learn more from people by reading what they write than by listening to them talk. Recently developed learning materials, which provide for a lot of responding by the learner, indicate that teaching is better defined as the arrangement of information for learning, rather than the physical presence of a human being (Skinner, 1965).

Thus, learning takes place in the presence of information and in the behaving organism. John Dewey (1916) was correct; learning *is* doing and, in general, the more we do, the more we learn. If, with an interactive computer, information could be presented to students in such a way that they could do more and thus learn more, then computer-assisted instruction would be a welcome innovation.

This does not mean that students would be deprived of human interaction. On the contrary, the faster the learning is accomplished, the more time remains for interaction between persons, and that interaction can be enhanced by greater learning. Implicit in this concept is the idea that any function that can better be performed by some automatic medium should be — that it is degrading for a human being to perform any task that a machine can do better. As every student knows, teachers, as human beings, are not at their best while performing routine functions of drill, clerking, and discipline. Our memories of inspiration by fine teachers are largely memories of after-school sessions; only then did the teacher convey a sense of what it all meant. Those rare moments created a nagging demand for more learning, and the demand persisted despite further accomplishment.

Good teachers inspire, counsel, guide, entertain, manage, relate, organize, and provide evidence of the glories of attainment and knowledge. It is materials, on the other hand, that instruct, promote learning, require continual response, and instill Krebs' cycle and the brachial plexus into the student's repertoire of skills. One doesn't learn to read by listening to a teacher read. One doesn't learn to write by watching a teacher write. One may be inspired to imitate the teacher as a shining example, but the mechanics of learning are most efficiently guided by well-written workbooks.

Efficiency is as desirable in education as it is in any other activity. The same content may be displayed to the learner in the pages of a book or on a cathode-ray tube. The computer can store responses electronically and branch contingent upon them to text of particular relevance to an individual student. But in principle, it doesn't matter whether a student responds by writing in a workbook or by typing answers into a computer terminal. Computers cannot teach any more than can teachers. They are, like books, transmission systems that convey information. The medium is not the message, and no learning is possible with a computer unless it is possible without it.

Which of the teacher's functions can the computer replace? At present, teachers take responsibility for seeing to it that materials are placed in the hands of students: in elementary school, teachers pass out the lessons; in medical school, they call the bookstore and put in their orders. These functions can readily be replaced by the computer. No less readily, the computer can record responses and, in many cases, judge correctness. In all cases, the computer can store information about the progress of the learner and make planned decisions as to the sequence of presentation of materials. The teacher counts hands to find how many students think a particular answer is correct. The computer could more efficiently perform this function, and do so on a continual basis, providing further guidance for the student and teacher.

The teacher checks the progress of each student (often while the others must wait) to see whether the student should "go on" or "go back" and relearn. The computer can perform this function in a small fraction of the time, with no waiting on the part of the other students. The teacher tries to discover and remember what errors a student has made and prescribes practice according to the amount of difficulty. The computer can do this in elegant detail, so that the more difficult content can receive more opportunity for practice.

With computer instruction, students can proceed in their own way in private and without embarrassment if they are progressing slowly or making mistakes (Seltzer, 1971). For teachers of good will who are more interested in accomplishment than test scores, there is hope that the bell-shaped curve may be redistributed along with the profits from tests that are used to exclude students rather than help them.

Whether the computer will, in fact, be generally used in the process of education has yet to be determined. Much of the responsibility for any future success will fall on the shoulders of the lesson writers. If the computer is to help students in their quest for information, and we think it will, lesson writers will have to generate good self-instructional materials that effectively use the machine's ability to individualize the dialogue. Unfortunately, such good materials are still scarce. All too often the computer is merely a fancy medium for presenting bad textbooks, page after page, to unwary students who are eager to partake of educational technology. The computer may be the most expensive page-turner in history, but it has yet to successfully replace the oppositional digit of the sixth-grader. Of course, much of this has been said before, many times over many years. With computer-assisted instruction, there has been a tendency for prophecy to substitute for accomplishment. We believe that educators should press on with the task of preparing materials that teach concrete objectives – the specifiable tools with which students want to be prepared. The better informed the students, the better the dialogue with the teachers. Let us find out whether the computer can, in fact, become an effective, economical provider of information.

Can Computers Teach Patients?

Some computer-assisted instruction has been written for student professionals in the health fields, but the patient, who is also in need of assistance, has received little attention. Dialogue between doctor and patient is a time-honored process revered by the medical profession. During conversation with the patient, the doctor can establish rapport, evaluate the patient's ability to engage in productive discussion and collect historical information of clinical relevance. In addition, the doctor can dispense useful information and assess the patient's understanding. Medical interviewing and teaching go hand-in-hand, yet doctors as interviewers are busy, expensive, and sometimes hard to find. They have little time to spend on instructing their patients in matters of health. It seems reasonable, therefore, to consider using computers to serve at least some of the purposes of medical interviewing in widespread and inexpensive ways. (Slack *et al.*, 1966).

Like the student, the patient can interact with the computer by means of a cathode-ray screen and a keyboard that are attached directly to the machine or located remotely as a terminal. The computer communicates with the patient by means of text (questions, explanations, and requests) displayed on the screen, and the patient communicates with the computer by means of the typewriter-like keyboard. Rapport is established by the program with opening statements of welcome. Words of instruction teach patients how to respond with the keyboard. The computer branches to new questions contingent upon responses to previous ones and, in this way, can collect historical information in detail, teach the meaning of concepts not understood, give advice and provide words of encouragement and humor.

Principles of patient–computer interaction have already been applied with some success in efforts to help patients teach themselves about matters of importance to their health (Slack, 1967a; Van Cura *et al.*, 1975; Witschi *et al.*, 1976). We believe that it is important for patients to be encouraged to make their own clinical decisions (Slack, 1972) and to provide more and more medical care for themselves and their families. In the long run, the computer may be of more direct help to the patient than to the doctor, who already benefits (profits) from knowledge that is unavailable to the patient. By helping future patients learn to assume more control over their own medical destinies, computers can help doctors indirectly, by freeing them to engage in more productive dialogue with their patients.

The computer, as a "thinking machine" with its human-like qualities of memory and logic, is challenging our beliefs in human uniqueness. By now doing things that once only people could do, the computer is forcing us to new conceptions of the relationship between man and machine. At one and the same time, the computer provides an opportunity for enhancing human endeavors and gives the humanist a chance to ponder new concepts of uniqueness. Certainly, there is more room for full professorships, journal articles, and books with computers than without them.

References

Dewey, J., 1916. *Democracy and Education. An Introduction to the Philosophy of Education*, pp. 194–197, Macmillan, New York.

Scheffler, I., 1965. *Conditions of Knowledge. An Introduction to Epistemology and Education*, pp. 10–13, Scott Foresman and Company, Glenview, Illinois.

Seltzer, R. A., 1971. Computer-assisted instruction – What it can and cannot do, *Am. Psychol.* 26: 373–377.

Skinner, B. F., 1965. The technology of teaching, *Proc. Roy. Soc. B* 1962: 427–443.

Slack, W. V., 1967a. Computer-based instruction as an adjunct to computer-based medical interviewing, *in Proceedings of the Annual Conference on Engineering in Medicine and Biology, Vol 9*, The Conference Committee for the 20th Annual Conference on Engineering in Medicine and Biology, Boston.

Slack, C. W., 1967b. The truth about computerized instruction, *Educational Technology* Oct. 15: 8–14.

Slack, W. V., 1972. Patient power: A patient-oriented value system *in* John A. Jacquez, (Ed.), *Computer diagnosis and diagnostic methods*, Charles C. Thomas, Springfield, Illinois.

Slack, W. V. and Slack, C. W., 1972. Patient–computer dialogue, *N. Engl. J. Med.* 286: 1304–1309.

Slack, W. V., Hicks, G. P., Reed, C. E. and Van Cura, L. J., 1966. A computer-based medical-history system, *N. Engl. J. Med.* 274: 194–198.

Van Cura, L. J., Jensen, N. M., Greist, J. H., Lewis, W. R. and Frey, S. R., 1975. Venereal disease: Interviewing and teaching by computer, *Am. J. Public Health* 65: 1159–1164.

Witschi, J., Porter, D., Vogel, S., Buxbaum, R., Stare, F. J., and Slack, W. V., 1976. A computer-based dietary counseling system, *J. Am. Dietetic Assoc.* 69: 385–390.

MERIT — An Application of CASE

William G. Harless, Nancy A. Farr, Marcia A. Zier, and John R. Gamble

This appendix is, essentially, a description of an application of CASE (Computer-Aided Simulation of the Clinical Encounter) (Harless *et al.*, 1971), which had its origin at the University of Illinois Medical School and subsequently was moved to The Ohio State University School of Medicine. CASE was developed as a natural-language simulation of a complete patient with a specific health problem (or problems), primarily for use in medical student education. Although this purpose is still being pursued by Ohio State and by other medical schools via the Health Education Network, the simulation shows great promise for evaluation of some dimensions of clinical competence.

Specifically, there has been an intensive effort at Pacific Medical Center in San Francisco to ultilize CASE as a part of the American Board of Internal Medicine (ABIM) recertification procedure. This effort has been financially supported by ABIM through a contract which stated the following project task:

> to conduct a pilot study which utilizes an existing technological development to establish a continuing education–evaluation model which focuses on the real health care delivery situation of the physician and the needs therein. (*Project Proposal to Committee on Recertification*, American Board of Internal Medicine, February 5, 1973, p. 3)

The project, which has assumed the acronym MERIT (Model for Evaluation and Recertification through Individualized Testing), began July 1, 1973. Specifically, the MERIT Project was designed to investigate:

1. An approach to recertification whereby the specific patient problems of each internist will be the basis for the evaluation of his skills, knowledge, and clinical judgment
2. The use of an advanced computer simulation of the physician–patient encounter (CASE) as the examination instrument for the individualized evaluation
3. The development of a scoring system for CASE to assess various dimensions of clinical behavior

William G. Harless, Nancy A. Farr, Marcia A. Zier · University of the Pacific, Forest Grove, Oregon. *John R. Gamble* · University of the Pacific Medical Center, Forest Grove, Oregon.

4. The involvement of each participating internist in an evaluation process which will help him to identify deficiencies and thus allow him to plan for more meaningful individualized continuing education.

5. Attitudes of practicing internists toward a recertification process that embraces the preceding components.

The MERIT evaluation process was first pilot-tested in San Francisco in 1974 with 28 local practicing internists. After continued refinement of the process, MERIT was utilized in a pilot test among 90 practitioners in nine sites throughout Ohio in April, 1976.

Each participating physician maintained a diary of 100 patients seen in his practice so that the CASE exam could be individualized and relevant to the professional demands made on him. The diary data were summarized into an individualized practice profile.

The practice profiles of the internists participating in the two pilot tests established needs for the following types of CASEs which comprise the current MERIT CASE library:

Diagnostic area	Number of CASEs
Infectious Disease	1
Oncology	1
Endocrinology	4
Hematology	2
Mental Disorders	1
Cardiology	6
Pulmonary Disease	3
Gastroenterology	5
Rheumatology	1

The distribution of diagnoses shown above reflects only the primary problems in each CASE. However, like many real patients, many of the CASE patients have health problems in several diagnostic areas.

The three CASEs for each physician's exam are selected from this library to represent, as closely as possible, the types of patient problems seen in his practice. For his exam session, each participant has the option to: (1) type for himself, (2) bring a typist, or (3) request typing help. Having made this choice, he sits at a terminal and is presented with a computerized, interactive orientation to using CASE. Following this, the examinee is presented with a brief description of the three CASEs he will see and chooses his first patient. He is then presented with a paragraph or two describing the clinical setting, some physical characteristics of the patient, and the circumstances of his visit. From this point, the examinee has complete control over the course of the interaction. He conducts an unstructured interview with the patient, asking medical and personal-history questions, and at any time he may request specific physical exam findings and order particular laboratory tests. Excerpts from one participant's interaction with the CASE Al Cole appear in Figure 1.

HISTORY

   IS YOUR FATHER STILL ALIVE?
BOTH OF MY PARENTS ARE STILL LIVING . . .

   HOW IS YOUR FATHER'S HEALTH?
GENERALLY SPEAKING, MY FATHER IS NOT IN VERY GOOD HEALTH. I DON'T
KNOW . . . HE HAD A HEART ATTACK 8 YEARS AGO, AND HE HAS CATARACTS, TOO.
HE ALSO HAS HIGH BLOOD PRESSURE, GOUT, AND DIABETES.

   HOW IS YOUR MOTHER'S HEALTH?
MY MOTHER IS IN GENERALLY GOOD HEALTH EXCEPT THAT SHE HAS PSORIASIS.
SHE HAS HAD IT FOR MANY YEARS.

   ARE THERE ANY OTHER FAMILY MEMBERS WITH DIABETES?
BOTH MY FATHER AND MY PATERNAL GRANDFATHER HAD DIABETES.

   ARE YOU MARRIED?
RITA AND I WERE MARRIED JUST BEFORE I WENT INTO THE ARMY . . . WE'VE BEEN
SEPARATED NOW FOR THREE MONTHS, MAINLY BECAUSE SHE SAYS SHE CAN'T
TAKE MY DRINKING ANYMORE. THERE'S NOT MUCH LEFT OF MY MARRIAGE BUT I
DO CARE ABOUT MY KIDS. IT'S FRUSTRATING TO WATCH THEM GROW UP AND
LEAVE HOME. . . .

   HAVE YOU EVER HAD ANY HEAD INJURIES?
I RAN MY HEAD THROUGH THE WINDSHIELD OF MY CAR WHEN I HAD A WRECK ON
NEW YEAR'S EVE 3 YEARS AGO. I DIDN'T HAVE A CONCUSSION OR HEAD INJURY
EXCEPT FOR CUTTING UP MY FACE. I HAD PLASTIC SURGERY TO TAKE CARE OF
THE SCARS AROUND MY EYE. . . .

   DO YOU HAVE ANY PROBLEM WITH YOUR VISION?
I'M EXTREMELY NEARSIGHTED. IT'S SO BAD, IN FACT, THAT I ALMOST DIDN'T
GET INTO THE ARMY . . . THEY LET ME IN, THOUGH.
            (CONTINUED AT PHYSICIAN DISCRETION)

PHYSICAL EXAMINATION
   GENERAL APPEARANCE
THE PATIENT IS SHORT, OBESE, ACNE-SCARRED AND HAS A MELANCHOLY
APPEARANCE. HE IS IN NO ACUTE DISTRESS.

   ABDOMEN
ABDOMEN (INSPECTION) – INCREASED GIRTH, DISTENDED WITH SLIGHT FLANK
BULGING. DILATED VEINS VISIBLE, DISTENDED WITH NORMAL FLOW PATTERN. A
WELL-HEALED 6 CM. SCAR IN RIGHT LOWER QUADRANT. NO OTHER ABNORMALI-
TIES.

   PALPATE ABDOMEN
ABDOMEN (PALPATION) – MINIMAL ABDOMINAL TENDERNESS WITH NON-
LOCALIZED REBOUND. NO MASSES FELT. PALPABLE FLUID WAVES PRESENT.
SPLEEN, KIDNEYS NOT PALPABLE. LIVER PALPABLE 3 FINGER BREADTHS BELOW
RIGHT COSTAL MARGIN. NO EVIDENCE OF HERNIA.
            (CONTINUED AT PHYSICIAN DISCRETION)

LABORATORY
   FASTING BLOOD SUGAR
FASTING BLOOD SUGAR: 160 MG/100 ML

BUN
BLOOD UREA NITROGEN: 40 MG/100 ML

GASTROSCOPY
GASTROSCOPY: DIFFUSE GASTRIC INFLAMMATION AND SUPERFICIAL ULCERA-
TIONS. NO EVIDENCE OF ACTIVE ULCER. NO EVIDENCE OF ESOPHAGEAL VARICIES
OR MUCOSAL TEARS.

GASTRIC ASPIRATION
GASTRIC ASPIRATION: BRIGHT RED BLOOD
(CONTINUED AT PHYSICIAN DISCRETION)

Figure 1. Excerpts from a physician's interaction with Al Cole.

After acquiring sufficient information about the patient, the physician may
proceed to the diagnosis and management phase of the CASE. First, he provides
his diagnoses; then he describes his short-term management plan, including medications, procedures, referrals, and instructions to the patient.

The scoring of the CASE exam is designed to provide the Board with data for decisions about recertification and to provide the individual examinee with information
about his performance that will be useful to him in planning continuing education.

Detailed feedback and summary scores are provided to the Board and to the
examinee reflecting his diagnostic correctness, the appropriateness of his management plan, his thoroughness and efficiency throughout the entire CASE, and a
danger-and-discomfort index which reflects the number and severity of any contra-
indicated procedures he ordered or performed.

A great majority of the participants in the two field tests have had a satisfying
exam experience. The average appropriate response rate for the two field tests in
each CASE was between 90% and 96%. This means that in the average interaction
with a CASE, the computerized patient responded appropriately to 90%–96% of
the physician's inquiries.

The average length of time required to complete the exam comprised of three
CASEs is just over 3 hours. A postexam questionnaire regarding the examinees'
reactions revealed 91% of the participants rated the CASE simulation as an appropriate and desirable testing mechanism for recertification, 93% felt the CASEs in
their exam were representative of the patients in their practice, and 84% felt their
performance with the CASEs was similar to their behavior with actual patients.

A representative sample of medical records has been audited during the two
field tests to determine the similarity of behavior of a physician while dealing with
actual patients with a particular diagnosis, and with the computerized patients
(having the same diagnosis) which comprised his exam. The results of the comparison show a high degree of similarity in terms of the kind of information gathered
and management plans offered.

The Future of MERIT

Negotiations are currently underway to develop a plan whereby the MERIT
process, which includes access to the CASE system, can be managed by the office

of the Director of Evaluation of ABIM and integrated into the recertification process.

Many of the unique and promising aspects of the MERIT process stem from (1) the capabilities of CASE to respond to natural-language inquiries and, therefore, allow a candidate to be assessed according to the things *he* determines to be important in making clinical decisions about a patient; and (2) a generating system (GENESYS) which allows relatively rapid creation of CASEs representing a wide variety of patients with varying disease situations. Two papers have been published in *Computers in Biology and Medicine* that provide detailed descriptions of CASE as a natural-language model and GENESYS as a system to create CASEs (Harless *et al.*, 1973a, b).

References

Harless, W. G., Drennon, G. G., Marxer, J. J., Root, J. A., and Miller, G. E., 1971. CASE: A computer-aided simulation of the clinical encounter, *J. Med. Educ.* **46**:443.

Harless, W. G., Drennon, G. G., Marxer, J. J., Root, J. A., Wilson, L. L., and Miller, G. E., 1973a. GENESYS – A generating system for the CASE natural language model, *Comput. Biol. Med.* **3**:247–268.

Harless, W. G., Drennon, G. G., Marxer, J. J., Root, J. A., Wilson, L. L., and Miller, G. E., 1973b. CASE – A natural language computer model, *Comput. Biol. Med.* **3**:227–246.

Evaluation of the Experimental CAI Network (1973–1975) of the Lister Hill National Center for Biomedical Communications, National Library of Medicine

Martin L. Rubin, Beverly Hunter, and Marilyn Knetsch

[*Editor's Note*: During the course of the Lister Hill Center's Experimental CAI Network project (detailed in Chapter 8) the Human Resources Research Organization was asked to perform an evaluation of the Network. The report of that work was submitted to the Lister Hill Center at the National Library of Medicine in January, 1975, entitled the same as this chapter. Here, we present excerpts from that report, in particular the *Introduction* and *Chapter II, Impact of The Network Experiment*. The Introduction includes a listing of the several categories evaluated. The complete report may, of course, be obtained for further perusal.]

Introduction

Purpose of the Study

This report, undertaken by the Human Resources Research Organization in May, 1974, summarizes the findings of the evaluation of the Lister Hill Center Experimental Computer-Assisted Instruction (CAI) Network (referred to in this report as the "Network Experiment"). The purposes of the study were to describe and analyze the impact and experience of the Network Experiment in ways that would assist decision makers in planning future mechanisms for distributing biomedical CAI, and to identify additional research and development needs.

This report is addressed not only to the sponsors and participants of the Network Experiment, but also to educators and technologists who have an interest in sharing learning resources through technology-based distribution systems. Much of what was learned in the biomedical Network Experiment has general applicability to other educational networking efforts and attempts to share CAI materials.

Martin L. Rubin, Beverly Hunter, and Marilyn Knetsch · Human Resources Research Organization, Alexandria, Virginia.

Description of the Network

The Lister Hill Center Experimental CAI Network was established in July, 1972. Its purpose was to test the feasibility of sharing CAI learning materials through a national computer network.

Soon after the establishment of the Lister Hill Center, Dr. Martin M. Cummings, Director of the National Library of Medicine, asked the American Association of Medical Colleges (AAMC) to take a leadership position in involving the academic medical community in Network plans. A conference was held in February, 1969 to consider the educational services that a network might provide (Smythe, 1969). Subsequent to this conference, the AAMC was asked to recommend more specific plans, which resulted in the production of a report from the Steering Committee, Council of Academic Societies, Association of American Medical Colleges (Stead *et al.*, 1971). This report covered the state-of-the-art of instructional technology, the need for a biomedical community network, factors governing selection of materials, organization and administration, evaluation, and staff. The Steering Committee report included many recommendations, one of which is covered in the following statement:

> The Steering Committee advocates the organization of a biomedical communications network designed to meet some of the needs of medical education and medical practice and to capitalize on the current state of development of various phases of communications and computer technology. Of primary importance is the requirement to maintain a high level of learning experiences for growing numbers of students to whom medical, dental, nursing and other health career schools are committed.

The AAMC report was presented to members of the Board of Regents of the National Library of Medicine. The Board appointed a Priorities Review Committee to study the report. This committee presented four recommendations which were adopted unanimously by the Board of Regents. One of the four recommendations read:

> The Committee advocates the organization of a biomedical communications network fundamentally conceived as providing the mechanism by means of which interinstitutional cooperation and sharing of resources will *be used to meet some of the needs* of medical education. Implementation of this goal began in September 1971.

The original Network was based on four contracts with the National Library of Medicine (NLM): one with a commercial time-sharing service and three with institutional centers having CAI expertise. The three institutions are Massachusetts General Hospital, the University of Illinois Medical Center, and Ohio State University College of Medicine.

Course material from Massachusetts General Hospital (MGH) is primarily intended for supplemental use by medical students and physicians involved in continuing education and contains programs in Abdominal Pain, Coma, and Jaundice, among others. The University of Illinois Medical Center

(UIMC)* offered two types of material: (a) a computerized random item bank (CRIB) and (b) a computer-aided simulation of the clinical encounter (CASE). The programs from Ohio State University College of Medicine (OSU) cover a broad spectrum of health problems and were written for many different educational levels (Wooster and Lewis, 1973).

The purpose of the Network Experiment was not to establish an operational distribution mechanism for CAI libraries, but rather, to provide an experiential setting for evaluating the new medium and the problems and prospects for national distribution. Formal NLM support for the Network itself is programmed to terminate in May, 1975.

Description of the Evaluation Study

The focus of the Network Evaluation Study is on the institutions and people who use the Network. Information was gathered from four main sources:

1. Field trips to selected user and contractor institutions to interview administrators, faculty, library and media center personnel, and students.
2. Bimonthly reports to the Lister Hill Center from user institutions. These reports address a wide range of technical, educational, financial, and administrative matters which were encountered in the Network Experiment.
3. Data from contractors on CAI program usage by user institutions.
4. Meetings of the Health Education Network Users' Group (HENUG) of the Association for Development of Computer-Based Instructional Systems (ADCIS).

The information gathered from these sources was interpreted and organized into several categories of study. This report is organized around the following categories:

Impact of the Network Experiment on users
    Institutions
    Curricula
    Faculty
    Students
    Libraries and media centers
Institutional variables affecting utilization of network
Evaluation of CAI materials
Cost/benefit analysis
What was learned from the Network Experience
    Materials
    Development of materials

---

*The University of Illinois withdrew from the Network Experiment in February 1974. Its CRIB system was not considered to be a cost-effective use of computers. The CASE system, however, was transferred to the Ohio State University computer.

Distribution mechanisms
Evaluation methods
Functional requirements of a CAI distribution system
User tailoring
Feedback-revision process
Support services
User documentation
Peer review
People networks
Recommendations for future distribution mechanisms

Impact of the Network Experiment

Qualitative and quantitative indicators of the impact of the Network Experiment or users are organized into five categories:

Institutions
Curricula
Faculty
Students
Libraries and media centers

Impact on Institutions

A total of 95 institutions had participated at some time in the Network Experiment as of October 1, 1974. A breakdown by type of institution follows:

Medical schools	65
Teaching hospitals	9
Research institutes and associations	7
Health science centers	2
Continuing education centers	5
Schools of dentistry	2
Schools of nursing	2
Other	2
Total	95

Fifty institutions have participated in the Network Experiment for a year or longer; 21 institutions participated for 3 months or less, and then dropped out. As of December, 1974, there were approximately 65 active institutional Network users.

At the beginning of the Network Experiment, users were designated "trial" or "operational," with operational users having greater responsibility to contribute evaluative data. It was also anticipated that operational users would contribute to the network CAI library. This designation was dropped in February, 1974 when usage charges were initiated.

Dr. Harold Wooster and Ms. Jinnet Lewis of the Lister Hill Center conducted a statistical analysis of the significance of the presence of an Office of Medical Education on the incidence of institutional participation in the Network Experiment (Wooster and Lewis, 1974). Using a chi-square analysis, they found that institutions that have an Office of Medical Education were much more likely to participate in the Network Experiment. Of the three components of a medical institution (i.e., education, research, and service), it is presumed that the presence of an Office of Medical Education is an indication of the degree of emphasis placed on the educational component. It also means that there is an individual with the time and interest to help investigate and nurture a new learning modality.

The participating institutions varied widely in the extent to which they used the Network. (See Table 1 for lists of Network users and dates and amount of time used.)

By August, 1974, Network users had logged a total of 11,090 hours on the Ohio State University (OSU) system. Of the 72 institutions which have used OSU's system, six institutions accounted for approximately 60% of the usage hours: University of California at Los Angeles (UCLA), University of Washington, George Washington University, University of Oregon School of Nursing, University of the Pacific, and Fort Worth Osteopathic Hospital. Twenty of the institutions using Ohio State's program library used a total of less than 10 hours each.

By August, 1974, Network users had logged a total of 21,220 hours on the Massachusetts General Hospital (MGH) system. Of the 90 institutions which have used the system, six of them accounted for 37% of the total usage hours: UCLA, University of Pennsylvania, Harvard, Medical College of Virginia, University of Arizona, and George Washington University.

By February, 1974, when the University of Illinois Medical College (UIMC) left the Network, Network users had logged a total of 5144 hours on the UIMC system. Of the 63 institutions which used the system, six of them accounted for 54% of the total usage hours: UCLA, University of Pennsylvania, Medical College of Virginia, University of Texas at San Antonio and Galveston, and Stanford University. Twenty-four institutions used the UIMC materials for a total of less than 10 hours each.

Most institutions made some modifications to the physical plant in order to accommodate the computer terminals. Study carrels were built in media labs and libraries. Most large institutional users built or designed special facilities to house the computer terminal. At UCLA, special soundproof rooms were constructed so that students working in small groups would not disturb other library users. Stanford University had a unique CAI study area. The terminal was located in the Media Center, in front of a comfortable couch where small groups of students could easily work together. The terminal was connected to a large video display monitor which provided a large screen image of the text. The typical Lister Hill user had one terminal but some of the larger users had as many as four terminals.

Table 1. Summary of Network Use

| User | Usage period | | Time used | | Mean hours/ month usage |
	Start	Continuing[a], or ending date[b]	Months[c]	Hours	
Alabama, Univ. of–School of Medicine, Birmingham	11/72	C	22	483.9	22.0
Albany Medical College of Union University, Albany, N.Y.	4/73	C	17	546.5	32.2
American Academy of Ortho- pedic Surgeons, Chicago, Ill.	6/74	7/74	2	8	4
American College of Radiology, Boston, Mass.	3/73	C	2	38.2	19.1
American Heart Association, Brookline, Mass.	11/72	12/72	2	5/5	2.7
Arizona, Univ. of – Arizona Medical Center, Tucson	10/73	C	11	1264.2	114.9
Augusta General Hospital, Augusta, Me.	11/72	12/73	14	72.5	5.2
Baylor Univ., Waco, Tex.	11/72	12/72	2	3.1	1.5
Beth Israel Hospital, Boston, Mass.	1/73	9/73	9	93.0	10.3
Bird, Kenneth T., M.D., Massachusetts General Hospital, Boston	4/74	C	3	18.4	6.1
Boston Univ. Medical Center, University Hospital	1/73	5/74	11	24.5	2.2
Brown Univ., Providence, R.I.	2/73	C	7	167.2	23.9
CAPO (Bolt, Beranek, and Newman)	11/72	12/72	2	4.4	2.2
California, Univ. of, Davis	11/72	C	20	328.1	16.4
California, Univ. of, Los Angeles	11/72	C	22	3235.1	147.1
California, Univ. of – Los Angeles, Cedars–Sinai Medical Center	1/74	C	8	40.1	5.0
California, Univ. of – Los Angeles, Harbor General Hospital	1/74	C	8	112.0	14.0
California, Univ. of, San Diego	6/73	C	15	162.5	10.8
Case Western Reserve Univ., Cleveland, O.	1/73	C	19	682.2	35.9
CBX Project, National Board of Medical Examiners	11/72	10/73	12	318.6	26.6
Chicago, Univ. of	8/73	9/73	2	19.8	9.9
Cincinnati, Univ. of	4/74	6/74	3	1.4	.5
Columbia Univ., New York – College of Physicians and Surgeons, Medical Library	5/73	C	16	461.8	28.9
Columbia Univ., New York – College of Physicians and Surgeons, Dept. of Pathology	3/73	C	13	186.1	14.3

Connecticut, Univ. of – Health Center, Farmington	5/73	C	16	621.8	38.9
Emergency Medical System Medical Group, Palo Alto, Calif.	9/73	6/74	5	23.6	4.7
Florida, Univ. of – J. Hilli Miller Health Center, College of Dentistry, Gainesville	6/73	1/74	8	39.1	4.9
Fort Worth (Texas) Osteopathic Hospital	4/73	C	17	611.9	36.0
George Washington Univ., Washington, D.C.	11/72	C	22	1513.4	68.8
Georgia, Medical College of Augusta	12/72	12/73	13	278.2	21.4
Hahnemann Medical College of Philadelphia	9/73	C	12	665.7	55.5
Harvard Medical School – Francis A. Countway Library of Medicine, Boston, Mass.	11/72	C	23	1599.5	69.5
Howard Univ., Washington, D.C.	7/73	C	14	131.8	9.4
Kentucky, Univ. of, Lexington	11/72	2/74	16	29.8	1.9
Loma Linda Univ., Loma Linda, Calif.	9/73	C	6	70.9	11.8
Los Angeles County (Calif.) Medical Association	12/72	1/74	14	115.3	8.2
Louisville (Ky.), Univ. of – Health Sciences Center	4/73	10/73	4	9.8	2.5
Maryland, Univ. of – School of Medicine, Baltimore, Md.	2/73	C	19	296.1	15.6
Massachusetts General Hospital, Boston, Mass.	8/73	C	11	40.4	3.7
Massachusetts General Hospital – Continuing Education	10/73	C	11	549.4	50.0
Massachusetts, Univ. of, Boston	6/74	C	3	13.2	4.4
Matthew Thornton Health Plan, Nashua, N.H.	1/73	6/74	18	73.0	4.1
Mayo Foundation, Rochester, Minn.	11/72	8/73	10	142.5	14.3
McGill Univ., Montreal, Canada	9/73	12/73	4	104.5	26.1
Michigan State Univ., East Lansing	11/72	C	22	327.2	14.9
Michigan, Univ. of – School of Nursing, Ann Arbor	3/73	C	18	154.8	8.6
Michigan, Univ. of –School of Dentistry, Ann Arbor	5/73	8/73	4	23.1	5.8
National Institutes of Health, Clinical Center, Bethesda, Md.	1/73	6/73	3	25.4	8.5
National Library of Medicine, Lister Hill Center	11/72	C	22	167.1	7.6
Naval Medical Research Institute, National Naval Medical Center, Bethesda, Md.	11/72	C	23	125.2	5.4
Nebraska, Univ. of, Medical Center, Omaha	11/72	C	22	226.8	10.3
New England Deaconess Hospital, Boston	11/72	C	22	146.7	6.7

Table 1 (*continued*)

User	Usage period		Time used		Mean hours/ month usage
	Start	Continuing[a], or ending date[b]	Months[c]	Hours	
New York, State Univ. of, Buffalo	4/73	C	15	228.5	15.23
New York, State Univ. of – Children's Hospital, Buffalo	8/74	C	1	2.2	2.2
New York, State Univ. of, Downstate Medical Center, Brooklyn	11/72	C	22	927.9	42.2
New York, State Univ. of, Stony Brook	11/72	C	22	152.7	6.9
New York, State Univ. of, Upstate Medical Center, Syracuse	11/72	C	22	407.7	18.5
Northwestern Univ., Chicago	11/72	1/74	15	573.3	38.2
Ohio, Medical College of, Athens	11/72	12/72	2	1.3	.7
Ohio State Univ., Medical School, Columbus	11/72	C	17	36.5	2.2
Oklahoma Univ., Norman	5/74	5/74	1	45.2	45.2
Oregon, Univ. of – School of Medicine and School of Nursing, Portland	3/73	C	14	1117.4	79.8
Pacific, Univ. of – Pacific Medical Center, San Francisco	2/74	C	7	28.7	4.1
Pennsylvania, Medical College of, Philadelphia	3/74	C	88	44.6	5.6
Pennsylvania, Univ. of – School of Medicine, Philadelphia	11/72	C	22	2583.7	117.5
Pittsburgh, Univ. of – School of Medicine, Eye and Ear Hospital	3/72	C	18	517.4	28.7
RAND Corporation, Santa Monica, Calif.	3/74	5/74	3	8.3	2.8
Rochester, Univ. of, Rochester, N.Y.	11/72	1/74	15	391.1	26.1
Rush Medical College, Chicago	4/73	8/73	5	83.7	16.7
Rutgers Univ., New Brunswick, N.J.	5/74	C	4	27.7	6.9
South Carolina, Medical Univ. of, Charleston	5/73	C	16	654.6	40.9
Southern California Univ. of, Los Angeles	11/72	1/74	15	531.2	35.4
Southern Illinois Univ., Carbondale	5/73	C	16	530.2	33.1
Stanford Univ. – School of Medicine, Stanford, Calif.	11/72	C	22	1033.0	46.9
Texas College of Osteopathic Medicine, Fort Worth	8/73	C	13	466.0	35.7
Texas Tech Univ., Lubbock	10/73	12/73	3	16.0	5.3

Texas, Univ. of, San Antonio	11/72	C	22	1121.1	51.0
Texas, Univ. of, Galveston	3/73	1/74	11	317.4	28.9
Texas, Univ. of, Houston	9/73	1/74	5	162.4	32.5
Texas, Univ. of – Southwestern Medical School, Dallas, Tex.	11/72	1/74	16	517.4	32.3
Tufts Univ., Medford, Mass.	5/73	C	16	170.8	10.7
Utah, Univ. of, Salt Lake City	1/73	C	18	389.1	21.6
Vanderbilt Univ., Nashville Tenn.	6/73	8/73	3	17.1	5.7
Virginia Commonwealth Univ. – Medical College of Virginia, Richmond	1/73	7/74	19	1913.2	100.7
Washington Hospital Center, Washington, D.C.	11/72	C	22	335.5	15.3
Washington Univ., St. Louis, Mo.	11/72	C	22	961.6	43.7
Washington, Univ. of, Seattle	11/72	C	22	3662.2	166.4
Wayne State Univ., Detroit, Mich.	3/73	4/73	2	64.9	32.5
Wisconsin, Medical College of, Milwaukee	1/73	C	18	473.6	26.3
Wisconsin, Univ. of, Madison	6/74	C	3	4.3	1.4

[a]Continuing participants are indicated by a C.
[b]Cut-off date for data analyzed is August 31, 1974.
[c]Based on number of months of actual usage rather than a straight calculation of start and end dates. If there were three or more consecutive months of nonusage, these were not counted.

The University of Connecticut's School of Medicine has adopted the portable terminal concept in addition to having several terminals within their center. In the short time that these terminals have been in use, they have become very popular. There have been recent requests by physicians to borrow a terminal for trial use in their offices.

The user institution's Network funds came from outside sources, such as grants, donations, and special funds. In some cases support came from funds from the dean's office but not from the operational departmental budgets. Institutions were required to pay for their own terminals. Many schools purchased the terminals since they were a relatively small, one-time cost. The schools also were required to pay the local charges for linking into the nearest TYMSHARE communications node. If the school was at some distance from the nearest node, phone charges for this hook-up could amount to as much as $1000/month. However, if the institution was in a TYMSHARE node city such as Los Angeles, there were no local phone charges.

Initially, the Network service itself was free to users. It was later decided to have Network users pay an increasing portion of the cost. The initial charge was $2.50/ hour as of February, 1974. In July, 1974, the charge was raised to $5.00/hour. Since total Network costs range between $16 and $20 an hour, depending on total usage, Lister Hill is still subsidizing the major portion of the Network cost.

While the Network provided an entirely new learning modality to many user institutions, it did not affect the overall educational philosophy and program as much as could have been anticipated. Although the learning resource was much in demand, it failed to stimulate any broad curriculum reform.

However, the CAI Network utilization did benefit greatly from curricular reforms and educational innovations that were already in place in many user institutions. Many of the user institutions had previously shifted from a high lecture orientation to a high emphasis on self-directed study. These institutions had excellent facilities for self-directed learning, and were anxious to provide still another modality in addition to videocassettes, audiotapes, heart-sound synthesizers, and other devices.

Institutions with a traditional lecture-oriented, lock-step curriculum reported difficulty in scheduling CAI usage. The computer tutorials were in no case used as final examinations. Therefore, the utilization of CAI did not have any effect on established procedures for grading.

The Network Experience has exposed administrators, faculty, staff, and students to the possibilities of the computer as a learning medium. When individual institutions made a decision to terminate Network involvement, students invariably were vociferous in their objections to losing this learning tool.

Faced with the termination of the experimental Network in May, 1975, faculty members have been asked to review their thinking and to establish long-term policies toward this new media. However, only a few schools have made firm alternative plans for continuing CAI without the availability of the national Network. Many of them hesitate to make the heavy capital outlay for equipment and staff required to run their own facility.

Some institutions are developing network substitutes. The University of Washington is working with the University of California at Davis on the use of a Meta compiler to translate their WISP COURSEWRITER programs to a language of the PDP-10 which is on order. George Washington University has acquired a mini-computer system and is gradually translating some programs in the CAI library to that system.

Impact on Curricula

The CAI materials were used, with few exceptions, as a supplementary learning resource. While the CAI learning materials were perceived by both faculty and students to be a valuable educational addition, as measured by student usage and opinion surveys, they did not bring about any major changes in course objectives or content. The CAI materials served mainly as enrichment, or supplements, to their regular programs. Third-year and fourth-year students had an opportunity to diagnose medical problems in coma, jaundice, abdominal pain, diabetes, heart irregularities, and other diseases. Computer simulations guarantee that students will "see" a large variety of cases with different symptoms and prognoses.

At the University of Pennsylvania the discussion of the CAI clinical diagnostic exercises was a major component of a course on the introduction to clinical medicine. These programs enabled the students to develop problem-solving skills in a way not possible in the traditional "making-the-rounds" with a faculty member.

While the CAI programs do not supplant the rounds-making experience, they have demonstrated their ability to augment this method.*

Most student usage of the CAI library was strictly voluntary. That is, on their own initiative they sought the use of the CAI library. (This practice supports the fact that students are highly goal-oriented and self-motivated by the time they reach medical school.)

Ohio State's tutorial learning units are most effectively used in conjunction with specific courses. Many of the CAI learning modules, when used in conjunction with textbooks, could substitute for lectures. However, few institutions revised curricula to make use of the OSU materials in this way. At the Medical College of Wisconsin, a series of Ohio State's anatomy modules was made an integral component of the gross anatomy course unit.

In summary, the CAI library was used (a) as an augmentation of clinical experience, (b) as a self-assessment tool in basic science subjects, and (c) as a supplement to regular coursework.

Impact on Faculty

Demonstrations were carried out in over a hundred institutions, at which time faculty had an opportunity to try out the learning materials. Many of the faculty members were so intrigued that they spent hours at the terminal going through the materials. While they were quick to point out deficiencies, they generally reported favorably on overall quality.

Ohio State requested that its users evaluate the suitability of its learning modules prior to initiating use. The college counseled the user institution to establish faculty committees to review learning objectives of the learning units. Therefore, many faculty members were brought in on some aspect of the program even though they were not active creators of CAI materials.

As a condition for receiving use of the Network facilities, user institutions were asked by the Lister Hill Center to prepare CAI materials to be added to the library. The medical school faculty was expected to develop these materials. It was hoped that they would become involved with the total process. However, the faculty at most institutions maintained a hands-off attitude toward CAI. They generally endorsed the idea of using the learning resource but left it up to the students as to how they would use it.

In many of the schools that were the largest users (e.g., UCLA and Stanford), faculty members were not interested in becoming CAI developers, since research was their primary interest.

Only in the final year of the experiment has an interest developed in authoring materials. Ohio State University has worked closely with the University of

---

*A future direction may be the development of a clinical core curriculum which is performance-based (i.e., the student's ability to diagnose and treat medical problems is measured) and uses the computer as a major educational tool.

Pittsburgh Eye and Ear Hospital to develop learning units on diseases of the eye. CAI course content is being developed at the University of Pittsburgh, and the programming is taking place at Ohio State. In December, 1974, Ohio State University reported that a total of 53 instructional units were being developed by Lister Hill Network users.

The Network Experiment did not provide funds for faculty release time to perform development activities such as authoring course materials or devising new computer-oriented curricula. These activities are extremely time consuming and, in addition, require specialized computer skills. Therefore, the lack of faculty involvement was not surprising.

Typical faculty attitudes regarding the Network Experiment and CAI materials are reflected in the following excerpts from copies of the Bimonthly User Report:

> Demonstrations to faculty have, for the most part, been met with varying degrees of interest but as yet little commitment. However, there has been one encouraging development. A neurologist, the chairman of the second year Neural Sciences Group, who has been a leader here in innovative teaching, is prepared to utilize CAI heavily in his course. Since he plans the development of a modular sequence of course topics with student self-pacing, he would like to use a program such as UIMC's CRIB to store a large number of test items which students could use both to monitor their own progress through material and approach as a criterion test at the completion of each course module.
>
> *Letter from Paul L. Grover, Jr., PhD., Assistant Professor, Division of Medical Education and Communication, University of Rochester, School of Medicine and Dentistry, March 6, 1973*

> Most faculty members agree that time is the greatest factor in *requiring* use of CAI. With the present curriculum load for first- and second-year students, it is difficult to find a block of time to take advantage of those programs considered valuable. There have been few who have found no merit in the system at all, and the verbal consensus of the faculty seems to be in favor of a teaching tool so well accepted by the students.
>
> *Texas College of Osteopathic Medicine, Experimental Network Users Report, March 1, 1974, for the period January 1–February 28, 1974*

> Although thirty of these letters were sent out, unfortunately the faculty response has been poor and the materials have only been demonstrated to approximately ten faculty members.
>
> *Letter from Robert F. Johnston, M.D., Director, Division of Pulmonary Diseases, The Hahnemann Medical College and Hospital of Philadelphia, November 6, 1973*

> Faculty usage has declined as most have had one or more demonstrations. Several instructors have returned to the terminal on their own and it is this group that I hope to interest in more substantive CAI input.
>
> *Trial Users Report from Marilyn Margon, Staff Development Specialist, Department of Educational Resources and Development,*

Southern Illinois University, School of Medicine, December 26, 1973

Up to this time we have interviewed all faculty . . . users of the programs.

The Pharmacology faculty has indicated that, in their view, several of the MGH programs provide an excellent means of bridging the disciplines of pharmacology and therapeutics.

Introduction to the Patient (Physical Diagnosis): the faculty has expressed some interest in considering UIMC CASE as a means of introducing students to the experience of interviewing patients.

Faculty of the Department of Medicine concerned with the clinical clerkships and third- and fourth-year electives are enthusiastic about the capability of the programs to instruct the students in the approach to the management of disease processes (MGH programs).

College of Physicians and Surgeons of Columbia University, August 3, 1973, Report on use from Norman Kahn, D.D.S., PhD., Pharmacology and J. Thomas Bigger, Jr., Associate Professor of Medicine and Pharmacology

Impact on Students

Network materials received the most usage from students, usually on their own initiative. It was evident from this heavy continuing use that students perceived the learning experience to be important.

Some user institutions attempted to keep data on number and types of students using the resource, but had difficulty getting users to complete survey forms. Data on system usage, however, are available from the contractors. Massachusetts General Hospital was the only Network node which gathered usage data by type of student. The Massachusetts General data cannot indicate how many students used its system, since individual students did not have unique identifiers. Its data show how many times a particular category of student used the programs.

Table 2 shows the usage time of the Massachusetts General Hospital system, by class of user at UCLA and Stanford, two major user institutions.

No provision was made in the Network Experiment for a systematic assessment of the impact of the materials on student learning. Each user institution was expected to provide its own evaluation of the materials and their use. However, only a few institutions were able to complete any kind of systematic study. Furthermore, each institution that performed some kind of study performed it in its own way. Objective summary data regarding student learning are available for only a few institutional evaluations.

Surveys of faculty and student opinion were conducted by five institutions: Medical College of Virginia, Mayo Foundation, Albany Medical College, State University of New York Downstate Medical College, and the University of Pittsburgh. Findings were submitted to the Lister Hill Center.

Students at Albany Medical College were specifically asked to rate the educational value of specified CAI materials. Summary results of this study are shown in Table 3.

Table 2. *Time of Massachusetts General Hospital System, by Class of User (11/1/72–10/1/74)*

Institution/class of user	Usage time[a]
UCLA	
Med 1 (preclerkship)	747
Med 2 (clerkship)	631
House physician	299
Nonmedical	128
Auxiliary medical	79
Physician	55
Nurse	22
Fellow	11
Stanford	
Med 2 (clerkship)	254
Med 1 (preclerkship)	235
Nonmedical	45
House physician	29
Physician	22
Auxiliary medical	14
Fellow	6
Nurse	0

[a]Rounded to the nearest hour.

Table 3. *Ratings by Albany Medical College Students on Educational Value of Specified CAI Materials (October, 1973)*

Program number and name	Number of times used	Average rating (scale, 1–10)[a]
1. Abdominal Pain	3	7.67
2. Anticoagulant Simulation	5	8.40
3. Cardiac Simulator	1	4.00
4. Cardiopulmonary Resuscitation	15	8.67
5. Coma	4	9.00
6. Diabetic Ketoacidosis	8	8.63
7. Digoxin Dosage Adviser	1	6.00
8. Idiopathic Respiratory Distress in the Newborn	2	8.00
9. Jaundice	3	8.33
10. Pediatric Cough and Fever	1	9.00
11. A Bird's-Eye View of Pediatrics	6	7.50
12. Acid–Base Balance	5	8.70
13. Anticoagulant Meditation	2	8.50
14. CAI Demonstration Games	6	2.00
18. Introduction to CAI	1	3.00
20. Juvenile Diabetes	1	8.00
30. Reading the Medical Record	1	2.00
37. CASE	12	9.08
38. CRIB	8	8.00

[a]Highest possible score, 10.

Controlled experiments to determine the effects on student performance were too costly in faculty time to be carried out at most institutions. One study was conducted with 34 resident nurses at Cape Cod Hospital (Hoffer *et al.*, 1975). In this study, 22 nurses using 90 hours of computer time made statistically significant improvements in a test of their knowledge of cardiopulmonary resuscitation. A control group of 12 nurses who had no access to the computer programs showed no improvement in knowledge.

Impact on Libraries and Media Centers

The Lister Hill Network terminals were located in a variety of places (emergency rooms, hospital corridors, hospital wards, libraries, learning resource centers, medical association headquarters, student and faculty lounges, laboratories, etc.).

When terminals were moved from inconvenient places into a conspicuous location in the library, their usage greatly increased. A list of terminal locations by type and number is provided below:

Biomedical libraries — 25
Student biomedical labs (planned) — 17
Learning resources centers (multidisciplinary lab) — 16
Computer laboratories and centers — 12
Medical school departments (Surgery; Pathology; Ear, Nose and Throat) — 16
Terminal rooms — 5
Conference rooms — 4
Offices of medical education — 4
Student study areas — 3
Emergency rooms — 3
Offices of continuing education — 3
Resident lounges — 2
Ward rooms — 2
Cardiac care units — 2
Hospital library — 1
Family practice clinic — 1
Health testing unit — 1
Unspecified — 29

Individual librarians interviewed (e.g., Gloria Werner, Assistant Biomedical Librarian, UCLA) were very enthusiastic about the potential of CAI service. The UCLA library constructed special facilities for CAI library use — soundproofed enclosed study areas where groups of students could work at the terminals without disturbing other library activities.

Ms. Louise Darling, Biomedical Librarian at UCLA, recognizes CAI as an important service of the library but also feels that it is not the library's role to become involved with curriculum matters that inevitably arise whenever CAI is used to augment traditional instruction. Because of this problem, UCLA established a special CAI Faculty Curriculum Committee to review UCLA's long-term commitment to CAI.

When librarians and media center directors were questioned about their interest in having their own local system (desktop computer or intelligent terminal) they liked the concept but were somewhat apprehensive about possible technical problems and the availability of instructional programs. The idea of a CAI program cassette library was particularly appealing to the librarians since they were already using cassettes for video and tape instruction.

References

Hoffer, E. P., Mathewson, H. D., Loughrey, A., Barnett, G. D., 1975. Use of computer-aided instruction in graduate nursing education: A controlled trial, *Jen.* 1(2):2709.

Smythe, C. McC., 1969. Potential Educational Services from a National Biomedical Communications Network. Association of American Medical Colleges, Washington, D.C.

Stead, E. A., Jr., Smythe, C. McM., Gunn, C. G., and Littlemayer, M. H., 1971. Educational technology for medicine: Roles for the Lister Hill Center, *J. Med. Educ.* 46(7): Part 2 (July), 97 pp.

Wooster, H., and Lewis, J. F., 1973. Distribution of computer-assisted instruction materials in biomedicine through the Lister Hill Center Experimental Network, *Comput. Biol. Med.* 3:319–323.

Wooster, H., and Lewis, J. F., 1974. The utility of computer-assisted instruction – An experimental network, *in* P. L. Zund (Ed.), *Information Utilities – Proceedings of the 37th ASIS Annual Meeting*, pp. 213–217, American Society for Information Science, Washington, D.C.

Bibliography

Christopher R. Brigham, Edward C. DeLand,
Richard B. Friedman, and M. Kamp

Aberg, H., Johansson, R., and Michaelsson, M., 1974. Phonocardiosimulator as aid in teaching auscultation of the heart, *Br. J. Med. Educ.* 8(4):262–266 (December).

Abrahamson, S., Denson, J. S., and Wolf, R. M., 1969. Effectiveness of a simulator in training anesthesiology residents, *J. Med. Educ.* 44:515–519.

Abrahamson, S., and Hoffman, K. I., 1974. Sim One: A computer-controlled patient simulator, *Lakartidningen* 71(47):4756–4758 (November 29).

Adams, E. N., 1972. Technical Considerations in the design of a CAI system, *Programmed Learning* 9(5):256–271 (September).

Alpert, D., and Bitzer, D. L., 1970. Advances in computer-based education, *Science* 167: 1582–1590 (March).

Anastasio, E. J., and Morgan, J. S., 1972. *Inhibiting the Use of Computers in Instruction*, EDUCOM, Interuniversity Communications Council, Inc., Princeton, N.J.

Anderson, J., and Tomlinson, R. W., 1974. Teaching the uses of computers within the clinical course, *Proc. R. Soc. Med.* 67(9):948–950 (September).

Andrew, B. I., 1972. An approach to the construction of simulated exercise in clinical problem solving, *J. Med. Educ.* 47(12):952–958 (December).

Appleton, D. R., 1973. Interactive use of computer models in teaching population genetics, *Am. J. Phys. Anthropol.* 39(21):267–277 (September).

Apter, J. T., and Berman, S. A., 1977. Medical students time-sharing: An analog computer to learn physiology, *IEEE Trans. Biomed. Eng.* 19:82–88.

Atkinson, R. C., and Wilson, H. A. (Eds.), 1969. *Computer-Assisted Instruction, A Book of Readings*, Academic Press, New York.

Attia, R. R., Miller, E. V., and Kitz, R. J., 1975. Teaching effectiveness: Evaluation of computer-assisted instruction for cardiopulmonary resuscitation, *Anesth. Analg. (Cleve.)* 54(3): 308–311 (May–June).

Barnet, G. O., 1973. Strategies, potentials, and problems of computerized assisted instruction, *Physiologist* 16(4):621–625 (November).

Barnett, M., 1971. *An Introduction to FOIL Programming in MTS*, Center for Research on Learning and Teaching, University of Michigan, Ann Arbor, Mich.

Bates, F., and Douglas, M. L., 1967. *Programming Language/One*, Prentice-Hall, Englewood Cliffs, N.J.

Bergen, S. S., Jr., 1973. The computer as a tool in medical instruction, *J. Med. Soc. N.J.* 70(4):327 (April).

Christopher R. Brigham · Family Practice Center, Eastern Maine Medical Center, Bangor, Maine.
Richard B. Friedman · Department of Medicine, University of Wisconsin, Madison, Wisconsin.
Edward C. DeLand · Division of Thoracic Surgery, Health Science Center, University of California, Los Angeles, California. *M. Kamp* · Scientific Computing Services, University of California School of Medicine, San Francisco, California.

Bitzer, M. D., 1966. Clinical nursing instruction via the PLATO simulated laboratory, *Nurs. Res.* 15(2):144–150.

Bitzer, M. D., and Bitzer, D. I., 1973. Teaching nursing by computer: An evaluative study, *Comput. Biol. Med.* 3(3):187–204 (October).

Bitzer, M. D., and Boudreaux, M. D., 1969. Using a computer to teach nursing, *Nurs. Forum* 8:234–254.

Bitzer, M. D., Boudreaux, M., and Avner, A., 1973. Computer-based instruction of Basic Nursing Utilizing Inquiry Approach, CERL Report Z-40, University of Illinois, Urbana, Ill.

Bleich, H. L., 1971. The computer as a consultant, *N. Engl. J. Med.* 284:141–147.

Bleich, H. L., 1972. Computer-based consultation: Electrolyte and acid–base balance, *Am. J. Med.* 53:285–291.

Bleich, H. L., 1974. Computerized Clinical Diagnosis, *Fed. Proc.* 33(1):2317–2319 (December).

Bless, S. R., and Riflind, R. A., 1973. Computer-assisted medical instruction, *N.Y. State J. Med.* 73(18):2252–2255 (September 15).

Blomme, R., Parry, J., Sherwood, B., and Tenczar, P. PLATO IV System Software, Computer-Based Education Research Laboratory, University of Illinois, Urbana, Ill.

Bowden, D. H., 1967. Computer-assisted instruction in pathology, *Can. Med. Assoc. J.* 97:739–742.

Bowden, J. M., 1972. Digital computer applications in pharmacologic teaching and research, *Am. J. Vet. Res.* 33:227–233.

Brandt, E. N., 1966. Electronic computers in medical education of the future, *Clin. Anesthesia* 1:125–136.

Brandt, E. N., Jr., 1971. Role of the computer in continuing medical education, *Tex. Med.* 70(1):43–46 (January).

Brandt, E. N., Harless, W. G., and Lynn, T. N., 1967. Some experiences with computer aided instruction in a medical center environment, *Proceedings of the 8th IBM Medical Symposium*, pp. 133–140, IBM, White Plains, N.Y.

Brigham, C. R., 1973a. Programming Languages Used for Health Sciences Computer Assisted Instruction, Report No. PB 224 421/AS. National Technical Information Service, U.S. Dept. of Commerce, Springfield, Va.

Brigham, C. R., 1973b. Mini-Computers in Health Sciences Instruction, Report No. PB 224 397/AS, National Technical Information Service, U.S. Dept. of Commerce, Springfield, Va.

Brigham, C. R., and Kamp, M., 1973a. A selected bibliography to computerized instruction in the health sciences, *Comput. Biol. Med.* 3(3):337–342 (October).

Brigham, C. R., and Kamp, M., 1973b. Introduction to special issue on computer-assisted instruction in the health sciences, *Comput. Biol. Med.* 3(3):183–186 (October).

Brigham, C. R., and Kamp, M., 1974. The current status of computer-assisted instruction in the health sciences, *J. Med. Educ.* 49(3):287–289 (March).

Brigham, C. R., Kamp, M., and Cross, R. J. (Eds.), 1973. A Guide to Computer-Assisted Instruction in the Health Sciences, Report No. PB 241 351, National Technical Information Service, U.S. Dept. of Commerce, Springfield, Va.

Brody, H., Lucaccini, L., Kamp, M., and Rozen, R., 1973. Computer based simulated patient for teaching history-taking, *J. Dent. Educ.* 37(8):27.

Brown, D. W., Groome, D. S., Niehoff, R. D., and Cleaveland, J. D., 1968. Computer-assisted instruction in nuclear medicine, *J.A.M.A.* 206:1059–1062.

Brown, T. C., McCleary, L. E., Stencheuer, M. A., and Poulson, A. M., Jr., 1973. A Competency-based educational approach to reproductive biology, *Am. J. Obst. Gynecol.* 116(7):1036–1042 (August 1).

Brudner, H. J., 1968. Computer-managed instruction, *Science* 162:970.

Budkin, A., and Warner, H. R., 1968. Computer-assisted teaching of cardiac arrhythmias, *Comput. Biomed. Res.* 2:145–150.

Burford, H. J., and Stritter, F. T., 1974. Evaluation of a teaching program in medical pharmacology, *J. Med. Educ.* 49(3):236–244 (March).

Cassidy, R., *et al.*, 1972. Computer-assisted instruction for diagnostic problem solving of toothache, *J. Dent. Educ.* 36:46–59.

Carroll, J., and Becker, S., 1975. The paucity of course work in medical care evaluation, *J. Med. Educ.* 50(1):31–37 (January).

Chansky, L., 1972. An Analytical Study of Computer-Based Clinical Cases for Medical Education, *University of Microfilms*, Ann Arbor, Mich.

Clark, D. E., 1970. Computers and medical education, *Manchester Med. Gaz.* 49:8–11.

Clark, R. R., 1974. The impact of computerized peer review system on continuing medical education, *Ohio State Med. J.* 70(12):748–751 (December).

Colby, K. M., and Enea, H., 1967. Heuristic methods for computer understanding of natural language in context-restricted on-line dialogues, *Math. Biosci.* 1:1–25.

Cole, J. R., Tornton, J. A., Whelpton, D., and Wilson, A. M., 1968. Some applications of analogue computers to teaching, *Br. J. Anaesth.* 40:373–382.

Collart, M. E., 1973. Computer assisted instruction and the teaching–learning process, *Nurs. Outlook* 21:527–532 (August).

Computer Applications in Dental Education: A Conference Report, 1971. *Dental Health Center*, University of California, San Francisco.

Computer-assisted instruction: Two major demonstrations, 1972. *Science* 176:1110.

Computer-assisted programs in pediatrics, 1973. *Ariz. Med.* 30(11):792 (November).

Computer-Assisted Instruction in Medical Education, 1966. *Educ. Technol.* 6:16–17.

COURSEWRITER III, Version 3 Application Description Manual, GH20-0987-2, 1971. International Business Machines Corporation, White Plains, N.Y.

Culbertson, L. B., 1974. CAI – Beneficial teaching tool at Texas School for the Deaf, *Am. Ann. Deaf* 119(1):34–40 (February).

Culbertson, L., 1975. "Statewide project for the deaf, *J. Computer-Based Instruction* 1:127.

DeDombal, F. T., Hartley, J. R., and Sleeman, D. H., 1969. A computer-assisted system for learning clinical diagnosis, *Lancet* i:145–148.

DeDombal, F. T., Horrocks, J. C., Staniland, J. R., and Gill, P. W., 1971a. Simulation of clinical diagnosis – A comparative study, *Br. Med. J.* 2:575–577.

DeDombal, F. T., Horrocks, J. C., Staniland, J. R., and Guillou, P. J., 1971b. Production of Artificial 'Case Histories' by Using a Small Computer, *Br. Med. J.* 2:578–581.

Denson, J. S., and Abrahamson, S., 1971. A Computer-Controlled Patient Simulator, *J.A.M.A.* 208:504–508.

DeTornyay, R. J., 1970. Instructional technology and nursing education, *J. Nurs. Educ.* 9:3–8.

Diamond, H. S., Weiner, M., and Plotz, C. M., 1974. A computer assisted instructional course in diagnosis and treatment of the rheumatic diseases, *Arthritis Rheum.* 17(6):1049–1055 (November-December).

Dickinson, C. J., 1974. Letter: Trendiness in the biomedical computer biz. *Can. Med. Assoc. J.* 111(1):16–17 (July 6).

D'Ivernois, J. F., and Marquis, Y., 1975. Letter: Computers and the recycling of physicians, *Nouv. Presse Med.* 4(16):1210 (April 19).

Dockstader, J., Hepburn, B., Strauss, R., Lynborg, M. D., 1974. Guidelines for developing socially beneficial medical computer systems, *Med. Instrom.* 8(5):269–273 (September–October).

Dywer, J. M., and Schmitt, J. A., 1969. Using a computer to evaluate clinical performance, *Nurs. Forum* 8:266–275.

Editorial: Plastic patients, 1975. *Br. Med. J.* 1(5960):703–704 (March 29).

Einstein, S., 1974. Drug abuse training and education: The physician, *Int. J. Addict* 9(1):81–99.

Entwisle, G., and Entwisle, D. R., 1963. The use of a digital computer as a teaching machine, *J. Med. Educ.* 38:803–812.

Ertel, P. *et al.*, 1972a. Learning from the computer: What every health care administrator should know, *Mod. Hosp.* 119:103–107 (November).

Ertel, P., *et al.*, 1972b. CAI can provide both: Repaid reviews and specific answers, *Mod. Hosp.* 119:107 (November).

Farnsworth, J., CAMP: Computer and Me: Psycotherapeutically, *J. Nurs. Educ.* 13(4):26–29 (November).

Farquhar, B. B., Barnett, G. O., Goldfinger, S. E., and Dinnen, J. J., 1973. Computer-based examination; A technique to evaluate clinical competence, *in* J. P. Lysaught (Ed.), *Self-Instruction in Medical Education*, University of Rochester, Rochester, N.Y.

Feingold, S. L., 1968. PLANIT – A language for CAI, *Datamation* 14(9):41–47 (September).

Feurzeig, W., Munter, P., Swets, J. A., and Breen, M., 1964. Computer aided teaching in medical diagnosis, *J. Med. Educ.* 39:746–754.

Fiege, H. R., Smith, R. S., Palit, D., and Kruger, E., 1969. An experimental anatomy system, *Comput. Biomed. Res.* 2:373–384.

Fitzgerald, W. F., 1973. The instructional use of computers in dental education, *Comput. Biol. Med.* 3(3):307–318 (October).

Flandrin, G., *et al.*, 1972. Computer assisted teaching of hematology, I. Application to the teaching of blood cytology, *Nouv. Presse Med.* 1:2369–2371 (October 14) (Fre) (Eng. abst.).

Fonkalsrud, E. W., Hammidi, I. B., and Maloney, J. V., 1967. Computer-assisted instruction in undergraduate surgical education, *Surgery* 62:141–147.

Forsythe, A. B., Freed, J. R., Frey, H. S., 1975. Programmed instruction nucleus (PIN): A simplified author-language for computer-aided instruction, *Comput. Biol. Med.* 5(1)2: 77–88 (June).

Frazier, D. T., 1972. Computer-assisted self-evaluated tests for medical physiology, *Physiologists* 15(4):360–367 (November).

Freed, J. R., Forsythe, A. B., Bleich, D. R., Knutson, J. W., 1975. Computer-aided instruction in dental education: Application to an introductory statistics course, *J. Dent. Educ.* 39(5):284–291 (May).

Frenkel, L. D., 1973. An evaluation of the application of computer technology to medical education, *J. Med. Educ.* 66(4):433–438 (April).

Friedman, R. B., 1973. A computer program for simulating the patient–physician encounter, *J. Med. Educ.* 48(1):92–97 (January).

Frye, C. H., 1968. CAI languages: Capabilities and applications, *Datamation* 14(9):34–37 (September).

A Functional Specification for a Programming Language for Computer-Aided Learning Applications, 1972. Associate Committee on Instructional Technology, National Research Council of Canada, Ottawa, Ontario (July).

Gadd, A. S., 1973, Educational aspects of integrating social sciences in the medical curriculum, *Soc. Sci. Med.* 7(12):975–984 (December).

Gale, J., Anderson, J., Freeling, P., Pettingale, K. W., and Tomlinson, R. W., 1974. Planning of educational courses – A model of the management of an educational workshop for teachers of medicine, *Br. J. Med. Educ.* 8(2):87–91 (June).

Gaston, G. W., 1971. Computer assisted instruction in dental education, *J. Dent. Educ.* 35: 283–288.

Gaston, G. W., and Griesen, J. V. (Eds.), 1970. *Proceedings of the Ohio State Regional Medical Program CAI Conference*, Ohio State Regional Medical Program Press, Columbus, Ohio.

Geis, G. L., 1967. Computer assisted instruction: Current applications, *in* J. P. Lysaught (Ed.), *Self-Instruction in Medical Education*, pp. 193–196, University of Rochester, Rochester, N.Y.

Gilchrest, B. A., *et al.*, 1972. A computer-based teaching program in hemostasis. *Blood* 40:560–567 (October).

Goldberg, M., Green, S. B., Moss, M. L., Marbach, C. B., and Garfinkel, D., 1973. Computer-based instruction and diagnosis of acid–base, a systemic approach, *J.A.M.A.* **223**:269–275.

Gordon, M. S., 1974. Cardiology patient simulator-development of an animated manikin to teach cardiovascular disease, *Am. J. Cardiol.* **34**(3):350–355 (September).

Gregory, D. H., Wilkins, I., and Cufley, G. A., 1974. Model for postgraduate medical education: Study of Crohn's Disease in New Mexico, *J. Med. Educ.* **49**(6):612–615 (June).

Greist, J. H., Gustafson, D. H., Stauss, F. F., Rowse, G. L., Laughren, T. P., Chiles, J. A., 1973. A computer interview for suicide-risk prediction, *Am. J. Psychiatry* **130**(12):1327–1332 (December).

Griesen, J. V., 1970. Computer-Assisted Independent Study, *in: Proceedings of the Conference on Information Systems for Health Sciences Centers.*

Griesen, J. V., Beran, R. L., Folk, R. L., and Prior, J. A., 1971. A pilot program for independent study in medical education, *in* J. P. Lysaught (Ed.), *Self-Instruction in Medical Education,* University of Rochester, Rochester, N.Y.

Grimes, G. M., Rhoades, H. E., Adams, F. C., and Schmidt, R. V., 1972. Identification of bacteriological unknowns: A computer-based teaching program, *J. Med. Educ.* **47**:289–292.

Grisell, J. L., Beckett, P. G. S., and Gudobba, R., 1967. Teaching diagnostic strategies with a computer, *J. Med. Educ.* **42**:275.

Grubb, R. E., 1971. Computer-assisted instruction – The technology, *in* J. P. Lysaught (Ed.), *Self-Instruction in Medical Education*, University of Rochester, Rochester, N.Y.

Hagamen, W. D., Linden, D., Leppo, M., Bell, W., and Weber, J. C., 1974. Arts in exposition, *Comput. Biol. Med.* **3**(3):205–226 (October).

Hagamen, W. D., Weber, J. C., Linden, D. J., and Murphy, S. S., 1971. A tutorial system (ATS): Concepts and facilities, Cornell University Medical College, New York.

Hall, P., and Sebag, J., 1974. Decision-making in clinical practice and medical research: A theoretical analysis of predicators, indicators and health indices, *Int. J. Biomed. Comput.* **5**(4):301–309 (October).

Harless, W. G., 1967. The development of a computer-assisted instruction program in a medical center environment, *J. Med. Educ.* **42**:139–145.

Harless, W. G., Lucas, N. C., Cutter, J. A., Duncan, R. C., White, J. M., and Brandt, E. W., 1969. Computer-assisted instruction in continuing medical education, *J. Med. Educ.* **44**:670–674.

Harless, W. G., Drennon, G. G., Marxer, J. J., Root, J. A., and Miller, G. E., 1971. CASE: A computer-aided simulation of the clinical encounter, *J. Med. Educ.* **46**:443–448.

Harless, W. G., Drennon, G. G., Marxer, J. J., Root, J. A., Wilson, L. L., and Miller, G. E., 1973a. CASE – A natural language computer model, *Comput. Biol. Med.* **3**(3):227–246 (October).

Harless, W. G., Drennon, G. G., Marxer, J. J., Root, J. A., Wilson, L. L., and Miller, G. E., 1973b. GENESYS – A generation system for the CASE natural language model, *Comput. Biol. Med.* **3**(3):246–268 (October).

Hellerstein, E. E., Mast, T. A., and Stolurow, L. M., 1968. CAI: Socratic dialogue and laboratory simulation in pathology, *Technical Report AD 667 657*, Harvard Computing Center, Cambridge, Mass.

Herrick, M. C., 1970. A new approach to computer assisted instruction in health science education, *Ala. J. Med. Sci.* **7**:172–174.

Hesselbart, J. C., D'Arms, T., and Zinn, K. L., 1969. *A Manual for FOIL In Two Volumes*, Center for Research on Learning and Teaching, University of Michigan, Ann Arbor, Mich.

Hickey, A. R., 1968. *Computer-Assisted Instruction – A Survey of the Literature* (3rd Ed.), Entelek, Newburyport, Mass.

Higginson, J., 1973. Role preparation: Disease priorities in medical education, *J. Med. Educ.* **48**(12):95–101 (December).

Hillman, R. G., 1971. The teaching of psychotherapy problems by computer, *Arch. Gen. Psychiat.* **25**:324–329.

Hoffer, E. P., 1973. Experience with the use of computer simulation models in medical education, *Comp. Biol. Med.* **3**(3):269–280 (October).

Hoffer, E. P., 1975. Computer-aided instruction in community hospital emergency departments: A pilot project, *J. Med. Educ.* **50**(1):84–86 (January).

Hoffer, E. P., Barnett, G. O., and Farquhar, B. B., 1972. Computer simulation model for teaching cardiopulmonary resuscitation, *J. Med. Educ.* **47**:343–348.

Hoffer, E. P., Barnett, G. O., Farquhar, B. B., Prather, P. A., 1975a. Computer-aided instruction in medicine, *Ann. Rev. Biophys. Bioeng.* **4**:103–118.

Hoffer, E. P., Mathewson, H. D., Loughrey, A., Barnett, G. O., 1975. Use of computer-aided instruction in graduate nursing education: A controlled trial, *Jen.* **1**(2):2709 (March–April).

Holm, C., Thompson, W. M., Wilber, M. C., and Wells, C. H., 1973. CAISYS-8: A CAI language developed for a minicomputer, *Compt. Biol. Med.* **3**(3):261–291 (October).

Hoover, L. W., and Moore, A. N. N., 1974. Dietetic Com-Pak, an educational model simulating computer-assisted dietetics, *J. Am. Diet. Assoc.* **64**(5):500–504 (May).

Hubbard, J. P., Levit, E. J., Barnett, G. O., Goldfinger, S. E., Dinnen, J. J., Farquhar, B. B., and Schumacher, C. F., 1970. Computer-Based Evaluation of Clinical Competence, *ACP Bull.* 502–505.

Hunka, S., Hudson, B., and Gilbert, J., 1968. Computer assisted instruction and testing in medical education, in: *Proceedings of the 9th IBM Medical Symposium*, pp. 33–39, IBM, White Plains, N.Y.

Hyatt, G. W., and Avner, R. A., 1973. Interactive teaching modules for animal behavior on the PLATO IV system, *Physiologist* **16**(4):649–657 (November).

Hyatt, G. W., Eades, D. C., and Tenczar, P., 1972. Computer-based education in biology, *BioScience* **22**:401–409.

If the simulator would be interesting it should be better than the real situation, 1974, *Lakartidningen* **71**(47):4760–4762 (November 20).

Johnson, D. C., 1973. Three 10-minute presentations of application programs, I. A program to teach and demonstrate cardiovascular control through simulation, *Physiologist* **16**(4): 636–643 (November).

Kagen, N. I., 1974. Teaching interpersonal relations for the practice of medicine, *Lakartidningen* **71**(47):4756–4758 (November 20).

Kahn, N., and Bigger, J. T., Jr., 1974. Instruction in pharmacokinetics: A computer-assisted demonstration system, *J. Med. Educ.* **49**(3):292–295 (March).

KaLache, A., Coelho, M. A., 1974. The use of computers in educational evaluation, *Educ. Med. Salud.* **8**(2):191–204 (April).

Kamp, M., 1971. Evaluating the operation of interactive free-response computer programs, *J. Biomed. Systems* **2**:31–44.

Kamp, M., 1975. *Index to Computerized Teaching in the Health Sciences*, Health Sciences Interest Group of the Association for the Development of Computer-based Instructional Systems, Kentfield, Ca.

Kamp, M., and Buyrnside, M., 1974. Computer-assisted learning in graduate psychiatric nursing, *J. Nurs. Educ.* **13**(4):18–25 (November).

Kamp, M., and Starkweather, J. A., 1973. A return to a dedicated machine for computer-assisted instruction, *Comput. Biol. Med.* **3**(3):293–298.

Katzenberger, K., 1975. Computers in medicine: IV. First results, *Med. Welt.* **22**:1110–1113 (May 30).

Kemeny, J. G., and Hurtz, T. E., 1967. *BASIC Programming*, John Wiley and Sons, New York.

Killip, D. E., 1968. Innovation in education – Computer-assisted instruction, *J. Dent. Educ.* **32**:110.

Kirsch, A. D., 1963. A medical training game using a computer as a teaching aid, *Methods Inform. Med.* 2:138–143.

Kowalski, C. J., 1972. Computer-aided instruction of statistics to dental students, *J. Dent. Educ.* 36:68–73.

Lekan, H. (Ed.), 1971. *Index to Computer Assisted Instruction*, Harcourt Brace Jovanovich, New York.

Letter: Trendiness in the biomedical computer biz, 1974, *Can. Med. Assoc. J.* 110(6):618 *passim* (March 16).

Levine, D. Z., 1973. Computer-aided instruction at the Ottawa General Hospital, *Can. Med. Assoc. J.* 108(4):486 *passim* (February 17).

Levine, D., and Wiener, E., 1975. Let the computer teach it, *Am. J. Nurs.* 75(8):1300–1302 (August).

Levine, L., 1975. The use of previously administered examinations for computer-assisted instruction, *Am. J. Optom. Physiol. Opt.* 52(7):497–501 (July).

Levy, J. P., *et al.*, 1972. Computer assisted teaching of hematology, evaluation of an experiment, *Nouv. Presse Med.* 1:2367–2368 (October 14) (Fre).

Lobo, L. C., 1974. Use of new educational technology in the development of human resources, *Educ. Med. Salud.* 8(2):140–149 (April).

Lower, S. *A CAI System Based on APL*, Simon Fraser University, Burnaby, British Columbia.

Lower, S. K., and Arsenault, G. *A Functional Evaluation of COURSEWRITER III*, Simon Fraser University, Burnaby, British Columbia.

Luskin, B. J., Gripp, T. J., Clark, J. R., and Christianson, D. A., 1972. Sharing Programs and Selecting a Language, *in Everything You Always Wanted to Know About CAI*, Computer Uses in Education, Huntington Beach, Ca.

Mapleson, W. W., 1971. The use of analogs in teaching of the pharmacokinetics of the inhalation anesthetic agents, *Int. Anesthesiol. Clin.* 9:65–97.

Marchand, E. R., and Steward, J. P., 1974. Trends in basic medical science instruction affecting role of multidiscipline laboratories, *J. Med. Educ.* 49(2):171–175 (February).

Marple, D. P., 1973. Comment on E. Van De Walle and J. Knodel's teaching population dynamics with a simulation exercise, *Demography* 10(1):123 (February).

Maxman, J. S., 1975. Forecasting and medical education, *J. Med. Educ.* 50(1):54–65 (January).

Mayor, S. J., 1973. The assay of medical student performance using a minicomputer, *J. Med. Educ.* 48(1):100–101 (January).

McAlister, N. H., 1973. Trendiness in the biomedical computer biz, *Can. Med. Assoc. J.* 109(12):1195 (December).

McGown, H. L., and Faust, G. W., 1971. Computer-assisted instruction in physical therapy – a pilot program, *Phys. Ther.* 51:1113–1120.

McGuire, C. H., 1973. Educational program research and development, *J. Med. Educ.* 48(4) Suppl: 137–143 (April).

McGuire, C. H., and Solomon, L. M. (Eds.), 1971. *Clinical Simulations*, Appleton-Century-Crofts, New York.

McKnown, R., and Barr, I., 1973. TV simulation of excitable membrane experiments, *Physiologist* 16(4):626–630 (November).

McLeod, J. (Ed.), 1968. *Simulation*, McGraw-Hill, New York.

Mead, C. F., 1973. IX. Guess the animal, *Physiologist* 16(4):669–673 (November).

Meadow, R., and Hewitt, C., 1972. Teaching communication skills with the help of actresses and video-tape simulation, *Br. J. Med. Educ.* 6(4):317–322 (December).

Meyer, J. H., and Beaton, G. R., 1974. An evaluation of computer-assisted teaching in physiology, *J. Med. Educ.* 49(3):295–297 (March).

Miller, J. G., 1968, Computer-based and computer-planned continuing medical education for the future, *J.A.M.A.* 206:621–624.

Nishimoto, G. M., and Walters, R. F., 1972. A simplified method for computer-based student self-evaluation, *J. Med. Educ.* 47:487–488.

Nunnery, A. W., 1969. Computer-assisted pediatric instruction of medical students, *Southern Med. J.* 62:1542.

Nystrup, J., 1974a. Simulation and Play in Medical Education, *Nurs. Med.* 89(1):20–23 (January).

Nystrup, J., 1974b. Simulating – An old concept with a new meaning, *Lakartidningen* 71(47): 4753–4755 (November 20).

Olde, G. L., and Luebke, R. G., 1969. Application of computer techniques in a dental clinical teaching program, *J. Dent. Educ.* 33:119–126.

Orf, H. W., 1975. Computer-assisted instruction in organic synthesis, *J. Chem. Educ.* 52(7): 464–467 (July).

Osbaldenston, L. W., 1974. CBI in medicine at the University of Alberta, *J. Computer-Based Instruction* 1:64.

Ovenstone, J. A., 1966. Computer assisted instruction in undergraduate and post-graduate medicine, *Med. J. Aust.* 2:487–491.

Partridge, L. D., 1972. Simulation in biomedical teaching: Introduction, *IEEE Trans. Biomed. Eng.* 19:78–81.

Pascoe, J. E., 1974. Teaching the uses of computers to medical students, *Proc. R. Soc. Med.* 67(9):946–948 (September).

Patton, D. D., 1971. Computer-assisted instruction in the radiological sciences using a desk-top computer, *Radiology* 100:553–559.

Paxton, H. T., 1970. The electronic patient, *Hospital Physician* 6(5):57–64.

Penta, F. B., and Kofman, S., 1973. The effectiveness of simulation devices in teaching selected skills of physical diagnosis, *J. Med. Educ.* 48(5):442–445 (May).

Pentico, D. W., and Barnhill, B., 1975. A technique for scheduling medical clerkships, *J. Med. Educ.* 50(1):89–91 (January).

Petrova, T. R., Iagodkin, S. I., and Pavlishchok, S. A., 1973. Elements of programmed instruction at the department of facultative therapy, *Zoravookhr Ross Fed.* 17(3):25–27 (March).

Pilot 1.6 Guide, 1973. Office of Information Systems Report, UCS 03.01.01, University of California, San Francisco.

Pinkerton, M., Hamilton, J., and Steinrauf, L. K., 1974. A course for teaching medical computer applications to medical students, *J. Med. Educ.* 49(3):284–285 (March).

Prather, P., 1973. *Teaching Program Drivers*, Laboratory of Computer-Science, Massachusetts General Hospital, Boston, Mass.

Proceedings of the Conference of the Use of Computers in Medical Education, 1968. University of Oklahoma Medical Center, Oklahoma City.

Raeside, D. E., and Traub, S. P., 1974. A note on a Monte Carlo approach to scheduling, *Radiology* 110(3):735 (March).

Rauitch, M. M., 1974. Editorial: A computer logic program in the operating room, *Surgery* 76(2):202–203 (August).

Reed, F. C., *et al.*, 1972. Computer assisted instruction for continued learning, *Am. J. Nurs.* 72:2035–2039 (November).

Reinecke, R. D., 1968. Computer-assisted instructional entry and exit systems to an information center data bank, *in* J. P. Lysaught (Ed.), *Individualized Instruction in Medical Education*, pp. 128–133, University of Rochester, Rochester, N.Y.

Rupeiks, I., 1972. Computer-aided medical instruction using an interactive graphics model of the normal and congenitally defective heart, *IEEE Trans. Biomed. Eng.* 19:88–96.

Saffir, A. J., and Myers, H. M., 1972. A modern statistics course for dentists using a time-sharing computer, *J. Dent. Educ.* 36:26–30.

Sajid, A., Lipson, L. F., and Telder, V., 1975. A simulation laboratory for medical education, *J. Med. Educ.* 50(10):970–975 (October).

Sammet, J. E., 1969. *Programming Languages: History and Fundamentals*, Prentice-Hall, Englewood Cliffs, N.J.

Sammet, J. E., 1972. Programming languages: History and future, *Communications of the A.C.M.* **15**(7):601–610 (July).

Schneiderman, H., and Muller, R., 1970. The diagnosis game: A computer-based exercise in problem solving, *J.A.M.A.* **219**:333–335.

Schorow, M., 1967. Problem-solving theory and the practice of clinical medicine, *Can. Med. Assoc. J.* **97**:711–716.

Seidel, R. J., 1973a. II. Challenges of CAE development: I. Introductory remarks, *Physiologist* **16**(4):610–616 (November).

Seidel, R. J., 1973b. II. Hardware technology for computers in education: One of the solvable problems, *Physiologist* **16**(4):610–616 (November).

Sheretz, D. D., 1972. *MUMPS Reference Manual*, Laboratory of Computer Science, Massachusetts General Hospital, Boston, Massachusetts.

Siegel, B., 1972. The Stony Brook authoring system – How it facilitates curriculum development, *ACS SIGCUE Bulletin* **6**(4):25–26 (October).

Simulated patients, (Editorial), 1974. *Br. Med. J.* **2**(916):399–400 (May 25).

Slack, W. V., Hicks, G. P., Reed, C. E. and Van Cura, L. J., 1966. A computer-based medical-history system, *New Engl. J. Med.* **274**:194–198.

Smith, L. C., 1974. The medical librarian and computer-assisted instruction, *Bull. Med. Libr. Assoc.* **62**(2):92–94 (April).

Smith, S. G., and Sherwood, B. A., 1976. Educational uses of the PLATO computer system, *Science* **192**:344.

Sobotik, Z., *et al.*, 1973. Modelling of a disease on a computer for teaching purposes, *Cas. Lek. Cesk.* **112**:139–144 (February 2) (Cze) (Eng. Abst.).

Sokolow, S., and Solberg, W., 1971. Computer-assisted instruction in dental diagnosis: A product development, *J. Dent. Educ.* **33**:349–355.

Sorlie, W. E., and Jones, L. A., 1975. Description of a computer-assisted testing system in an independent study program, *J. Med. Educ.* **50**(1):81–83 (January).

Spencer, R. P., 1969. The analog computer as a training aid in nuclear medicine, *J. Nucl. Med.* **10**:660.

Spivak, A. P., and Miller, D. K., 1967. The arrhythmia trainer; a small computer for training in the recognition and electrical treatment, *J.A.M.A.* **202**:299–301.

Spivey, B. E., 1971. The computer's impact in education, *Trans. Am. Acad. Ophthalmol. Otolaryngol* **75**:1132–1138.

Starkweather, J. A., 1965. Computest: A computer language for individualized testing, instruction and interviewing, *Psychol. Rep.* **17**:227–237.

Starkweather, J. A., 1967a. Computer-assisted learning in medical education, *Can. Med. Assoc. J.* **97**:733–738.

Starkweather, J. A., 1967. Educational use of computer assisted instruction, *Proceedings of the 8th IBM Computing Symposium*, pp. 141–142, IBM, White Plains, N.Y.

Starkweather, J. A., Kamp. M., and Monto, A., 1967. Psychiatric interview simulation by computer, *Methods Inform. Med.* **6**:15–23.

Stead, E. A., Smythe, C. McM., Gunn, C. G., and Littlemeyer, M. H., 1971. Educational technology for medicine: roles for the Lister Hill Center, *J. Med. Educ.* **46**(7):Part 2 (July), 97 pp.

Stetten, K. J., 1972. *Toward a Market Success for CAI – An Overview of the TICCIT Program*, MITRE Corporation, Washington, D.C.

Stolurow, L. M., Peterson, T. I., and Cunningham, A. C. (Eds.), 1970. *Computer-Assisted Instruction in the Health Professions*, Entelek, Newburyport, Mass.

Suppes, P., and Morningstar, M., 1969. Computer-assisted instruction, *SCIENCE* **166**:343.

A supplement: Undergraduate medical education: Elements, objectives, costs; A report by the Committee on the Financing of Medical Education of the Association of American Medical Colleges, 1974, *J. Med. Educ.* **49**(1):7–128 (January).

Swain, R. W., Lynn, W. R., Hodgson, T. A., Becker, N. G., and Johnson, K. G., 1972. Epidemic simulation for training in public health management, *IEEE Trans. Biomed. Eng.* **19**: 120–125.

Swets, J. A., and Feurzeig, W., 1965. Computer-aided instreuction, *Science* **150**:572–576.

Tennyson, R. D., 1973. II. Applications of computers in education, *Physiologist* **16**(4):595–599 (November).

Teuscher, G. W., 1971. Editorial: Education and the computer, *J. Dent. Educ.* **35**:338.

Thies, R., Harless, W. G., Lucas, N. C., and Jacobson, E. D., 1969. An experiment comparing computer-assisted instruction with lecture presentation in physiology, *J. Med. Educ.* **44**:1156–1160.

Thompson, D. M., 1974. Computer training of medical students in statistical analysis, II. Comparison of standard errors of the means of data from small and large classes, *J. Am. Osteopath. Assoc.* **75**(5):413–414 (January).

Tidball, C. S., 1973a. II. Challenges of CAE development, I. Introductory remarks, *Physiologist* **16**(4):595–599 (November).

Tidball, C. S., 1973b. VII. MEDLEARN: An orientation to MEDLINE, *Physiologist* **16**(4): 669–673 (November).

Tidball, C. S., 1973c. II. Operating systems and computer languages for educational applications, *Physiologist* **16**(4):617–621 (November).

Tobias, S., 1973. Distraction, response mode, anxiety and achievement in computer-assisted instruction, *J. Educ. Psychol.* **65**(2):233–237 (October).

Trzebiatowski, G. L., and Ferguson, I. C., 1973. Computer technology in medical education, *Med. Prog. Technol.* **1**(4):178–186 (February).

USA Standard FORTRAN, 1966. *USAS X3.9–1966*, United States of America Standards Institute, New York (March).

Valish, A. U., and Boyd, N. J., 1975. The role of computer assisted instruction in continuing education of registered nurses: An experimental study, *J. Cont. Educ. Nurs.* **6**(1): 13–32 (January–February).

Van Cura, L. J., Jensen, N. M., Greist, J. H., Lewis, W. R., and Frey, T. I., Sr., 1965. Venereal Disease, interviewing and teaching by computer, *Am. J. Public Health* **65**(11):1159–1164 (November).

Van De Walle, E., and Knodel, J., 1970. Teaching population dynamics with a simulation exercise, *Demography* **7**:433–448.

Vanselow, N. A., 1975. Computer assisted instruction in pharmacology at the University of Arizona Medical School, *Ariz. Med.* **32**(8):633–634 (August).

Wakefield, J. S., 1971. Review of two years' experience with CAI, *Computer Medicine* **1**:10–11.

Warner, H. R., 1968. A link trainer for the coronary-care units, *Comput. Biomed. Res.* **2**:135–144.

Weber, J. C., and Hagamen, W. D., 1969. Medical education – A challenge for natural language analysis, artificial intelligence and interactive graphics, *AFIPS Conference Proceedings* **35**:307–318.

Weber, J. C., and Hagamen, W. D., 1972. ATS – A new system for computer-mediated tutorials in medical education, *J. Med. Educ.* **47**:637–644 (August).

Weinberg, A. D., 1973. CAI at the Ohio State University of Medicine (1973), *Comput. Biol. Med.* **3**(3):299–305 (October).

Weizenbaum, J., 1967. Contextual understanding by computers, *ACM* **10**(8):474–480.

Wells, C. H., Thompson, W. M., and Holm, C. S., 1973. X. Instruction in renal physiology on a minicomputer-based educational system, *Physiologist* **16**(4):678–683 (November).

Williams, T. E., Jr., Beran, R. L., Folk, R. L., Prior, J. A., and Zollinger, R. M., 1971. The Ohio State University Pilot Medical School, *Surgery* **70**:47–52.

Wilson, A. M., The use of analogs in teaching, *Int. Anesthesiol. Clin.* **9**:1–37.

Woods, S. M., 1974. A computerized self-assessment examination for residents, *Am. J. Psychiatry* **131**(11):1283–1286 (November).

Wooster, H., 1973. The Lister Hill Experimental CAI Network – A progress report, *Physiologist* **16**(4):621–625 (November).

Wooster, H., and Lewis, J. F., 1973. Distribution of computer-assisted instructional materials in biomedicine through the Lister Hill Center Experimental Network, *Comput. Biol. Med.* 3(3):319–323 (October).

Zinn, K. L., 1969. *A Comparative Study of Languages for Programming Interactive Use of Computers in Instruction*, EDUCOM, Boston, Mass.

Zinn, K. L., 1970. *Requirements for Programming Languages in Computer-Based Instructional Systems, Technical Report CERI/CT/70.62,* Centre for Educational Development, Paris.

Zinn, K. L., 1973. Instructional software, *in* K. Zinn, M. Refice, and A. Romano (Eds.), *Computers in the Instructional Process: Report of an International School*, Elsevier.

Zuckerman, A., DeLand, E. C., Dell, R., and Winters, R. W., 1972. Fluidmod: A Program for Computer-Based Instruction in Clinical Fluid Therapy, *Rand Corp. Publication* No. P-4799.

Index